Neuropsychological Evaluation of the Child

Neuropsychological Evaluation of the Child

IDA SUE BARON

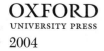

OXFORD
UNIVERSITY PRESS
2004

OXFORD
UNIVERSITY PRESS

Oxford   New York
Auckland   Bangkok   Buenos Aires   Cape Town   Chennai
Dar es Salaam   Delhi   Hong Kong   Istanbul   Karachi   Kolkata
Kuala Lumpar   Madrid   Melbourne   Mexico City   Mumbai Nairobi
São Paulo   Shanghai   Taipei   Tokyo   Toronto

Copyright © 2004 by Oxford University Press, Inc.

Published by Oxford University Press, Inc.
198 Madison Avenue, New York, New York 10016
http://www.oup-usa.org

Library of Congress Cataloging-in-Publication Data
Baron, Ida Sue.
Neuropsychological evaluation of the child / Ida Sue Baron.
p. ; cm.   Includes bibliographical references and index.
ISBN 0-19-514757-X (cloth)
1. Psychological tests for children.
2. Pediatric neuropsychology.
3. Brain damage—Diagnosis.
I. Title.
[DNLM: 1. Neuropsychological Tests—standards—Child.
2. Pediatric neuropsychology.
3. Brain damage—Diagnosis.
I. Title.
[DNLM: 1. Neuropsychological Tests—standards—Child.
2. Brain Diseases—diagnosis—Child.
3. Child Development.
4. Mental Disorders—diagnosis—Child.
5. Statistical Distributions.
WS 340 B265n 2003]   RJ486.6.B37 2003   155.4′1828—dc21   2003043354

9 8 7 6 5 4 3

Printed in the United States of America
on acid-free paper

To my mother,
Mollie W. Baron
with infinite love and respect

Preface

This book had its genesis in the mounting frustration I share with many child neuropsychologists as we, individually, try to determine what tests are available for children of different chronological ages and what normative data can be responsibly applied. Scoring a child's test protocol often results in a cumbersome and time-consuming procedure that depends on a search for elusive data sets buried in diverse journals and texts. A compilation of normative data specific to children was sorely needed, although some authors had begun to include child data on selected tests, along with more comprehensive consideration of adolescent and adult results (Lezak, 1995; Spreen and Strauss, 1998; Mitrushina, Boone et al., 1999). Toward this end, I began to collate published data for individual tests for my own use, and this book took shape.

Test manuals and test batteries that contain large normative data sets already fill our bookshelves, our choices dependent on our theoretical bent and practical patient concerns. Several of these test instruments and batteries are briefly noted in this volume because of their inherent historical and practical interest to child neuropsychologists. My main focus, however, was directed to highlighting available *individual* data sets and with specifying their demographic information when available.

Along with the major purpose of compiling available child normative data in one reference book, additional goals evolved in the course of its writing. These included drawing attention to the often-deficient state of child normative data and the imperative need for well-executed normative studies across populations, ages, cultural groups, and gender. I hope that the reader's awareness of the range of available tests will increase and that some will undertake empirical study of the applicability of specific tests with both normal children and clinical populations.

In compiling these data, it quickly became evident that there also existed research results that were relevant but unpublished for a variety of reasons. Some of these were collected for regional use and published locally, such as those graciously offered for inclusion in this volume by Vicki Anderson, Genevieve Lajoie, and Richard Bell (Anderson, Lajoie et al., 1995). The existence of unpublished meta-normative neuropsychological data for 3225 children was also brought to my attention (Findeis and Weight, 1993), and permission was granted for publication.

Through the generosity of several researchers cited throughout these chapters, a number of master's theses, doctoral dissertations, and scientific presentations that were obscure but highly relevant to practitioners were collected and are included in this volume. These individuals deserve special mention and are cited in the Acknowledgments, along with those persons who were especially helpful in the preparation of this volume. Their generosity and that of many test publishers also helped to fulfill the goals of this volume.

The absence of a consistent collection of sufficiently well-stratified normative data to support interpretive conclusions is striking in our current child neuropsychology literature. Yet, tests are a core responsibility of neuropsychologists. They serve as a major means to test theories as well as individuals, to formulate and change hypotheses, to examine with statistical rigor, and to introduce and amend treatments. These steps are taken in an effort to expand our knowledge about brain mediation of behavior. Fortunately, tests are now being developed that correct past weaknesses, standardization samples are more appropriate and often census based, models of child development are given priority in test development, and age-based norms rely on respectable sample size (Ns). These steps are essential if interpretation based on data acquisition is to have the highest likelihood of leading to meaningful recommendations and treatments.

Normative data guide decisions, but often in child neuropsychology, these data are not as well disseminated for individual tests constructed by researchers as they are for test batteries sponsored by publishing houses. Thus, it seemed important to me to compile several of these tests along with their respective child normative data. This book presents a selective review that is heavily based on my own interests and practice. It is not intended to diminish the substantial and, in some instances, seminal contributions of those given only cursory attention. As in any undertaking that attempts to locate and compile dispersed normative data, and to include a limited but important range of such data, it is to be expected that some omissions will occur. In some instances, such an omission resulted from practical considerations, such as a failure to obtain permission from the copyright holder, rather than the author's intention. Newer tests and their data were also emphasized whenever possible, especially those based on child development theory instead of downward extensions from original adult versions. In many instances, older tests have a substantial and easily accessed literature and detailed test manuals that could not be concisely summarized. In these cases, the data for the tests or batteries are referenced rather than reproduced. Although the reader may note some omissions, these are not intended as a rejection of a specific theoretical orientation or approach.

This book has 11 chapters, divided into three parts. In the first part, the introductory chapter reviews the current status of child neuropsychology, discusses the contributions made by child neuropsychologists to child evaluation, notes common reasons for referral, and emphasizes the importance I place on convergence profile analysis as a desirable outcome of a child neuropsychological evaluation. There is a brief discussion of alternate test forms and practice effects linked to the consideration of test choice and application, along with a mention of ways to detect significant change over time. The chapter concludes with a discussion of the ideals and realities of the current state of normative data in child neuropsychology. Part II includes Chapters 2 and 3 that discuss practical aspects related to the direct assessment of a child and communication through the interpretive session and written report. These chapters draw heavily from Chapters 5 and 6 of a previous book of which this author was senior author (Baron, Fennell et al., 1995) and have been concisely adapted and updated. These discussions were judged important enough to repeat in a volume focused on child neuropsychology assessment, individual tests, and their normative data. For more detailed information, the practitioner is encouraged to review the 1995 text.

In addition, Chapter 2 presents a sampling of some of the behavioral measures that may be crucial for a complete child neuropsychological evaluation. These tests have detailed test manuals and, often, computerized scoring programs to assist the clinician. Thus, the many existent measures that would serve these purposes were not a focus in this volume.

In Part III, Chapter 4 is concerned with brief assessment and classification instruments related to child evaluation. This chapter provides a personal example of methods to screen a child preliminarily as the initial part of a comprehensive evaluation. It concludes with a summary of a screening instrument currently nearing publication. Chapter 5 briefly discusses the history of intelligence testing and raises issues related to general intelligence tests, including a discussion of their positive aspects and their inherent limitations. Some of the more widely used intelligence tests are listed and briefly summarized. Despite occasional mention of academic achievement tests, it was determined that these testing instruments are best omitted from this book as their normative data are easily accessed in their respective test manuals. It was also not my intent to address any intelligence test in great detail since they are comprehensively covered in numerous other sources.

Chapters 6 through 11 were the principal motivation for this book and include a compilation of tests and their associated published and unpublished normative data. While recognizing the possibility for overlap, tests were assigned in a reasoned manner among specific cognitive domains: executive function, attention, language, motor and sensory-perceptual evaluation, visuoperceptual, visuospatial and visuoconstructional function, and learning and memory.

While this volume is not intended to be inclusive of all relevant child neuropsychology tests, procedures, and normative data, it is certainly intended to be a useful desk reference with easily accessed normative data for a variety of specific child neuropsychological tests. I hope the reader finds this book as useful in his or her clinical practice as I have in my own during its development.

Potomac, Maryland   I.S.B.

REFERENCES

Anderson, V., Lajoie, G., & Bell, R. (1995). *Neuropsychological Assessment of the School-Aged Child*. Melbourne: University of Melbourne.

Baron, I. S., Fennell, E. B., & Voeller, K. K. S. (1995). *Pediatric Neuropsychology in the Medical Setting*. New York: Oxford University Press.

Findeis, M. K., & Weight, D. G. (1994). *Meta-norms for Indiana-Reitan Neuropsychological Test Battery and Halstead-Reitan Neuropsychologial Test Battery for Children, ages 5–14*. Unpublished manuscript.

Lezak, M. (1995). *Neuropsychological Assessment,* (3rd ed.). New York: Oxford University Press.

Mitrushina, M. N., Boone, K. B., & D'Elia, L. (1999). *Handbook of normative data for neuropsychological assessment*. New York: Oxford University Press.

Spreen, O., & Strauss, E. (1998). *A compendium of neuropsychological tests: Adminstration, norms, and commentary* (2nd ed.). New York: Oxford University Press.

Acknowledgments

This book was made possible due to the enormous support of the following individuals and test publishers who contributed generously to the amassing of a variety of tests and normative data and who provided encouragement as well for this undertaking: Drs. Natasha Akshoomoff, Peter Anderson, Vicki Anderson, Marcia Barnes, William Barr, Richard Bell, Lynn Blackburn, Kathleen Brady, Erminio Capitani, William Culbertson, Martha Denckla, Jacobus Donders, Kimberly Espy, Philip Fastenau, Deborah Fein, Eileen Fennell, Michael Findeis, Alan Finlayson, Jack Fletcher, Rebecca Gaither, Gerry Gioia, Guila Glosser, Leslie Gonzalez-Rothi, Robert Gray, Kerry Hamsher, Naomi Harris, Jo Ann Hoeppner, C. Alan Hopewell, Janice Johnson, Betsy Kammerer, Lauren Kenworthy, Kimberly Kerns, Joel Kramer, Genevieve Lajoie, Glenn Larrabee, Harvey Levin, Muriel Lezak, Scott Lindgren, Ann Marcotte, Robert McInerney, Maura Mitrushina, Joel Morgan, Christopher Paniak, Marianne Regard, Jill B. Rich, Diana Robins, Caroline Roncadin, Joanne Rovet, Ronald Ruff, Elsa Shapiro, Paula Shear, Abigail Sivan, Gerry Stefanatos, Esther Strauss, H. Gerry Taylor, David Tupper, Deborah Waber, N. William Walker, Maryanne Wolf, and Eric Zillmer.
I also wish to thank the following book and journal publishers:

Elsevier Science

Hogrefe and Huber Publishers

Lawrence Erlbaum Associates

Masson Italia Periodici

Oxford University Press

Pergamon Press

PRO-ED

Psychological Assessment Resources, Inc.

Sage Publishing

Southern Universities Press

Swets and Zeitlinger

TEA Ediciones, S. A.

Thames Valley Test Center, Ltd.

The Psychological Corporation

The Stoelting Corporation

Western Psychological Services

I am indebted to Lynda Crawford, Production Editor at Oxford University Press; her professionalism and guidance were instrumental in bringing this book to completion. Special personal mention is due my editors with whom it was once again a great pleasure to work and learn, Fiona Stevens and Jeffrey House of Oxford University Press. Their support for providing this book to the child neuropsychology community preceded my involvement by many years, and I am grateful to them for allowing me to take on this task. It was a wonderful experience.

Contents

III. DOMAINS AND TESTS

I

CHILD NEUROPSYCHOLOGY: CURRENT STATUS

1

Introduction

The specialty of neuropsychology includes individuals employed in varied clinical and research settings who have diverse educational and training backgrounds. This diversity of conceptual perspectives, theoretical biases, and practical experiences strengthens the field and provides strong clinical and empirical bases for advancing research and improving clinical proficiency. Within the broader field of neuropsychology are those who share a common desire to contribute to the understanding of neurobehavioral functions of the infant, child, and adolescent. For these *child neuropsychologists,* developmental issues are of central importance, along with an appreciation for the genetic, medical, environmental, behavioral, and sociocultural influences that determine how a child matures.

The responsibilities of clinical child neuropsychologists extend well beyond an early primary role as technicians collecting data on the cognitive consequences of brain injury or disease in neurological populations. It was not until the 1960s that interest in the behavioral sequelae of cerebral dysfunction in children began to thrive (Benton, 2000). Clinical practice, research participation, academic responsibilities, and consultative liaison roles have broadened as the science and practice of child neuropsychology has advanced. *Clinical practice* roles include the care, treatment, management, and rehabilitation of children with psychological, psychiatric, neurological, or other medical conditions or diseases. An emphasis on

the need to better understand normal brain development has seen a surge in research on normal populations as well. The child neuropsychologist might function as an independent provider or participate as a multidisciplinary team member, but he or she always brings an unique medical-psychological perspective to the multifactorial assessment of a child's neurocognitive functioning.

A substantial *research* role has advanced our understanding of neurodevelopment and contributed to investigations about a wide spectrum of disorders, besides the more common neurological, neurosurgical, or psychiatric conditions that characterized early practice and research. Neuropsychologists are increasingly involved in clinical trials, assisting in the design and implementation of protocols that are intended to improve or prolong life and/or minimize late effects of adjuvant therapies for systemic disease as well as central nervous system disease. They contribute to retrospective or prospective studies about the long-term consequences of prenatal insult and innovative postnatal medical procedures. They are engaged in assessing the impact of neurological conditions, such as monitoring the consequences of traumatic brain injury, at different developmental stages. Their interests extend to systemic, noncentral nervous system, disorders that influence higher cerebral function, such as congential cardiac conditions and metabolic disorders. They examine the reliability and validity of test instruments for different clinical populations and attempt to make discriminations between the profiles of co-morbid disorders, such as for Attention Deficit Hyperactivity Disorder (ADHD) and Tourette syndrome. They recognize the relevance of evidence-based medicine and possess the tools to further such research. Child neuropsychology practice is more diverse than ever before.

Importantly, the linkage between brain function evaluation and the development of practical and effective rehabilitation techniques is more visible today, and is steadily growing, although the literature remains sparse compared to that for adults. For instance, while the efficacy of cognitive rehabilitation with brain-injured adults and the adjunct use of computer rehabilitation techniques along with conventional therapy techniques was reviewed (Cicerone, Dahlberg et al., 2000), evidence-based cognitive rehabilitation techniques with children are currently less well described. Developing effective treatment programs is one of neuropsychology's greatest challenges, but progress in the area of remediation is occurring, for example, as attested to in the literature on children with cancer.

Baseline neuropsychological evaluation, obtained early in the disease course or soon after injury, aids the identification and monitoring of neurodevelopmental deficits and allows for intervention in a timely and effective manner. However, the inadvisability of interpreting individual tests for their functional implications in daily living skills without examining their construct validity has been pointed out (Johnstone and Wilhelm, 1997). One must understand what a test actually measures in order to make such judgments. A test does not always measure what its authors or publisher intend, and rigorous scientific investigation is needed to verify underlying factor structure before one accepts the validity of claims.

The advances in *academician and consulting roles* are made evident by the prominent positions held by colleagues in medical centers, higher academic institutions, the corporate world, and on nonprofit advisory panels. The Houston Conference on Specialty Education and Training in Clinical Neuropsychology, a conference to specify education and training guidelines, highlighted the ability of the profession's diverse membership to achieve consensus and respect differences in order to issue an unified visionary statement for the specialty of neuropsychology (Hannay, Bieliauskas et al., 1998). The current availability of training opportunities in neuropsychology contrasts markedly with what was available only three decades ago, and training issues continue to be prominent. Guidelines that resulted from a task force on test-user qualifications are now the policy of the American Psychological Association (Turner, DeMers et al., 2001). These specify the combination of knowledge, skills, abilities, training, experience, and practice credentials for responsible use of psychological tests.

The contributions of child neuropsychologists are explicit in an expanded literature that has depth, as well as breadth, of influence. This literature includes information about normal brain development, cognitive sequelae of brain insult, new ecologically more valid tests, expanded clinical population data, more sophisticated experimental designs, cross-cultural studies, new medical diagnostic techniques and procedures, improved treatment protocols and rehabilitative techniques, forensic neuropsychology, and the focus of this book, normative data. Ecological validity simulation tests have begun to be investigated in adult populations. Some studies report that ecological simulation tasks do serve as predictors of real world functioning (Nadolne and Stringer, 2001).

Such studies have yet to be reported for child populations, although there is considerable interest in the applicability of such tasks. There is increasing recognition of cross-cultural issues in neuropsychology, and the literature has begun to keep pace with issues specific to neuropsychology across cultural and racial groups (Ardila, 1995; Campbell, Rorie et al., 1996; Pontón, Satz et al., 1996; Artiola i Fortuny and Mullaney, 1997; Fletcher-Janzen, Reynolds et al., 2000; Manly and Jacobs, 2002). There is also an increased emphasis on theory and empirical testing of brain development models and testing models, along with greater attention directed to the pertinent contributions made by developmental, educational, and cognitive science colleagues. More sophisticated statistical techniques allow for more reliable and valid testing of assumptions about developmental brain pathology, behavioral disorder, and normal development (Ivnik, Smith et al., 2001). Computerized testing is increasingly being utilized, along with computerized scoring programs, and the advantages and disadvantages are weighed on an individual basis. There is variability in how well tests are converted to computerized formats, but it may be that the most successful are those that were computerized with minimal change in task demands. One example of the application of computerized tests in child evaluation is the Cambridge Neuropsychological Test Automated Battery (CANTAB) for young children (Luciana and Nelson, 1998).

Together, these many advances provide child neuropsychologists with the resources that enable them to contribute effectively to the investigation of normal and abnormal brain-behavior relationships in children and adolescents across socioeconomic and ethnic groups.

THE CONTRIBUTION OF NEUROPSYCHOLOGY TO CHILD EVALUATION

A distinction between clinical psychology and neuropsychology can be made, although many aspects of education and training overlap for these two specialty areas. A difference lies in the emphasis in the science of neuropsychology on the study of brain-behavior relationships and in the practice of neuropsychology on the application of brain–behavior relationships to individual patients (Adams, 1996). This concern with the linkage between behavior, or neurocognitive function, and the brain substrate defines the field of neuropsychology. Neuropsychologists are engaged in active exploration to authenticate their impressions about brain function through hypothesis testing at both an individual and broader level. This knowledge might arise from clinical examination of an individual patient or from experimental investigation of clinical or normal populations.

Age at injury and lesion severity continue to be the deserved subject of many investigations due to the prominence of these variables on outcome following brain insult. The idea that the earlier the insult, the better the child will function cognitively is now recognized as the myth that it is (Anderson and Moore, 1995; Taylor and Alden, 1997; Ewing-Cobbs, 1998). Some outcome and longitudinal studies of early focal lesions found less cognitive deficit than after later focal lesions (Dennis, 1980; O'Gorman et al., 1985; Aram, 1988; Vargha-Khadem, Carr et al., 1997; Stiles, Bates et al., 1998). It is also apparent that early diffuse lesions can have pervasive effects, even more than later diffuse lesions (Ewing-Cobbs, Levin et al., 1987) (Ewing-Cobbs, Fletcher et al., 1997).

The effects of closed-head injury (CHI) severity on cognitive function appeared most apparent in children younger than 10 years old (Levin, Culhane et al., 1993), although greater verbal learning and memory impairment was found for adolescents with severe CHI than for the children (Levin, High et al., 1988). There is also report of difficulty in acquiring reading skills after traumatic brain injury (TBI) in the preschool population (Anderson, Catroppa et al., 2000). Children with early-age, severe TBI were more severely impaired in spatial learning and orientation than older children (Lehnung, Leplow et al., 2001). In general, and of related interest, an imaging activation study finds that children demonstrate more diffuse cognitive activity than adults (Casey, Giedd et al., 2000).

Neuropsychological assessment is only one component of neuropsychological practice. It provides standardized, objective, and reliable measures of diverse aspects of human behavior, allowing for the specification of each individual's unique profile (Ivnik, Smith et al., 2001). With the addition of unique qualitative data, a full assessment adds substantially to our understanding of the child. Adult and child neuropsychology practice require some similar, but also some different, skills. These are described in comprehensive detail elsewhere (Baron, Fennell et al., 1995). To summarize, brain-behavior relationships in a developing child are both qualitatively and quantitatively different than those for an adult. It is crucial that the child neuropsychologist be familiar with the range of normal variation at each age level and be knowledgeable about how to adjust his or her clinical impressions for the child's developmental stage. Such knowledge is essential if one is to avoid misidentification of a normally developing child as one who is impaired or developmentally delayed.

It is also essential to comprehend better how neurological insult impacts on behavior and how behavior evolves in response to critical influences encountered at each developmental stage. Maturation is a variable, producing enormous complexity, and maturational level will affect the choice of test instrumentation and the evaluation of success or failure on any behavioral measure chosen. Maturation affects the breadth of behavioral measures that can be employed and validly assessed and necessitates the independent evaluation of a child's results, irrespective of any group considerations. The decision-making process about therapy, intervention, and management options is also influenced by maturational level.

The potential for plasticity, that is, the capacity for reorganization associated with an immature brain, must be considered. Plasticity, and the potential for dramatic change, is unlikely to be as relevant a factor in an adult examination as it is a child's. The child neuropsychologist must also consider differing diagnostic considerations between adults and children, and the various influences these diagnoses may have on the child compared to an adult. There is a greater potential for more unreliable assessment in the young age groups, and the examiner's expertise in eliciting optimal behavior becomes particularly crucial. Finally, restraint is required before adult rules of brain-behavior function are liberally applied to children since these may not apply or may need to be modified (Baron, Fennell et al., 1995).

Increasingly, child neuropsychologists are appropriately concerned with effective intervention for documented disorders of brain function, and optimal application of techniques that enhance the likelihood that the child will pass through a normal developmental sequence. Their interest in distinguishing between brain-based and psychological conditions parallels an interest in defining the range of neurocognitive strengths and weaknesses in order to facilitate appropriate treatment recommendations. Importantly, there is also increased sensitivity to the environmental and socioeconomic influences in recovery from brain disorder and how these directly affect outcome (Broman, Nichols et al., 1987; Taylor, Wade et al., 2002).

REASONS FOR REFERRAL

Referral to a child neuropsychologist is appropriate for diverse clinical, research, and/or academic reasons. Neuropsychological evaluation has progressed considerably from obsolescent "organicity" evaluations, when a single test instrument was often considered a sufficient screening for brain damage. The inaccuracy of that assumption is now well recognized by most clinicians (Bigler and Ehrfurth, 1981), along with the limitations inherent in the singular use of any one test instrument. Rather than test score–brain anatomy correlations, it is the overall profile that emerges in an evaluation that includes test results as one component that is critical (see discussion of convergence profile analysis below). Test results are considered, along with a careful history taking, keen clinical observations, and respect for the sociocultural context, in order to best understand the individual's neurocognitive function. This multistep evaluative process is especially critical since neuropsychological evaluation has predictive value for a child and will often serve as a basis for academic or vocational decisions and implementation of therapeutic options.

Commonly encountered are referral requests for information about the child's behavioral and emotional functioning in order to understand existing learning or behavioral problems and to develop a treatment plan and/or educational intervention strategy. Evaluation may be requested to document whether a profile of central nervous system disorder exists or to anticipate the late effects of a known early insult. The clinical course of a child, whose disease or disorder, or its treatment, might influence brain function differently at different developmental stages, needs to be established with a baseline evaluation and monitored over time. Interest in conducting a clinical trial or longitudinal research investigating developmental maturation may initiate a series of referrals.

In clinical practice, precedence should be given to the identification of the child's strengths as well as weaknesses in order to (1) make practical and meaningful recommendations to ameliorate the presenting problem and (2) better educate the school and family about the child's needs. While rare reasons for referral might emerge in the course of one's practice, the reasons specified below arise for either inpatients or outpatients and are especially common across many practice settings:

Referrals from School

Children experiencing learning or behavior problems in the academic setting represent a substantial number of outpatient child neuropsychology referrals. These children typically are referred when prior medical and/or psychological consultations do not sufficiently explain their observed behavior. Sometimes, parents are reluctant to accept a school committee's explanation and request an independent consultation, or second opinion, before accepting the school's decision. At other times, the neuropsychologist may be among the first to be consulted when the wide range of potential etiological factors has yet to be considered. Helping parents choose the needed consultations and effectively advocate for their child then comes under the purview of the neuropsychologist, who now is in a position to guide the family toward the resources that will best address the issues raised in evaluation.

Obviously, school problems can result for markedly diverse reasons. Not all of these are primarily neuropsychological in nature, but neuropsychological evaluation often contributes to better understanding true etiology. For example, observed academic failure or behavioral displays that seem out of the ordinary for the child's chronological age and contextual circumstances may initiate an evaluation to confirm or disconfirm an assumption of learning disability (LD). The neuropsychologist has the resources to consider the presumptive LD diagnosis while determining whether another explanation makes more sense. At the evaluation's conclusion, the neuropsychologist can place the child along a continuum, from intact function without evidence of LD, at one extreme, to subtle findings characteristic of the child with LD, to clear and specific LD, to complex or multiple learning disabilities, at the other extreme. Even more importantly, the evaluation that rejects LD as explanatory is likely to provide a revised framework in which to understand the child, one that may be inconsistent with the presumptive reason for referral but consonant with the behaviors that brought the child to the clinician's attention.

One must proceed cautiously when a referral includes a presumptive diagnosis based solely on observed behavior. The overt behavior might mask another relevant contributory problem that will be exposed with careful consideration of all relevant personal, historical, contextual, and medical factors. Thus, while diagnosis is rarely the intent of child neuropsychological evaluations, it might well result. For example, a presumed LD may in fact be symptomatic of another underlying neuropsychological etiology not yet considered by parents or teachers.

J. S. was an 11-year-old boy referred by his teacher for a "learning disability." The neuropsychological profile was clearly abnormal and revealed strongly focal, lateralized, right cerebral hemisphere dysfunction, with parietal lobe functions prominently impaired. Magnetic resonance imaging (MRI) of the brain was therefore recommended, and it revealed right parietal cortical malacia, likely due to an old ischemic etiology. Thus, in this instance, neuropsychological data compelled further investigation and led to recognition of a disabling, but heretofore unconsidered, neurological condition that also negatively affected school performance. The ostensibly clear LD "diagnosis" made by his teacher was actually behavior symptomatic of an unknown, but prepotent, neurological condition that, in turn, affected specific abilities important for academic performance.

Children whose atypical or idiosyncratic classroom behavior bewilders teachers or parents and who are resistant to the usual structured attempts to modify their behavior are also commonly referred for evaluation. Emotional maladjustment or primary emotional disorder might certainly be responsible. However, a presumption of a primary emotional etiology might not be satisfactory or sufficient. Referral is appropriate to allay concern about the reasons for associated academic problems, underachievement, or behavioral abnormality. It is important to clarify the child's cognitive strengths and weaknesses in order to better explain the child's atypical behavior.

Referrals from Family

Perplexing behavior, demonstrated at home or in other environmental contexts but not observed at school, might lead a parent to seek a neuropsychological evaluation. The evaluation is useful to examine neuropsychological integrity of function, primary psychological factors, acquisition of developmental milestones and level of maturity, or parenting skill effectiveness. It is sensitive to deviations from expectation. For instance, an evaluation might suggest a contributory seizure disorder, major mood disorder, neurodevelopmental delay, or late effects of an acquired condition such as an earlier traumatic brain injury. It might also highlight the inconsistency between parents in setting limits on a child's behavior as contributing to the problem.

While not uncommon, discrepancy between parent and teacher report requires clarification. Genuine differences might exist within each setting, but often, parents and teachers view similar behaviors quite disparately. The two very different settings can produce radically different behavioral presentations. Factors such as subject area proficiency, chronological age, class size, or the child's temperament affecting interpersonal relationships and learning style might influence teachers' perceptions. For example, a child with calculation weakness might behave better in English than in mathematics class; a middle school child's disruptive behavior might be attributed to "raging hormones" and inappropriately minimized; a child's intrusive behaviors might be better tolerated in a small class where there is more one-to-one attention than in a large class that has no teacher aides; or, an introverted, but learning-disabled, child might escape notice while an assertive, but normally maturing, child's antics might bring unwarranted attention.

Additional modulating variables must be considered when interpreting the child's behavior in any setting. These include age, family circumstances, and dynamics (Yeates, Taylor et al., 1997; Taylor, Yeates et al., 2001; Taylor, Wade et al., 2002); cultural and socioeconomic status (Broman, Nichols et al., 1987; Pérez-Arce, 1999; Kirkwood, Janusz et al., 2000); identifiable trauma or stressors, developmental maturity level, medical status, general intelligence, and overall adaptive ability. For instance, a young child might not easily respond to a teacher's demand to stay in her seat, follow the structure of set rules, or join a group cooperatively. The child's customary role within the family dynamic might be inappropriately transferred to the school setting.

A child living in poverty and a child from a wealthy family have quite different experiential histories, and the associated cognitive implications may vary. Emotional trauma cannot be easily blocked from intruding once the child enters the classroom. Medical illness or injury may result in school absence that further complicates the child's progress, and intellectual potential and emotional intelligence can affect the ease of adaptability across different settings.

Neurological Disease, Disorder, or Injury

The need to document cognitive consequences of disease, disorder, or injury on brain function in the developing child has not diminished over the years. However, our ability to understand these negative influences, and their impact on cognition, is enabled by increasingly more sophisticated means. Neuroimaging advances and other neurodiagnostic methods (Bigler, 1997) allow for a better understanding of structure-function relationships and make detection of neuropsychological deficit or preserved function all the more verifiable and intriguing. Yet, interpretive caution is needed since activation studies on clinical populations do not explain whether an activated area is critical for function or represents activation secondary to recruitment of that brain region in the face of the acquired insult.

Commonly, referral is initiated to characterize the current neurobehavioral effects of a known brain or systemic disorder. When a disease or disorder is as yet unknown, an evaluation might be requested to elicit behavioral elements that might contribute to a better understanding of the clinical behavioral pattern. In both instances, the neuropsychologist formulates conclusions based on knowledge of likely associated cognitive effects, potential influences of prescribed medications, typical course, associated known late effects, and the treatment regimen's potential impact on brain function.

There are special challenges in child neuropsychology, and several of these arise out of the intricacy of monitoring and predicting developmental course and maturation. The timing of the course of disease or disability on a developmental spectrum is a challenge particularly suited to child neuropsychologists who are well trained in normal and abnormal development, in general, and in the diverse effects on brain maturation, specifically. Among these considerations are the child's age at the time of insult, location and severity of a lesion, the focal or diffuse nature of the lesion, and the impact of acute insult and its possible evolution over time into a chronic condition (see Baron, Fennell et al., 1995, for a detailed discussion).

Prognosis after childhood disease or injury is often severely restricted. This is due, in part, to an inability to predict the extent of dynamic brain plasticity for any one individual and, therefore, a limitation in understanding how normal development will be affected by early and specific brain insult. Other considerations include genetic factors, the influential impact of time and experience, and the important influences of personality and motivation. As a result, optimism about eventual outcome is not irresponsible, but must be tempered with the facts that comprise the individual case.

The neuropsychologist often has a greater awareness of the potential for the persistence of cognitive interference and deficit than someone who erroneously views disease resolution or injury recovery as a sign of a eventual return to a normal functional level. An appreciation for the profound behavioral implications of early brain insult and for the limitations of brain plasticity is important. This is based on both clinical experience and empirical evidence. For example, peak cerebral metabolism declines after age 9 in children who had a temporal lobectomy at an earlier age, possibly indicative of already reduced plasticity at this young age (Chugani, Chugani et al., 1999). Also, regional measurements of the corpus callosum found cross-sectional reduction following pre- and perinatal brain injury (Moses, Courchesne et al., 2000). While focal cortical lesions in vascular insult have been the basis for the concept of greater plasticity in young children compared to adults, diffuse axonal injury and multiple ischemic injury associated with severe TBI represent quite different mechanisms (Di Stefano, Bachevalier et al., 2000). These authors suggest that disruption of white matter maturation has adverse effects on cognitive development and prevents recovery to normal levels.

Parents, too, are sometimes under the mistaken impression that resolution of the short-term effects of neurological insult parallels neurocognitive recovery, when, in fact, residual deficits can be far more persistent and intrusive on behavior and academic achievement. Typical clinical prediction is of at least a two-year course of recovery following an insult such as traumatic brain injury. It is useful to explain to parents that the initial rapid recovery is usually followed by a less rapid, but definite, course of improvement, and then by a more subtle period of resolution and accommodation that can extend even beyond the 2-year period. However, there is also evidence that while some children achieve stability or improve, others may worsen over time for a variety of reasons, e.g., in TBI populations (Brown, Chadwick et al., 1981; Jaffe, Plissar et al., 1995; Kinsella, Prior et al., 1995).

The suggestions of full, or nearly complete, recovery after early focal left or right hemisphere damage support hypotheses of neural plasticity of the young brain. It has been suggested that the right hemisphere has the ability, albeit less efficient, to mediate language for the very young child with left hemisphere damage. Brain activation studies of children who had very early focal brain injury have shown this more clearly (Müller, Rothermel et al., 1998; 1999; Booth, Macwhinney et al., 1999). Of related interest, left hemisphere activation for a spatial task normally mediated by the right cerebral hemisphere was found in a teenager who had right parietal and right temporal lesions at 7 months old (Levin, Scheller et al., 1996). The circumstances under which adaptation of the young brain occurs are not yet fully known. Language delays and deficits do result after left hemisphere damage, but not all aspects of language development are affected (Thal et al., 1991).

These observations appear to support the notion that the left hemisphere has a special role in language acquisition at the very earliest ages. Thal and colleagues conducted a longitudinal, prospective study of infants with focal brain injury. They found delayed lexical development in comprehension and production and a holistic approach to language learning. The latter was interpreted as characteristic of slower language learning rates and suggestive of a right hemispheric learning style. Lesion size did not appear to affect the linguistic measures. They also reported that left posterior cortical lesions resulted in slower rates of recovery from expressive delays but did not affect lexical comprehension.

Referral from Psychiatric and Other Medical Specialties

Concern about the child's ability to self-regulate behavior or about specific manifestations of psychiatric symptomatology are also prominent reasons for referral. Referral might be initiated to determine if measureable neuropsychological deficit coexists with the behavior of concern, and if the data provide further insight into etiological factors, such as, a profile consistent with temporal lobe epilepsy, a cerebral neoplasm, or hydrocephalus. A neuropsychologist might be requested to expand upon the consequences of either prescribed (iatrogenic) or abused substances, since a therapeutic medication regimen can carry unintended cognitive consequences as can incidental substance abuse during gestation or toxic exposure (Pérez-Arce, Johnson et al., 1989; Heffelfinger, Craft et al., 2002).

Referrals are also made by medical specialists not primarily concerned with the central nervous system but whose patient base holds interest for neuropsychologists. For example, some metabolic or endocrine disorders are of particular interest because disorders such as these result in a significant early insult to the developing nervous system. One of these, phenylketonuria, is especially associated with

prefrontal cerebral dysfunction, and the developmental trajectory of children with this disorder may hold potential for understanding the acquisition of mature working memory systems (Brunner, Jordan et al., 1983; Welsh, Pennington et al., 1990).

Data from such clinical populations are useful in examining differences between the course of a developmental deficit and a developmental delay, as when the deficit is not apparent in a young cohort but evident in the older children (White, Nortz et al., 2002). A focused series of studies are also reported for hypothyroidism (Rovet, 1992), hormone insufficiency (Gearing, Kalin, et al., 1992), diabetes (Northam, Bowden et al., 1992; Ryan, Vega et al., 1984; Rovet, Ehrlich et al., 1988), and renal failure (Davidovicz, Iacoviello et al., 1981; Fennell, Rasbury et al., 1984; Morris, Fennell et al., 1985). Organ transplantation has also come under some scrutiny (Stewart, Silver et al., 1991).

Referrals for Longitudinal Developmental Study

Longitudinal study and serial clinical evaluation of a developmental course are valuable but not always practical. These are not easily accomplished in the clinical setting due to a number of intrusive factors, including patient transience, acute medical conditions overwhelming psychological and academic interest, economic constraints, and the rarity of some disorders of interest. Despite these obstacles, examples of early brain disorder longitudinal studies include those of children with hydrocephalus (Brookshire, Fletcher et al., 1995), traumatic brain injury (Ewing-Cobbs, Fletcher et al., 1997), frontal lobe damage (Eslinger, Grattan et al., 1992), *Haemophilus influenzae* meningitis (Taylor, Schatschneider et al., 2000), pre- and perinatal focal brain injury (Stiles, Bates et al., 1998), and low birth weight (Vohr and Garcia Coll, 1985). There is recognition that age-related changes in the neuropsychological sequelae of early onset disease or disorder will be best understood with rigorous longitudinal studies of clearly defined cohorts of children with diffuse brain insult (Taylor, Schatschneider, et al., 2000). Longitudinal study, rather than cross-sectional study, is optimal to investigate developmental maturation and patterns of developmental change (Francis, Fletcher et al., 1991; Francis, Shaywitz et al., 1994).

Some correlate behavioral data with neuroimaging data in systematic and specific ways (Stiles, Moses et al., 2003). Such studies have the potential to provide valuable insight into the course of brain development following lesion. Neuroimaging data offer valuable insight into normal development as well. For example, positron emission tomography (PET) scans of infant brains found that the thalamus and brain stem had high rates of activity by 5 weeks, the cerebral cortex and outer portion of the cerebellum were still immature until approximately 3 months, and it was not until about 7 to 8 months that the frontal lobes showed more than minimal signs of activity (Chugani and Phelps, 1986).

In a study of the relation between brain maturation and cognitive development using event-related brain potentials (ERPs), it was concluded that cognitive transition, using Piagetian conservation tasks, was related to new neurocognitive mechanisms emerging during childhood (Stauder, Molenaar et al., 1999). These authors suggested that there is an important qualitative shift in the processing of information by the brain during middle childhood. Further, these authors made the interesting point that sudden qualitative changes in neurocognitive development should lead to rejection of the common use of chronological age for comparison to a child's reference group during these middle childhood years. Rather, they propose that both chronological age and level of cognitive development should be considered in choosing a norm group for certain tests, especially executive function tests that rely on evaluation of complex situations, like the Wisconsin Card Sorting Test (WCST) and Tower of London (TOL).

Children for whom a significant change in performance is expected (those with medical conditions that often result in cognitive deterioration or that have a potential for decline over time) are prime candidates for baseline and serial evaluation of neurobehavioral course. Serial evaluation also makes it possible to monitor recovery, document stability of function, and give insight into the individually determined clinical course and residual neurobehavioral profile, as well as contribute to updated educational and treatment recommendations.

Examination of the predictive validity of tests or outcome efficacy of treatment is only recently being given an increased emphasis. It is now well recognized that some long-term survivors of previously terminal childhood diseases will not escape late effects of their illness (Fletcher and Copeland, 1988). Longitudinal follow-up studies document the impact of the disease and/or treatment on the developing nervous system, even of some systemic and not primarily central nervous system diseases. Our knowledge of brain function in response to direct insults at different maturational times increases beneficially as a result of such studies. It is still necessary to investigate whether there are even more effective interventions that might ameliorate these expected late effects.

Along with disease and treatment factors, the important influences of family environment, as well as injury severity, are recognized as influential determinants of long-term outcome after childhood injury (Yeates, Taylor et al., 1997) and serve as the basis for current research. For example, social disadvantage was associated with poorer outcome and more adverse behavioral sequelae in a prospective study of outcome that extended for a mean of 4 years after traumatic brain injury (Taylor, Wade et al., 2002).

It is also recognized that parent attitude relates to parenting behavior and, thus, to parental competence (Miller-Loncar, Landry et al., 1997). The parenting attitudes of mothers of children with a complicated medical course have been shown to differ from those who have healthy children (Greenberg and Crnic, 1988). Not infrequently, history taking finds that a parent is reluctant to relinquish parental responsibility or to encourage the child to manage independently. A parent might psychologically hover over the child from a natural feeling of overprotectiveness that is no longer adaptive for either the child or the parent.

Referrals of Normal Children

Clinical referral intended merely to provide greater understanding of a child's capabilities is sometimes requested by parents. Despite the seemingly stable or intractable nature of a child's problem, some parents might request such an evaluation in the absence of precipitating school or medical problems. They might do so to aid in resolving persisting concern about a gestational or birth complication, a medication the mother took during pregnancy, or an early acquired childhood condition that they suspect has been the source of long-term negative cognitive effects. For example, a parent of a teenager who has always fared poorly academically and been intractable to the usual interventions may search for a medically based explanation. One aim may be to alleviate concern that a preexisting medical or psychological condition had placed the child at risk; another may be to obtain supplemental information when prior consultations seen insufficient to explain a child's behavior. Greater appreciation of the child's strengths and weaknesses is a most useful neuropsychological evaluation outcome and a valid precipitating reason for referral in selective instances.

Referrals Due to the Presence of Neurological "Soft Signs"

Children who exhibit neurological "soft signs," such as mild memory changes, mild personality or mood changes, borderline or abnormal electroencephalograph (EEG) without overt behavioral manifestation, attention lapses, speech disturbances, and motor dysfunction such as below-age gait or posture, involuntary movements, and asymmetrical motor-overflow movements, make neurological problems suspect (see Chapter 9 for discussion and normative data related to motor soft signs). The presence of soft signs can be a marker for an as yet unrecognized cognitive disorder. When soft signs are detected, a neuropsychological evaluation may be helpful to gain a better understanding about the extent of any associated neurocognitive problem.

Scientific Research Referrals

Empiricism provides an exciting opportunity for child neuropsychologists. The relatively young field of child neuropsychology, while maturing, still offers extensive research possibilities. Among these are the opportunity to in-

vestigate normal and abnormal development as a consequence of congenital conditions, disease, or injury, in context with the multiplicity of factors that affect outcome (Taylor and Schatschneider, 1992). Retrospective data collection was employed most commonly in the early child neuropsychology literature. However, well-timed and methodologically rigorous prospective studies will add most to our understanding of neurodevelopmental outcome after early neurological insult.

Prospective, longitudinal research designs, intended to follow developmental trajectory after congenital or acquired brain dysfunction, have been somewhat limited in child neuropsychology. Serial study to observe the developmental impact of an illness or injury, and the outcome of medical, rehabilitative and educational interventions is clearly desirable. Neuropsychologists are increasingly participating actively in clinical trial protocols evaluating neurocognitive outcome, correlating developmental brain pathology and behavioral pathology, researching treatment effectiveness and efforts to minimize consequent late effects of therapy, investigating differential function between clinical and normal groups, validating assessment instruments, and determining efficacy of rehabilitative efforts.

Referrals for Treatment, Management, and Rehabilitation Recommendations

Specific recommendations for instructional and rehabilitative strategies are the intent of a well-developed and well-conducted child neuropsychological evaluation. The clinician perspective makes the blending of medical concerns and psychological issues extremely valuable. The child neuropsychologist is well trained to assume a consultative or direct therapeutic role to formulate and/or apply a treatment/rehabilitation program. Early empirical studies including neuropsychological data rapidly led to the recognition that these data were unique and could be applied to developing more efficacious treatment and rehabilitation protocols.

It has been suggested that beliefs about cognitive rehabilitation may be summarized by four principles: basic science is the foundation for rehabilitation; cognitive rehabilitation success is dependent on rehabilitation techniques; recovery will be multiply determined and is not specific to the rehabilitation treatment; and outcome assessment must be evaluated in real-world situations (Stuss, Winocur et al., 1999).

CONVERGENCE PROFILE ANALYSIS

Convergence profile analysis is a term I use to explain to parents what it is that I do in a neuropsychological evaluation. It is profile analysis, supplemented by consideration of all relevant data acquired about the child. Along with knowledge of the available range of test instruments, statistical properties of tests, and available and appropriate normative data for each test, there are other important considerations if one is to best differentiate neurocognitive strengths and weaknesses. Profile, or pattern analysis, after administration of multiple test instruments, typically refers to interpretation after raw scores are converted to uniform standardized scores in those instances when this conversion is possible. This is a limited step, however, that does not completely capture the neuropsychologist's full contribution.

Why one neuropsychologist might be better able to make diagnostic formulations than another has been formally investigated. In a study of the relationship of neuropsychologists' cognitive complexity, ability to interpret behavior in a multidimensional way, and the validity of their diagnostic judgments, cognitive complexity was not significantly related to validity. The authors hypothesized that it may be the neuropsychologists' reliance on normative data that allowed them to make valid clinical judgments, independent of whether they had high or low cognitive complexity (Garb and Lutz, 2001).

As anyone familiar with the seminal work of Alexandr Luria can appreciate, however, normative data are not always required for valid conclusions to be reached about neuropsychological function. For the majority of current practitioners who ascribe to testing and use normative data, it is apparent that analyzing quantitative features with respect to appropriate normative data needs to be supplemented by integration of qualitative observations about the child's individual style and temperament. These impressions must then be weighed in comparison to the overall database of knowledge about the child.

I, therefore, refer to the additional steps taken beyond a standard profile or pattern analysis as *convergence profile analysis,* an expanded analysis of the entire spectrum of information about the child. It demands that suppositions based on one data point be matched or correlated sensibly with others before their import is overstated. Heavy emphasis is therefore placed on the neuropsychologist's clinical judgment. Certainly, in child evaluation, strict rules of interpretation, especially those originally based on adult models, are easily broken in consideration of the individual child. Rule breaking is often required in child evaluation since typicality within a homogeneous clinical subgroup is often not possible. Thus, while a hypothesis based on a single test result or an outlier score or performance, may be tentatively entertained, all such conjecture requires solid back-up. Clinical impressions cannot be considered definitive conclusions without such strong evidential support, that is, *convergence* within the full data spectrum.

This lesson was highlighted years ago when I supervised someone who administered the Tactual Performance Test and found marked left-upper-extremity impairment that contrasted with normal right-upper-extremity function for a supposedly normal adolescent. The pattern was sufficiently severe to raise concern about possible right cerebral hemisphere dysfunction, if one viewed only this single result as diagnostic. However, the adolescent was a perfectly normal well-functioning individual who agreed to be tested for practice. Questioning and some further investigation revealed that she always had difficulty with spatial directions, but there was no further history that raised concern about neurological status. Thus, a match between behavior and a test result was indeed present, but was not indicative of identifiable neurological impairment. The test result indicated only an interesting variation of normal development and made this individual's reported minimal spatial difficulty even more understandable.

It should also be emphasized that included within the full data spectrum are those critical qualitative performance features that must be scrutinized for their relevance to any explanation offered for the child's behavior. A mismatch between the child's behavior and neuropsychological results suggests something may have been overlooked, either in the test data, history, or real-world setting and experiences. While often implied, specific examples of overt recognition of the importance of such convergent data are occasionally encountered in the literature. While most normative data refer only to a total score as the value of interest for the Category Test, for example, despite there being multiple subtest scores, there are clinically evident differences in functioning across the subtests, with some proving easy and others troublesome.

Similarly, the possibility that poor performance on subtests IV and V of the Children's Category Test-2 suggests a perceptual organization deficit may be entertained. The authors of one study pointed out that solid back-up with some other measures of similar abilities, such as the Tactual Performance Test Localization Index (Nesbit-Greene and Donders, 2002) is required before one may make this assertion. In essence, they remind the reader that these data must converge from different sources, and only with back-up lines of evidence, can one be sure that the correct etiology for the behavior has been determined. Seeking confirmation from objective and/or subjective data sources is an active part of convergence profile analysis.

Qualitative observations to supplement normative data and aid interpretive conclusions contribute heavily to accurate convergence profile analysis. The very recent emphasis on quantifying qualitative observations in newly constructed tests, or as modifications of older, more established tests, is a most positive development, although the highlighted observations more often tend to be negative rather than positive ones. Unfortunately, a focus on negatives or deficit promotes a continued emphasis on what the child cannot do rather than what he or she can. Repetitious responses, perseverative responding, intrusion errors, a wide range of motor abnormalities, and an inability to sustain responding across a time interval are a few examples of such observations that deserve quantification. For example, failure to self-monitor performance or effectively maintain an on-line editing process may be reflected in perseverative responding on word list learning tasks. A difference in functioning was found when repetitious responses were quantified in a study of adults with right, left, or bilateral frontal lesions. Organizational strategies on word list learning tasks were examined for individuals with stable lesions, while excess intralist repetitions characterized the performance of patients with right frontal injuries. These repetitions were greater over longer periods of time, possibly related to an impaired ability to sustain attention that has been associated with right frontal pathology. Significant intrusion errors (confabulations) were not found for any group (Stuss, Alexander et al., 1994).

Persistence in attempting difficult tasks, engaging in an organized search, and exhibiting careful planning and placement on a work sheet are examples of positive observations, some of which are now being quantified in order to evaluate strategic choices. The latter may provide additional clarity about how the child masters a task or succeeds most readily, but too often these are not quantified, standardized, or emphasized by test developers. Both the errors and positive constituent behaviors are expected to lead to a more complete understanding of the child's information-processing style as well as enhance the recognition of why he or she might fail to succeed or, in contrast, achieve up to or beyond expectation. Yet, it is the strengths that will especially assist in determining appropriate interventions, and that have influential predictive value.

As alluded to above, formal application of standardized test procedures to qualitative behavioral features is now being addressed in newer adult tests (Stern, Singer et al., 1994; Stern, Javorsky et al., 1999), including normative data on intrasubtest scatter to highlight arousal level, attention, and motivational variability (Kaplan, Fein et al., 1991). Unfortunately, the same rigor is rarely directed to the evaluation of qualitative features of children's test performances, although this is changing and there is a new emphasis on quantifying some error types (Waber and Holmes, 1985; 1986; Bernstein and Waber 1996; Delis, Kaplan et al., 2001). Child clinicians have traditionally had to develop individualized ways to reach their conclusions, which are heavily dependent on their clinical judgment and years of experience. Informal techniques sometimes require deviation from standardized procedures, while maintaining sufficient rigor to score standardized tests validly. For example, it is useful to compare scores calculated under standardized time constraints to those obtained when time limits are extended beyond the cut-off-time limits.

Careful note taking also helps to document problem-solving strategies. Administration of items beyond the "discontinue" point helps gauge the true extent of competence. Provision of a multiple-choice format helps test the limits of a child's knowledge while also assessing retrieval and recognition memory. How varying clinical populations respond differentially is also an area of interest to those who consider qualitative features of a child's performance. For example, children with orbitofrontal or inferior frontal lesions had difficulty using error feedback from prior trial performances to correct their actions. They had difficulty making choices and evaluating risks associated with divergent possibilities (Levin, Song et al., 2001). Such interest in error, as well as intact performance patterns, is evident in the adult literature as well; for example, the error types on the Trail Making Test that were defined and examined in a dementia population may be of interest to child neuropsychologists as well (Cahn, Salmon et al., 1997). It is expected that such attention to finer details about adult performance will continue to expand to childhood populations.

What is normal and what is abnormal may be more difficult to dissociate for children than for adults. For example, an adult's inability to inhibit perseveratory responses is a classic sign of abnormality. However, it is not until 10 years of age that the ability to inhibit attention to irrelevant stimuli and reduce perseveratory responses is almost sufficiently matured, with complete mastery generally achieved by age 12 (Passler et al., 1985). Since a range of acceptable normal variability exists for each develop-

mental skill acquisition, determination of the boundaries of acceptable responding can be especially difficult to discern for a child whose chronological age bridges the age range cited for maturation. The statistical boundaries of normality are, as a result, often wider for a child than an adult. What represents normality may have a wider range of acceptability and will be reflected by larger standard deviations for a particular test score.

It is useful to develop a framework for examining test data. Three common approaches to interpreting neuropsychological test data use cross-sectional data: absolute scores, difference scores, and profile variability. One approach uses longitudinal data, or change scores. Absolute scores refer to a single score from each test that might best differentiate each diagnostic group. Difference scores refer to a comparison of performance on tests sensitive to neurocognitive dysfunction with that on tests resistant to these effects. Profile variability is based on an assumption that impairment will affect performance variability across a range of tests. Change scores refer to longitudinal data obtained at test–retest intervals (Ivnik, Smith et al., 2001). Interestingly, when these were applied to an adult database, it was concluded that difference scores were not supported for diagnosis over cut-scores. These authors also found that measures of intraindividual test score variability and test-retest change were not diagnostically useful and that positive and negative predictive values and likelihood ratios provided information better able to quantify the probability that diagnostic conclusions were accurate (Ivnik, Smith et al., 2000). The reader is referred to these articles for greater definition, discussion, and a schematic for understanding the diagnostic capabilities of clinical tests in adults and a heuristic for consideration of the diagnostic potential of clinical tests in children.

TESTING MODELS

Much has been written, and even debated, about testing models and strategies. Strong opinions may be expressed by proponents of the different models: fixed battery, flexible battery, process approach, personal core battery, and dynamic models. The conceptualization of, and need for, a personal model should not be minimized. Yet, as clinicians search for the model most congruent with their own style of practice, they recognize that the model cannot be held responsible for less than stellar professional practice. Therefore, perhaps a basic consideration is not which testing model one philosophically endorses, but whether one follows a logical and justifiable path to best answer a referral question and comprehensively understand the range of psychological, medical, and sociocultural issues impacting on the individual being assessed.

An experienced practitioner, using a repeatable fixed-battery approach, may be equally as capable of detecting and interpreting the broader range of characteristics and nuances of neuropsychological function that explain a child's behavior as the practitioner who endorses a flexible battery, although the routes to reaching that conclusion diverge. While the neuropsychologist's education, training, and practice may be highly determinant of capability, the ability to integrate a fundamental and sensible model appears crucial for the ability to appreciate the broader perspective. Thus, despite having an excellent education and training, clinicians who follow a restrictive or flawed model may never achieve the degree of proficiency that may result if an alternative, more appropriate model is their theoretical context.

Given this perspective, it is relevant to note that there are some significant differences among well-recognized models that the clinician may consider. The early fixed- or core-battery approach was developed with the recognition that a single test result was not sufficient for the broader purpose (Ernhart, Graham et al., 1963). Yet, despite the profound simplicity of that sentiment, fixed-battery advocates often administered specific tests to each child, independent of incidental behavioral observations, diagnostic considerations, or the utility of the tests within that battery for the deficits observed or suspected.

The fixed-battery model, therefore, led many to search for, elucidate, and endorse alternative models. Despite the fixed battery's added merit over single test administration, and its perceived usefulness in obtaining nor-

mative and research data, an inflexible fixed-battery approach often proved insensitive to individualized referral concerns across diagnostic populations and was often limited when one needed to better understand the diverse concomitants of brain dysfunction. For example, someone following a fixed-battery model, such as the original Halstead Reitan Neuropsychological Test Battery (HRNTB), but evaluating individuals with traumatic brain injury, quickly recognizes this battery's weakness with respect to this population's behavioral concomitants. The HRNTB is weak with respect to examining attentional subcomponents, learning, free recall and recognition memory, and critical aspects of executive function. This was certainly my experience early in my professional career when I was assigned to a neurosurgical service with responsibility for evaluating all children admitted to the hospital following a traumatic brain injury. It quickly became apparent that there was a serious disconnection between the questions I was being asked by physicians and family and what answers I could produce using only a fixed battery.

The adult literature provides some perspective in this regard. Factor analysis of the HRNTB, Wechsler Adult Intelligence Scale (WAIS), and Wechsler Memory Scale-Revised (WMS), found that the HRNTB tests loaded with WAIS factors of Perceptual Organization and Processing Speed, and with a WAIS/WMS attention factor, but found no support for a HRNTB memory component. In fact, the adult literature has repeatedly determined that the HRNTB and the WAIS had equivalent sensitivity to brain damage and appear to be measuring the same constructs (Kane, Parsons et al., 1985). Such failure reinforces clinical impressions of the model's weaknesses.

Practitioners are therefore more in control of their practice when they chose to modify test selection and exhibit greater flexibility. Cognitive testing that uses multiple measures differentiates normal from impaired cognitive states better than when there is reliance on individual scores (Ivnik, Smith et al., 2001). The solution for some practitioners was to avoid the fixed battery or move from a fixed battery to the flexible battery approach. A flexible battery approach meant that tests were added to a fixed battery or their own personal core battery, based on individual need. It was intended that by so tailoring the evaluation, one would better evaluate domains or subdomains omitted in the rigidly structured battery. This procedure resulted in considerably less dependence on a core fixed battery and made acceptable greater interest in the available and expanding range of measures that would best answer the clinical questions. These additional measures, for example, may be older test instruments developed for adults, downward extensions of adult tasks for children, newly developed tests, or modifications of experimental procedures from allied areas such as developmental or cognitive psychology. Procedural variation to explore how and when a child will function optimally placed central importance on educated test selection, and tests with limited clinical utility could be dropped and alternative tests added and tried.

The emphasis on qualitative observation of a person's particular cognitive style was always recognized as influential and necessary for good clinical practice, but was not quantified formally in standard testing until highlighted in the adult literature as the Process Approach (Kaplan, 1988). The importance of considering the individual's process, or individual style, received even greater exposure as clinical observations became formalized routinely and as new adult tests and methods were constructed with requirements that the examiner directly quantify such observations. This practical and efficient approach has particular salience in child evaluation. For example, a study of executive function in unmedicated children with Tourette syndrome or attention deficit hyperactivity disorder provided data supporting the use and analysis of process variables, especially those related to inhibition and intrusion errors (Mahone, Koth et al., 2001). Yet, one should recognize that the recommended procedural modifications may alter what is being measured as well as affect the ability to refer to standardized normative data for the specific test being modified. A focus on process can be a time-intensive procedure that provides multiple data points that are unequal in their relevance or applicability to the child in question.

Currently, our available tests do not fully assess the diverse ways brain disease can affect a child's cognitive capacities (Taylor and Schatschneider, 1992), nor do we fully understand the influence of learning on functional organization of the brain (Castro-Caldas, Petersson et al., 1998). We understand or analyze existing data incompletely or fail to obtain data that will be most elucidating without recognizing that what is omitted may be most illuminating. Due to considerable methodological and technological limitations inherent to child evaluation, our knowledge of structural-behavioral correlation in childhood still lags way behind advances reported for adults.

A Pragmatic Approach

My own step-by-step evolution with respect to which test model might best serve my needs continues to be modified, even after three decades of child evaluation. I began with a fixed battery, but, for the reasons noted above, found its limitations exceeded its usefulness far too often to merit continuing its use. I moved toward a flexible battery approach around a core and appreciated the greater latitude it provided. But, as many of the fixed-core tests had limited clinical utility, the time spent administering them consistently across diverse populations appeared inappropriate. The range of child tests began to burgeon, and I began a trial-and-error test selection around a personal core battery.

Careful observation and note taking about qualitative and performance style features became even more critical in influencing my evaluation summaries, paralleling the formalization of the Process Approach from the adult literature. Yet, none of these models sufficiently met all my needs. My evolution led me to what seemed to fit my patient base best, a model that built on the pragmatic importance of always seeking knowledge about a child's strengths in order to understand the observed weaknesses. I am not suggesting that this is radically different from the conceptual thinking that any clinician may advance, but it is the model I use, and I therefore present it as an example. This emphasis on strengths became a prominent focus of each evaluation.

Detailing the child's strengths during testing also became a clear focus in interpretive sessions. The search for and identification of strengths enabled me to be more specific and practical with parents and sharpened my ability to make appropriate home and school recommendations. Pointing out what their child could do and placing the weaknesses in appropriate context seemed to be something that was often forgotten or overlooked as attention centered on deficits and weaknesses. Yet, this perspective was necessary to optimize interpretive discussion and intervention planning and to provide a framework for an eventual plan of action toward the desired outcome.

Following this pragmatic approach, I choose each test or subtest depending on the moment-to-moment decisions I make about the child while engaged in the dyadic test interaction. In essence, this approach is a non-battery model. It is a continuous application, testing a fluid train of thought. This pragmatic approach is one that is easily understood by parents, teachers and other nonneuropsychologists, and thus the interpretive sessions are made more practical as well. An overemphasis on deficit seems limiting in child assessment where deficit is linked to developmental maturity. Such a focus on negatives necessitates structured reminders to integrate the enormously important evidence of the child's strengths and to remember to communicate these data to those involved in the child's care.

To some extent, my approach most closely shares features described for dynamic models, which also place emphasis on knowing what a child can accomplish. In both, one investigates what works and what doesn't, with the intention of finding these strengths and interpreting and using them effectively. The identification of these strengths, in turn, has the remarkable ability to change the perspectives of those involved in the child's care and may lead to different interpretive conclusions than would have resulted had they not been detected and incorporated. For example, a child is referred because of poor handwriting, and the teacher suspects a learning disability. Evaluation finds the child indeed has a very poor handwriting, but in all other respects is a normal, well-functioning individual with some normal-range relative weaknesses as well as more highly developed capacities. The problem that initiated referral is not an issue at home but one that is prominent at school, due to the teacher's emphasis on neatness in written production. As a

result, her constant criticism results in the child's negative self-perception and an increase in inattentive and acting out behaviors.

The neuropsychological evaluation results enable communicating the child's range of strengths, provide a developmental perspective for poor handwriting, and place its importance in a new and more realistic context. Without focusing on the child's inherent strengths, one may incorrectly conclude there is "dysfunction" when, in fact, the child possesses genuine strengths reflecting cognitive efficiency in all domains assessed. For this child, the parents need to be reminded that, in maturity, their child may choose to print rather than write in cursive, may have exceptional keyboarding skill, obviating the need for extensive written production, or may even have a secretary. Technology will evolve and provide other means of delimiting the emphasis on writing in real-world situations. The focus of the interpretive session shifts from the intended referral for recommendations for ameliorating a weakness to recognizing normal variation and emphasizing the child's strong cognitive capacities, along with specific recommendations that will make demands for written production less stressful. In view of the teacher referral, the parents need to be encouraged to schedule a conference with the school where they can provide evidence of their child's neurocognitive strengths. They also need to be assured that their child will regain the positive self-image he possessed before writing became a source of contention in the academic setting.

Most importantly, the pragmatic approach is acutely sensitive to the import and dynamic nature of maturation that must be addressed in every test choice and for each interpretative conclusion. By virtue of its attention to this dynamic behavioral sampling process, the model is sensitive to the needs of special populations and cross-cultural assessment issues. Admittedly, it may depend less on normative data than some models, not lessening the importance of normative data when they are available and applicable. The approach supports assessment within the immediate context with examination of whether underlying assumptions about the observed behaviors are generalizable to the external context, ecologically valid, and/or insightful for prediction of future behavior. To date, it is this pragmatic approach that I am most comfortable with and which allows me to define a logical and justifiable strategy in testing both children and adults.

ALTERNATE TEST FORMS

Included in this volume are several tests that have alternate (parallel) forms. These forms were developed for use when reevaluation is required or when the primary form is invalidated for any number of reasons outside the examiner's control. Caution is in order when one uses an alternate form on a repeat administration. Alternate forms are not always proven to be of equal difficulty. Also, the existence of an alternate form does not imply that a novel test administration will result on retesting. In fact, the child may recall the initial test form or procedure, remember procedural conditions making the novelty factor moot, adapt behavior to accommodate the now-familiar test condition, or even retreat emotionally from full participation on a test that was difficult on its initial presentation. For example, when incidental recall is required on a novel word list-learning test, one cannot presume that recall is not anticipated on readministration with an alternate form. As a result, clinical interpretation needs to consider these and other possibilities. An "incidental" immediate recall of the Rey-Osterrieth Complex Figure Test immediately after the copy trial depends on the child not knowing a recall drawing will be requested. On a second evaluation the child will often recall the request for another drawing, even when an alternate form is presented. The procedural requirement will no longer be novel, and practice effects can be presumed to be operating.

Of interest in this regard, the reliability of Trail Making Test alternate forms was examined, and subjects did better on the second trial regardless of whether an original form or alternate form was given first (Franzen, Paul et al., 1996). Also, subjects significantly improved their verbal fluency over a 6-month, test-retest period using the Controlled Oral Word Association Test (COWAT) alternate forms (Ruff, Light et al., 1996). Improved COWAT performance and a large practice effect were found despite the use of alternate forms over a 2-month, test–retest interval (Barr, 2003). It is apparent that in many instances the examiner cannot ensure the absence of practice effects between test session 1 and 2 and should be alert to their possible influence, even when using alternate forms. Determinations about change need to be based on knowledge about the reliability of the test instrument, the extent that novelty affects performance, and the magnitude of any practice effects.

In contrast, some tests that do not have alternate forms do appear to have limited practice effects, although these are relatively few. Minimal practice effects were reported in an adult study of two different verbal list-learning tests administered in the same test battery (Crossen and Wiens, 1994), suggesting there may be times when procedures from one test do not generalize to another test with similar procedures. Clinical impressions that motor tests, such as the Finger Tapping Test, the Grooved Pegboard Test, and the Purdue Pegboard Test, are less likely to show improvement with repeat evaluation are in fact finding support in the literature (Barr, 2003).

However, a psychomotor problem-solving test, the Tactual Performance Test (TPT), has potentially significant practice effects, and it does not require empirical data to recognize the impact this test has on a child the first time it is administered. The TPT evokes especially strong emotion in children who consider it aversive due to the requirement that they be blindfolded and rely on only tactile and kinesthetic cues. Attempts to reevaluate someone who experienced difficulty on the TPT will often produce an immediate negative response, thus reducing its effectiveness in serial evaluation or longitudinal study. Some attention test results appear to be minimally affected by practice, such as digit span (Barr, 2003), other verbal and nonverbal span tests, and some visual search cancellation tests. Test–retest reliability data are not always available for a specific instrument to enable the neuropsychologist to make a more accurate judgment about the potential for practice effects or to aid in the evaluation of reliable change. Further, alternate forms represent two separate instruments with different propensities for regression to the mean, making interpretation of test-retest change scores even more difficult.

Whenever one readministers a test, the conceptual issues for evaluating poor performance are necessarily different than they were for the baseline administration. This holds true whether it is a clinical examination or an experimental study. As noted above, administration of alternate forms does not eliminate the need for consideration of practice effects. As a result, in consideration of the issues associated with test–retest reliability, stability of test scores with serial study, regression to the mean, the use of alternate forms, and the emphasis on outcome study, there is increasingly greater importance placed on calculating "change" scores.

Tests discussed in this volume that have alternate forms are listed in Table 1.1. COWAT requires production of words in response to the letters C, F, and L. The alternate version uses P, R and W. There are six word lists for the Hopkins Verbal Learning Test (Brandt, 1991; Benedict, Schretlen et al., 1998). Various forms of the Selective Reminding Test exist for different ages (see Chapter 11). The Judgment of Line Orientation Test (Benton, Varney et al., 1978; Benton, Hamsher et al., 1983) has two forms with the items arranged in different order. There are Forms A and B for the Test of Everyday Attention for Children (Manly, Robertson et al., 1999). Commonly, one will administer the Taylor Complex Figure when

Table 1–1. Examples of Tests with Alternate Forms

Controlled Oral Word Association Test
Hopkins Verbal Learning Test-Revised
Verbal Selective Reminding Test
Peabody Picture Vocabulary Test-III
Judgment of Line Orientation Test
Benton Visual Retention Test-5th Ed.
Rey-Osterrieth Complex Figure Test
Test of Everyday Attention for Children
Multilingual Aphasia Examination Sentence
  Repetition Test
Token Test
Test of Nonverbal Intelligence–3
Porteus Maze Test
Rivermead Behavioural Memory Test for Children
  Aged 5 to 10 Years Old

---

the Rey-Osterrieth Complex Figure Test has been initially administered (Taylor, 1959). The Multilingual Aphasia Test has two sentence memory stimuli lists (Benton and Hamsher, 1976). The Test of Nonverbal Intelligence–3 has two equivalent forms (Brown, Sherbenou et al., 1997). A supplemental series provides additional stimuli for retesting with the Porteus Mazes Test. The Rivermead Behavioural Memory Test for Children Aged 5 to 10 years has four parallel forms (Wilson, Ivani-Chalian et al., 1991).

DETECTING SIGNIFICANT CHANGE

The recent literature expands discussion about detecting significant intraindividual change, focusing on determinations about whether an individual's change over time (test-retest score difference) is in fact meaningful. Determination about change is often needed in the absence of any comparison group, for example, in clinical practice when reevaluation is requested to monitor neurodevelopment following a course of treatment or subsequent to an acquired brain injury. Among the relevant statistical procedures to accomplish these analyses are the Reliable Change Index (RCI) and RCI with adjustment for practice effect (Jacobson and Truax, 1991; Chelune, Naugle et al., 1993; Sawrie, Chelune et al., 1996). The RCI establishes significance of any change on the difference between initial and retest scores for the normative subject sample. A change score is considered significant if it falls outside the standard deviation of the test-retest difference in the norming sample, multiplied by the z-score cutoff point that defines a specified percentile of the normal distribution. For example, using a 95th percentile cutoff point, the resulting z-score cutoff will be ± 1.645. The resulting prediction or confidence interval will include 90% of normative sample individuals.

A second model, proposed as an improvement to the RCI model, recommended the use of the RCI with practice effects (Chelune, Naugle et al., 1993). In this model the predicted retest score is the baseline score plus the mean practice effect for the normative sample. The RCI with practice model suggests the comparison value is exceeded by chance only 10% of the time if assumptions used in its derivation are true (Dikmen, Heaton et al., 1999). It is also assumed that the changes follow a normal distribution and that variability in retest changes is the same for all subjects (Dikmen, Heaton et al., 1999). However, as practice effects are not constant for all subjects and different practice effects may be based on initial performance level, age, education, or other variables, these assumptions may be inaccurate.

Linear regression of retest scores on initial scores in a norming sample is a third model. This model uses correction for practice effects and regression to the mean to predict a future score based on initial score. This model is exemplified by "T scores for change" (McSweeny, Chelune et al., 1993.). A significant retest score is thus one that differs from its predicted value by greater than the standard deviation from the norming sample, multiplied by 1.645, the above noted z-score cutoff point. These authors recommended norms for change that are population-specific and a regression approach that is continuous rather than categorical (indicating gain, loss, or no change). They presented the results in a familiar context for psychologists by converting the change score norms to standardized T scores with a mean of 50 and SD of 10.

Stepwise linear regression is also suggested as a fourth model. In this model, multiple factors enter into consideration to determine whether a predicted retest score is significant. Included are the test–retest temporal interval, demographic characteristics, and general neuropsychological competence. This model uses a method for determining significant deviation similar to the linear regression model noted above. It also considers the possibility of a nonlinear relationship between scores (Temkin, Heaton et al., 1999).

These statistical procedures regarding change over time are of special interest to child neuropsychologists, who must frequently make determinations about a child's developmental progression and comment on any deviation from the expected course observed with serial evaluation over an extended time. These are always complicated judgments that must be made with knowledge of the enormous dynamic influences associated with maturational change and, therefore, with full knowledge of normal child development principles and milestones.

CHILD NEUROPSYCHOLOGICAL NORMATIVE DATA: SOME IDEALS AND THE REALITIES

A principal impetus for this volume was to compile a selective summary of normative data for individual child neuropsychology tests. Normative data provide a distribution of test scores in a particular sample from the population (Turner, DeMers et al., 2001). Child neuropsychologists are especially cognizant of the importance of using reliable and valid tests with appropriate normative data for their population (American Psychological Association, 1985). Yet, despite such awareness, there is wide disparity in the availability and applicability of such data across tests. While many researchers focused on the clinical trajectory associated with normal brain development, the increasing proficiency with increased age, and the deviations associated with abnormal development, such investigations often neglected the importance of using tests that have reliable and valid normative data. As a result, major omissions in the acquisition of applicable normative data remain.

Even when data are available, their application can be limited. This is due, in part, to limited regional rather than population-based sampling, procedural and methodological inconsistencies within and across tests, pooled rather than stratified groups, small Ns that become even smaller when stratified by age or grade, data variance reflected in large standard deviations, heterogeneous, rather than homogeneous, sampling, and poor interrater reliability. Further, summary standardized scores might obscure important clinical features, thereby limiting interpretive conclusions. While test batteries require inspection of their factor structure in both clinical and normal populations to determine if they measure what they purport to measure, such research is not always available for some of our older—but still standard—measures. The importance of confirmatory factor analysis during test development is now well recognized.

It cannot be stated too often that children may not be conceptualized as very young adults and that the brain-behavior rules associated with adults will not necessarily apply to the child. Attempts to extend knowledge of brain-behavior relationships established in adult neuropsychology downward have often proved inadequate and inappropriate (Baron, Fennell et al., 1995) but their use has persisted in the absence of empirical studies to the contrary. Appropriate validation of adult test instruments adapted for use with children is not always available, raising serious concern about a particular instrument and its applicability to children at different developmental stages.

Even older-child tests cannot be confidently applied to younger children (Kaspar and Sokolec, 1980). The dynamic nature of maturation makes such application highly questionable. Both qualitative and quantitative differences exist and require greater attention. The recognition of "pastel" versions of adult-acquired deficits (Denckla and Cutting, 1999) nicely underscores the subtle manifestations of childhood deficit compared to the more overt symptoms commonly seen in adults. Also, symptoms of brain insult in childhood can be far more transient than those observed in adulthood. To best evaluate a child's performance, one must choose the most appropriate normative data. It is therefore highly desirable that demographic data be complete and reported to assist in that choice.

Subject variables need to be accounted for in interpretation. In fact, child neuropsychology normative data do not always identify the sample's demographic characteristics sufficiently well. Expected reports include such features as intelligence, educational level, cultural background, race/ethnicity, socioeconomic status (SES), and gender as these variables can be influential (Amante, VanHouten et al., 1977; Halpern, 1992; Kimura, 1999). Higher diagnostic classification accuracy is associated with the use of demographically adjusted neuropsychological summary scores in adult studies (Vanderploeg, Axelrod et al., 1997). Performance on the Luria Nebraska Neuropsychological Battery (LNNB) and HRNTB is signif-

icantly related to intelligence (Golden, Kane et al., 1981; Chelune, 1982; Seidenberg, Giordani et al., 1983; Reitan, 1985).

Performance can be strongly related to age and education, with education effects often quite robust (Matarazzo and Herman, 1984; Heaton, Grant et al., 1986). As a result, tests that utilize cutoff scores might misidentify someone whose particular demographics are not characteristic of those in the utilized normative data base, e.g., a lower intelligence, less-educated person might be mistakenly identified as cognitively impaired (Marcopulos, McLain et al., 1997). The development of culturally appropriate test batteries with normative data from individual tests to full batteries continues. These are intended to enable more reliable and valid investigation of brain-behavioral functional relationships without dependence on data from an inappropriate reference group (Nielsen, Knudsen et al., 1989; Pontón, Satz et al., 1996; Agostini, Metz-Lutz et al., 1998; Ostrosky-Solis, Ardila et al., 1999; Reye, Feldman et al., 1999). Many tests, however, lack adequate specificity for ethnic minorities, and this is an area of continuing concern in test construction and standardization sampling. Cultural experiences need to be accounted for, and literacy levels are not routinely noted. Study of the impact of requirements for speeded performance, familiarity with the test items, attention to detail, along with consideration of diverse language and educational factors and acculturation, is also needed (Manly and Jacobs, 2002).

It has been pointed out that one should consider using literacy to equate ethnic groups and that test relevance will supersede cultural group with respect to the individual's motivation (Manly and Jacobs, 2002). Since reading level attenuates differences in neuropsychological test performance between African American and white elders, the clinician should recognize that years of education is an inadequate measure of educational experience among multicultural elders. Adjusting for quality of education is more likely to improve the specificity of certain neuropsychological measures (Manly, Jacobs et al., 2002). These findings have relevance for child and adolescent clinicians as well. Using separate ethnic norms may leave observed ethnic differences unexplained and therefore subject to misinterpretation if one does not examine the individual's cultural and educational experiences. Assumptions about the "culture-free" features of some tests may also be erroneous; for example, cancellation tests, digit span length, timed tests, reasoning tests, nonverbal tests, and simple reaction-time tests may all be affected by cultural factors, although they frequently are considered more culture-free than other tests. Thus, one must define, measure, and adjust for racial/cultural group rather than merely assigning an individual to a race/ethnicity group and making a judgment without consideration of other relevant and more pertinent factors.

Gender differences may prove especially pertinent since studies often highlight differential function of male and female subjects (Halpern, 1997). For example, early investigations documented female superiority on verbal tasks and male superiority for visuospatial function and calculation, and recent adult studies reinforced these findings. Female superiority in verbal production tasks and on some episodic memory tests with a visuospatial component was found, while male superiority was found on a mental rotation task (Herlitz, Airaksinen et al., 1999). With attention to more specific behavioral concerns, it was also found that the female advantage on episodic memory tasks was not found on tasks of semantic memory, primary memory, priming, or procedural memory (Herlitz, Nillson et al., 1997). Wechsler scale digit symbol superiority of females is also documented (Kaufman, 1990; Jensen and Reynolds, 1983). These differences need to be considered also with respect to biological factors, such as neuroanatomical differences or hormonal influences, and psychosocial factors, such as environment and the influences imposed by stereotypes (Steele, 1997).

Gender differences highlighted in the child literature often parallel those reported in the adult literature. Early developmental memory studies found girls more proficient in verbal memory than boys (Maccoby and Jacklin, 1974). Female over male superiority was found for word fluency at ages 9 to 13 years and spelling written names at ages 7, 9, 10, and 11 years (Gaddes and Crockett, 1975). Girls generated more names than boys on a semantic fluency test (Harris, Marcus et al., 1999). Developmental studies found the female over male advantage in episodic memory evident as early as age 5 (Kramer, Delis et al., 1997; 1998). The gender differences favoring girls were found on the California Verbal Learning Test for Children (CVLT-C), but with small effect sizes and significance for age clusters but not individual age groups (Kramer, Delis et al., 1997). Female adolescents surpassed males in long term retrieval of a word list (Levin, Benton et al., 1982). An adolescent female over male advantage was also found for information processing (WISC-III digit symbol subtest), mental tracking (Trail Making Test), and verbal initiation (verbal fluency) (Barr, 2003). Besides study of normal children, gender influences in clinical populations are also explored. For example, the influence of gender in a learning disability population received detailed attention in a series of seminal studies (Geschwind and Galaburda, 1985a; 1985b; 1985c). In study using the CVLT-C, it was concluded that male gender was associated with an increased risk for retrieval deficits after pediatric TBI, possibly due to a reduced speed or efficiency of information proessing (Donders and Hoffman, 2002). Gender differences were found after treatment for acute lymphoblastic leukemia, with females being especially vulnerable to late effects (Waber and Mullenix, 2000). It was pointed out that some degree of conservativism should be maintained when considering whether valid gender differences exist for specific tests of cognitive functions or for the behavioral effects of a disease due to methodological flaws inherent to many studies, including statistical shortcomings and failure to define the construct being investigated sufficiently well (Caplan, MacPherson, & Tobin, 1985). Despite the increased methodological sophistication of more recent studies, alternative explanations may explain some gender differences better. For example, the influence of gender-related sociocultural influences may be especially pertinent and explanatory.

In compiling data for this book, the extent of the problems within our field with respect to availability of reliable and valid child neuropsychology normative data were made manifest. The problems seem considerable and need to be addressed if we intend to improve our ability to generalize results from the test environment to the real-world environment. In considering the reasons for infrequent attention to standardization of test procedures, failure to obtain appropriate population-based normative data, inconsistent methodological and procedural applications, and the limitations of studies comparing individual tests with respect to their purported reliability and validity, a number of conclusions emerged that contrasted with the ideal.

Ideally, for example, normative data are obtained on a large, representative number of individuals, based on appropriate population demographic data. Yet, sometimes the only normative data available are for a population that is not a match for the individual being evaluated. Thus, normative data from North America might be the principal source for a child from another continent, and confirmatory studies of the applicability of these data across populations often are lacking. The need for data appropriate across the demographic spectrum and for the development of regional norms is apparent.

Also, tests may be applied to clinical groups without a normative (normal) sample database available to ensure appropriateness of any comparisons made. In the absence of such a study for single tests developed locally, the reality is that many of our most used tests are based on small subject numbers, local/regional sampling, and confounding variables are not uniformly examined or excluded. Large variances in studies with small sample size are evident on inspection of the standard deviations across many of these insufficient normative studies. Further, partitioning is of little help when cell sizes are small. This is particularly evident in early normative studies, many of which we depended on in the absence of more thorough studies. Age-based norms are more common in recent reports, but collapsing large age ranges in the past obviously complicated attempts to examine the impact of normal developmental maturity.

Ideally, cultural and ethnic appropriate subject selection is conducted and reported. In reality, the examiners of subjects from diverse groups are often faced with limited resources

and therefore refer to data normed on North American (United States and Canada) populations by default. There are an increasing number of exceptions in recent years. This is evidenced in this book by recent data for Italian (Immediate Span, Judgment of Line Orientation Test), Mexican (Stroop Color Word Test), German (d2 Test of Attention), and Spanish (Symbol Digit Modalities Test) children. Data for children from the Netherlands (Facial Recognition Test and Judgment of Line Orientation Test) are also included, along with numerous normative studies for children from Australia. Additional references for data sets from non-North American countries are also noted. Further, many countries have their own preferred tests (some translated for the local population) and normative data sources. These data, however, are often obtained for a specific test, or a few tests, with dependence on an inappropriate broad database for other tests still a concern for interpretation. Also, the language reference group of one country might not generalize to other similar linguistic groups. For example, normative data from one Spanish-speaking country are not applicable to all Spanish speakers because of language differences across countries.

Ideally, reported details about demographic characteristics of the normative sample are sufficiently complete to allow for determination of how appropriate the data are for application to another population. Data stratification for age, grade or education, and gender are desirable. Available age-based norms for some of our tests do not capture age effects because they are not sufficiently stratified or robust (Kizilbash, Warschausky et al., 2001). Some studies include intelligence data while others omit them. In reality, demographic characteristics such as age, education, socioeconomic status, race/ethnicity, handedness, intelligence level, and gender are often incompletely specified, merged, or even omitted. An additional complication is that inclusion and/or exclusion criteria across studies with the same instrument are often inconsistent.

Ideally, the reported age or grade range would be complete and inclusive within a study. In reality, these data might be constricted to certain selected consecutive years, or to a range of nonconsecutive years. Gaps are prominent in many data sets. Adolescent norms are especially lacking, and this absence has long been a burden for practitioners evaluating these young adults. Recently, adolescent normative data are being reported, sometimes along with reliable change indices for test-retest situations (Barr, 2003). Culturally appropriate adolescent data are also reported in the recent literature. For example, normative data for tests of fluency (Word Fluency Test and Design Fluency Test), attention (Digit Span, Symbol Digit Modalities Test, Stroop Colour-Word Test, Trail Making Test), and memory (Chinese Rey Auditory Verbal Learning Test and Aggie Figure Learning Test) were reported for 341 Cantonese Chinese adolescents in grades 7, 9, and 11 (Lee, Yuen et al., 2002) (see Table 1–2 for adolescent normative data included in this volume). Prefrontal maturation continues until midadolescence (Huttenlocher, Dabholkar et al., 1997), and a thorough evaluation of neurocognitive functioning often contributes to fractionating which behaviors of concern have a basis in neuropsychological developmental delay and which are best ascribed to other psychological factors.

Ideally, multiple measures are normed on a single representative population. In reality, many single tests are normed on one small, restricted population sample. Importantly, exceptions to this have been published recently, and these are the current subject of validity studies. The Test of Everyday Attention for Children (TEA-Ch; Manly, Robertson et al., 1999), Delis-Kaplan Executive Function System (Delis, Kaplan et al., 2001), and Rivermead Behavioural Memory Test (Wilson, Ivani-Chalian et al., 1991) are examples of what happens when different subtests are combined within one large battery to aid comparisons of distinct subdomains of broader cognitive function.

Ideally, normative data are both reliable and valid. In reality, the small *N*s of many studies do not contribute to sound normative data, statistical practice, or interpretation. Data indicating that the test is measuring what it purports to measure (construct validity) and assessing a function distinct from that measured by another test (convergent and divergent validity) are often not available.

Ideally, definitions of constructs and choice of instruments would be specific and uniform

Table 1–2. Adolescent Normative Data Presented in this Volume

Age	Test
13 years	Boston Naming Test
	Tower of London
	Porteus Mazes
	Cancellation of Targets
	Digit and Block Span
	Story Recall
	Rey Auditory Verbal Learning Test
13–14 years	Wisconsin Card Sorting Test
	Multilingual Aphasia Examination
	Repeated Patterns Test
	Judgment of Line Orientation Test
	Semantic Fluency
	Benton Visual Retention Test
	Benton Facial Recognition Test
	Ruff Figural Fluency Test
13–15 years	Rapid Automatized Naming/Rapid Alternating Stimulus
	Concept Generation Test
	Rey-Osterrieth Complex Figure Test
	Wechsler Memory Scale-Revised
	Grooved Pegboard Test
	Continuous Visual Memory Test
13–16 years	Contingency Naming Test
	Cognitive Estimation Test
	Verbal Selective Reminding Test
	Nonverbal Selective Reminding Test
13–17 years	Symbol Digit Modalities Test
	Sentence Repetition
	Timed Motor Examination
	Finger Tapping Test
13–18 years	Continuous Recognition Memory Test
	Extended Complex Figure Test
	Category Test
13–19 years	Paced Auditory Serial Addition Task
	Children's Paced Auditory Serial Addition Task
	d2 Test of Attention
	Trail Making Test
	Speech Sounds Perception Test
	Rhythm Test
	Auditory Consonant Trigrams Test
	Grip Strength
	Tactual Performance Test
15 years	Hopkins Verbal Learning Test
15–20 years	Verbal Fluency (oral and written)

across studies. In reality, these often are not. While two investigators might use the same construct term, their definitions vary, making comparisons inappropriate. Also, comparisons occur between tests for which the presumptive construct is variously defined, or alternative terms confound understanding of what is being measured by a specific instrument. For example, different test versions might be labeled measures of "sustained attention" without confirmatory comparison across the many versions. Data are thus obtained for many different versions for supposedly the same construct, and a uniform study of one instrument across normal and clinical populations is not conducted.

Ideally, we would use the same measurement parameters and our administration procedures and scoring rules would be invariable for the same test. In reality, this has been an enormous complicating factor. Single tests are often administered and scored in different ways (Baker, Segalowitz et al., 2001). Different versions of the same test exist, such as for the Stroop Color-Word Test and Tower of London Test. Specific test instructions and/or scoring rules may vary considerably or even be left unspecified. The Finger Tapping Test studies alone are overwhelming in the numbers of ways the test has been administered and differentially scored by numerous investigators who were trained in different laboratories (Snow, 1987; see Chapter 9). Surprisingly, some studies recommend use of a deficit scale based on raw scores for some tests, without consideration of age (Reitan and Wolfson, 1992). Clinical experience would suggest the importance of considering age, and other studies provide support for these clinical impressions (Forster and Leckliter, 1994; Kizilbash, Warschausky et al., 2001).

And finally, ideally, there *will* be normative data for normal and clinical populations, and these data will extend through the age range for which the test is applicable and link to criterion measures. In reality, there may be an absence of such data, and one then relies on clinical judgment that by necessity supersedes a desired statistical basis. For example, tests such as the Halstead-Wepman Screening Test, some sensory-perceptual tests, and some go-no go tests do not always lend themselves to normative data comparisons. This is understandable and acceptable in some cases, as one must examine test data from a qualitative perspective and consider the specific indications of abnormality that, when present in themselves, are major signs of dysfunction, i.e., often referred to as pathognomonic signs. However, even use of a pathognomonic sign approach can present interpretive difficulty since such signs may not be consistently present on examination or may be identified or interpreted similarly by different examiners (Kaspar and Sokolec, 1980).

CONCLUSION

The course of the normally developing child and the child with abnormal brain function is a primary focus within child neuropsychology. The child neuropsychologist contributes precise, yet practical, information that is not easily obtained in any other way. Such an evaluation needs to be considered as a multistep process that is a result of a thorough history taking, records review, behavioral observations, formal testing, and supplemental data acquisition from the school, pediatrician, or others familiar with the child.

Challenges remain in child neuropsychology. Efforts need to be taken to provide appropriate developmental norms for our tests. Greater attention needs to be paid to discriminating between the applicability of varying tests across domains and how these tests will differ in the presence of selective dysfunction. Empirical data supporting assignation of a test to its most relevant domain is needed. Data are needed that compare how clinical subgroups fare with the same test instrument or how a homogenous clinical sample will respond across different measures. Failure to obtain support for commonly accepted clinical assumptions with methodologically strong research data has perpetuated myths that persist in clinical practice. Common among these are the impressions that less dysfunction will result if the child is younger at the time of the neurological insult, that a focal lesion will result in less damage than a generalized insult, and that IQ subtests localize to specific brain regions.

The practice of neuropsychological assessment is evolving rapidly. Reliance on tests constructed long ago has not necessarily proved successful, with some notable exceptions. As the research for this book made clear, there is a heavy dependence on old and inadequate norms in child neuropsychology. The attempts to downwardly extend tests to young age ranges is not altogether acceptable. There is a misapplication of cognitive constructs and models that makes such revision unacceptable when concerned about the child's developing brain and the influence of neurological insult on its development. There is a need to look at lessons learned from cognitive and experimental psychology in order to apply principles and models to both normal and neurologically impaired children. Such an approach may be especially constructive with regard to understanding brain development and treatment applications. These investigations have begun, but require further attention, development, and rigorous empirical investigation.

It is understandable from a practical point of view that there is a history of reluctance to pursue child normative data study. This is likely due to the excessive time demands inherent in developing and executing a study, the large expense involved, methodological complications, and the need to obtain as homeogeneous a "normal" population as possible. However, failures in this respect have left the field open to criticism and our clinical interpretation to suspicion when we are obligated to depend on normative data to reach our conclusions. It is hoped that this volume will stimulate the reader to consider critically the state of our normative data and contribute fundamentally to ensuring that the decisions we make are based on sound principles, techniques, and appropriate normative data comparisons. Because these goals are attainable, child neuropsychologists need to face this challenge.

It is beyond the scope or intent of this book to review the wide range of intelligence tests and academic achievement tests that are available and used for ability-achievement comparison. These are the subjects of intensive review and critique in other texts. Due to their prominence in the experience of child neuropsychologists, some mention of specific tests occurs in this book. There are detailed manuals for these standardized measures, including extensive normative data often stratified by age. Their inclusion in this volume would be redundant, and I decided to focus on the specific individual tests and their available normative data instead.

Similarly, this book's focus precludes detailed discussion of the history and use of neuropsychological test batteries such as the HRNTB and the Luria Neuropsychological Test Battery. Norms for these batteries have long been available (Reitan and Davison 1974; Golden 1981a; 198b; Golden, Kane et al., 1981; Reitan and Wolfson, 1985), and data are presented in this volume for a number of component tests within the appropriate domain chapters. These batteries have a rich literature to which the reader is referred for further information.

It is important to recognize that there is a changing emphasis in neuropsychological practice from localizing brain lesions to assessing change in cognitive functioning over time. This represents a change from the study of group difference to the analysis of intraindividual change. As a result, the component tests of the earlier-designed batteries served a purpose of documenting brain dysfunction that is less salient now that measuring change over time is in demand (McSweeny, Chelune et al., 1993.).

REFERENCES

Adams, R. L. (1996). Introduction. In R. L. Adams, O. A. Parsons, J. L. Culbertson & S. J. Nixon (Eds.), *Neuropsychology for clinical practice* (pp. 1–5). Washington, DC: American Psychological Association.

Agostini, M., Metz-Lutz, M. N., Van Hout, A., Chavance, M., Deloche, G., Pav„o-Martins, I., et al. (1998). Batterie d'evaluation du language oral de l'enfant aphasique (ELOA): Standardization Française (4–12 ans). *Revue de Neuropsychologie, 8,* 319–367.

Amante, D., VanHouten, V. W., Grieve, J., Bader, C. A., & Margules, P. H. (1977). Neuropsychological deficit, ethnicity and socioeconomic status. *Journal of Consulting and Clinical Psychology, 45,* 524–535.

American Psychological Association. (1985). Standards for educational and psychological testing, Washington, DC: American Psychological Association.

Anderson, V., Catroppa, C., Morse, S., Haritou, F., & Rosenfeld, J. (2000). Recovery of intellectual ability following traumatic brain injury in childhood: Impact of injury severity and age at injury. *Pediatric Neurosurgery, 32,* 282–290.

Anderson, V., & Moore, C. (1995). Age at injury as a predictor of outcome following pediatric head injury: A longitudinal perspective. *Child Neuropsychology, 1,* 187–202.

Aram, D. (1988). Language sequelae of unilateral brain lesions in children. In F. Plum (Ed.), *Language, Communication, and the Brain* (pp. 171–197). New York: Raven Press.

Ardila, A. (1995). Directions of research in cross-cultural neuropsychology. *Journal of Clinical and Experimental Neuropsychology, 17,* 143–150.

Artiola i Fortuny, L., & Mullaney, H. A. (1997). Neuropsychology with Spanish speakers: Language use and proficiency issues for test development. *Journal of Clinical and Experimental Neuropsychology, 19,* 1–9.

Baker, K., Segalowitz, S. J., & Ferlisi, M.-C. (2001). The effect of differing scoring methods for the Tower of London task on developmental patterns of performance. *The Clinical Neuropsychologist, 15,* 309–313.

Baron, I. S., Fennell, E. B., & Voeller, K. K. S. (1995). *Pediatric Neuropsychology in the Medical Setting.* New York: Oxford University Press.

Barr, W. B. (2003). Neuropsychological testing of high school athletes: Preliminary norms and test-retest indices. *Archives of Clinical Neuropsychology, 18,* 91–101.

Benedict, R. H. B., Schretlen, D. J., Groninger, L., & Brandt, J. (1998). Hopkins Verbal Learning Test-Revised: Normative data and analysis of inter-form and test-retest reliability. *The Clinical Neuropsychologist, 12,* 43–55.

Benton, A. L. (2000). Foreward. In K. O. Yeates, M. D. Ris & H. G. Taylor (Eds.), *Pediatric Neuropsychology: Research, theory, and practice* (pp. xv). New York: Guilford Press.

Benton, A. L., Varney, N. R., & Hamsher, K. (1978). Visuospatial judgment: A clinical test. *Archives of Neurology, 35,* 364–367.

Benton, A. L., & Hamsher, K. (1976). *Multilingual Aphasia Examination.* Iowa City: University of Iowa.

Benton, A. L., Hamsher, K., Varney, N. R., & Spreen, O. (1983c). *Contributions to neuropsychological assessment: A clinical manual.* New York: Oxford University Press.

Bernstein, J. H., & Waber, D. P. (1996). *Developmental scoring system for the Rey-Osterrieth Complex Figure. Professional Manual.* Odessa, FL: Psychological Assessment Resources, Inc.

Bigler, E. D. (1997). Brain imaging and behavioral outcome in traumatic brain injury. In E. D. Bigler, E. Clark & J. E. Farmer (Eds.), *Childhood traumatic brain injury* (pp. 7–29). Austin, TX: PRO-Ed.

Bigler, E. D., & Ehrfurth, J. (1981). The continued inappropriate singular use of the Bender Visual Motor Gestalt Test. *Professional Psychology, 12,* 562–569.

Booth, J. R., Macwhinney, B., Thulborn, K. R., Sacco, K., Voyvodic, J., & Feldman, H. M. (1999). Functional organization of activation patterns in children: Whole brain fMRI imaging during three different cognitive tasks. *Progress in Neuro-Psychopharmacology and Biological Psychiatry, 23,* 669–682.

Brandt, J. (1991). the Hopkins Verbal Learning Test: Development of a new memory test with six equivalent forms. *The Clinical Neuropsychologist, 5,* 125–142.

Broman, S., Nichols, P. L., Shaughnessy, P., & Kennedy, W. (1987). *Retardation in young children: A developmental study.* Hillsdale, NJ: Lawrence Erlbaum Associates, Inc.

Brookshire, B. L., Fletcher, J., Bohan, T. P., Landry, S. H., Davidson, K., & Francis, D. J. (1995). Verbal and nonverbal skill discrepancies in children with hydrocephalus: A five-year longitudinal follow-up. *Journal of Pediatric Psychology, 20,* 785–800.

Brown, G., Chadwick, O., Shaffer, P., Rutter, M., & Traub, M. (1981). A prospective study of children with head injuries: III. Psychiatric sequelae. *Psychological Medicine, 11,* 63–78.

Brown, L., Sherbenou, R. J., & Johnsen, S. K. (1997). *Test of Nonverbal Intelligence-Third Edition.* San Antonio, TX: The Psychological Corporation.

Brunner, R. L., Jordan, M. K., & Berry, H. K. (1983). Early-treated phenylketonuria: Neuropsychologic consequences. *Journal of Pediatrics, 102,* 831–835.

Cahn, D. A., Salmon, D. P., Bondi, M. W., Butters, N., Johnson, S. A., Wiederholt, W. C., et al. (1997). A population-based analysis of qualitative features of the neuropsychological test performance of individuals with dementia of the Alzheimer type: Implications for individuals with questionable dementia. *Journal of the International Neuropsychological Society, 3,* 387–393.

Campbell, A., Rorie, K., Dennis, G., Wood, D., Combs, S., Hearn, L., et al. (1996). Neuropsychological assessment of African Americans: Conceptual and methodological considerations. In R. Jones (Ed.), *Handbook of Tests and Measurement for Black Populations* (pp. 75–84). Berkeley: Cobb and Henry.

Caplan, P. J., MacPherson, G. M., & Tobin, P. (1985). Do sex-related differences in spatial abilities exist? *American Psychologist, 40,* 786–799.

Casey, B. J., Giedd, J. N., & Thomas, K. N. (2000). Structural and functional brain development and its relation to cognitive development. *Biological Psychology, 54,* 241–257.

Castro-Caldas, A., Petersson, K.-M., Reis, A., Sonte-Elander, S., & M., I. (1998). Learning in childhood determines the functional organization of the adult brain. *Brain, 121,* 1053–1063.

Chelune, G. J. (1982). A reexamination of the relationship between the Luria-Nebraska and Halstead-Reitan Batteries: Overlap with the WAIS. *Journal of Consulting and Clinical Psychology, 50,* 578–580.

Chelune, G. J., Naugle, R. I., Lüders, H. O., Sedlak, J., & Awad, I. A. (1993). Individual change after epilepsy surgery: Practice effects and base-rate information. *Neuropsychology, 7,* 41–52.

Chugani, H. T., Chugani, D. C., & al., e. (1999). Basic mechanisms of childhood epilepsies: Studies with positron emission tomography. *Advances in Neurology, 79,* (883–891).

Chugani, H. T., & Phelps, M. E. (1986). Maturational changes in cerebral function in infants determned by [18] FDG positron emission tomography. *Science, 231,* 840–843.

Cicerone, K. D., Dahlberg, C., Kalmar, K., Langenbahn, D., Malec, J. F., Bergquist, T. F., et al. (2000). Evidence-Based Cognitive Rehabilitation: Recommendations of the Cognitive Rehabilitation Committee of the Brain Injury-Interdisciplinary Special Interest Group, American Congress of Rehabilitation Medicine. *Archives of Physical Medicine and Rehabilitation, 81,* 1596–1615.

Crossen, J. R., & Wiens, A. N. (1994). Comparison of the Auditory-Verbal Learning Test (AVLT) and Calfornia Verbal Learning Test (CVLT) in a sample of normal subjects. *Journal of Clinical and Experimental Neuropsychology, 16,* 190–194.

Davidovicz, H., Iacoviello, J., & McVicar, M. (1981). Cognitive functions in children on chronic intermittent hemodialysis. *Pediatric Research, 15,* 692.

Delis, D., Kaplan, E., & Kramer, J. (2001). *The Delis-Kaplan Executive Function System: Examiner's Manual.* San Antonio, TX: The Psychological Corporation.

Denckla, M. B., & Cutting, L. E. (1999). History and significance of rapid automatized naming. *Annals of Dyslexia, 49,* 29–42.

Dennis, M. (1980). Capacity and strategy for syntactic comprehension after left or right hemidecortication. *Brain and Language, 10,* 287–317.

Di Stefano, G., Bachevalier, J., Levin, H. S., Song, J., Scheibel, R. S., & Fletcher, J. (2000). Volume of focal brain lesions and hippocampal formation in relation to memory function after closed head injury in children. *Journal of Neurology, Neurosurgery and Psychiatry, 69,* 210–216.

Dikmen, S., Heaton, R. K., Grant, I., & Temkin, N. R. (1999). Test-retest reliability and practice effects of Expanded Halstead-Reitan Neuropsychological Test Battery. *Journal of the International Neuropsychological Society, 5,* 346–356.

Donders, J., & Hoffman, N. A. (2002). Gender differences in learning and memory after pediatric traumatic brain injury. *Neuropsychology, 16,* 491–499.

Ernhart, C. B., Graham, F. K., Eichman, P. L., Marshall, J. M., & Thurstone, D. (1963). Brain injury in the preschool child: Some developmental considerations: II. Comparison of brain-injured and normal children. *Psychological Monographs. 11,* 17–33.

Eslinger, P. J., Grattan, L. M., Damasio, H., & Damasio, A. R. (1992). Developmental consequences of childhood frontal lobe damage. *Archives of Neurology, 49,* 764–769.

Ewing-Cobbs, L. (1998). Attention after pediatric traumatic brain injury: A multidimensional assessment. *Child Neuropsychology, 4,* 35–48.

Ewing-Cobbs, L., Fletcher, J., Levin, H. S., Francis, D. J., Davidson, K., & Miner, M. E. (1997). Longitudinal neuropsychological outcome in infants and preschoolers with traumatic brain injury. *Journal of the International Neuropsychological Society, 3,* 581–591.

Ewing-Cobbs, L., Levin, H. S., Eisenberg, H. M., & Fletcher, J. M. (1987). Language functions following closed-head injury in children and adolescents. *Journal of Clinical and Experimental Neuropsychology, 9,* 593–621.

Fennell, R. S., Rasbury, W. C., Fennell, E. B., & Morris, M. K. (1984). The effects of kidney transplantation on cognitive performance in a pediatric population. *Pediatrics, 74,* 273–278.

Fletcher, J. M., & Copeland, D. R. (1988). Neurobehavioral effects of central nervous system prophylactic treatment of cancer in children. *Journal of Clinical and Experimental Neuropsychology, 10,* 495–538.

Fletcher-Janzen, E., Reynolds, C., & Strickland, T. L. (2000). *Handbook of Cross-Cultural Neuropsychology.* New York: Plenum Press.

Forster, A., & Leckliter, I. (1994). The Halstead-Reitan neuropsychological test battery for older children: the effects of age versus clinical status on test performance. *Developmental Neuropsychology, 10,* 299–312.

Francis, D. J., Fletcher, J., Steubing, K. K., Davidson, K., & Thompson, N. (1991). Analysis of change: Modeling individual growth. *Journal of Consulting and Clinical Psychology, 59,* 27–37.

Francis, D. J., Shaywitz, S. E., Steubing, K. K., Shaywitz, B. A., & Fletcher, J. (1994). The measurement of change: Assessing behavior over time and within a developmental context. In G. R. Lyon (Ed.), *Frames of reference for the assessment of learning disabilities* (pp. 29–58). Baltimore: Paul H. Brookes.

Franzen, M. D., Paul, D., & Iverson, G. L. (1996). Reliability of alternate forms of the Trail Making Test. *The Clinical Neuropsychologist, 10,* 125–129.

Gaddes, W. H., and Crockett, D. J. (1975). The Spreen-Benton aphasia tests: Normative data as a measure of normal language development. *Brain and Language, 2,* 257–280.

Garb, H., & Lutz, C. (2001). Cognitive complexity and the validity of clinician's judgments. *Assessment, 8,* 111–115.

Gearing, M. A., Kalin, G., Rose, S., Small, B., Kamp, G., & Mohr, E. (1992). Neuropsychological consequences of insufficient sex hormone exposure at adolescence. *Journal of Clinical and Experimental Neuropsychology, 14,* 113.

Geschwind, N., & Galaburda, A. (1985a). Cerebral lateralization. Biological mechanisms, associations, and pathology: I. A hypothesis and a program for research. *Archives of Neurology, 42,* 428–459.

Geschwind, N., & Galaburda, A. (1985b). Cerebral lateralization. Biological mechanisms, associations, and pathology: II. A hypothesis and a program for research. *Archives of Neurology, 42,* 521–552.

Geschwind, N., & Galaburda, A. (1985c). Cerebral lateralization. Biological mechanisms, associations, and pathology: III. A hypothesis and a program for research. *Archives of Neurology, 42,* 634–654.

Golden, C. J. (1981). The Luria-Nebraska Children's Battery: Theory and formulation. In G. W. Hynd & J. E. Obrzut (Eds.), *Neuropsychological assessment and the school-age child* (pp. 277–302). New York: Grune & Stratton.

Golden, C. J. (1981b). A standardized version of Luria's neuropsychological tests. In S. Filskov & T. Boll (Eds.), *Handbook of Clinical Neuropsychology*. New York: Wiley-Interscience.

Golden, C. J., Kane, R., Sweet, J., Moses, J. A., Cardellino, J. P., Templeton, R., et al. (1981). Relationship of the Halsted-Reitan Neuropsychological Battery to the Luria-Nebraska Neuropsychological Battery. *Journal of Consulting and Clinical Psychology, 49,* 410–417.

Greenberg, M., & Crnic, R. (1988). Longitudinal predictors of developmental status and social interaction in preterm and full-term infants at age 2. *Child Development, 59,* 554–570.

Halpern, D. F. (1992). *Sex differences in cognitive abilities (2nd ed.).* Hillsdale, NJ: Erlbaum.

Halpern, D. F. (1997). Sex differences in intelligence: Implications for education. *American Psychologist, 52,* 1091–1102.

Hannay, H. J., Bieliauskas, L., Crosson, B. A., Hammeke, T. A., Hamsher, K. d., & Koffler, S. (1998). Proceedings of The Houston Conference on Specialty Education and Training in Clinical Neuropsychology. *Archives of Clinical Neuropsychology, 13,* 157–250.

Harris, N. S., Marcus, D. J., Rancier, S. A., & Weiler, M. D. (1999). First name fluency in learning disabled children vs. controls. [Abstract]. *The Clinical Neuropsychologist, 13,* 226.

Heaton, R. K., Grant, I., & Matthews, C. G. (1986). Differences in neuropsycholgical test performance asociated with age, education, and sex. In I. Grant & K. M. Adams (Eds.), *Neuropsychological assessment of neuropsychiatric disorders* (pp. 100–120). New York: Oxford University Press.

Heffelfinger, A. K., Craft, S., White, D. A., & Shyken, J. (2002). Visual attention in preschool children prenatally exposed to cocaine: Implications for behavioral regulation. *Journal of the International Neuropsychological Society, 8,* 12–21.

Herlitz, A., Airaksinen, E., & Nordström, E. (1999). Sex differences in episodic memory: The impact of verbal and visuospatial ability. *Neuropsychology, 13,* 590–597.

Herlitz, A., Nillson, L.-G., & Bäckman, L. (1997). Gender differences in episodic memory. *Memory and Cognition, 25,* 801–811.

Huttenlocher, P. R., Dabholkar, A. S., & al., e. (1997). Regional differences in synaptogenesis in human cerebral cortex. *Journal of Comparative Neurology, 387,* 167–178.

Ivnik, R. J., Smith, G. E., Cerhan, J. H., Boeve, B. F., Tangalos, E. G., & Petersen, R. C. (2001). Understanding the diagnostic capabilities of cognitive tests. *The Clinical Neuropsychologist, 15,* 114–124.

Ivnik, R. J., Smith, G. E., Petersen, R. C., Boeve, B. F., Kokmen, E., & Tangalos, E. G. (2000). Diagnostic accuracy of four approaches to interpreting neuropsychological test data. *Neuropsychology, 14,* 163–177.

Jacobson, N. S., & Truax, P. (1991). Clinical significance: A statistical approach to defining meaningful change in psychotherapy research. *Journal of Consulting and Clinical Psychology, 59,* 12–19.

Jaffe, K. M., Plissar, N. L., Fay, G. C., & Liao, S. (1995). Recovery trends over three years following pediatric traumatic brain injury. *Archives of Physical Medicine and Rehabilitation, 76,* 17–26.

Jensen, A. R., & Reynolds, C. (1983). Sex differences on the WISC-R. *Personality and Individual Differences, 4,* 223–226.

Johnstone, B., & Wilhelm, K. L. (1997). The construct validity of the Hooper Visual Organization Test. *Assessment, 4,* 243–248.

Kane, R., Parsons, O. A., & Goldstein, G. (1985). Statistical relationships and discriminative accuracy of the Halstead-Reitan, Luria-Nebraska, and Wechsler IQ scores in the identification of brain damage. *Journal of Clinical and Experimental Neuropsychology, 7,* 211–223.

Kaplan, E. (1988). A process approach to neuropsychological assessment. In T. Boll & B. K. Bryant (Eds.), *Clinical neuropsychology and brain function: Research, measurement, and practice* (pp. 143–155). Washington, D. C.: American Psychological Association.

Kaplan, E., Fein, D., Morris, R., & Delis, D. C. (1991). *WAIS-R as a neuropsychological instrument.* San Antonio, TX: The Psychological Corporation.

Kaspar, J. C., & Sokolec, J. (1980). Relationship between neurological dysfunction and a test of speed of motor performance. *Journal of Clinical Neuropsychology, 2,* 13–21.

Kaufman, A. S. (1990). *Assessing adolescent and adult intelligence.* Needham Heights, MA: Allyn and Bacon, Inc.

Kimura, D. (1999). *Sex and cognition.* Cambridge, MA: MIT Press.

Kinsella, G., Prior, M., Sawyer, M., Murtaugh, D., Eisenmajer, R., Anderson, A., et al. (1995). Neuropsychological deficit and acdemic performance in children and adolescents following traumatic brain injury. *Journal of Pediatric Psychology, 20,* 753–767.

Kirkwood, M., Janusz, J., Yeates, K. O., Taylor, H. G., Wade, S. L., Stancin, T., et al. (2000). Prevalence and correlates of depressive symptoms following traumatic brain injuries in children. *Child Neuropsychology, 6,* 195–208.

Kizilbash, A., Warschausky, S., & Donders, J. (2001). Assessment of speed of processing after paediatric head trauma: need for better norms. *Pediatric Rehabilitation, 4,* 71–74.

Kramer, J., Delis, D., & Daniel, M. (1998). Sex differences in verbal learning. *Journal of Clinical Psychology, 44,* 907–915.

Kramer, J., Delis, D., Kaplan, E., O'Donnell, L., & Prifitera, A. (1997). Developmental sex differences in verbal learning. *Neuropsychology, 11,* 577–584.

Lee, T. M. C., Yuen, K. S. L., & Chan, C. C. H. (2002). Normative data for neuropsychological measures of fluency, attention, and memory measures for Hong Kong Chinese. *Journal of Clinical and Experimental Neuropsychology, 24,* 615–632.

Lehnung, M., Leplow, B., Herzog, A., Benz, B., Ritz, A., Stolze, H., et al. (2001). Children's spatial behavior is differentially affected after traumatic brain injury. *Child Neuropsychology, 7,* 59–71.

Levin, H. S., Benton, A., & Grossman, R. G. (1982). *Neurobehavioral consequences of closed head injury.* New York: Oxford University Press.

Levin, H. S., Culhane, K. A., Mendelsohn, D., & al., e. (1993). Cognition in relation to magnetic resonance imaging in head-injured children and adolescents. *Archives of Neurology, 50,* 897–905.

Levin, H. S., High, W. M. J., Ewing-Cobbs, L., Fletcher, J. M., Eisenberg, H. M., Miner, M. C., et al. (1988). Memory functioning during the first year after closed head injury in children and adolescents. *Neurosurgery, 22,* 1043–1052.

Levin, H. S., Scheller, J., Rickard, T., & Grafman, J. (1996). Dyscalculia and dyslexia after right hemisphere injury in infancy. *Archives of Neurology, 53*(1), 88–96.

Levin, H. S., Song, J., Ewing-Cobbs, L., & Roberson, G. (2001). Porteus maze performance following traumatic brain injury in children. *Neuropsychology, 15*(4), 557–567.

Luciana, M., & Nelson, C. A. (1998). The functional emergence of prefrontally-guided working memory systems in four- to eight-year-old children. *Neuropsychologia, 36,* 273–293.

Maccoby, E. M., & Jacklin, C. N. (1974). *The psychology of sex differences.* Palo Alto: Stanford University Press.

Mahone, E. M., Koth, C. W., Cutting, L. E., Singer, H. S., & Denckla, M. B. (2001). Executive function in fluency and recall measures among children with Tourette syndrome or ADHD. *Journal of the International Neuropsychological Society, 7,* 102–111.

Manly, J. J., & Jacobs, D. (2002). Future directions in neuropsychological assessment with African-Americans. In R. Ferrarro (Ed.), *Minority and Cross-Cultural Aspects of Neuropsychological Assessment* (pp. 79–96): Swets & Zeitlinger.

Manly, J. J., Jacobs, D., Touradji, P., Small, S. A., & Stern, Y. (2002). Reading level attenuates differences in neuropsychological test performance between African American and White elders. *Journal of the International Neuropsychological Society, 8,* 341–348.

Manly, T., Robertson, I. H., Anderson, V., & Nimmo-Smith, I. (1999). *The Test of Everyday Attention for Children: Manual.* Bury St. Edmunds, UK: Thames Valley Test Company Ltd.

Marcopulos, B., McLain, C. A., & Giuliano, A. J. (1997). Cognitive impairment or inadequate norms? A study of healthy, rural, older adults with limited education. *The Clinical Neuropsychologist, 11,* 111–131.

Matarazzo, J. D., & Herman, D. O. (1984). Relationship of education and IQ in the WAIS-R standardization sample. *Journal of Consulting and Clinical Psychology, 52,* 631–634.

McSweeny, A. J., Chelune, G. J., Naugle, R. I., & Lüders, H. O. (1993.). "*T* Scores for change": An illustration of a regression approach to depicting change in clinical neuropsychology. *The Clinical Neuropsychologist, 7,* 300–312.

Miller-Loncar, C. L., Landry, S. H., Smith, K. S., & Swank, P. R. (1997). The role of child-centered perspectives in a model of parenting. *Journal of Experimental Child Psychology, 66,* 1–21.

Morris, M. K., Fennell, E. B., Fennell, R. S., & Rasbury, W. C. (1985). A case study of identical twins discordant for renal failure: Long-term neuropsychological deficits. *Developmental Neuropsychology, 1,* 81–92.

Moses, P., Courchesne, E., Stiles, J., Trauner, D., Egaas, B., & Edwards, E. (2000). Regional size reduction in the human corpus callosum following pre-and perinatal brain injury. *Cerebral Cortex, 10,* 1200–1210.

Müller, R. A., Rothermel, R. D., Behen, M. E., Muzik, O., Chakraborty, P. K., & Chugani, H. T. (1999). Language organization in patients with early and late left-hemisphere lesion: A PET study. *Neuropsychologia, 37,* 545–557.

Müller, R. A., Rothermel, R. D., Behen, M. E., Muzik, O., Mangner, T. J., & Chugani, H. T. (1998). Differential patterns of language and motor reorganization following early left hemisphere lesion: A PET study. *Archives of Neurology, 55,* 1113–1119.

Nadolne, M. J., & Stringer, A. Y. (2001). Ecologic validity in neuropsychological assessment: Prediction of wayfinding. *Journal of the International Neuropsychological Society, 7,* 675–682.

Nesbit-Greene, K., & Donders, J. (2002). Latent structure of the Children's Category Test after pediatric traumatic head injury. *Journal of Clinical and Experimental Neuropsychology, 24,* 194–199.

Nielsen, H., Knudsen, L., & Daugbjerg, O. (1989). Normative data for eight neuropsychological tests based on a Danish sample. *Scandinavian Journal of Psychology, 30,* 37–45.

Northam, E., Bowden, S., Anderson, V., & Court, J. (1992). Neuropsychological functioning in adolescents with diabetes. *Journal of Clinical and Experimental Neuropsychology, 14,* 884–900.

Ostrosky-Solis, F., Ardila, A., & Rosselli, M. (1999). Neuropsi: A brief neurpsychological test battery in Spanish with norms by age and educational level. *Journal of the International Neuropsychological Society, 5,* 413–433.

Passler, M., Isaac, W., & Hynd, G. W. (1985). Neuropsychological development of behavior attributed to frontal lobe functioning in children. *Developmental Neuropsychology, 4,* 349–370.

Pérez-Arce, P. (1999). The influence of culture on cognition. *Archives of Clinical Neuropsychology, 14,* 581–592.

Pérez-Arce, P., Johnson, C. B., Rauch, S., Bowler, R. M., & Mergler, D. (1989). Neuropsychological screening of 6– to 15–year-old children exposed to neurotoxins while in-utero. *Clinical Neuropsychologist, 3,* 280.

Pontón, M. O., Satz, P., Herrera, L., Ortiz, F., Urrutia, C. P., Young, R., et al. (1996). Normative data stratified by age and education for the Neuropsychological Screening Battery for Hispanics (NeSBHIS): Initial report. *Journal of the International Neuropsychological Society, 2,* 96–104.

Reitan, R. (1985). Relationships between measures of brain functions and general intelligence. *Journal of Clinical Psychology, 41,* 245–253.

Reitan, R., & Davison, L. (1974). *Clinical neuropsychology: Current status and applications.* New York: Hemisphere.

Reitan, R., & Wolfson, D. (1985). *The Halstead-Reitan Neuropsychological Test Battery.* Tucson, AZ: Neuropsychological Press.

Reitan, R., & Wolfson, D. (1992). *Neuropsychological Evaluation of Older Children.* South Tucson, AZ: Neuropsychology Press.

Reye, G. J., Feldman, E., Rivas-Vasquez, R., Levin, B. E., & Benton, A. (1999). Neuropsychological test development and normative data on Hispanics. *Archives of Clinical Neuropsychology, 14,* 593–601.

Rovet, J. (1992). The effect of neonatal thyroid hormone deficiency on motor development. *Journal of Clinical and Experimental Neuropsychology, 14,* 113.

Rovet, J., Ehrlich, R., & Hoppe, M. (1988). Specific intellectual deficits in children with early onset diabetes mellitus. *Child Development, 59,* 226–234.

Ruff, R. M., Light, R. H., & Parker, S. B. (1996). Benton Controlled Word Association Test. Reliability and updated norms. *Archives of Clinical Neuropsychology, 11,* 329–338.

Ryan, C. M., Vega, A., Longstreet, C., & Drash, A. (1984). Neuropsychological changes in adolescents with insulin-dependent diabetes. *Journal of Consulting and Clinical Psychology, 52,* 335–342.

Sawrie, S. M., Chelune, G. J., Naugle, R. I., & Lüders, H. O. (1996). Empirical methods for assessing meaningful neuropsychological change following epilepsy surgery. *Journal of the International Neuropsychological Society, 2,* 556–564.

Seidenberg, M., Giordani, B., Berent, S., & Boll, T. (1983). IQ level and performance on the Halstead-Reitan neuropsychological test battery for older children. *Journal of Consulting and Clinical Psychology, 51,* 406–413.

Snow, W. G. (1987). Standardization of test administration and scoring criteria: Some shortcomings of current practice with the Halstead-Reitan Test Battery. *The Clinical Neuropsychologist, 1,* 250–262.

Stauder, J. E. A., Molenaar, P. C. M., & van der Molen, M. W. (1999). Brain activity and cognitive transition during childhood: A longitudinal event-related brain potential study. *Child Neuropsychology, 5,* 41–59.

Steele, C. M. (1997). A threat in the air: How stereotypes shape intellectual ability and performance. *American Psychologist, 52,* 613–629.

Stern, R. A., Javorsky, D. J., Singer, E. A., Singer Harris, N. G., Somerville, J. A., Duke, L. M., et al. (1999). *The Boston Qualitative Scoring System for the Rey-Osterrieth Complex Figure.* Odessa, FL: Psychological Assessment Resources, Inc.

Stern, R. A., Singer, E. A., Duke, L. M., Singer, N. G., Morey, C. E., Daughtrey, E. W., et al. (1994). The Boston qualitative socring system for the Rey-Osterrieth Complex Figure: Description and interrater reliability. *The Clinical Neuropsychologist, 8,* 309–322.

Stewart, S. M., Silver, C. H., Nici, J., Waller, D., Campbell, R., Uauy, R., et al. (1991). Neuropsychological function in young children who have undergone liver transplantation. *Journal of Pediatric Psychology, 16,* 569–583.

Stiles, J., Bates, E., Thal, D. J., Trauner, D., & Reilly, J. (1998). Linguistic, cognitive, and affective development in children with pre-and perinatal focal brain injury: A ten-year overview from the San Diego Longitudinal Project. In C. Rovee-Collier, L. P. Lipsitt & H. Hayne (Eds.), *Advances in infancy research* (pp. 131–163). Stamford, CT: Ablex Publishing Corporation.

Stiles, J., Moses, P., Roe, K., Trauner, D., Hesselink, J., Wong, E., et al. (2003). Alternative brain organization after prenatal cerebral injury: Convergent fMRI and cognitive data. *Journal of the International Neuropsychological Society.*

Stuss, D. T., Alexander, M. P., Palumbo, C. L., Buckle, L., Sayer, L., & Pogue, J. (1994). Organizational strategies of patients with unilateral or bilateral frontal lobe injury in word list learning tasks. *Neuropsychology, 8,* 355–373.

Stuss, D. T., Winocur, G., & Robertson, I. H. (1999). *Cognitive neurorehabilitation.* Cambridge, UK: Cambridge University Press.

Taylor, E. M. (1959). *Psychological appraisal of children with cerebral deficits.* Cambridge, MA: Harvard University Press.

Taylor, H. G., & Alden, J. (1997). Age-related differences in outcomes following childhood brain insults: An introduction and overview. *Journal of the International Neuropsychological Society, 3,* 555–567.

Taylor, H. G., & Schatschneider, C. (1992). Child neuropsychological assessment: A test of basic assumptions. *Clinical Neuropsychologist, 6,* 259–275.

Taylor, H. G., Schatschneider, C., & Minich, N. (2000). Longitudinal outcomes of *Haemophilus influenzae* Meningitis in School-age children. *Neuropsychology, 14,* 509–518.

Taylor, H. G., Wade, S. L., Stancin, T., Yeates, K. O., Drotar, D., & Minich, N. (2002). A prospective study of short- and long-term outcomes after traumatic brain injury in children: Behavior and achievement. *Neuropsychology, 16,* 15–27.

Taylor, H. G., Yeates, K. O., Wade, S. L., Drotar, D., Stancin, T., & Burant, C. (2001). Bidirectional child-family influences on outcomes of traumatic brain injury in children. *Journal of the International Neuropsychological Society, 7,* 755–767.

Temkin, N. R., Heaton, R. K., Grant, I., & Dikmen, S. (1999). Detecting significant change in neuropsychological test performance: A comparison of four models. *Journal of the International Neuropsychological Society, 5,* 357–369.

Thal, D. J., Marchman, V., Stiles, J., Aran, D., Trauner, D., Nass, R., et al. (1991). Early lexical development in children with focal brain injury. *Brain and Language, 40,* 491–527.

Turner, S. M., DeMers, S. T., Fox, H. R., & Reed, G. M. (2001). APA's guidelines for test user qualifications: An executive summary. *American Psychologist, 56,* 1099–1113.

Vanderploeg, R. D., Axelrod, B., Sherer, M., Scott, J., & Adams, R. L. (1997). The importance of demographic adjustments on neuropsychological test performance: A response to Reitan and Wolfson (1995). *The Clinical Neuropsychologist, 11,* 210–217.

Vargha-Khadem, F., Carr, L. J., Isaacs, E., & Brett, E. (1997). Onset of speech after left hemispherectomy in a nine-year-old boy. *Brain, 120*(1), 159–182.

Vargha-Khadem, F., O'Gorman, A., & Watters, G. (1985). Aphasia and handedness in relation to hemispheric side, age at injury, and severity of cerebral lesion during childhood. *Brain, 108,* 677–696.

Vohr, B. R., & Garcia Coll, C. T. (1985). Neurodevelopmental and school performance of very low-birth weight infants: A seven year longitudinal study. *Pediatrics, 76,* 345–350.

Waber, D. P., & Holmes, J. M. (1985). Assessing children's copy productions of the Rey-Osterrieth Complex Figure. *Journal of Clinical and Experimental Neuropsychology, 7,* 264–280.

Waber, D. P., & Holmes, J. M. (1986). Assessing children's memory productions of the Rey-Osterrieth Complex Figure. *Journal of Clinical and Experimental Neuropsychology, 8,* 563–580.

Waber, D. P., & Mullenix, P. J. (2000). Acute lymphoblastic leukemia. In K. O. Yeates, M. D. Ris & H. G. Taylor (Eds.), *Pediatric neuropsychology: Research, theory and practice* (pp. 300–319). New York: Guilford.

Welsh, M. C., Pennington, B. F., Ozonoff, S., Rouse, B., & McCabe, E. R. B. (1990). Neuropsychology of early-treated phenylketonuria: Specific executive function deficits. *Child Development, 61,* 1697–1713.

White, D. A., Nortz, M. J., Mandernach, T., Huntington, K., & Steiner, R. D. (2002). Age-related working memory impairments in children with prefrontal dysfunction associated with phenylketonuria. *Journal of the International Neuropsychological Society, 8,* 1–11.

Wilson, B. A., Ivani-Chalian, R., & Aldrich, F. (1991). *The Rivermead Behavioural Memory Test for Children Aged 5–10 years: Manual.* Bury St. Edmunds, Suffolk, UK: Thames Valley Test Company, Ltd.

Yeates, K. O., Taylor, H. G., Drotar, D., Wade, S., Stancin, T., & Klein, S. (1997). Preinjury family environment as a determinant of recovery from traumatic brain injury in school-age children. *Journal of the International Neuropsychological Society, 3,* 617–630.

II

CLINICAL ISSUES

2

Behavioral Assessment

What a child neuropsychologist needs to know for competent clinical practice is learned, in part, through academic pursuits, externship experiences, clinical internship, and postdoctoral training. These are all immensely valuable in building the skills required for effective practice. However, it is often the day-to-day experiences gained over time as a practicing professional that expose the nuances and realities of clinical neuropsychology practice that greatly influence the clinician's competence. The discussion below reviews some basic and often necessary steps at different stages of the neuropsychological evaluation, for consideration and adaptation by practitioners to fit their own practice needs.

The intake interview preceding appointment scheduling, records review, and history taking are each important early steps in the neuropsychological evaluation of both inpatient and outpatient children. These steps are then followed by test selection, test administration and scoring, interpretation, an interpretive interview, formulation of final treatment recommendations, report writing, and perhaps other consultations with parent authorization, as needed. Together these components comprise a comprehensive neuropsychological evaluation that has a high probability of resulting in a meaningful profile of the child's neuropsychological strengths and weaknesses.

INTAKE INTERVIEWING AND SCHEDULING

The telephone intake interview for an outpatient evaluation helps determine whether the referral is indeed appropriate. A clinician needs to be assured that she can assess the child within proscribed ethical responsibilities for psychologists that specify that one not examine or treat outside the bounds of one's own competence. Also, she needs to determine that the referral is justified since it is a time-intensive and costly evaluation. While it is intended to add essential information relevant to the child's care, not all referrals are appropriate nor should a referral be accepted just because it is recommended. A parent needs to understand the procedures associated with a neuropsychological evaluation and what the likely outcome will be. It is helpful to explain the ways in which a neuropsychological evaluation differs from other psychological evaluations and describe the noninvasive techniques, domains to be assessed, time involved for the one-to-one testing, and likely number of visits needed, along with the purpose of the evaluation individualized for the referral reason.

Also, parents often need guidance about what to tell their child prior to evaluation in preparation for the test session. The intake interview provides this opportunity to assure parents that a simple explanation is sufficient, provide some examples tailored to the child's chronological age, and indicate that discussion about why their child is being tested will also occur directly with the child before formal assessment begins to ensure optimal cooperation. Parents may be encouraged to emphasize in their description to the child the play aspect of testing for a young child. For an older child or adolescent, who likely will be more cognizant of the reasons for such an evaluation, they can take the opportunity to emphasize the test session will examine both strengths and overall competencies, along with any potential weaknesses.

REVIEWING RECORDS

The child's historical records are valuable but not always easily obtainable. Educational and medical records allow for preliminary judgment about test selection and are subject to modification as the evaluation progresses. Supplementary records, including information about socioeconomic and environmental variables, also provide useful data about family relationships and dynamics, the child's coping strategies and behavior across varying settings, and factual detail about the developmental and medical course, educational placement, and achievement to compare with oral reports in interviews. Prior medical consultations, diagnostic procedures, treatment regimens, and any psychological or psychiatric reports are desirable. There might be parent reluctance to release prior psychological data since the parent hopes for an unbiased assessment and worries about the influence of prior testing.

Offering the parent assurance that there will be independent judgment and emphasizing the importance of the prior records to better understand the child's developmental course often are sufficient to learn of, and obtain the release of, these previously withheld or forgotten data. A practitioner is dependent on the parents' formal authorization for release of relevant records for the outpatient. However, an inpatient child's medical chart contains nursing notes, progress notes, and daily behavioral observational notes for staff review and can be easily consulted. Some skepticism is wise in reviewing records since they can be misleading. For example, a lenient report-card grade may have been given to a child absent due to serious illness in order to offer encouragement on reentry into school, or a conclusion may have been reached based on incomplete information.

HISTORY TAKING

The *critical* importance of a thorough history taking cannot be overstated. Information revealed in history taking inevitably influences the final interpretive conclusions. It serves as a double-check on the history taken by others and as an opportunity to obtain information not previously reported to the child's pediatrician, teacher, or others involved in the child's care. Parents do not always appreciate the extent of their knowledge about their child and, therefore, might omit critical information, thinking it unimportant unless there is direct and focused inquiry. What they recall about early risk factors, deviations from normal development, relevant family history, or prior illness, injury, or treatment regimens that can result in late cognitive or behavioral effects needs to be systematically reviewed. The neuropsychologist's facility for listening is essential in reviewing the important topics in a child history taking: pregnancy and delivery, peri-and neonatal course, language, motor, and social development, medical history, family history, educational history, prior consultations, and extracurricular interests. Appendix 2–A presents a sample history questionnaire that serves as a stimulus for further direct inquiry about history.

Special attention should be given to the medically unsophisticated parent who might not understand medical terminology and, therefore, unintentionally omits important information. For example, one father of a child with a seizure disorder said "no" when asked whether anyone else in the family had a history of seizures. But with further questioning, he revealed that three family members would say, "Here it comes!." He then began to shake his limbs to indicate what occurred next, having obviously witnessed their seizures. In another example, a mother denied anyone in the family had a "neurological problem." But when then asked,

"Does anyone have a problem with their brain?" she replied, "Oh yes, my mother and her sister both have something called a Chiari malformation, and my mother had brain surgery last year."

A parent's reluctance, unwillingness, or inability to comply can also complicate history taking. For example, the parent of a child involved in a custody battle might be unwilling to divulge information freely, a parent suspected of neglect might withhold information, or a parent of a hospitalized child may be at work and unavailable for interview. A more complete history occurs with a combination of questionnaire, parent interview, child interview and/or records review with signed authorization. The reader is also referred to discussion of informed consent in neuropsychological practice (Johnson-Greene, Hardy-Morais et al., 1997).

PREPARATORY STEPS FOR TESTING

Testing is expected to proceed smoothly, but to ensure this, a number of obstacles to optimal test administration need to be anticipated. Preparing the tests, forms, and testing room in advance of the child's arrival fosters the examiner's ability to actively encourage the child without the distraction of routine administrative matters. Given the wide variety of test equipment and supplemental forms from which to choose, it is useful to plan on an initial screening across domains of particular concern and then administer a more focused investigation as the testing proceeds (see Chapter 4). Prepared folders containing age-appropriate scoring forms, and alternate forms, are therefore useful.

A checklist of potential tests helps to monitor those completed (I draw a line through each test name as the test is completed) and those intended for administration (I circle the test name I wish to add). Such a list also serves as a quick visual survey of the tests sampled in each domain. The face sheet I use lists tests by general behavioral domain, but clearly, a test may have greater implication for another domain than the one under which it is listed (a sample face sheet checklist is presented in Ap-

pendix 2–B). The face sheet notes tests that have no accompanying forms as well, for example, the draw-a-person test, alphabet and number writing, and incidental drawing tests. Plenty of extra paper, sharpened pencils, colored pens, batteries, a stopwatch, and the presence of any other needed technical equipment are obvious necessities, especially when multiple examiners test concurrently and share equipment.

Test choice and administration order are influenced by chronological age, functional level, referral questions, the child's cooperation, and a need to challenge the child to better understand complex cognitive capabilities. New hypotheses are developed during testing and these expand initial choices. However, external conditions beyond the examiner's control can complicate planned test administration, for example, an immobility of the inpatient's preferred upper extremity due to an intravenous line, medications that result in lethargy, distractions within the room, or intermittent interruption by medical staff. As a result, flexibility is essential and extends to versatility with test materials.

Test order can directly affect the overall results. One, therefore, needs to consider a child's strengths and weaknesses in determining the optimal test order. Repeated failure on a sequence of similarly difficult tests might result in the child attempting to terminate a test session prematurely. Interspersing easy and hard tests generally encourages continued cooperation. It is especially useful to administer an easy task after particularly hard tasks to counter feelings of failure or frustration. Test order might also be dictated by a medical contingency such as the need for urinary catheterization or medication. Planned interruption can be used advantageously—for example, for tests with a delayed retrieval condition. Personality characteristics or temperament can also influence test order. For example, relatively nonthreatening tests are best administered early to a child subject to aggressive outbursts or temper tantrums, while harder tasks likely to stimulate a negative response are best left for later in the test session. Manipulative tests can be given to a reticent child, and verbal expression tests delayed until the child appears more comfortable and willing to communicate freely.

BEHAVIORAL OBSERVATIONS

Although critically important information can be obtained by clinical observation, this information does not always receive the emphasis it deserves. A thorough neuropsychological evaluation always considers clinical observations along with quantitative data. Such observation begins in the waiting room. For the outpatient and mobile inpatient, the waiting room more closely approximates a natural environment than will the testing room and incidental observations can be highly informative about parent-child and parent-parent interactions. Waiting-room play may provide clues about the child's emotional state. The ways in which parent and child separate for testing or greet each other when reunited in the waiting room are also of interest. Information can be gained from observation of the parent-child interaction at the start of testing, at breaks, and at the conclusion of testing. Nonverbal signals between a parent and child should be attended to as well as the child's attitude about returning to the parent, e.g. pleasure at being reunited, concern about punishment for doing poorly. The child's interactions with siblings or other children in the waiting room are also informative with respect to his or her ability to socialize.

Observations by office staff can contribute useful information. Office staff members are often invisible to the waiting family, and thus have an unique observational role. Anecdotes about waiting-room behavior can reveal interpersonal dynamics otherwise missed by the examiner. Differences in behavior between occasions when the examiner is present and absent are of particular interest. For example, a parent may speak sharply to the child or threaten punishment before the examiner appears, but not when the examiner is actually present. Or, parents who offer each other limited support may visibly reveal such feelings in the waiting room by sitting separately, remaining silent, or bickering, but attempt to hide these reactions in the presence of the profes-

sional. Such observations may be integrated into the overall case formulation and explored further in the interpretive session when communicated by the staff.

Observation continues in the testing room. Children who find it hard to express concerns and fears verbally might reveal important information indirectly. Drawings and puppet play are useful for a child who cannot easily verbalize. Informal conversation about family or friends might contain references to details not available in the history or elicited from the parents with direct questioning. Children unwilling or unable to freely tell what they know might draw their problem in response to "draw-a-person" or "draw-a-family doing something" screening tests. Asking for their "three wishes" is another useful, nonthreatening technique.

How a child responds to the stress of testing should be closely monitored. Sometimes children verbalize how much they like the examiner or what fun they are having. They may express enthusiasm for taking tests they perceive as difficult, seeking reassurance. Such comments often link to areas of weaker function or cumulative feelings of distress and should be viewed in context as a sign of potential need for extra reassurance. Sometimes it is tears welling up in the child's eyes that are the first sign of the discomfort they are experiencing. Because a child may attempt to hide a weakness, it is important to be observant when they evade a task. Children naturally shy away from or refuse to engage in activities if they believe they will fail. They may attempt to deflect the examiner by engaging in actions that have proved successful in other settings such as the classroom. In this way, their evasive strategies are of great interest.

Signs and symptoms of dysfunction may be missed if one depends on test results without considering incidental behaviors. For example, perfect performance on formal language tests might lead one to conclude that language function is intact. Yet, incorrect word retrieval, echolalia, circumlocutory speech, auditory perceptual errors in response to verbal directions, or any number of subtle language errors might only emerge in informal clinical observation of spontaneous language. The examiner's impressions, therefore, may undergo modification throughout the evaluation in response to these direct observations. These observations help guide the process of test selection and behavior sampling.

Behavioral observations should be made about specific physical attributes or mannerisms, including height and weight estimates, body type, hair, blemishes, birthmarks, scars, and other distinctive physical features, even what clothing is worn. The child's activity level should be noted, along with how it varies in response to task requirements, test difficulty level, and with and without examiner structure. Instances of hyperactivity, such as frequent out-of-seat behavior, persistent reaching for desk top articles, hanging over the chair, or otherwise moving about in the middle of a task, or hypoactivity, such as slumping over as if exhausted, apathy, lethargy, or general slowed responding, should be noted.

Observations of the child's ability to reason and plan allows for preliminary determination about whether a child responds in a rigid, inflexible, or stimulus-bound way or is adept at developing alternative strategies. The examiner can investigate executive functions more thoroughly with specific tests and in interviews with the parent. It is important to be alert for signs or symptoms of anxiety, reluctance to respond, distractibility, medication effects, effects of current illness, any influence of recent family trauma, fatigue, impeding cultural factors, and failure to maintain rapport.

Motor function needs to be attended to, including choice of preferred upper extremity, lateral dominance consistency, and right–left discrimination, gross and fine motor function, gait and balance, and examples of unusual motor activity level. History taking will review acquisition of motor developmental milestones such as crawling, sitting alone, walking, and riding a bicycle (see Appendix 2–A). Pencil grip position and how the child places the paper when writing (i.e., normal, rotated or awkward) should be noted, along with any attempt at bilateral use on unilateral trials that might signal a stronger upper extremity attempting to assist a weaker one. Letter formation and line quality in written productions should also be appraised. Other body actions may reflect a ha-

bitual response, a stereotypic mannerism or specific neurological dysfunction. These include tics, twitches, and involuntary movements. For example, hand-washing movements are associated with Rett syndrome, a disorder that affects females after normal development over the first year of life; stereotypic hand movements are associated with autism and pervasive developmental disorder; and mouth movements such as chewing or licking may precede an epileptic seizure. Motor overflow activity is also of interest, for example, when the contralateral finger or hand mimics the activity of the ongoing ipsilateral body movement. Compensatory actions that reflect sensory disturbance might be observed, such as a move closer to the examiner to hear more accurately, reaching for the wall while walking in order to maintain balance, or turning the head to compensate for hemispatial visual neglect.

Sensory impairment may be overlooked, and therefore, confirmation of vision and hearing screenings is necessary. Differential function in response to verbal or nonverbal instructions may suggest a problem with either hearing or vision, respectively. Useful questions for the parent include whether the child talks loudly compared to other family members, does not answer soft-spoken questions, turns the volume of a television up high, sits too close to the television, or holds the head close to the paper when writing. Tactile, auditory, and visual imperception testing can establish gross integrity of response to unilateral stimuli and double simultaneous stimulation testing.

Observations of language should note inflection, articulation, volume, rate, and rhythm of speech, vocabulary use, and grammar. Written letter or number reversals and rotations, or mirror-image writing need to be evaluated with respect to developmental level. Such errors normally disappear by 7 years of age, and their persistence beyond this age deserves particular attention. Speech hesitations, a stammer, or a stutter should be noted along with missed or misperceived verbal commands, word retrieval difficulty, or impaired naming. Irrelevancies or confabulation might be indicators of psychiatric disorder or aphasia and need to be recorded. Some speech patterns are of particular diagnostic significance. For example, monosyllabic speech may reflect test anxiety, may mask expressive speech impairment, or may be associated with a specific diagnosis, for example, Asperger's syndrome.

Nonverbal behaviors should be observed, including body position, ability to maintain eye contact, and responsiveness to nonverbal cues and gestures. Duration of attention span and any obstacles to full attention should be monitored along with how well the child functions over the time course of the test session. Evidence of a preferential modality (i.e., auditory, visual, tactual, or kinesthetic) should be documented, and compared with formal test results. Appropriateness of the child's sense of humor is also of interest.

THE TESTING ENVIRONMENT

The outpatient setting should be a visually appealing and comfortable environment that limits the potential for distraction. Familiar items such as colorful toys that clean easily between visits, age-appropriate books and magazines, and manipulative toys support a comfortable setting. The office should include appropriately sized furniture with a smooth writing surface and stable chairs that do not swivel but do adjust for height. The floor may be used as a testing surface when a child is not comfortably seated at a desk, and may be most effective for some physically handicapped children. A small pad or area rug tucked away in a closet may be brought out if the room is uncarpeted.

The examiner has less influence over the inpatient test setting. A child's medical condition has priority, and testing must be adapted according to the medical schedule. There is less time to build rapport, less opportunity to meet parents before testing, and imposed time constraints that make advance preparation that much more important. A hospitalized child's mood can seriously interfere with testing. If possible, the child should be removed from the hospital room and taken to more pleasant surroundings. An office can be a welcome change in surroundings for the hospitalized child. If transport is not approved, the examiner can bring clean test materials to the bedside. Frequent interruptions at the bedside by medical personnel might invalidate test results, and the examiner needs to be flexible in adjusting to the vagaries of the hospital setting. The examiner's attitude influences the child's performance. Therefore, it is desirable to be perceived as relaxed and comfortable rather than harried, distressed, or irritated by such interruptions. Notes about the timing of interruptions aid in determining whether there was a negative influence on performance.

A visit to the child to introduce oneself helps gauge the child's mental and physical capabilities. A puppet or other appealing toy can be used to initiate the relationship. For the actual testing it can be helpful to have a parent or favorite nurse present initially to reduce fearfulness. Since an ill child might require more frequent rest breaks than a healthy child, the inpatient testing may need to be completed in segments over days.

The examiner needs to avoid negative nonverbal facial and body language when faced with a very ill or injured child. A nonpunitive, unconditional acceptance of the child or adolescent should be communicated. Since an ill or uncomfortable child may not respond optimally, it is best to acknowledge this and obtain the best sample of behavior that is possible under these adverse testing conditions. A minimum number of tests to answer a referral question should be administered and a recommendation made for future comprehensive evaluation under more favorable circumstances, if judged appropriate.

ESTABLISHING RAPPORT

Good rapport is a prerequisite for a reliable and valid evaluation. It is especially important for a young child, but is essential for an examinee of any age. The examiner must be ready with a variety of behavioral techniques appropriate for different chronological and mental ages to reinforce continued attention across the test session's complete time course. Initial cooperation from the child is aided by parent acceptance of testing. Thus, the examiner's self-introduction to the child and family in the waiting room offers the first opportunity to set a positive tone that, hopefully, will persist through the entire assessment.

For the young child, the examiner's introduction (accompanied by a warm smile) should be directed first to the parent, along with a statement about looking forward to working (playing) with their child. With obvious parent acceptance, it is easier to introduce the child to the examiner or have the examiner directly face the child, make eye contact, and, introduce oneself. The examiner can kneel down to reduce the physical size disparity for very small children and become less physically threatening. Saying "Did you come to *play* with me today?" can reduce anxiety through the use of the word "play." A more direct welcome is appropriate for the older child, e.g., "I am so glad you are taking the time to work with me today." The examiner needs to observe the child's comfort level at the introduction. Some children will be confident and demonstrate their independence by easily separating from the parent. Others, particularly young children, may need their parents to accompany them to the testing room and remain with them briefly before they feel comfortable. These children will therefore need a longer warm-up period before formal testing begins.

Chronological age influences decisions about direct parent involvement in testing. While infants are best assessed in the presence of a parent, preschool-aged children may require a parent present for only a brief period of time and rarely for an extended period. By 3 years of age, children have experience in preschool settings and more easily leave their parent for a new environment. They may respond best with their parent nearby, but can often be expected to confidently separate. By age 4, most children separate successfully. Separation provides another opportunity to observe the child's self-confidence, ease around new adults, and degree of eagerness in approaching new situations. An unusual degree of dependence on the parent or separation anxiety is clinically notable.

Extra time for contact with the parent may be necessary, as well as verbal acknowledgment of a child's concerns about leaving the parent. The examiner can encourage the child to view and explore the testing room while offering reassurance. The examiner can clearly indicate when the child can return to the parent, by saying, "We'll be out when it is time for lunch, but now we have a lot to do. Your mother is going to be here in the waiting room while we are in my play (testing) room. Let's go see what special things I've brought to show you. What's your favorite kind of toy? Let's go see if I have anything close to that." Then, the examiner should confidently guide the child to the testing room.

A child can be expected to employ many strategies to lessen the anxiety and stress associated with being tested. These are especially notable at times of fatigue or when a test is especially hard. The temporal connection between a task and its associated negative behavior needs to be observed. For example, when does a child put his head down on the desk, ask to see the parent, request a bathroom break? Instead of agreeing to a request for a break, the examiner may propose one more short task before a brief break to establish control over the order of events and limit the frequency of such requests.

Physical surroundings may need to be adjusted. The examiner may choose to rearrange the furniture in the testing room if warned about a child's likely unwillingness to cooperate. Outbursts of physical acting out can be better controlled by repositioning furniture to restrain a child and to manage more easily a physical confrontation, for example, by seating the child against a wall and with the table placed to confine. This also gives the examiner sitting across the table convenient access to outside assistance.

Parent participation in testing may be an asset when evaluating an infant or very young child due to the child's greater cooperation and parents' ability to supply additional information about performance not achieved in testing but apparent at home. The parent must remain neutral but observant while the examiner tests the child, despite how difficult this can be for the parent. A parent's presence often comforts the child, and when seated out of view, she can often extend a test session when the child balks at continuing to cooperate since the child will be aware of her presence. While the parent's physical presence alone as a silent observer will often encourage the child to cooperate, a very young child may need to sit in the parent's lap.

Since parents find it difficult to remain silent while watching their child make errors, the examiner should stress the rules for maintaining standardized testing procedures and ask the parent to remain unobtrusive, refrain from providing verbal or nonverbal cues, and avoid prompting the child unless asked to by the examiner. As parents will often observe their child failing tasks they believe could be passed, the examiner should provide a means for them to record their observations during testing for later discussion.

INITIATING AND SUSTAINING TEST-TAKING BEHAVIOR

Testing produces anxiety even for a well-prepared child, especially at the beginning when the structure of the situation is still unfamiliar. Reassurance that no medical procedures are involved might need to be said clearly, especially for a young child, but even for older children who can more readily mask their discomfort. As noted above, initial test choice is influenced by perceived anxiety level, with more challenging tasks deferred until a more ideal comfort level is reached. Child examiners quickly learn to avoid physical or verbal associations with physician visits, such as wearing a white coat. The reason for the testing can be addressed directly. Children offer interesting insights about the reason for referral and should be asked to explain what they understand to be the reason they are being tested. Inquiring why the child believes the visit is necessary and then providing a simple explanation of the purpose of testing will often be sufficient to allay some anxiety.

While some children are prepared well by their parents, some are not given an explanation for their visit, and therefore a reason is imagined. Clarification is important to avoid unreasonable distortions. For example, "You are here today so I can see what kinds of things you do very well and where, if any, you have difficulty. Do you do certain things very well? Do you have special areas of difficulty?" The examiner might add, "I am a play doctor and that is very different than the other doctors you see," while pointing out the colorful boxes of games. A drawing is often an icebreaker since some feelings are more easily expressed nonverbally. It is up to the examiner to judge how much needs to be said to the child to increase comfort, to counter distortions, and foster the best possible testing.

Informal conversation at the beginning of a test session about a favorite game or activity, special interests, best friends, or upcoming events provides an opportunity for the examiner to formulate initial clinical impressions. Such discussion provides information about receptive and expressive language and familial and social relationships. One needs to avoid probing too deeply initially, and sensitive topics are best left until rapport is stronger. Nonjudgmental questioning is often effective. For example, asking a teenager about substance abuse or sexual conduct among friends is less threatening than a direct question about personal use.

Children need clear guidelines about what is expected during the session. Even though a child is reassured early in the test session, additional supportive comments may be needed at later times. Testing is aided procedurally by avoiding initial tasks that emphasize a known weakness, determining the optimum test administration order, liberal nonjudgmental feedback, anticipation of behavioral variability, and by not accepting nonparticipatory responding such as "don't know". The first test should ease the child into the testing situation. Knowing the child's limitations from the history taking allows an examiner to choose a test for which the child has a high likelihood of early success. For example, a young child without visuomotor integration problems generally enjoys drawing, so a shape-drawing test or a draw-a-person or a simple verbal task such as reciting the alphabet might be selected. One would not immediately administer a verbal list-learning test to a highly anxious or shy child. Positive reinforcement throughout the test session is important, as is balancing tests that are easy with those that are hard. For example, a difficult verbal learning test may be followed by an easy shape-drawing task to avoid persistent failure that will sabotage the positive momentum of the test session. Test choice should be parsimonious but inclusive of enough measures to answer the referral question and any additional hypotheses generated while working with the child.

The form of reinforcement is adjusted for age. For example, effusive physical responses such as clapping and smiling broadly will please a young child while older children may find verbal encouragement of their efforts more satisfying. Reiteration that no test is of a pass/fail nature is appropriate for all ages. Fear of failure might prevent a child from making an educated guess, and reassurance that there is no failing can be encouraging. The examiner must avoid a scoring pattern that can be interpreted by the child, such as smiling or saying "very good" every time a correct answer is given. Random reinforcement, for both good and poor responses helps. Well-timed rest breaks are advantageous, and these can include merely stretching and moving about in the testing room or a bathroom break without there being a need to remove the child from the testing environment or return to the parent.

Behavioral management principles and techniques include a consistent and systematic application of positive reinforcement contingencies. For example, young children may work very hard for a small sticker, shiny star, or token prize. Tokens may be collected along the way, with any number achieved sufficient to earn a final reinforcement. An appealing desktop item or the stopwatch can be used effectively as a reinforcer.

A long test session provides opportunity to see how a child responds to both success and failure. Testing will often elicit negative behavior as the difficulty level increases. Many hard items in close temporal proximity might result in avoidance actions. Negative behavior might parallel that reported by a parent or teacher, but since testing takes place in a highly structured, one-to-one setting, there is opportunity to permit a wider range of behaviors as long as they do not interfere with the testing.

To engage the child actively again, it is helpful to identify which tasks elicit the negative behavior and document them to reveal any pattern that emerges. The child should be reminded that many tests are deliberately designed to push the test-taker to her limits, and it is not possible to always be correct. Children are often reassured when told that a hard item is actually intended for an older child. Often, withdrawal and avoidance behaviors are a normal reaction to a stressful condition.

A child may also test limits or seek to terminate administration of a particularly difficult task. How a child responds in the testing room can reveal patterns common in the home or at school. Firm limits need to be set when manipulation is suspected. Informing the child that if tests are not completed, there will be a return visit might sufficiently motivate a child to cooperate for a longer period of time. With clear rules, a child is often better able to accept the conditions of the test setting. Instances of overt defiance in the presence of an authority figure are rare occurrences, but they do occur. These actions signal the need for further exploration of relevant cognitive and personality factors, parent and teacher effectiveness, and adequacy of school placement.

A reliable and valid assessment implies that a child has put forth appropriate effort. If an examiner suspects that motivation is limited, the conclusions will be in doubt, and the purposes of testing unmet. Sometimes, the confidence gained through early success will foster a motivation to succeed sufficiently well even for a difficult task. The Finger Tapping Test is one measure that allows an examiner to offer considerable praise since a child with normal or abnormal motor function cannot judge his level of success and will be guided by the examiner's verbal interpretation.

Motivational problems may be especially evident for children with psychiatric histories, such as conduct disorder, anxiety disorder, or clinical depression. A history of emotional problems alone is not fully predictive of what will ensue in testing. Any child is subject to moments of motivational loss, due to fatigue, hunger, anxiety, insecurity, or distress over preceding performances. Extreme resistance to being tested can be especially challenging. Such behavior can be demonstrated by a young child as well as an older child or adolescent. Highly active children might require considerable structure from the examiner but are often capable of cooperating for the testing without the initiation of specific techniques to reduce their activity level. Establishing rapport and administering the most critical tests early might be effective when it is anticipated that a child will not cooperate for a full test session.

Frequent requests for rest breaks to leave the testing room, to go to the bathroom, or to get a drink of water, and somatic complaints are generally cues that the child is feeling stressed. While a break is acceptable, one should be cautious about allowing a child to see the parent early in the testing. It is not uncommon for a child to refuse to return to the testing room or to return with a different, often reduced, level of cooperation. Rest breaks that encourage stretching, moving about, exploring the test room, or brief but active calisthenics are favored. The task immediately preceding a break should be one that has a high likelihood of success to instill confidence and acceptance of a return to formal testing.

Self-paced tasks frequently present problems for active children or those with an attentional deficit, and a child may skip questions or a test section. Redirection of the child, if in compliance with standardized test instructions, will be useful. Extension of time limits to gauge how well the child can function outside the bounds of standardized test constraints will add to knowledge about whether it is the task content that is problematic or the test conditions.

Certain behaviors are of special interest with respect to a child's ability to signal a neurological disorder. Inconsistent behavior or inattentive episodes might be evidence of a seizure disorder. For children with known seizure disorders, the timing and duration of blank staring spells or brief episodes of drifting or altered consciousness should be recorded along with the test being attempted at the time these behaviors occur. For example, complex partial seizures, unlike simple partial seizures, are associated with an alternation of consciousness. The examiner should also note whether the child responds during the altered state and how easily he or she returns to full responsiveness. Testing needs to be postponed in the postictal period when confusion or lethargy often occurs. Every once in a while, these observations will be the first time anyone has documented behaviors indicative of a likely seizure disorder. A clinician, therefore, needs to be sure the referring physician is contacted and the parents

consulted to obtain more information regarding the true implications of the observed behaviors.

Unusual or infrequently noted behaviors that require further exploration include, but are not limited to, extreme affection, overt aggression, self-determined termination of a test session in defiance of the examiner, mutism, rocking or head-banging, periods of staring, report of auditory or visual hallucinations, echolalia, bizarre or confabulatory speech, verbal or motor perseverations, singular attachment to an object or intense discussion about one, and idiosyncratic motor movements.

RECOGNIZING BEHAVIORAL AND PERSONALITY DISORDER

The possibility that there is a contributory behavioral or personality disorder is a significant consideration in any neuropsychological evaluation. Evaluation will often routinely include formal investigation of mood, personality, and/or adaptive behavior, and a number of helpful instruments are noted below in this discussion. A child neuropsychologist's strength is the ability to combine behavioral observations, direct testing, history review, and a reservoir of didactic knowledge about normal and abnormal brain development in order to make an informed clinical judgment about a child's current neurodevelopmental level, adaptive ability, and behavioral and social adjustment.

The focus of this volume is to compile and publish normative data for individual neuropsychological tests. Only a few examples of behavioral instruments commonly relied on by child neuropyschologists are summarized in this chapter since the normative data for many of these tests are not easily reproducible. The reader is encouraged to explore the many options, and the far wider array of instruments, as relevant for their particular clinical populations.

Circumstances associated with some clinical subgroups will especially test the neuropsychologist's acumen. Additionally, any child may present enormous obstacles to reliable and valid evaluation in the confines of a structured one-to-one testing session. While it may be anticipated that a child diagnosed as having autism, pervasive developmental disorder, elective mutism, conduct disorder, or another psychiatric disorder is untestable, rarely is this the case. It may take some creative solutions to conduct a valid testing, but often a behavioral sampling is entirely possible and can be expected to add to the already documented clinical knowledge about the child. While severely impaired children, or those highly resistant to testing, may seem to be unsuitable candidates for formal evaluation, in many cases, the obstacles can often be overcome, compliance achieved, and valuable data obtained.

Useful questionnaires are also available for some of these disorders that add substantially to the clinical knowledge, some sampling a broad range of problems and some more narrow in their focus. For example, the Diagnostic Interview for Children and Adolescents (4th ed.) (Reich, Welner et al., 1997; Welner, Reich et al., 1987) is a semistructured interview for past or current psychiatric diagnoses. The Conners' Parent Rating Scale–48 (PRS–48) is a 48-item rating scale that aids in identifying and rating the severity of behavior. The scales are Conduct Problems, Learning Problems, Psychosomatic Symptoms, Impulsivity/hyperactivity, and Anxiety. A Hyperactivity Index is also calculated. There is the Children's Yale-Brown Obsessive Compulsive Scale, and Symptom Checklist (Goodman, Price et al. 1989; Scahill, Riddle, et al. 1997) and the Leyton Obsessional Inventory–Child Version (Berg, Rapoport et al., 1985) when concern is raised about an obsessive compulsive disorder. The Checklist for Child Abuse Evaluation is an individually administered survey to evaluate symptomatology associated with neglect or abuse appropriate for children and adolescents (Petty, 1990). Parent attitudes toward child rearing can be explored further with the Parent Attitudes Toward Childrearing Questionnaire (Easterbrooks and Goldberg, 1984). The Warmth and Aggravation scales of this questionnaire were examined in a study of children with extracorporeal membrane oxygenation (ECMO), respiratory problems, and normal controls (Landry, Knowles et al. 1998).

Numerous instruments were developed to assist in making the diagnosis of autism. Older instruments specific for autism include the E-2 form of the Diagnostic Checklist for Behavior-Disturbed Children (Rimland, 1964), the Behavior Rating Instrument for Autistic and Atypical Children (Ruttenberg, Dratman et al., 1966), and the Behaviour Observation Scale for Autism (Freeman, Ritvo et al., 1978). The Autism Behavior Checklist (ABC) (Krug, Arick et al., 1980) was developed before the Diagnostic and Statistical Manual of Mental Disorders, 4th ed. was published. This behavior checklist has 57 items apportioned to five categories: sensory, body and object use, language, social, and self-help. Diagnostic usefulness is lessened by its low sensitivity but it has usefulness in research on intervention strategies (American Academy of Pediatrics, 2001). The Childhood Autism Rating Scale (CARS; Schopler, Reichler et al., 1988) was also developed before the DSM-IV was published. It rates behavioral characteristics after observation of children who are 2 years old and older and requires appropriate training for correct administration. The CARS consists of a 15-item structured interview that takes approximately 30 minutes, with each item scored according to a 7-point scale that indicates how deviant the child is from a normal same-aged child. An overall score is computed based on the ratings of each item and a cut-off score is used for categorization. The scale distinguishes between mild-to-moderate and severe autism, referenced to assessments of about 1500 children.

The Wing Autism Diagnostic Checklist (Wing, 1985; Rapin, 1996) items that best discriminated between pervasive developmental disorder subgroups were published (Fein, Stevens et al., 1999). One may also wish to review, and compare the usefulness of the Schedule of Handicaps, Behaviors, and Skills teacher report instrument, (Rapin, 1996), the Social Abnormalities Scales (Rapin, 1996), a Screening Test for Autism in Two-Year-Olds (Stone and Ousley, 1997), and the Infant Behavioural Summarized Evaluation (Adrien, Barthelemy et al., 1992). The Gilliam Autism Rating Scale (GARS) is a brief checklist based on DSM-IV criteria defining autism. The test is subdivided into four subtests with frequency based ratings. There are three core subtests: Stereotyped Behaviors, Communication, and Social Interaction. A fourth subtest, Developmental Disturbances, allows parents to provide information about their child's early development (Gilliam, 1995). The GARS is intended for those 3- to 22-years-old and was normed on 1092 individuals with autism from 45 states, Puerto Rico, and Canada.

The Checklist for Autism in Toddlers (CHAT) was developed as a screening for young children between 18 months and 3 years of age (Baron-Cohen, Allen et al., 1992), and data were obtained on more than 16,000 children. The CHAT consists of 14 questions (9 from parent history and 5 from observation by the home health visitor, a public health role in Britain) assessing joint attention, imitation, and pretend play. Five items are considered critical and indicative of severe risk for autism: history Q no. 5, 7, and observation Q no. 2, 3, and 4. These items were predictive of an autism diagnosis between 20 and 42 months when all were failed twice, at a one-month interval (Cox, Klein et al., 1999). Failure of protodeclarative pointing (history no. 7) and producing a point (observation no. 4) are indicative of a mild risk

for autism. More than three failures on any item places the child at risk for a different developmental disorder. Normal limits are considered when there are less than three failures on any item.

An extension of the CHAT, the Modified-CHAT or M-CHAT, was developed to address the issue of the CHAT's poor sensitivity. The M-CHAT has 23 yes/no parent report items (Robins, Fein et al., 2001) (see Table 2–1), including the first 9 items of the CHAT but eliminating the home healthcare observer items. A subset of six most discriminating items was found, i.e., questions 7, 14, 2, 9, 15, and 13 in descending order according to the standardized canonical discriminant function coefficients obtained for each item. The M-CHAT instructions are:

Please fill out the following about how your child usually is. Please try to answer every question. If the behavior is rare (e.g., you've seen it once of twice please answer as if the child does not do it.

Table 2–1. The Modified Checklist for Autism in Toddlers (M-CHAT)

1. Does your child enjoy being swung?	Yes	No
2. Does your child take an interest in other children?	Yes	No
3. Does your child like climbing on things, such as up stairs?	Yes	No
4. Does your child enjoy playing peek-a-boo/ hide-and-seek?	Yes	No
5. Does your child ever pretend, for example, to talk on the phone or take care of dolls, or pretend other things?	Yes	No
6. Does your child ever use his/her index finger to point, to ask for something?	Yes	No
7. Does your child ever use his/her index finger to point, to indicate interest in something?	Yes	No
8. Can your child play properly with small toys (e.g., cars or bricks) without just mouthing, fiddling, or dropping them?	Yes	No
9. Does your child ever bring objects over to you (parent) to show you something?	Yes	No
10. Does your child look you in the eye for more than a second of two?	Yes	No
11. Does your child ever seem oversensitive to noise? (e.g., plugging ears)	Yes	No
12. Does your child smile in response to your face or your smile?	Yes	No
13. Does your child imitate you? (e.g., you make a face-will your child imitate it?)	Yes	No
14. Does your child respond to his/her name when you call?	Yes	No
15. If you point at a toy across the room, does your child look at it?	Yes	No
16. Does your child walk?	Yes	No
17. Does your child look at things you are looking at?	Yes	No
18. Does your child make unusual finger movements near his/her face?	Yes	No
19. Does your child try to attract your attention to his/her own activity?	Yes	No
20. Have you ever wondered if your child is deaf?	Yes	No
21. Does your child understand what people say?	Yes	No
22. Does your child sometimes stare at nothing or wander with no purpose?	Yes	No
23. Does your child look at your face to check your reaction when faced with something unfamiliar?	Yes	No

Bold = most discriminating items

Source: Courtesy of the authors; © 1999 Diana Robins, Deborah Fein, & Marianne Barton.

There is a Spanish version of the M-CHAT. There is also reference to the CHAT and M-CHAT in the American Academy of Pediatrics policy statement regarding the pediatrician's role in the diagnosis and management of Autistic Spectrum Disorder (American Academy of Pediatrics, 2001).

Other more current and related instruments often apply to older children and/or require supervised training for proper administration and interpretation. The Autism Diagnostic Observation Schedule–Generic (ADOS; Lord, Rutter et al., 1997) is a standardized semistructured observation of a range of activities that enables an assessment of social behavior in natural communicative contexts. The stimuli are designed to elicit abnormal behavior or to illustrate occasions when normal behavior may not be exhibited. It has several modules that can assess social, communicative, and language behaviors in verbally fluent children.

Different tasks are administered depending on the child's age and language abilities. Module 1, for children with little language, will give information about ways to engage the child in interaction and how the child initiates adult involvement. There is a Pre-Linguistic ADOS for young children who do not yet speak (DiLavore, Lord et al., 1995), and this was combined with the ADOS to provide information for a wider age range and across greater developmental levels (Lord, Risi et al., 2000). The Autism Diagnostic Interview-Revised (ADI-R; Lord, Rutter et al., 1994) is a complementary interview instrument also requiring training for effective use that yields scores based on history. There are both clinical and research forms. These are lengthy assessments, taking approximately 45 minutes for the observation and 90 minutes for the interview. Both operationalize DSM-IV and International Classification of Diseases, 10th Revision criteria.

Certainly, compliance may be limited for more profound neurodevelopmental disorders, and in these cases the examiner's observational and clinical skills are especially challenged. Sometimes, it is a matter of overt willful control on the child's part. In such a case, the child attempts to wield ultimate control of the testing situation and the examiner must establish and make clear their authoritative role before expecting the child's cooperation. This can often be accomplished in subtle but effective ways and is necessary if testing is to proceed toward its intended goal.

It was recognized early that depression and central nervous system damage can interact and suppress intelligence test results (Black, 1973). Clear and direct effects of depression on attention and concentration are often clinically evident. Commonly used tests that may reveal impairment related to such mood disorder and its associated effects on attention and concentration include, among other measures, the Wechsler Intelligence Scale for Children–3rd ed. Digit Span and Coding subtests, Trail Making Test, and Continuous Performance Tests or other tasks requiring sustained attention. Tests requiring immediate recall of novel encoded information and recall of previously learned complex information are also subject to disruption in the presence of such disorder, due to the importance of concentrating on the novel stimuli on their initial presentation. While a relationship has long been reported between left cerebral function and depression (Starkstein & Robinson, 1991), a correspondence also appears to exist between depression and right hemisphere function, i.e., right dorsolateral prefrontal cortex, with this neocortical region being a critical convergence zone (Liotti and Mayberg, 2001). The data also support linking negative mood with the dorsal anterior cingulate cortex, which aids in monitoring conflict and inhibition of action, such as assessed with the Stroop Color-Word Test and go-no go tests (Pardo, Pardo et al., 1990).

While a mood disorder, such as childhood depression, has the potential to reduce an intelligence score, this possibility is not always considered (Cotton, Crowe et al. 1998). A general lowering of test scores may be observed or, a lowered verbal intelligence quotient compared to Performance intelligence quotient may be an important marker of a mood disorder, and not of lateralized brain dysfunction. In contrast, in many cases where there is documented neurological impairment, it is often the subtest scaled scores contributing to the nonverbal, performance IQ that are lowered, in part due to the requirements for speeded performance and focused attention to details. The presence of a mood disorder is also commonly reflected on tests of motor function and other speeded measures, with generalized slowing evident.

Generally lethargic production in association with flat affect also signals the importance of attending to possible emotional concomitants. Personality assessment is an important part of the neuropsychological evaluation, providing data that maximize the ability to predict real-world behaviors relevant to independent and socially responsive functioning in young adults (Ready, Stierman et al., 2001). These authors found neuropsychological measures to be predictors of achievement and work-related behavior, while personality measures were associated with disinhibited, risk-taking, and aggressive behaviors.

Of particular interest, was the finding that neuropsychological measures (Controlled Oral Word Association, Trail Making Test, and Wisconsin Card Sorting Test) and personality measures of executive functions were not significantly correlated. Thus, different types of information contribute to our knowledge about the individual. Sometimes, substitution of one test for another is not going to result in an equivalent assessment. What each test offers may be a matter of some variability from individual to individual, but it is important to have a fundamental knowledge about what each test or procedure one administers contributes to an assessment to maximize the clinical information obtained from each measure.

Since children with a history of mood disorder present special obstacles to neuropsychological evaluation, and as cognitive functions are directly influenced by mood, certain cognitive tests are especially likely to reflect this influence, as noted above. Also, there are a number of measures that explore mood more specifically. Among these are narrow-band, self-report inventories for depressive symptomatology. The Children's Depression Inventory (CDI) is appropriate for children aged 7 to 17 years old (Kovacs, 1992). Normative data were collected on 1266 Florida public school children in grades 2 through 8 (592 boys aged 7 to 15 and 674 girls aged 7 to 16). Race and ethnicity data were not reported, but it was estimated that there were 77% Caucasian and 23% African American, American Indian, and Hispanic, mostly middle-class children. About 20% came from single-parent families. The test has 27 items, with responses indicated on a 3-point scale, i.e., $0 =$ symptom absent, $1 =$ mild symptom, and $2 =$ definite symptom. The questionnaire items are read easily by even young children. The test is divided into five subscales: negative mood, interpersonal problems, ineffectiveness, anhedonia (physical effects of depression), and negative self esteem. A total CDI score is also calculated.

The five primary factors are significantly intercorrelated; they intercorrelate in the .34 to .59 range and are correlated .55 to .82 with the total CDI. Internal consistency reliability in the normative sample resulted in a Cronbach's alpha of .86. Alpha coefficients for the factors ranged from .59 to .68. There is also a 10-item short form that does not include the suicide question. However, use of the short form does not allow for calculation of the five subscales.

The short form correlated $r = .89$ with the full test. Its alpha reliability coefficient was .80. Raw scores are converted to T-scores, and graphed by gender and age, i.e., for girls or boys 7 to 12 years old and girls or boys 13 to 17 years old. A T-score of 65 or greater is considered clinically significant, although it is recommended that a T-score of 70 be used to indicate problems if one is doing a routine screening for a child believed not likely to have problems.

Another measure, the Reynolds Child Depression Scale (Reynolds, 1989) is also a brief screening measure written at a second grade level and appropriate for children in grades 3 to 6. It consists of 30 items rated on a 4-point scale and can be administered individually or to a group. Reliability coefficients range from .87–.91. There is also a Reynolds Adolescent Depression Scale (Reynolds, 1987).

The influence of anxiety needs to be carefully considered during an evaluation, and behavioral responses suggesting anxiety recorded. Anxiety questionnaires and self-report inventories are available for more formal assessment. The State-Trait Anxiety Inventory for Children (STAIC) is a self-report measure of anxiety in 9- to 12-year old children in Grades 4, 5, and 6 (Spielberger, Edwards et al., 1973). The STAIC was normed on 737 males and 814 females. It can be administered individually or to a group. It is also recommended for children with average or above reading ability or older below average children. Separate self-report scales measure state anxiety (A-State) and trait anxiety (A-Trait). There are 20 statements for the A-State, inquiring about subjective consciously perceived feelings. There are also 20 statements for the A-Trait scale. The STAIC is appropriate for adolescents and adults (Spielberger, 1983). The Anxiety Disorders Interview Schedule (ADIS) for DSM-IV (Silverman and Albano, 1996) has both a parent version and a child version, for separate interviews. The ADIS specifically identifies targets for intervention.

The Multidimensional Anxiety Scale for Children (MASC) (March, 1997) is a self-report inventory for those 8 to 19 years old. It assesses of a range of anxiety symptoms. It provides information about four scales: physical symptoms, harm avoidance, social anxiety, and separation/panic. It also provides an Anxiety Disorders Index, Total Anxiety Index and Inconsistency Index. The Revised Children's Manifest Anxiety Scale (RCMAS; Reynolds and Richmond, 1985) is a brief self-report inventory of 37 yes-no items for those 6 to 19 years old. A Total Anxiety score is obtained along with four subscales: Worry/Oversensitivity, Social Concerns/Concentration, Physiological Anxiety, and a Lie Scale. There are gender-specific norms for almost 5000 individuals, including children in gifted and learning disabled classes. Separate African American population norms are available.

Even children without known significant psychological or psychiatric contributions to their behavior may react negatively to the testing environment. It is not unusual for a child to exhibit a temper tantrum, become tearful, pout, become sullen, reach for and/or throw available items, become aggressive, whine, or otherwise attempt to deflect the examiner from the intended purpose of their time together. Child neuropsychologists are especially well-trained and capable of coping with these more difficult testing-the-limit circumstances, obstacles in test administration that rarely present similarly in an adult neuropsychological evaluation.

Neuropsychological and psychological tests may directly reflect a primary emotional basis

as a determining factor for the child's behaviors of concern. While these may be internally driven, there are times when external pressures may offer a better explanation. At some point in the testing session, negative behaviors may be precipitated when the test becomes especially difficult, when the child is becoming tired or hungry, or when the child believes his or her performance was inadequate. For example, a child may be responding to unintentional but clear pressures from parents or a teacher to succeed at a higher level when there are genuine neuropsychological reasons why such success is tempered. In the absence of appropriate data highlighting the strengths and weaknesses sufficiently well, the child's reactive behavior may be evident in an exaggerated reaction to these parent- or teacher-driven pressures.

Instruments are also available to better appreciate the child's self-concept. Assisting in that determination is the Piers-Harris Children's Self-Concept Scale, a self-report inventory for those 8 to 18 years old (Piers and Harris, 1996). There are 80 yes–no items written at a third grade reading level that result in 6 subscales: Physical Appearance and Attributes, Intellectual and School Status, Happiness and Satisfaction, Anxiety, Behavior, and Popularity. Age-stratified normative data are provided for more than 1700 individuals. The Piers-Harris Children's Self-Concept Scale-Second Edition (Piers, Harris et al., 2002) reduced the length from 80 to 60 items. Normative data for the second edition were obtained from 1387 students across the United States, and the age range was extended downward to 7 years old. The Multidimensional Self Concept Scale includes six context-dependent self-concept domains: Social, Competence, Affect, Academic, Family, and Physical (Bracken, 1992). Total scale score reliability exceeds .97 for the total sample and each subscale coefficient alpha exceeds .90. The scale is appropriate for children and adolescents, and either individual or group administration is possible.

A considerable number of behavioral and personality measurement instruments are also available, including parent and teacher report inventories, self-report inventories, behavior rating scales, and structured interviews. Many of these behavioral and personality measures have detailed technical manuals that contain the relevant normative data. Several such tests are also have computerized scoring programs, and some will provide interpretive guidelines.

Among the adaptive behavior scales that are appropriate in childhood and adolescence are the American Association of Mental Retardation Adaptive Behavior Scales–School, (2nd ed.) (Lambert, Nihira et al., 1993). It was normed on children 3 to 18 years old, including over 2000 individuals with developmental disabilities and more than 1000 without documented disability. This is a two-part scale, one part concerned with personal independence and coping skills, and the second, related to social maladaptation. Five factors are identified: personal self-sufficiency, community self-sufficiency, personal-social responsibility, social adjustment, and personal adjustment.

The Vineland Adaptive Behavior Scales (VABS): Interview Edition, Survey Form (Sparrow, Balla et al., 1984) is a commonly used semistructured interview measure for assessing a child's social emotional development. The standardization was based on a representative national sample of 3000 children, from birth to 18 years, 11 months. There is also a classroom edition of 244 items to obtain the teacher's perspective about the child. These children were selected to correspond to 1980 U.S. census figures for age, gender, community size, 4 geographic regions, 4 levels of parent education, and 4 groups based on race/ethnicity. It included 100 subjects in each of 30 age groups subsequently reduced to 200 subjects in 15 age groups. The total sample was 1500 children. Of these, 719 (36%) participated in the standardization of the Kaufman Assesment Battery for Children (Kaufman and Kaufman, 1983). Standard scores are obtained for four adaptive behavior domains: Communication (receptive, expressive, written), Daily Living (personal, domestic, community), Socialization (interpersonal relationships, play and leisure time, coping skills) and Motor Skills (gross and fine). There is an optional Maladaptive Behavior domain. An Adaptive Behavior Composite standard score with a mean of 100 and a standard deviation of 15 can be calculated.

The VABS has supplemental norms for a variety of populations, including samples from institutional versus community settings. The Scales of Independent Behavior-Revised (SIB-R) can be completed by the parent independently or it can be administered in an interview format. The scale extends from infancy to adulthood and is useful for individuals both with and without disability. There is also a maladaptive behavior index. The SIB-R provides standard scores for the following areas: motor skills, social interaction and communication skills, personal living skills, community living skills, and broad independence (full scale). Further specification is possible for gross motor skill, fine motor skill, social interaction, language comprehension, language expression, eating and meal preparation, toileting, dressing, personal self-care, domestic skills, time and punctuality, money and value, work skills, home-community.

Among the most widely used psychological instruments that assess behavioral problems and personality is the wide-band Child Behavior Checklist (CBCL; Achenbach, 1991a; 1993), of the Achenbach System of Empirically Based Assessment (ASEBA). The CBCL is a behavioral rating scale for children and adolescents, based on parent ratings of children 4 to 18 years old, and, in its newest form, for children aged 1½ to 5 years old (Achenbach and Rescorla 2000). There are Spanish versions. The Teacher Report Form for ages 5 to 18 was normed on 1391 nonreferred students. There is also a Youth Self-Report for children aged 11 to 18, with fifth grade reading skill (or it may be administered orally). The latter scales were based on 1272 clinically referred individuals, and normed on 1315 nonreferred individuals. Thus, parent and child responses regarding the child's behavior and social competence can be directly compared, and computation of parent-teacher agreement by item scores intraclass correlation is possible.

The CBCL/4–18 was normed on 2368 nonreferred children, and 4455 clinically referred children were studied to validate the scales. The parent responds to a 100-item, 3-point scale, i.e., 0 = not true, 1 = somewhat or sometimes true; 2 = very true or often true. Test-retest reliability over one week was .90 for boys and .88 for girls. The CBCL is a well-validated measure for quantifying behavior (Cohen, Gotlieb et al., 1985). Reliability and validity are well established (Sattler, 1988; Ostrander, Weinfurt et al., 1998) along with validation for a Direct Observation Form of the Child Behavior Checklist (Reed and Edelbrock, 1983). The total score is based on assessment of multiple functional areas. The eight individual subscales include Withdrawn, Somatic Complaints, Anxious/Depressed, Social Problems, Thought Problems, Attention Problems, Delinquent, and Aggressive. Scores are also obtained for Activities, Social, School, and Total. The results of factor analysis with the Attention Problems Scale T-score as a dependent measures found a two-scale solution, i.e., externalizing and internalizing; T scores are calculated for both Internalizing and Externalizing summary scores. The Externalizing score consists of responses for items relating to delinquent behavior and aggressive behavior. The Internalizing score consists of responses for withdrawn behavior, somatic complaints, and anxious/depressed scales. Data can be compared to six taxonomic profiles: Somatic, Social, Withdrawn, Delinquent-Aggressive, Social-attention, and Delinquent.

In addition to 6 subscales (Emotionally Reactive, Anxious/Depressed, Somatic Complaints, Social, Withdrawn, Attention Problems, and Aggressive Behavior), the CBCL/1 1/2–5 has DSM-oriented scales for affective problems, anxiety problems, pervasive developmental problems, attention deficit/hyperactivity problems and oppositional defiant problems. There is a Sleep Problems scale. It also includes a Language Development Survey (LDS) for parent report of expressive vocabulary and word combinations, and screens for language delay risk factors. This measure was normed on a national sample of 700 children, and scales were based on ratings of 1728 children.

The Behavior Assessment System for Children (BASC) is a measure of emotional behavior problems, adjustment to home, school, and community that provides data based on parent report and student self-report ratings (Reynolds and Kamphaus, 1998a; 1998b). T-scores from 41 to 59 are average, typical or indicative of normal adjustment. An At-Risk score is a T-score of 60 to 69. Clinically significant ratings are T-scores of 70 or higher. A T-score of 65 for Anxiety scale is also signifi-

cant. An overall Behavioral Symptoms Index (BSI) is calculated. Parent ratings provide scores for clinical scales. An Externalizing Problems Composite based on subscale scores for hyperactivity, aggression, and conduct problems and an Internalizing Problems Composite based on Anxiety, Depression and Somatization subscale scores are calculated. There are also Clinical Scales for Atypicality, Withdrawal and Attention Problems.

An Adaptive Skills Composite score is derived from subscale scores for social skills and leadership. In contrast to the clinical scales, a higher T-score on the latter indicates better adjustment. Student report ratings result in a School Maladjustment Composite based on Attitudes to School, Attitude to Teachers, and Sensation Seeking Scales. A Clinical Maladjustment Composite is based on Atypicality, Locus of Control, Somatization, Social Stress and Anxiety Scales. The Depression and Sense of Inadequacy Scales provide additional data regarding emotional and behavioral functioning. An Emotional Symptoms Index is calculated. Also, the Personal Adjustment Composite is based on Relations with Parents, Interpersonal Relations, Self-Esteem and Self-Reliance scales. Validity data include those for children diagnosed as having Attention Deficit Hyperactivity Disorder (Ostrander, Weinfurt et al., 1998).

Learning to cope with these vagaries of testing is part of the child neuropsychologist's practical education in clinical practice. I offer a few suggestions that have served me well in observing behavior and taking notes, adapting the environment, using behavioral strategies, remaining in control, using parents wisely, starting easy and ending easy, providing feedback, and considering the options.

Observing Behavior and Taking Notes

One of the first things one learns is how easy it is to forget useful observational information once a lengthy test session has concluded. Therefore, taking sequential notes about the child's behavior and range of responses will later provide essential cues as to what may be influencing these behaviors. Formal recording rather than reliance on incidental recall also assists in documenting a wide range of responses that may not reveal their significance until the full test session is completed. For example, a word-finding problem noted early in testing may be excused as developmentally normal, be easily ignored, and not recorded. However, if other such word retrieval difficulties are evident throughout the test session and each is documented, the notes about each instance combine to result in a more stringent clinical judgment than would otherwise occur. The pattern can then be compared to other language data. As a result, the note taking may appropriately alter one's initial, perhaps erroneous, opinion and provide additional support for converging data.

Further, it is important to note the temporal relationship of a critical behavior to an activity. For example, when does the child become quiet and withdrawn, put her head down, become tearful, or otherwise react poorly to a specific type of task. Alternatively, an examiner should also carefully note when the child appears excited about a task and eager to cooperate. Whether a child's motivation to do well diminishes as the testing time increases is also of interest, as is whether a child appears refreshed after short but important rest breaks. Tracking and recording the examples of behaviors over the full time course makes it easier to later link a behavior with a task. For example, a young child with graphomotor delay may cooperate willingly for word games and a picture vocabulary test, retreat when faced with requests for a writing sample and a design drawing task, and then once again cooperate well when the task is once again verbal. Or, a child who experiences difficulty with visuoperceptual tasks may respond fluently and well in response to tests of expressive vocabulary and abstract verbal similarities but wiggle around and become overtly uncomfortable when faced with a request to construct block designs and judge line orientations.

An adolescent with anterior cerebral dysfunction secondary to bruising and shearing after a traumatic brain injury may respond well to concrete tasks that have specific and clear rules for performance, but become disorganized and ineffective when working on an abstraction task, such as card sorting or complex design replication. Obvious personality change in response to the increased task difficulty may be expected, particularly if problems with emotional regulation are another consequence of the injury. Intact function may be evident when simpler auditory/verbal tasks such as oral spelling and easy mental calculations are requested, but withdrawal behavior may be evident once again in response to requests for verbal or nonverbal recall of prior stimulus information or response to complicated commands. Thus, in addition to monitoring and recording data about accuracy, it is equally important to monitor and record data about behavioral and emotional reactions to specific stimuli and their temporal occurrence.

Observations not directly related to a formal test are equally as valuable as those obtained during traditional test administration. Such informal observations may even contradict test results. For example, how a child reaches for, grasps, and picks up a desired toy or object in a playroom may better confirm the level of motor skill acquisition and maturity of a pincer grasp than a requirement for similar behavior during testing when the child's cooperation is variable. Patiently watching the child and presenting stimuli as play objects—not as test items—may allow for more thorough "testing" than by only following formal administration procedures. It is then incumbent on the examiner to remain flexible and capable of recognizing those informal instances that capture critical information about the child's acquisition of developmental milestones, when these appear outside the usual testing structure.

Using Behavioral Strategies

Experience and theoretical orientation will dictate the clinician's specific approach to any child evaluation. Irrespective of one's academic knowledge and preferential evaluation style, it is particularly worthwhile to become familiar with the application of behavioral principles, even if these are not a primary orientation. Behavioral principles work exceptionally well in child testing circumstances. It has been my experience that knowledge of these behavioral techniques provides an especially useful pragmatic framework for working with difficult children. Importantly, these principles are equally applicable to all children confronted with the unusual demands inherent to the formal testing situation.

One effective strategy I often employ has its basis in behavioral principles: I ask a resisting or hesitant child to choose from among two choices for our next task. For example, "Do you want to work with colored blocks now or take a test involving words?" This question gives the objecting child a clear choice of options and seeming situational control, but it really demands a compliant response that advances the test session productively. In contrast, asking "Do you want to take a block test now?" or stating "Let's work on a block test now!" has a greater probability of resulting in "No!" and will provide the objecting child a basis for noncompliance and lead to continued poor cooperation. Such an application of behavioral principles may better encourage the establishment of a positive working relationship that optimizes the child's ability to demonstrate true competencies.

Behavioral principles also provide a substantial basis for positively guiding parents in the interpretive session about their options. Behavioral principles can be invoked to explain why their attempts to induce their child to behave better at home have not met with the success they expected. Even a few simple and fundamental behavioral shaping principles may be communicated effectively to parents requiring assistance in improving direct parent-child interactions. They are useful for developing interventions targeted to specific negative child behaviors. Techniques such as establishing a contract for a reinforcement contingency program, maintaining consistency between parents in application of reinforcement, and ignoring negative behaviors but reinforcing desired behaviors are valuable and universally applicable in all environments. These suggestions may presage the need for parents to receive more formal instruction through parent training sessions, or they may have the effect of making the parents more aware of how their usual actions encourage the continuation of some behaviors to which they object.

Remaining In Control

It becomes necessary to set firm boundaries overtly for some difficult children. While most children implicitly respect the authority figure, not all do. The child may attempt to have a test session proceed according to those contingencies typical within the child's family or those rules the child tries to personally impose during the test session, rather than according to the examiner's structure. This message, while often communicated subtly, should be clear and consistent. For example, rest breaks, repeated visits to the bathroom, and the timing of when the child returns to the parent all need to take place at the examiner's discretion. However, it is possible to negotiate these breaks judiciously with the child and reach mutually agreement about how many and when such breaks are acceptable. The child is then expected to honor the verbal contract to which they are now committed. Attempts to deflect tasks also need to be addressed directly. A surprisingly effective response for some noncompliant children who threaten imminent termination is a child-friendly restatement of the evaluation's importance, acceptance of the non-cooperation, emphasis on the session needing to continue, and casual comment about how failing to continue will only necessitate a return (horrors, a second!) visit.

Using Parents Wisely

Parent presence in the testing room should generally be avoided, but under extreme conditions, selective parent presence may be a sufficient stimulus to change a child from resistant to cooperative. Parents can be effectively involved in direct testing, but often only in specific and limited circumstances. When involved in testing, the parent should remain silent but be offered paper and pencil in order to take notes or write down questions that the neuropsychologist can later answer. The parent also needs to be instructed to remain seated out of view of her child. An exception is when an infant or very young child is most comfortable sitting in a mother's lap and can then better cooperate for the test items without stranger anxiety further complicating the interaction (see Baron and Gioia, 1998, for further discussion of the neuropsychology of infants and young children).

The proper timing of a parent's involvement is thus variable from child to child, with extensive involvement expected for infant assessment, a limited but carefully defined unobtrusive presence if needed for a noncompliant young child, and absence from the testing room, or an extremely rare presence, for older children or adolescents. Under rare circumstances, when a child does not separate easily from a parent, or is desolate about not seeing the parent, the parent will need to be instructed how to be a useful presence to better elicit on-task behavior. The American Academy of Clinical Neuropsychology policy statement regarding third-party observers comments on these exceptions (Hamsher, Lee et al., 2001). Empirical data suggest that the validity of neuropsychological test results may be compromised by an observer's presence (Kehrer, Sanchez et al, 2000).

Parents are the most knowledgeable informants about a child, and what they report needs to be taken most seriously. Yet, even the most well-intentioned parent may not recognize how well-informed they are about their child. Therefore, asking parents for any additional information they may have, even if they thought it too minor to mention to anyone, can be quite helpful and reveal previously unknown information. Parents report a wide range of relevant information when asked for any additional information they may have omitted from the history. There are many examples of surprisingly relevant information revealed with such questioning, including concussion, contributory family neurological or learning disorders, systemic medical problems not recognized as potentially influencing cognitive function, deaths, separations, substance abuse, potential child abuse, bullying at school, and periods of shaking or attentional lapses not recognized as seizure phenomena. It is also crucial, after spending time with the child in testing, to inquire further about the parent's ability to support or refute the neuropsychologist's own clinical observations about the child, to determine whether these impressions are compatible or inconsistent with what the parents recognize and report.

Starting Easy—Ending Easy

Easy and nonthreatening tasks need to be administered at the start of testing. The child needs to be actively engaged in the evaluation process. Presenting an initial task that taps into the child's area of weakness immediately creates a negative interaction that often will persist for the duration of testing. It is also helpful to move from the least to the most structured tasks over the testing time. Easing the child into the testing situation may require some initial relatively unstructured tasks. These can then be followed by the more challenging and highly structured tests that limit the child's ability to freely determine and manipulate the situation but for which full cooperation is required to avoid their being invalidated. As necessary, a return to an easier task may prolong a test session. Since the child should leave testing feeling confident and pleased as much as possible with his performance, an easily accomplished test at the conclusion of testing is recommended (see below).

Providing Feedback

Children may overtly, or even nonverbally, request information about their progress during testing. Reflection of the child's fears or concerns is a useful verbal technique. A child's perception of the examiner's empathy and understanding may be conducive to moving the evaluation process forward. Good communication may lead to greater trust and recognition that the examiner appreciates the child's feelings about such formal scrutiny in a relatively strange situation. It also reinforces the idea that working well and doing one's best will be the best way to aid the assessment process. Anticipation of a child's emotional or physical withdrawal is possible. For example, when those tears well up in the child's eyes, that is a time to immediately intervene, offer comfort, change the task, talk about the child's feelings, or otherwise engage in some action that will allow the child to continue with greater comfort.

Adapting the Environment

While a lenient attitude and approach may be entirely appropriate for a child, a more rigid structure may be required at some points during the testing session. This may extend to the physical environment. For example, the furniture may need rearrangement so an aggressive, acting-out child is confined behind a desk that limits out-of-seat behavior. The child with an attentional disorder may need window blinds drawn to reduce outside visual distractions or desktop items removed to limit their inherent attractiveness. The hyperactive child may need a chair with confining arms that does not swivel. A shy young child may find sitting across a desk intimidating and prefer testing on a carpeted floor; this may be possible for portions of the evaluation. Items in the room can be used as reinforcements. For example, the stopwatch is an attractive "toy" to a young child, and allowing some children to time the examiner clearing off one test and setting up another is a favored activity.

Considering the Options

The examiner needs to recognize that certain circumstances make children with behavioral problems especially unable or unwilling to cooperate. It is important to work with the child rather than engage in confrontational tactics or pedantic methods. The examiner should make conscious attempts to avoid engaging in those ineffective strategies that the parent may employ when faced with the same behaviors at home. These patterns are the child's context, and the examiner needs to protect himself or herself from being drawn into these nonconducive habitual interactions that are often sustained by intermittent reinforcement.

One option under extreme conditions may be to terminate testing and reschedule for another session. This is perfectly acceptable and may be the best choice for a number of reasons. For example, if the child is easily fatigued, the remaining testing will stress the child too much, and there is a strong risk the child will fail to continue cooperating. Perhaps the child arrives for testing feeling ill. Or, the current session is not judged to be a valid assessment, and a second visit may better help sort out the relevant contributions.

CONCLUDING THE TEST SESSION

Difficult tests need to be saved for late in the testing session because they have a high probability of leading to termination of the testing. The highly threatening Tactual Performance Test (TPT) that requires being blindfolded for an extended period of time or the mentally taxing 128-card Wisconsin Card Sorting Test are examples of tests that might bring a session to an early conclusion and are likely to be remembered should a child return for reevaluation. In contrast, the examiner should plan to administer a final test that is relatively easy in order to give the child an opportunity to leave with a sense of successful accomplishment. The examiner should acknowledge the efforts made by the child over the testing time, for example, saying, "I'm so pleased with how well you worked, even for the hard tests." Expressing appreciation for the child's cooperation by praising the child in the parents' presence is especially important. Offering a token toy or sticker to the young child should not be contingent on performance.

The conclusion of the test session can focus on the child if the parent has been told in advance that a meeting to review results will take place at a future date. On occasion, it may be important to talk to the parent privately at the conclusion of the testing. It is a delicate matter to accomplish this consultation without upsetting the child. Excusing oneself and the parent for a brief time "in order to fill out some routine paperwork" presents a rationale for the child to feel less threatened by the ensuing private conversation.

CONCLUSION

Child neuropsychologists apply knowledge about normal child development along with information obtained through a thorough history taking and astute clinical observation to evaluate efficiently a child's behavior in the clinical setting. The result of these many valuable information sources is an evaluation that leads to practical and meaningful recommendations for treatment or management, the purpose of a well-conceived clinical neuropsychological evaluation. Children with behavioral or personality problems present special circumstances, but there are many objective test instruments that supplement carefully observed and recorded subjective data to assist in fractionating the relevant contributions to the child's overall behavioral profile.

REFERENCES

Achenbach, T. M. (1991a). *Manual for Child Behavior Checklist 4–18 and 1991 Profile.* Burlington, VT: University of Vermont Psychiatry Department.

Achenbach, T. M. (1993). *Empirically based taxonomy: How to use syndromes and profile types derived from the CBCL/4–18, TRF, and YSR.* Burlington, VT: University of Vermont Department of Psychiatry.

Achenbach, T. M., & Rescorla, L. A. (2000). *Manual for the ASEBA Preschool Forms and Profiles.* Burlington, VT: University of Vermont, Department of Psychiatry.

Adrien, J., Barthelemy, C., Perrot, A., Roux, S., Lenoir, P., Hameury, L., et al. (1992). Validity and reliability of the Infant Behavioral Summarized Evaluation (IBSE). *Journal of Autism and Developmental Disorders, 22* (375–394).

Albano, A. M. & Silverman, W. (1996). *Anxiety Disorders Interview Schedule for DSM-IV.* Child version. San Antonio, TX: The Psychological Corporation.

American Academy of Pediatrics. (2001). The pediatrician's role in the diagnosis and management of autistic spectrum disorder in children (REO60018). *Pediatrics, 107,* 1221–1226.

Baron, I. S., & Gioia, G. A. (1998). Neuropsychology of infants and young children. In G. Goldstein, Nussbaum, P. D. and Beers, S. R. (Ed.), *Handbook of Human Brain Function: Assessment and Rehabilitation, Volume III: Neuropsychology* (pp. 9–34). New York: Plenum.

Baron-Cohen, S., Allen, J., & Gillberg, C. (1992). Can autism be detected at 18 months? The needle, the haystack, and the CHAT. *British Journal of Psychiatry, 161,* 839–843.

Berg, C. J., Rapoport, J., & Falment, M. (1985). The Leyton Obsessional Inventory—Children's Version. *Psychopharmacology Bulletin, 21,* 1057–1059.

Black, F. W. (1973). Intellectual ability as related to age and stage of disease in muscular dystrophy: A brief note. *The Journal of Psychology, 84* (333–334).

Bracken, B. A. (1992). *Multidimensional Self Concept Scale.* Austin, TX: PRO-ED.

Cohen, N. J., Gotlieb, H., Kershner, J., & Wehrspann, W. (1985). Concurrent validity of the internalizing and externalizing profile patterns of the Achenbach Child Behavior Checklist. *Journal of Consulting and Clinical Psychology, 53,* 724–728.

Cotton, S., Crowe, S., & Voudouris, N. (1998). Neuropsychological profile of Duchenne Muscular Dystrophy. *Child Neuropsychology, 4,* 110–117.

Cox, A., Klein, L., & Charman, T. (1999). Autism spectrum disorders at 20 and 42 months of age: Stability of clinical and ADI-R diagnosis. *Journal of Child Psychology and Psychiatry, 40,* 719–732.

DiLavore, P., Lord, C., & Rutter, M. (1995). The pre-linguistic autism diagnostic observation schedule. *Journal of Autism and Developmental Disorders, 25,* 355–379.

Easterbrooks, M. A., & Goldberg, W. A. (1984). Toddler development in the family: Impact of father involvement and parenting characteristics. *Child Development, 55,* 740–752.

Fein, D., Stevens, M., Dunn, M., Waterhouse, L., Allen, D., Rapin, I., et al. (1999). Subtypes of pervasive developmental disorder: Clinical characteristics. *Child neuropsychology, 5,* 1–23.

Freeman, B., Ritvo, E., Guthrie, D., Schroth, P., & Ball, J. (1978). The Behaviour Observation Scale for Autism: Initial methodology, data analysis, and preliminary findings on 89 children. *Journal of the American Academy of Child Psychiatry, 17,* 576–588.

Gilliam, J. E. (1995). *Gilliam Autism Rating Scale (GARS).* Austin, TX: Pro-Ed.

Goodman, W. K., Price, L. H., Rasmussen, S. A., et al. (1989). The Yale-Brown Obsessive Compulsive Scale: Vol. II. Validity. *Archives of General Psychiatry, 46,* 1012–1016.

Hamsher, K., Lee, G. P., & Baron, I. S. (2001). Policy Statement on the Presence of Third Party Observers in Neuropsychological Assessments: American Academy of Clinical Neuropsychology. *The Clinical Neuropsychologist, 15,* 433–439.

Johnson-Greene, D., Hardy-Morais, C., Adams, K., Hardy, C., & Bergloff, P. (1997). Informed consent and neuropsychological assessment: Ethical considerations and proposed guidelines. *The Clinical Neuropsychologist, 11,* 454–460.

Kaufman, A. S., & Kaufman, N. L. (1983). *Kaufman assessment battery for children: Interpretive Manual.* Circle Pines, MN: American Guidance Service.

Kehrer, C. A., Sanchez, P. N., Habif, U., Rosenbaum, J. G., & Townes, B.-D. (2000). Effects of a significamt—other observer on neuropsychological test performance. *The Clinical Neuropsychologist, 14,* 67–71.

Kovacs, M. (1992). *Children's Depression Inventory.* North Tonawanda, NY: Multi-Health Systems, Inc.

Krug, D., Arick, J., & Almond, P. (1980). Behavior checklist for identifying severely handicapped individuals with high levels of autistic behavior. *Journal of Child Psychology and Psychiatry, 21,* 221–229.

Lambert, N., Nihira, K., & Leland, H. (1993). *AAMR Adaptive Behavior Scales-School, Second Edition.* Austin, TX: PRO-ED.

Landry, S. H., Knowles, L. M., Miller-Loncar, C. L., Wildin, S. R., & Zwischenberger, J. B. (1998). Extracorporeal membrane oxygenation versus conventional treatment: neurodevelopmental and social outcomes at 24 months. *Child Neuropsychology, 4,* 118–130.

Liotti, M., & Mayberg, H. S. (2001). The role of functional neuroimaging in the neuropsychology of depression. *Journal of Clinical and Experimental Neuropsychology, 23,* 121–136.

Lord, C., Risi, S., Lambrecht, L., et al. (2000). The autism diagnostic observation schedule-generic: A standard measure of social and communication deficits associated with the spectrum of autism. *Journal of Autism and Developmental Disorders, 30,* 205–223.

Lord, C., Rutter, M., & DiLavore, P. (1997). *Autism Diagnostic Observation Schedule-Generic (ADOS-G).* New York: The Psychological Corporation.

Lord, C., Rutter, M., & Le Couteur, A. (1994). Autism Diagnostic Interview-Revised: A revised version of a diagnostic interview for caregivers of indivduals with possible pervasive developmental disorders. *Journal of Autism and Developmental Disorders, 24,* 659–685.

March, J. S. (1997). *Multidimensional Anxiety Scale for Children.* North Tonawanda, NY: MHS.

Ostrander, R., Weinfurt, K. P., Yarnold, P. R., & August, G. J. (1998). Diagnosing attention deficit disorders with the Behavioral Assessment System for Children and the Child Behavior Checklist: Test and construct validity analyss using optimal discriminate classification trees. *Journal of Consulting and Clinical Psychology, 66,* 660–672.

Pardo, J. V., Pardo, P. J., Janer, K., & Raichle, M. E. (1990). The anterior cingulate cortex mediates processing seletion in the Stroop attentional conflict paradigm. *Proceedings of the National Academy of Sciences, 87,* 256–259.

Petty, J. (1990). *Checklist for Child Abuse Evaluation.* Odessa, FL: Psychological Assessment Resources.

Piers, E. V., & Harris, D. B. (1996). *Piers-Harris Children's Self-Concept Scale.* Austin, TX: PRO-ED.

Piers, E. V., Harris, D. B., & Herzberg, D. S. (2002). *Piers-Harris Children's Self-Concept Scale,* 2nd Edition. Los Angeles, CA: Western Psychological Services.

Rapin, I. (1996). *Preschool children with inadequate communication: Developmental language disorder, autism, low IQ* (Vol. 139). London: Mac Keith Press.

Ready, R. E., Stierman, L., & Paulsen, J. S. (2001). Ecological validity of neuropsychological and personality measures of executive functions. *The Clinical Neuropsychologist, 15,* 314–323.

Reed, M. L., & Edelbrock, C. (1983). Reliability and validity of the Direct Observation Form of the Child Behavior Checklist. *Journal of Abnormal Psychology, 11,* 521–530.

Reich, W., Welner, Z., & Herjanic, B. (1997). *Diagnostic Interview for Children and Adolescents-IV (DICA).* Chicago, IL: Multi-Health Systems, Inc.

Reynolds, C., & Kamphaus, R. W. (1998a). *Behavior Assessment System for Children. Parent Rating Scale.* Circle Pines, MN: American Guidance Services, Inc.

Reynolds, C., & Kamphaus, R. W. (1998b). *Behavior Assessment System for Children. Self-report Version.* Circle Pines, MN: American Guidance Services, Inc.

Reynolds, C., & Richmond, B. O. (1985). *Revised Children's Manifest Anxiety Scale.* Austin, TX: PRO-ED.

Reynolds, W. M. (1987). *Reynolds Adolescent Depression Scale.* Odessa, FL: Psychological Assessment Resources.

Reynolds, W. M. (1989). *Reynolds Child Depression Scale.* Odessa, FL: Psychological Assessment Resources.

Rimland, B. (1964). *Infantile autism: The syndrome and its implications for a neural theory of behavior.* New York: Appleton-Century-Crofts.

Robins, D. L., Fein, D., Barton, M. L., & Green, J. A. (2001). The modified Checklist for Autism in Toddlers: An initial study investigating the early detection of autism and Pervasive Developmental Disorders. *Journal of Autism and Developmental Disorders, 31,* 131–144.

Ruttenberg, B., Dratman, M., Fraknoi, J., & Wenar, C. (1966). An instrument for evaluating autistic children. *Journal of the American Academy of Child Psychiatry, 5,* 453–478.

Sattler, J. M. (1988). *Assessment of children* (3rd ed.). San Diego, CA: Author.

Scahill, L., Riddle, M. A., & McSwiggin-Hardin, M. e. a. (1997). Children's Yale-Brown Obsessive Compulsive Scale: Reliability and validity. *Journal of the American Academy of Child and Adolescent Psychiatry, 36,* 844–852.

Schopler, E., Reichler, R., & Renner, B. R. (1988). *The Childhood Autism Rating Scale (CARS).* Austin, TX: PRO-ED.

Sparrow, S. S., Balla, D. A., & Cicchetti, D. V. (1984). *Vineland Adaptive Behavior Scales: Interview Edition.* Circle Pines, MN: American Guidance Service.

Spielberger, C. D. (1983). *State-Trait Anxiety Inventory*. Palo Alto, CA: Mind Garden.

Spielberger, C. D., Edwards, C. D., Lushene, R., Montuori, J., & Platzek, D. (1973). *State-Trait Anxiety Inventory for Children*. Redwood City, CA: Main Garden.

Starkstein, S. E., & Robinson, R. G. (1991). The role of the frontal lobes in affective disorder following stroke. In H. S. Levin, H. M. Eisenberg & A. L. Benton (Eds.), *Frontal lobe function and dysfunction* (pp. 288–303) New York: Oxford University Press.

Stone, W. O., & Ousley, O. (1997). *Screening test for autism in 2-year-olds.* Unpublished manuscript, University of Nashville, TN.

Welner, Z., Reich, W., Herjanic, B., Jung, K. G., & Amado, H. (1987). Reliability, validity, and parent-child agreement studies of the Diagnostic Interview for Children and Adolescents (DICA). *Journal of the American Academy of Child and Adolescent Psychiatry, 26,* 649–653.

Wing, L. (1985). *Autistic Disorders Checklist in Children.* Unpublished manuscript.

Appendix 2–A

SAMPLE: CHILD NEUROPSYCHOLOGY QUESTIONNAIRE

Child's Name: _____

Date of Birth: _____

Date of Evaluation: _____

Person who referred you for evaluation: _____

Name of person filling out this questionnaire: _____

Child's Pediatrician and address: _____

_____

Referral Information

Reason you are requesting this evaluation _____

_____

_____

Circumstances/factors you think are important regarding this reason _____

_____

_____

In my opinion, the major cause of my child's difficulties is _____

_____

_____

Describe some of your child's strengths _____

_____

_____

Describe some of your child's weaknesses _____

_____

_____

Do both parents agree about the nature and causes of the problem? _____

Family Information

Address _____

Telephone _____

Names of Parents

    Mother _____ age: ____ education: _____

    Occupation _____

    Father _____ age: ____ education: _____

    Occupation _____

Parents are married ___ separated ___ divorced ___ (Custody is with _____) re-married _____

deceased _____

Child is biological ____ adopted ___ (at age_____) foster _____

Does the child prefer one parent over the other? ____ which one? ____

    Siblings (name, age): _____

                 _____

                 _____

                 _____

    Others living in home_____

                 _____

Is child in Child Care? _____ How many hours/day? _____

Has your child experienced death or separation from a loved one? ____ Explain_____

Approximate Family Income

  0–15,000   _____

  15,000–35,000 _____

  35,000–55,000 _____

  55,000–75,000 _____

  75, 000 or higher _____

Are there any significant family or marital conflicts? (explain) _____

_____

Pregnancy and Birth History

Age of mother _____ and father _____ at delivery? _____ How many prior pregnancies? _____

How many prior miscarriages? _____ Was a fertility specialist consulted? _____ Procedures? _____

Any known health problems of mother during pregnancy? _____ vaginal bleeding? _____ toxemia? _____

hypertension? _____ gestational diabetes? _____ trauma? _____ fever/rash? (e.g., flu,measles?) _____

smoking? _____ alcohol? _____ illicit drugs? _____ antibiotics? _____

depression or other emotional problems? _____ blood incompatibility? _____ injury? _____ other?

_____

List any medications, tobacco use, alcohol use or drugs taken by mother during pregnancy _____

_____

Delivery was vaginal _____ Cesarean _____ (reason _____)

Baby was full term _____ or premature _____ (___ weeks gestation)

Birth Weight _____ lbs. _____ ozs.

Was labor prolonged? _____ (length of time = _____)

Any birth complications? (e.g., feet first/cord around neck/meconium staining/lacking oxygen-blue/jaundice-yellow)

_____

Did baby breathe spontaneously? _____ oxygen required? _____

Apgar scores if known _____ In Intensive Care Nursery? _____

How old was baby at discharge from the hospital after birth? _____

Medical problems after discharge (e.g., jaundice, fever, transfusion,surgery)

_____

Any problems in first few months? _____

Did you experience a postpartum (after birth) depression? _____

Developmental History

Motor

Age sat alone _____ crawled _____ stood alone _____ walked alone _____

Was your child slow to develop motor skills or awkward compared to siblings/friends (e.g., running, skipping,

climbing, biking, playing ball? _____

_____

Handedness: right _____ left _____ both _____ (explain) _____

Family history of left handedness (list relatives)? _____

Was physical therapy ever necessary? (when?) _____

Was occupational therapy ever necessary? (when?) _____

Speech/Language

Age spoke first word _____ put 2–3 words together _____

Speech delays/problems (e.g., stutters, difficult to understand)? _____

Oralmotor problems (e.g., late drooling, poor sucking, poor chewing)? (describe) _____

Was speech/language therapy ever necessary? _____

Was child slow to learn the alphabet? _____ name colors? _____ count? _____

Other language spoken at home (besides English)? _____

Besides English my child is fluent in _____

Toileting

Age when toilet trained _____

Problems with bedwetting?, urine accidents?, soiling? Until what age? _____

Any current problem? _____

Social Behavior

Does your child get along well with other children? _____ adults? _____ have friends? _____ keep friends? _____
understand gestures? _____ have a good sense of humor? _____
understand social cues well (e.g., knows when others are angry, in discomfort)? _____
have problems with peer pressure (e.g., alcohol or drug use) _____

_____

_____

Medical History

Has vision been checked? _____ Any problems: _____

Has hearing been checked? _____ Any problems: _____

CT __ or MRI __ obtained? _____ Results: _____

EEG obtained? _____ Results: _____

Other tests and results: _____

List serious illnesses/injuries/hospitalizations/surgeries

      date   incident (explain)

_____   _____

_____   _____

_____   _____

_____   _____

_____   _____

Is there a history of:

Failure-to-thrive?   _____

febrile seizures? (fever associated)   _____

epilepsy?   _____

staring spells?   _____

lead poisoning/toxic ingestion?   _____

meningitis or encephalitis?   _____

asthma or allergies?   _____

diabetes?   _____

loss of consciousness?   _____

abdominal pains/vomiting?   _____

    when do they occur?   _____

headaches?   _____

    when do they occur?   _____

frequent ear infections?   _____

    were ear tubes necessary?   _____

    age when tubes placed?   _____

sleep difficulties?   _____

eating difficulties or eating disorder?   _____

tics/twitching?   _____

repetitive/stereotypic movements?

    (e.g., hand flapping)   _____

impulsivity?   _____

temper tantrums?   _____

nail biting?   _____

clumsiness?   _____

head banging?   _____

self-injurious behavior?   _____

Describe head injuries: (e.g., date, type, loss of consciousness?, resulting changes in behavior?)

_____

_____

Current medications and reasons:

_____

Is there a history of learning difficulty in any family member?

_____

Is there a history of neurological illness in any family member?

_____

Is there a history of seizures in any family member?

_____

Is there a family history of psychiatric disorder?

_____

Does anyone else in the family have a problem similar to your child's reason for referral?

_____

Educational History

Current school and address: _____

Grade: _____ Placement: regular _____ resource _____ special education _____

other _____

Any grades that were skipped or repeated? _____

Teachers report problems in:

reading	_____	attention/concentration	_____
spelling	_____	behavior	_____
arithmetic	_____	social adjustment	_____
writing	_____		

Grade: Academic problems?

Nursery

Kindergarten

First

Second

Third

Fourth

Fifth

Sixth

Seventh

Eighth

Ninth

Tenth

Eleventh

Twelfth

Was your child unusually hyperactive? _____ inattentive? _____

Specific problems noted: _____

_____

Do teachers report problems that you do not notice? _____

My child's intelligence level is likely:

below average _____

average _____

high average _____

superior _____

His/her mother's intelligence level is likely:

below average _____

average _____

high average _____

superior _____

His/her father's intelligence level is likely:

below average _____

average _____

high average _____

superior _____

Prior Psychological History

Have you previously had direct contact with any social agency, psychologist, psychiatrist, clinic or private agency?

_____

Name of professional	Address	Dates

Any other comments you would like to make:

Appendix 2–B. Sample Face Sheet for Child Neuropsychological Evaluation

NAME   DOB   DOT   Age

GENERAL INTELLIGENCE
    WISC-III or WISC-IV
    WAIS-III
    DAS
    Bayley
    Mullen

ACHIEVEMENT
    WIAT Reading
    WIAT Spelling
    WIAT Arithmetic
    Woodcock-J

EXECUTIVE
    Wisconsin Card Sort
    Category Test
    Raven's Matrices
    Similarities
    Fluency—Design /Verbal (Phonemic/Semantic)
    Graphomotor Patterns
    Trail Making Test
    Go-NoGo
    BRIEF
    D-KEFS

LANGUAGE

Write name, address, phone number	Auditory Analysis Test
Peabody Picture Vocabulary Test-III	Aphasia Screening Test
Token Test	Boston Diagnostic Aphasia Exam
Paragraph Production	parts: _____
Vocabulary	RAN
Boston Naming Test	Multilingual Aphasia Exam
Spelling—written/oral/dictation	

    ABCDEFGHIJKLMNOPQRSTUVWXYZ (oral and written) JFMAMJJASOND (months)
    1,2,3,4,5,6,7,8,9,10 (count forwards);   Name colors
    20–19–18–17–16–15–14–13–12–11–10–9–8–7–6–5–4–3–2–1 (Count backwards)

SENSORY/MOTOR/TACTUAL-MOTOR

Sensory Testing:tactile, auditory, visual	Tapping
Finger Recognition	Grip
Number Writing/ Symbol Writing	Grooved Pegboard
Tactile Form Recognition	Purdue Pegboard
Left-Right-personal/extrapersonal	Lateral Dominance Exam
Luria Motor (3-part;reciprocal)	Apraxia Exam

NONVERBAL

Draw-a-person;-clock;-bicycle;-family   Facial Recognition
Rey-Osterrieth or Taylor Complex Figure   Road Map
Beery Developmental TVMI   Line Bisection
Judgment of Line Orientation   Hooper Visual Organization

LEARNING & RETRIEVAL

Selective Reminding Test & Delayed Recall
Nonverbal Selective Reminding Test & Delayed Recall
Verbal Paired Associates Immediate / Delayed Recall
Story Memory Paragraphs Immediate / Delayed Recall
Sentence Memory
Visual Reproduction Designs Immediate / Recall
Continuous Recognition Memory Test
Rey-Osterrieth (or Taylor) Immediate / Delayed recalls
Benton Visual Retention Test

ATTENTION/CONCENTRATION/ORIENTATION

Test of Everyday Attention for Children
Symbol Digit Modalities Test   Cancellation/Visual Search
WISC-III-Coding; Digit Span   Stroop Color Word Test
Trail Making Test   Money Road Map
Mazes   Continuous Performance
Consonant Trigrams Test   Letter Number Sequencing

PERSONALITY/DEPRESSION INVENTORY/MOOD

_____

_____

_____

3

Communicating Results: The Interpretive Session and the Written Report

The interpretive session and the written report are two important ways that the neuropsychological evaluation results and recommendations are transmitted. This chapter considers both of these communication methods.

THE INTERPRETIVE SESSION

The interpretive session is a time to review and clarify information obtained during the pre-testing clinical history taking, during records review and interviews with third parties, and during testing. The art of the interpretive session is to translate complex data into meaningful, clear, concise, and practical recommendations. An interpretive session might include parents, the child, and/or a teacher or other health professional to facilitate coordinated care. Results are therefore communicated directly to those most intimately involved in the child's care. Importantly, the session should be recognized as a time to acquire additional information in open discussion, and as a result of further questioning and the practitioner's observations. This is necessary in order to confirm initial impressions based on earlier stages of evaluation, that is, to explicate interpersonal relationships among family members and their potential influence on the child.

It is also a time to educate parents about how the brain influences their child's behavior and

cognitive function and about any correlation observed between a diagnosed medical or psychological condition and actual test performance or unique error pattern. It may also be an opportune moment to give a child or adolescent a direct but simple explanation of his or her cognitive strengths and weaknesses, relate these to the reason he or she was tested, and answer any questions he or she might be willing to ask.

Information Interchange

Hypotheses about a child's neuropsychological integrity are certainly generated before the interpretive session, but it is during this conversational session that these preliminary impressions can be validated. By reviewing and clarifying historical information and the reason for referral along with any available supplemental records, the child's behavior during the structured testing session can be compared with parent expectations, and a determination made about whether it diverges from their expectation or parallels their own observations.

The session becomes a final opportunity to probe for any preexisting conditions that might invalidate presumptive formulations and necessitate modification of one's conclusions. For example, finding a "deficit" profile, including calculation problems after head injury in a motor vehicle accident might lead one to conclude that the injury had a negative impact on this aspect of cognition, but not if the parents or teacher reported that the problem had been present before the accident. Not infrequently, parents may unintentionally omit valuable information from even the most thorough pre-testing history interview. For example, one parent denied her child had had any head injury despite a strong traumatic brain injury profile on evaluation. The parent finally responded to repeated questioning about whether there had ever been any car accidents, falls, or injury from an aggressive playmate by saying "Oh! there was the time she fell down a flight of stairs and was knocked unconscious, but the doctor found nothing wrong." The interpretive session is an essential time for further exploration of possibilities suggested by the neuropsychological profile.

A child's seemingly abnormal physical appearance, or behavioral idiosyncrasy, may lose its clinical significance when it is also observed in a parent or reported present in a sibling. The parent may also have a very large head, unusual voice quality, or odd facial feature, diminishing the concern raised by observation of a similar feature in the child. However, sharing a feature does not necessarily exclude its significance. For example, parent and child may both exhibit difficulty making eye contact, use monotonic speech, have limited interpersonal skill, and report motor awkwardness, characteristics also present in individuals diagnosed as having Asperger's syndrome (Wing, 1985).

The relative influences of genetic predisposition versus learned behavior also require consideration. For example, a parent's spelling errors on the intake questionnaire raise questions about the relative contribution of poor educational background or an inherited learning disability, as does evidence of writing dyspraxia. A child's singularly abnormal characteristic may actually represent normality in context with immediate family members. The interpretive session is the time to further consider all these possibilities.

Parent Education

A major goal of the interpretive session is to provide the parents with information that will make them even more effective advocates for their child than they currently are. Extensive objective, qualitative, and collateral data are collected in a neuropsychological evaluation, which then must be summarized succinctly if the lay person is going to understand and apply the information in a practical and meaningful way. Parents must first understand what is being communicated. Then, they must make the necessary intellectual and emotional adjustments to accommodate to the results. This then allows them to take positive steps in their child's best interest. Accomplishing these objectives within the interpretive session's time constraints is not always easy, but always necessary.

Professional terminology and unfamiliar concepts complicate communication in the interpretive session. Therefore, a practitioner should avoid technical jargon that is not clearly explained and should use simple language to convey complex information. The strategy of repeating the same information in different ways, and with different examples, is often especially useful. Some parents are reluctant to ask questions of the "doctor," and it is imperative that their questions be accepted, anticipated, and addressed. Asking a parent to "tell me what you have learned so far in this meeting" is revealing of the parent's acquisition of the new information and associated gaps. It is also useful to have one parent restate conclusions for the other, or for the child, to gain a better appreciation of what information has been integrated well and where there are lacunae in understanding or agreement.

In one of my interpretive sessions, the parents had widely divergent viewpoints. The father considered the child to be unmotivated but perfectly normal and had been unwilling to pursue neuropsychological evaluation. In contrast, his wife had a sensitive and knowledgeable appreciation of her son's deficits. She attributed their differences of opinion to the father's absence from the home, due to long work days and late returns home, sometimes when their son was already asleep. The mother, who was home when her son returned from school, saw directly her son's struggle with homework assignments and his consistently poor results. To explain the seriousness of his son's neurocognitive weaknesses and break the pattern of denial, the father was asked to pretend he was going to his job as he does every day, but to think aloud about how his son's identified specific problem areas would affect his on-the-job performance. Only in this context could the father relent and acknowledge that he might have failed to recognize the significance of his son's problems and that he might have contributed to the significant family stress as a result.

Concrete examples may be particularly helpful to parents. For example, a parent might focus on the Intelligence Quotient (IQ) to the exclusion of the other considerable neuropsychological data, thinking it a sufficient measure of their child's future success or failure. In such instances, the range of their child's strengths and weaknesses requires clarification to delimit the emphasis on an unitary global score to which they ascribe too much importance. Pointing out the profile of high and low scores, and stronger and weaker cognitive domains, and the specific implications of such scores for real-world experiences can make the "numbers" that much more meaningful to those with limited appreciation for test generalization and criterion-validity.

One score or one test result does not generally define a child's deficit and a multiplicity of factors typically influences the observed behavior. The importance of deriving a profile according to convergence profile analysis (see Chapter 1), based on qualitative and quantitative information, is relevant to further helping the parent understand his child's neuropsychological functioning.

Stages of the Interpretive Session

The neuropsychologist can learn substantial information about a child in a brief time, and the interpretive session is a time to convey what was learned. Early in the interpretive session, it may be evident that a parent is worried about the eventual results and perhaps skeptical about the process. Parents may be resistant to the idea that a relatively brief test session will result in sufficient dissection of their child's psychological function. Gaining parent acceptance of the evaluation conditions prior to communicating specific results is beneficial since the interpretive session will proceed more smoothly once parents recognize that valid impressions about their child are possible even in the context of such a time-limited evaluation. One means of accomplishing this is to ask parents to restate the reason for referral and their expectations for the evaluation at the beginning of the interpretive session to be sure that their primary concerns are addressed. Their response generally reveals the minimum knowledge they require, but may also highlight which central questions they should be asking that are not yet well formulated. Monitoring parents' verbal and nonverbal responses closely throughout the session helps to clarify their understanding about their child's situation and the full implications of the results being conveyed.

It is also useful to interpret one's own behavioral observations of the child early, by commenting on the child's interactive style and any idiosyncratic features that typified the child's performance. Such comments make it clear that there was sensitivity to the child's personality and temperament. For example, the clinician could comment about the child's resistance, shyness, high activity level, or low frustration tolerance, and the influence of such behaviors in the test session. Parents often visibly relax and more easily accept the validity of the evaluative process once they recognize that their child was seen as an individual. For instance, one could say, "Mollie seemed so worried at first. She kept her head down and only whispered answers to my questions. We needed to talk about her family and friends a bit before she felt comfortable enough to work with me on a test. Her caution can be a very good and protective response, and it did not interfere in this structured one-to-one testing, but let's talk a bit about how it can interfere in the school setting."

As the session progresses, the neuropsychologist must both guide and teach parents to prepare them for their advocacy role, that is, how to request special educational services, locate community rehabilitative services, obtain a consultation about a potential medical disorder or psychiatric condition, or expand their child's extracurricular experiences. Unfortunately, parents might not appreciate subtle symptoms of brain dysfunction that may be compromising their child's performances. For example, mild lateralized motor weakness may be ignored or right-left discrimination problems joked about despite their potential for highlighting subtle brain dysfunction that directly impacts on day-to-day function. The neuropsychologist plays a critically important role in helping parents recognize both their child's strengths and any discovered deficit or delay, along with their own advocacy role responsibilities.

Specific examples are often helpful, as long as a parent is not overwhelmed with unnecessary detail or complex vocabulary. It is important to seek a balance between the degree of detail offered and the nature of the child's needs. For example, ability–achievement discrepancy needs to be understood if the concern is about school placement and school-based intervention options, but perhaps unnecessary for the child whose medical condition raises more imminent questions about survival than late cognitive effects.

In the course of the interpretive session, an attempt should be made to recognize and address nonverbalized concerns. A parent may not initially reveal his or her concern about an incident that has, nonetheless, long been a source of worry. Surprisingly, parents may not raise their genuine concerns with their regular physicians, but worry silently instead. Common are longstanding concerns about an illness, medication, or diet during pregnancy, a long or complicated labor or other birth-related occurrence, a concussive event or illness their child had at an early age. A parent may be undereducated about the possible late effects of an illness or its treatment, particularly if the illness was not brain-related.

For example, parents may be unfamiliar with the late neurocognitive effects associated with acute lymphocytic leukemia and its treatment or cognitive consequences of cardiac abnormality and repair. Or, a parent may overemphasize a noncontributory factor and need advice about how to put that concern in perspective. A parent concerned that his or her child's problems are due to psychological factors and/or deficient parenting skills may be reassured, and also empowered, when the neuropsychological evalua-tion provides a specific "medically based" explanation that relates to the psychological features and abrogates her self-blame.

It is highly advantageous to have both parents present for the interpretive session, and it is simplistic (and often incorrect) to assume that both parents have parallel impressions of their child and similar goals and expectations. When both parents are present in the interpretive session, differences in their attitudes, opinions, and responses to their child's illness or injury may be discerned. For example, both parents may share a similar perspective about education but remain at odds over the best method to ensure academic attainment. Or, one parent may deny the existence of any brain-related problems, while the other acknowledges the full implications of how a neurological insult has affected the child's capabilities and self-image.

The verbal and nonverbal interactions between parents may reveal contradictory viewpoints or overt disagreement. The nonverbal indications of discordant thinking include, but are not limited to, obvious tension reflected in actions such as angry glances or physical distancing in their seating. Similarly, a sensitivity to signs of information overload such as gestures of discomfort, tensing of muscles, or change in eye contact might indicate that important information needs to be restated.

The interpretative session can also elicit feelings of blame rather than a realistic and concordant impression. Behavioral management techniques might be inconsistent, and thus, the parents find themselves working against each other. Problems within the marriage might be clearly expressed or suggested by their actions. Often, parents can once again work in concert on behalf of their child once the neuropsychological basis for the problem is recognized, and the impact of their actions better understood.

Both parents need to express their views in the interpretive session, even if, at first, one of the parents remains stoically silent. Specific inquiry, and follow-up questions as necessary, addressed to the silent parent may be necessary. Allowing only one parent to control the interaction is inadvisable. Parents' unrealistic concerns also need to be monitored. For example, test results obtained in childhood are but one tentative index of eventual adult function, and this sole performance does not allow for specific predictions about adult success or failure since so many other factors will be influential as the child matures. When parents nonetheless request such prognostication, their question needs to be reframed more appropriately, and the importance of life experiences, motivation, and opportunity emphasized, along with the impact of any needed interventions and how their own contribution as involved parents will shape their child's outcome.

A decision needs to be made about whether to include other professionals in the interpretive session. With the parents' consent, the results and recommendations can be communicated to multiple individuals simultaneously, thereby minimizing the potential for distortion of results through distant communication. The session should remain a personal time between the neuropsychologist and parents if it is anticipated that the third party presence may inhibit the work of the session. A second interpretive session may be needed for the parents and others directly involved in the child's care.

Teachers also need to be familiarized with the cognitive and behavioral impact of the child's illness or injury to the central nervous system and of any past or proposed treatment if they are to intervene and support the child effectively in the classroom. Certainly, a goal of the neuropsychological evaluation is to provide information that will enable a teacher to better address the student's learning capacity, and to bring attention to the child's existent strengths so they can be utilized to full advantage to ameliorate any weakness.

How much specific information can be communicated effectively varies. An open dialogue is more easily maintained with parents who communicate well. However, others may not express their concerns as freely. The process of obtaining multiple consultations and the need to take primary responsibility for juggling the sometimes contradictory messages from a variety of professionals may culminate in an overt expression of frustration during the interpretive session. Neuropsychological consultation obtained in a middle or late stage of a chain of referrals often requires the neuropsychologist to clarify the diverse data and place

them in a context whereby the parent can best meet their advocacy responsibility. Some parents struggle to accept the short- and long-term implications of their child's deficit, and concordance between parents might be lacking. The preliminary plan for presentation of results must change to accommodate the parents' sophistication and vary with any attempts to rationalize or suppress those findings that they find hard to hear.

The conclusion of the interpretive session is a time to summarize what was learned as a result of the full evaluation and to reiterate the concrete steps that need to be taken next. Hopefully, parents will leave the interpretive session able to link test data and simple brain-behavior lessons with an appreciation for how their child functions in real-life experiences. They can be reminded that the written report will recapitulate the interpretive session dialog and serve as a reference to which they or the teacher can consult and that they should feel free to call with any further questions related to the current evaluation.

Interpretive Session Strategies

As alluded to above, several interpretive session strategies prove especially useful, and these are highlighted below. These include communicating results simply, defining terminology, incorporating parent restatement, providing specific examples of strengths and weaknesses, encouraging questions and participation, and interpreting results directly to the child.

Communicating Results Simply

The neuropsychologist needs to communicate well-organized results simply and in a relatively brief time. This is especially important since there are limitations on how much anyone can integrate on first hearing new or unfamiliar information. Too much information will overwhelm parents, while insufficient information will provide them too little to use effectively on their child's behalf. Preplanning the main points one intends to convey, along with preparing potential treatment or intervention alternatives, produces an outline that then can be amended, based on information related during the interpretive session.

Defining Terminology

It often is necessary to introduce new terminology and unfamiliar concepts in the interpretive session, as well as to correct erroneous impressions resulting from limited parent integration of data from prior consultations or the unexplained use of professional jargon. Ideally, one avoids such jargon in favor of simple language, definition of terms, and provision of clarifying examples to promote optimal understanding. A complex vocabulary or rapid data presentation may leave parents bewildered, but reluctant to acknowledge their misunderstanding or misperception.

Concepts widely popularized by lay persons may not be fully understood or may be misleading with respect to the child's actual neuropsychological profile. For example, one cannot assume that highly educated parents will understand basic IQ concepts. Parents may assume that an IQ test allows for direct hypotheses about brain function and therefore provides a sufficient measure of the future success or failure their child will experience, even representing a critical determinant of their child's future potential. It is incumbent on the neuropsychologist to explain the full data set, dispute the decisiveness of one global score taken out of context, and emphasize that one score or one test is often insufficient as a prognostic indicator. It may be possible to explain how a profile emerges based on behavioral observations and results from many different tests. The neuropsychologist should reinforce, as necessary, the notion that any one test result often depends on a number of factors operating simultaneously, and among these are genetic, environmental, and socioeconomic contributions. The neuropsychological evaluation helps determine which factors may be most relevant to understanding a child's quality of response at this point in time.

Encouraging Parent Restatement

Having parents restate in their own words what the neuropsychologist has just communicated is a valuable technique that enables the neuropsychologist to gauge their level of understanding, pinpoint information that may have been missed or misinterpreted, and identify differences in comprehension between those present for the interpretive session. A parent who can correctly reiterate the key points would seem to be a step ahead of a resistant parent in implementing recommendations intended to rectify those specific aspects of their child's weakness and optimizing identified strengths. Restatement can be elicited in a one-to-one interpretation, by asking one parent to repeat the information to the other when both parents are present, and by asking either the child or parent to restate information to the other when the child is included at some point in the session.

Providing Examples of Strengths and Weaknesses

A need to focus on a deficit pattern should not negate a balanced presentation of the child's strengths and weaknesses. The neuropsychologist has a valuable opportunity to convey positive as well as negative features of the child's performance. Relative strengths are often overlooked, but they will aid the child and need to be incorporated in rehabilitation and treatment venues. It is easy to omit a discussion of strengths when one has identified and must explain dysfunction in a relatively brief time. The presentation and discussion of a child's clear strengths prior to the weaknesses often helps parents maintain a balanced perspective about the cognitive abilities that are functional and those which will require more focused attention.

Parents of a child with a nonneurological medical problem may be especially unprepared to hear of associated neurocognitive dysfunction, for example, that a brain dysfunction is a potential consequence of their child's illness and/or its treatment. Detection of deficit may evoke subtle to extreme reactions that cannot always be fully anticipated. By providing a balanced description of preserved and dysfunctional abilities, the neuropsychologist can help parents better comprehend the cognitive consequences and the diverse ways the problem might impact their child. Linking test behavior to academic performance may help in this regard, for example, "Your daughter had difficulty when tests required her to hold information in her mind in order to work simultaneously on something else. You recall that her teacher told you that her written work deteriorates when she has to listen to oral lectures. The neuropsychological evaluation results offer one possible explanation for why the teacher's observations may in fact be related to a true neuropsychological reason, and not to willful or defiant behavior, and what might need to be done to make it possible for your daughter to accomplish both tasks efficiently." Parents should be encouraged to relate actual anecdotal experiences that highlight their child's adaptation or reflect the disruption so that the neuropsychologist can then relate the test data to these real-world examples that are a focus of the parents' concern.

Encouraging Questions

The neuropsychologist should encourage interruptions and any questions that may arise during an interpretive session. This helps adjust the presentation level in direct response to the parents' comprehension level. Parents may feel that those health care professionals involved in their child's care too often restrict their time together, leading to a one-sided presentation that leaves them with questions remaining. If necessary, the length of an interpretive session should be extended to ensure comprehension of the important points resulting from the extensive evaluation. All present should be encouraged to participate, including a silent parent, as noted above. This will help confirm that there is parallel understanding of both results and recommendations, while providing the basis for further discussion between the parents later.

Parent interpretation of family dynamics before there is interpretation by the neuropsychologist may also be useful. This is accomplished, for example, when parents are asked to comment on what they see in their child's *kinetic family drawing*, of "a family doing something." For example, an 11-year-old boy, re-

ferred with a presumptive diagnosis of Attention Deficit Hyperactivity Disorder (ADHD) via teacher-reported inattentiveness at school, was asked to produce a kinetic family drawing as a screening measure. The child drew a detailed picture in which the parents were engaged in a vicious food fight. Fighter planes flew overhead and were dropping bombs. The patient was drawn in the center of the page holding an open umbrella over his head to protect himself, tears flowing down his cheeks. The emotional impact of the drawing, while clear, did not provide sufficient information for an outsider to understand its full significance.

In the interpretive session, both parents were shown the drawing without any interpretive conclusions and were asked to help me explain its meaning. The parents looked at each other, discomfited, and his mother said, "We are getting a divorce, but we didn't think he knew." In another example, the family drawing showed the mother in the kitchen, the child sleeping, and the father coming home from work through the front door. In this case, the child explained, "My dad always comes home late." In the interpretive session, the father quickly recognized the message conveyed by his child and acknowledged he was spending so much time at work that he had little time with his family and had neglected his child. He just did not realize how seriously his actions were affecting his child.

In yet another instance in which the father was perceived as away from home too often, the child omitted him entirely from the family drawing. This led to an interesting discussion in the interpretive session when the significance of his absence in the picture was explained and the father recognized what his son was communicating.

Parents may feel inadequate in their ability to explain test results to their child and may raise questions about how best to discuss such sensitive information with him or her. The interpretive session is a time to help guide parents about appropriate terminology and provide examples that are likely to be easily understood. Parents should be encouraged to explain results to their child in a way that is appropriate for the child's developmental or maturational level and that will serve to open the communication channel between parent and child that is so important at every developmental stage.

Interpreting to the Child

In some instances, interpretation to the child is beneficial. While not always possible due to age, logistical issues, or medical constraints, direct interpretation may be useful when the child is available, capable of communicating well, and when parent approval is obtained. Some children and adolescents favor direct feedback, while others may reject the evaluation process and its final interpretive session. When an interpretive session does proceed with the child, it is useful to recognize that the child's concerns and questions may be vastly different than those of their parents.

A session held with the child, with the child and parents together, or with the parents first and then the child brought in has several advantages. For example, the child can ask questions of an objective third person and hear answers to their own questions rather than those of interest to and raised by the parent. Also, the information is not secondarily translated by a parent, and it, therefore, may be more direct and complete. It provides an opportunity to correct some of the child's misperceptions and confirm their accurate impressions, while stressing those positive aspects that will support a strong self-image.

Consultation with the parent about inclusion or exclusion in interpretation may result in a determination that the child be excluded for any of a number of personal or situational reasons. The parent or neuropsychologist may suspect that the child's inclusion will be deleterious due to the discussion of medical or psychological matters that are best reserved for a time when the child is better able to integrate such information. It may be anticipated that the issues to be discussed with the parents will be sufficiently serious and too threatening for a child or that the child's emotional immaturity or intellectual deficiency will limit the usefulness of such a session. The child's resistance to evaluation may be extreme, and there may be refusal to return for the discussion. An addi-

tional visit may conflict with academic responsibilities. In such instances, the neuropsychologist can encourage the parents to allow the child future contact with the neuropsychologist. It is also possible to send a separate letter, appropriate for the child's developmental level, to the child that summarizes the results and reinforces the cooperation given for such an intensive test session.

Summary

The interpretive session is a crucial moment for providing a coherent and integrated profile of the child's cognitive and behavioral function. The session is an important time when disparate data can be integrated and translated into practical considerations and the parents can be better educated about their child and their advocacy role in supporting their child. It can be an emotionally intense time, as the information is sometimes quite serious or unexpected, but it is also an opportunity to help the parent assess the child's full range of abilities and support systems and plan productively for the necessary next steps.

THE WRITTEN REPORT

The written report combines all relevant observations into a succinct clinical analysis and interpretation of the child's neuropsychological functioning. The written report's form is influenced by the clinician's training, the target reader(s), and the purpose of the evaluation (Baron, Fennell et al., 1995), and these are subject to modification by the individual practitioner. The report is also influenced by the practice setting (Donders 2001a; Donders 2001b). Despite varying report preferences, there are certain commonalities in report preparation. Survey data suggests that most neuropsychologists will routinely include the referral source and reason for referral, a summary of the individual's clinical description obtained personally and through records, a list of tests administered, and a qualification of performance in descriptive terms (Donders 2001b), as often recommended (Axelrod, 2000).

The parents of a child seen in the outpatient setting may forget essential information once the interpretive session is concluded. The written report will serve as their tangible reminder and as an explicit explanation of the interpretive session discussion. It summarizes the test results and conclusions jointly reached by the neuropsychologist and the parents, including recommendations. It also specifies for the reader how the child may demonstrate deficit in real-world situations and describes in what ways the child can be expected to succeed or excel. As noted earlier, a child's strengths often receive less conference time than do the child's weaknesses. Parents naturally focus on deficits, wanting to understand them better as they seek advice about opportunities for remediation. The written report allows for an elaboration on the observed strengths, as well as for a clear restatement of the documented deficits.

My preference is to complete the written report after the interpretive session. This has the advantage of providing the lay reader—parents—with explanations that will enable a more sophisticated reading than if the report is prepared and provided without an opportunity for discussion and clarification. This order is also advantageous because final conclusions and recommendations may often be amended once the interpretive session is held and new information revealed. Of course, in some settings, the communication of results may need to be more immediate. This is likely when the child is hospitalized or in a rehabilitation facility. In such cases, the neuropsychologist is obligated to respond to the referral questions rapidly and without such additional communication, perhaps noting the initial summation as a preliminary impression in anticipation that a parent meeting will occur.

Since individuals with disparate perspectives about the child will likely read the report, one must consider how data is communicated for these diverse readers. While report style may vary for the intended reader, often a single written report is the only data summary of the child's evaluation, and it is intended for readers of varying technical sophistication. The language and terms selected need to be chosen with care since specialists in one discipline may find the terminology of another discipline puz-

zling or obscure, and since parents are often unprepared to understand a confusing, wordy, or insufficiently detailed report that is not written simply. Since consultation is often requested when a deficit is suspected but not confirmed and after other contributory consultations, it is also the responsibility of the neuropsychologist to integrate the range of previous data with those newly acquired into a reader-friendly report that parallels the communication that takes place in the interpretive session.

Report variables that may be directly affected by the intended readership include report length, lexicon, impressions of neurological course, and specificity of recommendations. Besides considering the inpatient or outpatient evaluation, the neuropsychologist may alter his or her report style, depending on whether the report is prepared for a treating specialist (e.g., neurosurgeon, neurologist), family pediatrician, parent, teacher, therapist, or attorney. Personal preference also affects inclusion of some features that others may exclude, for example, a list of tests administered, normative data citations, or an appendix of raw data.

Differing views on whether to append raw data are discussed in the literature along with ethical considerations (Matarazzo, 1995; Naugle and McSweeny, 1995), and this remains a controversial decision decided by the individual practitioner. The choice about whether the report should be divided into domain sections or written as a text letter without such division is also a personal choice. The report length, extent of history reiterated, inclusion of psychometric data, and preference for itemized or narrative recommendations also varies considerably.

Personal preference, combined with feedback from readers, often leads to the best report writing template for one's population. For example, in response to frequent physician based referrals, I often make a distinction in the test summary between neurological implications and neuropsychological implications. I may not make this distinction within the report for school or parent-based referrals that are unlikely to be read by a treating physician.

Neurological Implications is a section that is intended for the more medically sophisticated reader and, depending on the results, may relate test data to a specific incident, hypothesize brain regions implicated by poor performances, and highlight functional integrity. Medical terminology and assumptions about neuroanatomical correlation may be included in this paragraph, bridging other medical record sources when possible. Description of residual deficit, progressive disorder, and late effects is appropriate, along with discussion of likely permanence or transience of findings. This section is discussed with the parents as well, along with the qualification that some terminology may be included for the physician or other health professional that relates more to behavioral neurology.

The *Neuropsychological Implications* section captures the focus of the interpretive session and highlights all main points, translates the test results into functional behavior for all readers, links the objective measurement tests to real-life behavior, and includes specific recommendations developed as a result of the overall evaluation. It provides the opportunity to elaborate the recommendations into useful and practical steps in the child's best interest. Parents are advised to refer to this paragraph whenever they wish to review a summary. I include the following information in this section of the written report summary:

1. Evidence of abilities that reflect neurocognitive strength
2. Evidence of abnormal or delayed neuropsychological function
3. Functional brain systems implicated as impaired
4. A summary impression about whether, overall, the data correlate with normal range or abnormal brain function
5. Suggestions about how specific strengths can be used to strengthen any observed cognitive deficit
6. Options for therapeutic intervention or behavioral management

If parent permission is granted for report distribution, one must assume that the report may remain a part of the child's permanent medical and psychological records. It will influence current decisions affecting the child and potentially could be relied on again in the future. For ex-

ample, a hard-copy record is needed should there be a need for future reevaluation to assess interval change in response to an immediate treatment, when monitoring the success of a longer-term intervention program, and when tracking developmental progress and rate of maturation. The neuropsychologist needs to consider the report format and which data to include to ensure that valid comparisons will be accomplished should the child be seen by another neuropsychologist at some future time. Thus, report conclusions must be well-founded and clearly explicated. A poorly prepared report can lead to erroneous decision making and improper care, with an impact reaching across the years.

It may be desirable to follow up on one's recommendations, monitoring the success of an intervention program, recommending modifications of strategies that prove ineffective, and tracking progress and rate of maturation. This paragraph thus serves another reader as well, the neuropsychologist reading the report sometime in the future. Also, while a single-report format is often an efficient means of communicating neuropsychological conclusions and recommendations, an individual report for a single reader may also be appropriate at times. For example, a separate letter to the adolescent may simplify the results presented in greater detail to parents and highlight how these data relate to the individual's personal experiences, or a letter to the teacher can highlight the essential relationships between the child's test results and academic requirements.

Test Scores

Each neuropsychologist makes a determination about which and how many test scores are included in the written report. While in the past, raw scores were sometimes used for cutoff score determination of normal or abnormal function (Russell, Neuringer et al., 1970), such use is now uncommon and generally not recommended. Currently, protocol is to present the data as deviation IQs, standard scores, and percentiles. Descriptive labels about range are often used as well in addition. The size of the normative sample will affect such conversions.

A large normative data set lends itself to calculation of one or more of a number of standard scores, that is, the raw data are converted into standard measurement units for the performance of a standardization sample where there is an assumption of data that are normally distributed in the population. Thus, these data are commonly transformed into standard scores for comparability, such as a T score with a mean of 50 and standard deviation (SD) of 10 or z-score with a mean of 0 and a SD of 1.

The Wechsler series IQ scores are deviation IQs with a mean of 100 and SD of 15, not standard scores, and the subtest scaled scores have a mean of 10 and SD of 3. It should be noted that not all tests that use deviation IQs also use a SD of 15. Some tests scale the SD a few points lower or higher than 15, making interpretation of differences from the mean between these tests not directly comparable. As mentioned, scores can be converted into a nonstandard score such as a percentile. So, the neuropsychologist can present data in a variety of formats, for example, a T score of 44 falls within the average range, converts into a z-score of −0.6, and falls at the 27th percentile.

When a test is accompanied by a manual, there generally are tables for appropriate determination of performance using these standard units. By adding or subtracting the SD from the obtained score and comparing to the normative data one can determine how far above or below the mean the child's test result falls. Differences more than two standard deviations below the mean are especially notable. A score more than three standard deviations from the mean is particularly significant, at either end of the distribution. When a test is an individual performance measure unaccompanied by a manual, we have had to rely on the normative data published in journals, chapters, or left unpublished. Sometimes these tests provide data on both normal control subjects and clinical samples. Often, the number of subjects is small, and standard scores cannot be computed.

Mention of test scores requires noting the importance of knowledge about a test's sensitivity, specificity, positive predictive power, negative predictive power, and base rates. *Sensitivity* refers to the true positive rate and is calculated by the formula: true positive/true positive + false negative. It results in a figure for those correctly classified as impaired. *Specificity* refers to the true negative rate and is calculated by the formula: true negative/ true negative + false positive. It results in a figure for those correctly classified as unimpaired. *Positive Predictive Power* refers to the proportion of cases predicted by the model to be in the target group that were in the target group. It is calculated by the formula: true positive/ true positive + false positive. *Negative Predictive Power* is calculated by the formula: true negative/true negative + false negative. It refers to the proportion of cases predicted by the model to be in the non-target group that were in that group, or the probability that normal test performance indicates normal brain function.

With respect to IQ prediction formulas, for example, good positive predictive power suggests that a significant discrepancy from predicted IQ is probably meaningful. Poor negative predictive power suggests that a failure to find a significant discrepancy from predicted IQ is not necessarily informative. *Base rates* refer to essential information about the frequency with which a condition occurs, and knowledge of the base rate enables a practitioner to make a better judgment about the influence of a test finding for that specific individual (Chelune, Naugle et al., 1993).

Scores are ideally interpreted based on demographic information in addition to the obtained raw score. Age, gender, and education corrections, as appropriate, and as available for the individual instrument, provide a better context for evaluating the significance of an individual's performance. While the significance of an outlier score, or score profile, may be better appreciated when such conversions are possible, clinical interpretation also depends on the neuropsychologist's ability to substitute clinical judgment for a strict statistical interpretation. This is particularly true when it is recognized that there is an inadequate normative data set.

Scores are directly comparable within one test battery, or for a test composed of subtests, when the test was standardized on the same population sample. However, standard scores or percentiles are not directly comparable when they are derived from different tests, and these are obtained from different populations. For example, it is incorrect to compare a score that falls at the 92nd percentile with another score that falls at the 20th percentile and conclude that the difference between superior and low average function is significant. The assumption that all standard scores are directly comparable is inaccurate. Databases are based on samples having different demographic characteristics. Therefore, the uniformity desired may not be achieved (Axelrod and Goldman, 1996). Such statistical weaknesses may make clinical interpretation that much more complex, but not necessarily any less valid.

Not all relevant clinical data can be converted into standardized scores or into other designated statistical descriptors. Language screening tests provide a good example of when a specific error, or error pattern, may be sufficiently notable in the consideration of presence or absence of dysfunction, e.g., an aphasia. Certainly, pathognomonic errors require corroboration with other behavioral samples to determine their clinical significance. What is concluded with a clinical neuropsychological evaluation ultimately will depend on the neuropsychologist's interpretation of the individual child's performance in consideration of all relevant factors, not only on a comparison of that child to an existent normative standardization sample. Also, experimental techniques may be applied in the clinical setting although normative data are not available. Their cautious interpretation will also be based on factors other than those called upon with well-standardized tests, along with qualitative behavioral observations and error type and pattern analysis.

Is Average Really Average?

The clinical interpretation of test scores is the extended summary of all that was compiled and learned about the child. In this context, it is not the testing per se that ultimately matters, but the *evaluation* that is crucial. An overreliance on a test score or descriptive range may be risky and lead to erroneous conclusions. It is therefore important to consider the diverse interpretations that may result and to recognize, for example, that "average performance" is a generally meaningless description for either a single test score or a performance summary. A

child's average test score might, in actuality, represent a performance that is impaired, indicative of recovery, or reflects improvement, or it may actually be average and compatible with expectations for a child of the same chronological age. Thus, a child with a scaled score between 8 and 12 on the WISC-III, which descriptively falls within the average range, may in fact represent a significant decline from a higher range for a very bright child with a history of neurological insult. The same score may represent the recovery consequent to elapsed time since an injury or after a treatment regimen for another child, "average" thus being a positive gain from some prior lower functioning level. Similarly, for yet another child who might have previously scored below average, the score may represent the improvement resulting from an applied academic intervention, psychotherapeutic intervention, or medication trial. And finally, an average score may reflect accurately how that child generally functions on the specific subtest compared to age peers, neither below or above expectation for that specific test result.

Writing for the School

A well-written report aids in bridging the gap between teacher and parent. It is intended that the written report will help parents initiate an informed dialogue with school personnel about their child's cognitive status. I strongly encourage parents to make an appointment to take the report directly to the school for a parent-teacher conference, rather than having me mail it to the school directly. More personalized attention to the child's specific situation may result from a direct meeting, and the parents are better able to answer a teacher's questions, given what they learned at the interpretive session. Thus, they are better prepared to serve as the child's advocates.

Neuropsychological report conclusions are incomplete if they do not address recommendations for academic performance. An evaluation-based explanation for a child's problematic academic performances, hopefully, will enlighten a teacher about the child's real competencies and offer valid explanatory reasons that provide the teacher with a new perspective. The common situation in which a teacher has told a child, "You could do better if you just tried harder," when that child has already put considerable effort into a task and failed, remains a perception that must be balanced by discrimination of real strengths and weaknesses. That a child's efforts may not be rewarded by successful performance is too often underappreciated. Such teacher requests for greater effort only increase the child's emotional distress and a setting conducive to full effort is limited.

The written explanation of why a child may not be succeeding, along with the parent conference, may help the teacher make a better determination of how to teach the child. The report will provide valuable objective data justifying the need for special help, whether it be minimal assistance easily incorporated into a regular class setting or more intensive self-contained special educational services. The report should be a stimulus for the school system to provide appropriate modifications consistent with those mandated by federal law (Baron, 2002). A more positive interactive relationship is expected to develop between parent and teacher, once there are concrete data that explain, in large part, the child's true abilities.

The neuropsychologist, with the parents' written permission, can directly discuss the findings with school personnel. In some cases, a report may not seem to address a teacher's particular concerns or may receive less attention than it deserves because the teacher perceives it as too complex and overwhelming. In such an instance, a supplemental letter to the school may be useful. Parents should also discuss the link between documented test performances and observed academic performances directly with the school, using the written report as their resource. The child's learning style is expected to be better understood as a consequence of these steps. Caution against pressing a child in areas of identified weakness. Suggestions for compensatory actions that draw on the child's strengths may be better integrated as a result of more open communication.

Establishing and maintaining open channels of communication with the school may also be necessary to monitor the success of medical (e.g., drug) or psychological (e.g., behavioral

modification) interventions, placement changes or deferments, alternate courses, remedial learning techniques, or tutorial or other resource services. School recommendations are most helpful if specific, realistic, and novel. Repeating past recommendations that have been already tried and have proven unsuccessful does not serve the child well. School interventions that have been beneficial should continue to be supported.

A personal letter, written at the child's level of comprehension, that summarizes test results in simple language and highlights good capabilities can be mailed directly to the child or adolescent with parent approval. The letter can address the child's own concerns, which may differ from those stated by the parents. For example, a child may fear having a "bad brain," and a letter can address such concerns and offer him or her a better explanation. A personal letter may also remind the child of the need to take personal responsibility for overcoming cognitive obstacles. It may provide a way to reinforce messages that will also be conveyed from the parents and teachers, lending credence to interpretations made by the parents that the child might not otherwise fully believe. A child may also need encouragement to let teachers know more often when schoolwork becomes too difficult, when it is hard to follow along in class, or when the pressure of working within constricted time limits becomes overwhelming. Such a letter should also be an opportunity to thank the child for working so hard under such atypical circumstances.

Inpatient Notes

Before writing a note into the medical chart or preparing a full report, it is very helpful to read the existing medical chart carefully to review the impressions of other personnel in contact with the child. Nursing notes can often contain valuable documentation of behavioral observations about the inpatient. Such notes may offer clues to relevant diagnostic considerations, including observations whose neuropsychological significance may be missed by the nonpsychologist staff. For example, notes about "immature speech" or "refusal to talk" in a head-injured adolescent may be the unrecognized signs of the presence of aphasia. These data may also provide an opportunity to highlight the neuropsychological significance of a patient's behavior and to educate the staff further about the significance of complete neuropsychological data.

An inpatient note in the progress section of a child's medical record may precede the formal written report, or it may be the only report of the neuropsychologist's contact with the child. Staff may improve their attention to the child's specific situation if the range of capabilities that are preserved or compromised are better appreciated. The neuropsychologist may suggest practical guidelines for nursing personnel and others involved in the moment-to-moment care of a child. For example, suggestions about how to interact may be made for a child with receptive language problems. Such a child may need to have directions presented in brief but concrete phrases. An emotionally distressed child may not integrate well any information about what procedure he is being prepared for until calmed and instructed age appropriately.

A hemifield visual impairment may also go undetected. Once recognized, suggestions may be made that staff present themselves and visual material on the side of space to which the child is more attentive, that they encourage the child to monitor the full visual range, and that they use verbal and visual prompts to ensure full scanning to the neglected side of space, for instance, a colorful margin or bright stickers to which the child must refer when reading. The neuropsychologist may suggest positioning the child so that the busy hall or TV is not placed on the neglected side.

A Sample Report Format

As noted above, there is no definitive model for the written report. What follows is an example of my own practices with respect to report writing. This is not offered as a strict guideline but merely as an example of how I have resolved the issues related to report writing for multiple readers when a child is evaluated in the outpatient setting. Considering the preceding recommendations, however, a general format is outlined below. The reader is referred to Appendix 3–A for an example of a report about a young boy referred for presumptive ADHD.

Sample Outline

Neuropsychological Evaluation
Identifying Information
  Name
  Date of birth
  Date of testing
  Date of interpretation
  Chronological age
Reason for Referral
  Referral source
  Diagnosis (confirmed or presumptive)
  Specific clinical complaints that necessitated this referral
Relevant History
  Birth and developmental history
  Family and social history
  Personal medical history
  Educational background and current placement
  Previous psychological and psychiatric history
  Previous psychological or neuropsychological evaluations
  Other past interventions
Tests Administered
  Include test names, either by category of function and/or an itemized listing
Test Behavior and Results
  Behavioral Observations
    Orientation and Attention
    Mood and Affect
    Physical features and observed clinical behaviors (summarized succinctly with specific examples of particularly useful clinical observations included)
    Response to examiner's attempts to impose structure
    Ability to work for duration of the test session(s)
    Responses to reinforcement strategies employed
    Circumstances that were sources of particular stress
    Error patterns that may be significant
    Examiner's judgment about whether the testing was reliable and valid
  Test results (by domain):
    General Intelligence
    Academic Achievement
    Executive Functioning
    Attention/Concentration/Orientation
    Receptive and Expressive Language
    Sensory-Perceptual Examination
    Motor Examination
    Visuomotor Integration and Visuoperceptive Skill

Learning and Memory

Behavior and Emotional Integrity (such as personality inventories, mood questionnaires, projective drawings, and behavior rating scales)

Test Summary

General summary statement of patient's reason for referral

Overall conclusions about neuropsychological integrity

Neurological Implications

Written primarily for medical staff

Summary statement of test results

Applicable statements regarding:

Behavioral correlation with reason for referral

Behavioral correlation with other neurodiagnostic techniques

Likely etiology and differential diagnosis

Acuteness or Chronicity (whether a longstanding or a recent problem)

Diffuse or focal pattern

Stable or progressive profile (? needing follow-up)

Neuropsychological Implications

Written for all, but medical terminology limited

Intended to summarize findings at a less technical level

Practical implications of the results

Any implications for the child's future behavior

Applicable statements about learning or learning disability

Appliable statements about behavioral/emotional integrity

Needed modifications due to compromised cerebral functioning

Specific recommendations for the parents

Specific recommendations for the school

Summary of the child's strengths

CONCLUSION

A major focus of the neuropsychological process is to make meaningful recommendations that will positively affect the child's outcome. This is accomplished by collecting serial data to monitor the course of a medical therapy, evaluating changes consequent to a specific remediation, and making suitable recommendations for the inpatient stay, school placement, and academic interventions. These must be considered in light of documented neuropsychological strengths and weaknesses. The writ-

ten report is a central vehicle for communicating knowledge gained about a child in the evaluative process. It should be thorough and specific in delineating practical steps to follow for treatment purposes. Every clinician needs to determine the format that will be most useful in their practice and for their professional and lay readers. The report needs to include sufficient information so that another clinician can accurately assess any interval change in the event of a future reevaluation.

REFERENCES

Axelrod, B. N. (2000). Neuropsychological report writing. In R. D. Vanderploeg (Ed.), *Clinician's guide to neuropsychological assessment,* (2nd ed.) (pp. 245–273). Mahwah, NJ: Erlbaum.

Axelrod, B. N., & Goldman, R. S. (1996). Use of demographic corrections in neuropsychological interpretation: How standard are standard scores? *The Clinical Neuropsychologist, 10,* 159–162.

Baron, I. S. (2002). Learning disabilities. In B. L. Maria (Ed.), *Current Management in Child Neurology* (2nd ed.). (pp. 220–226). Hamilton, Ontario: Decker Periodicals.

Baron, I. S., Fennell, E. B., & Voeller, K. K. S. (1995). *Pediatric Neuropsychology in the Medical Setting.* New York: Oxford University Press.

Chelune, G. J., Naugle, R. I., L,ders, H. O., Sedlak, J., & Awad, I. A. (1993). Individual change after epilepsy surgery: Practice effects and base-rate information. *Neuropsychology, 7,* 41–52.

Donders, J. (2001a). A survey of report writing by neuropsychologists, I: General characteristics and content. *The Clinical Neuropsychologist, 15,* 137–149.

Donders, J. (2001b). A survey of report writing by neuropsychologists, II: Test data, report format, and document length. *The Clinical Neuropsychologist, 15,* 150–161.

Matarazzo, R. G. (1995). Psychological report standards in neuropsychology. *The Clinical Neuropsychologist, 9,* 249–250.

Naugle, R. I., & McSweeny, A. J. (1995). On the practice of routinely appending raw data to reports. *The Clinical Neuropsychologist, 9,* 245–247.

Russell, E. W., Neuringer, C., & Goldstein, G. (1970). *Assessment of brain damage.* New York: John Wiley & Sons.

Wing, L. (1985). *Autistic Disorders Checklist in Children.* Unpublished manuscript.

APPENDIX 3–A

IDA SUE BARON, PH.D., P.C.
NEUROPSYCHOLOGY CONSULTING

NEUROPSYCHOLOGICAL EVALUATION

NAME: B. B.
DOB: 00/00/0000
DATE OF TESTING: 00/00/0000
DATE OF INTERPRETATION: 00/00/0000
CHRONOLOGICAL AGE: 7 years 10 months
REASON FOR REFERRAL:

Neuropsychological evaluation of B. B. was requested to obtain detailed information about B. B.'s neurocognitive functioning. History was taken by interview with his parents and by questionnaire and will only be briefly summarized here. Full details are available under separate cover.

B. B. was born by Cesarean delivery due to failure to progress after a full term uncomplicated pregnancy. He weighed 7 lbs. No perinatal or neonatal complications were reported. Gross motor and language developmental milestones were achieved at age appropriate times. Social development was also normal, and B. B.'s relationships with peers and adults remain good. His hearing and vision were checked formally and are unimpaired. No medical problems were reported.

There is a strong family history of learning problems, with his mother, an older half-sister, and a maternal uncle all reported to have mild learning difficulty. Attentional problems were reported for his mother. There is no other contributory family history. His father earned a Ph.D., and his mother has a bachelor's degree. B. B. is in second grade. He is in a regular class, but experiences difficulty with reading, spelling, arithmetic, and writing. Developmental delays were observed as early as Kindergarten. Only recently did attention and concentration difficulties emerge.

TESTS ADMINISTERED

Neuropsychological evaluation was administered to assess the integrity of cerebral functions in the following broad areas: general intelligence, executive function, learning and memory, receptive and expressive language, lateral dominance and motor function, visual-motor integration and visuoperceptive skill, attention and concentration, and behavior.

Automatic Language Sequences and Mental Control Testing

Wechsler Intelligence Scale for Children-III

Wechsler Individual Achievement Test

Auditory Analysis Test

Boston Diagnostic Aphasia Examination Paragraph Production

Verbal Selective Reminding Test

Wide Range Assessment of Memory and Learning-Logical Memory

Trail Making Test-Delis-Kaplan Executive Function System

Draw-A-Clock Test

Beery Developmental Test of Visual Motor Integration

Draw-A-Person; Draw-A-Family

Luria Motor Evaluation

Apraxia Testing

Lateral Dominance Examination

Tapping Test

Grooved Pegboard Test

Cancellation of Targets Test

Test of Everyday Attention for Children

Behavior Rating Inventory of Executive Function

TEST BEHAVIOR AND RESULTS

B. B. was a handsome, well-dressed, right-handed boy, who appeared quite comfortable with the testing session. He engaged easily in lively conversation, and his spontaneous speech was entirely fluent and overtly intact. Subtle language errors are described below. There were no obvious gross or fine motor abnormalities. He demonstrated a good sense of humor, was very personable, and interacted well with the examiner throughout the lengthy test session.

A number of specific behaviors were observed during the evaluation that may have direct implications for his classroom behavior. These included his repeated attempts to see the examiner's answer sheets. He also made other attempts to take actions that would assist him when he was concerned he might not answer a question correctly. He had a slightly defiant attitude that was notable in his resistance to requests that he follow the instructions requested by the examiner. Also, on more than one occasion, he insisted that he had given a response that he had not actually given. He repeatedly said, "I said that!" hoping the examiner would believe him and score him higher. His concern about his performance was in itself considered a good quality, and he was sufficiently concerned to take the time to try to improve his performance when he judged his performance as weak. For example, he erased initial responses and successfully improved the quality of his response on more than one occasion.

Of great interest, given these observations, was the content of a letter mailed by one of his teachers following the test session. She wrote, "The inventory (referring to a questionnaire sent to her) did not cover one of B. B.'s biggest issues. B. B. goes to great lengths to avoid doing work that he does not feel successful with. B. B. can be very sneaky in his attempt to get out of work. B. B. is a very smart young man who does deal with some learning disabilities that make writing and reading difficult for him. But I am concerned at the length to which he will go to avoid work that he doesn't want to do. He is very young for the amount of avoidance behaviors he employs."

General Intelligence

The *Wechsler Intelligence Scale for Children-III* (WISC-III) was administered. B. B. obtained the following summary IQ scores, and associated percentiles, Confidence Intervals and descriptive ranges:

	IQ	C.I.	Percentile	Range
Verbal Scale =	107	(100–113)	68th	average
Performance Scale =	102	(94–110)	55th	average
Full Scale	105	(99–110)	63rd	average

B. B. obtained the following subtest scaled scores: (scaled scores range from 1 to 19; 8 to 12 = average).

Information =	14	Picture Completion =	11
Similarities =	12	Coding =	9
Arithmetic =	8	Picture Arrangement =	9
Vocabulary =	10	Block Design =	12
Digit Span =	8	(Symbol Search =	16)

The following additional Index scores were also calculated:

Verbal Comprehension	111	high average	77th percentile
Freedom from Distractibility	90	average	25th percentile
Processing Speed	114	high average	82nd percentile

Significant intrascale subtest scaled score scatter was noted within both the Verbal and Performance scales, but no subtest scaled score fell below the average range. Subtest scaled scores ranged as high as the very superior limits but the variability is important to note. To some extent, he demonstrated a pattern most closely associated with that found for children with documented attentional disorder. These individual subtest scaled scores are discussed below within the appropriate cognitive domains.

Academic Achievement

The Wechsler Individual Achievement Test was administered as a screening for basic academic achievement. B. B. earned the following standard scores, percentiles, and ranges:

Basic Reading	94	34th percentile	average
Mathematics Reasoning	111	77th percentile	high average
Spelling	98	45th percentile	average
Reading Comprehension	98	45th percentile	average
Listening Comprehension	138	99th percentile	very superior

As for the IQ test, his scores were at least within average limits, and they ranged as high as the very superior range. His reading and spelling academic achievement appeared either generally in line with prediction or slightly below expectation given his WISC-III summary IQ scores. However, there was clear elevation for mathematics reasoning and exceptionally elevated performance on a measure of his ability to comprehend what was read to him. The latter high score raises additional concern about the merely average performance on basic reading, spelling, and reading comprehension. He initially misunderstood the request on the first item of the basic reading section, when required to identify the picture that had the same beginning sound as the word spoken by the examiner. He incorrectly replied with the word having the same ending sound. With questioning he could correct this error. He also erred when he had to find the picture of the word with the same ending sound. These errors are of particular interest given the results of the Auditory Analysis Test noted below, and with clinical observation of other verbal errors. His earliest error type on the reading comprehension subtest was an inability to draw correct conclusions.

Executive Functioning

The Delis-Kaplan Executive Function System (D-KEFS) *Trail Making Test* was administered. This version includes a series of timed paper and pencil subtests. His time to completion on the first trial, when he had to scan an array for a target stimulus, fell within high average limits. On the next trial he had to draw a line in sequence between only numbers and his score also fell within high average limits. His ability to sequence only letters on the next trial fell within the superior range. On the difficult fourth trial, requiring number-letter switching, his performance fell only at the low end of the average range for his age. This performance represented a specific weakness. His time to completion on the fifth trial fell within the high average range, when he merely had to demonstrate his motor speed. Thus, these results attested to particular difficulty switching mental set between two automatic language sequences.

Abstract verbal reasoning, as assessed with the *WISC-III Similarities* subtest, found B. B. earning a subtest scaled score that fell at the upper end of the average range.

Questionnaires were given to his parents and teacher to obtain their impressions of B. B.'s behavior at home and at school, respectively. Parent report on the *Behavior Rating Inventory of Executive Function* indicated only one area of particular concern, i.e., organization of materials. Teacher report indicated no area of clinical concern and all subdomains fell within one standard deviation of the mean, although his ability to plan and organize and initiate action were relatively elevated. However, while the teacher did not find this questionnaire capturing the behaviors she was concerned about, her letter summarized above described some of her important observations of B. B. in the classroom setting.

Receptive and Expressive Language

B. B.'s spontaneous speech was fluent and articulate, and prosody and comprehension were intact. He demonstrated quite a good vocabulary during spontaneous speech. There were no clear paraphasic errors. *Automatic language sequences* were assessed; B. B. recited the alphabet and counted without error. He omitted May and October when reciting the months of the year. Expressive vocabulary was assessed with the *WISC-III Vocabulary* subtest, and his ability to orally define words fell within average limits.

The *Auditory Analysis Test* was administered, requiring B. B. to sort, order, and synthesize phonemic units. His score fell below the mean for a first grader, but within one standard deviation. He made early errors, such as removing the phoneme "car" from the word "carpet" and responding "bit." His difficulty perceiving some language units was also noted in his spontaneous conversation, by some comprehension errors for oral directions, and on academic achievement testing (as noted above).

Written formulation was assessed with a *Paragraph Production,* using the Boston Diagnostic Aphasia Examination Cookie Theft picture. His production was intact for linguistic aspects. His handwriting was enlarged. The paragraph was appropriate for content and he wrote complete, grammatically correct sentences. He had a tendency to overwrite in an attempt to improve on the form of the letters. Phonetic spelling errors were also noted, e.g., "duz" for "does."

Lateral Dominance and Motor Function

B. B., who is right handed, chose his right upper extremity for all unilateral motor actions, and there was no evidence of ideomotor dyspraxia. It was noted that he held his pencil awkwardly, with the middle finger over the pencil. He discriminated his right from left side correctly and made no errors when making extrapersonal discriminations. B. B. had adequate performance on tests of *rapid alternating movements,* screening tests of cerebellar integrity. B. B. did not yet perform *three-part sequenced motor actions* completely correctly.

B. B.'s right upper extremity performance on the *Finger Tapping Test* exceeded that of the left upper extremity on a measure of gross motor speed, as expected. His averaged tapping rate with each upper extremity fell within expected limits for his chronological age.

He also had better right than left upper extremity times-to-completion on a measure of motor dexterity, the *Grooved Pegboard Test.* Both upper extremities completed the task within expected time limits for his chronological age. There were no instances of peg dropping errors.

Visuomotor Integration and Visuoperceptive Skill

A variety of tests of nonverbal information processing and perceptual ability were administered, some but not all requiring paper and pencil production. B. B. inserted numbers in correct sequence and placement and set the hands correctly to the designated times on the *Draw-A-Clock* test, his performances appropriate for his chronological age on each portion. There was no evidence of conceptual or expressive difficulty.

B. B. was administered the *Beery Developmental Test of Visual-Motor Integration.* His design copying earned him a standard score of 108, which fell within average limits and was compatible with his summary IQ estimates. This score fell at the 70th percentile, and at a scaled score equivalent of 12.

His *WISC-III block design* construction subtest score fell at the upper end of the average range. His *WISC-III picture arrangement* subtest scaled score fell within average limits. These subtests assess visuoperceptual analysis and synthesis and visual sequencing of pictorial stimuli, respectively.

His *Draw-A-Person* was notable for the erasures and relative immaturity of the final production for his chronological age. The only facial features indicated were two filled-in dots for eyes, a single dot for a nose, and an upturned single line for the mouth. His *Draw-A-Family* was of only two figures that he would not identify. They were actively playing tennis.

Learning and Memory

B. B.'s fund of stored factual information was assessed in part with the *WISC-III Information* subtest. He earned a score that fell within high average limits, his highest Verbal subtest scaled score.

The *Verbal Selective Reminding Test* was administered. This test is a measure of verbal learning and memory for a novel lengthy word list. B. B. had an intact immediate recall on the first trial and he demonstrated adequate learning over the learning trials. His long term storage (LTS) score fell within expected limits for his chronological age as did his consistency of long term retrieval (CLTR) score. His delayed recall was also intact. Thus, there was no suggestion of impaired encoding, consolidation or storage. There was no evidence of rapid forgetting. A few intrusion errors were made, i.e., he recalled words that were not actually on the target list.

The *Wide Range Assessment of Memory and Learning Logical Memory* subtest was given. His immediate recall score fell within average limits for his chronological age. His savings score was average for his age. Thus, verbal learning of contextual novel information was intact, and decay of such meaningful verbal information over time was not observed.

Attention and Concentration

Clinically, B. B. appeared appropriately attentive throughout the testing session. However, he did not always remain seated, and in one instance he walked over to look out the window while continuing to respond to oral questions. There was repeated evidence that he could be easily distracted. He seemed entirely comfortable with the test session and, impressively, worked optimally for the duration of the testing. As noted above, his responses to mental control items such as stating the months of the year were unimpaired on a second attempt after an error on a first try.

The *Test of Everyday Attention for Children* (TEA-Ch) was administered and there was evidence of inconsistency in his performances. He experienced no difficulty maintaining his focus or selectively attending to a visual search task. He had high average performance scanning for repeated instances of a small target stimulus on a complex city map with many target foils. He had average performances when he had to engage in attentional control and shifting between two task requirements. However, when he had to sustain attention over time or engage in tests of divided attention his efficiency declined considerably. Some of his scores fell at the lowest possible scaled score and none fell above the low average range. Doing more than one thing at a time, persisting on a task over time when it is not inherently interesting, or engaging in competing dual tasks, reduced his efficiency from average or better limits to impaired limits. His confusion under competing circumstances was quite evident, and he stopped following directions on one dual task midway through the task, choosing to work on only one aspect rather than the two he had been working on.

Auditory attention for number sequences was assessed with the *WISC-III digit span* subtest. His score fell only at the lower end of average limits. He repeated 4 digits forward and 3 digits backward. He had similar relative weakness (low end of the average range performance) on the *WISC-III Arithmetic* subtest, which is also particularly sensitive to auditory attentional factors.

In marked contrast, his *WISC-III symbol search* subtest scaled score fell within very superior limits, and was his highest scaled score. His attention to essential visual detail, as measured by the *WISC-III picture completion* subtest, fell within average limits. The *WISC-III coding* subtest score also fell within average limits. This subtest measures the ability to code symbols in sequence and under timed circumstances, speed of information processing, psychomotor speed, and focused attention.

Nonverbal attention was also assessed with a paper and pencil *visual search cancellation test* requiring him to search for a target stimulus amid a competing visual array. B. B. had markedly poor performance. His ability to search for number or letter stimuli, or a target geometric stimulus, declined with each subsequent trial, suggesting his ability to sustain attention to an inherently non-interesting task is poor, even though it is of brief duration.

TEST SUMMARY

B. B. was a 7 years, 10-months-old right-handed, Caucasian boy in a regular second-grade class. B. B. was presumed to be a child of above average general intelligence, yet the current testing found that, despite a number of exceptionally good subtest performances, summary IQ estimates placed him consistently only within average limits. His Verbal Comprehension and Processing Speed factor scores were within high average limits. There were clear weaknesses evident on subtests especially dependent on attentional capacity, and his scores were sufficiently lowered on these subtests to diminish the potential suggested by his elevated performances on other subtests.

This degree of performance variability and his failure to reach above average or higher IQ estimates can be partially explanatory for academic problems in classrooms with a challenging academic curriculum. For example, the reading problems may, in part, be secondary to a developmental delay or a mild language learning disability but with some average capacities, he may find himself unable to successfully master the demands placed on him. Also, he likely experiences frustration with his academic work when many of his peers are instead ready for a more challenging academic curriculum, resulting in the less desirable behaviors observed during this evaluation and reported by his teacher.

Despite reports of school delay, some academic achievement scores obtained on this evaluation were consistent with his general intellectual level, falling within at least average limits for reading, spelling, and reading comprehension. However, these scores appeared low when compared to his other scores. His score for mathematics reasoning fell within high average limits, an area of apparent relative strength. He was also exceptionally capable on the listening comprehension subsection, obtaining an elevated score and demonstrating excellent performance when he had to integrate what he hears.

B. B. did exhibit weakness in phonological processing, a precursor skill for how well a child will read or master written language. Auditory analysis of speech sounds was below age level expectation, and such a finding is also highly correlated with reading delay. Specific tutorial assistance in mastering sound-symbol associations would appear helpful, and this might be best obtained through private channels. It was also noted that mental switching between two language sequences caused him great difficulty while performance on easier trials was unimpaired, and in fact elevated in most instances.

Strengths were apparent in a number of areas. Aside from some referral concerns about his ability to organize, many executive function subdomains were not perceived to be problematic by either his parents or teachers. His fund of stored factual information was elevated, and his ability to match symbols was exceptionally strong. He had intact motor function, and sensory screening was intact. Reading comprehension fell within average limits, despite concerns about his achievement in this area, and listening comprehension was excellent. Visuoperceptual and visuoconstructional skills were intact. Learning and memory for novel contextual verbal information and new unrelated verbal information were intact.

It does appear that he can convey information better through the oral channels rather than through written production. The following recommendations might therefore prove useful at school, and can be adjusted as he moves from grade to grade:

- extend time limits for examinations and written productions
- encourage one-word responses, true/false formats or multiple-choice responses, rather than lengthy essay-type questions
- encourage examination and essay production through dictation on an audiocassette recorder or to another individual
- record teacher's oral presentations for later replay to minimize the need for rapid or extensive written transcription during class time
- decrease demand for copying from the chalkboard
- increase provision of written handouts
- decrease emphasis on written production, e.g. by grading content separately from neatness and form of written production
- extend time limits or eliminate these constraints
- decrease repetitive writing
- increase use of a computer keyboard to replace laborious written formulation

The profile of highly variable attention is important to note. He was inconsistent on tests of the ability to selectively attend to and focus on information, sustain responding over a period of time, and shift between two competing mental tasks and therefore divide his attention. B. B. also has difficulty planning and organizing action, according to parent report. The family history of mild learning and attentional problems is likely highly relevant. Accommodations that are made for children with attentional disorder can be implemented. Among these are the following:

- Confirm B. B.'s understanding of verbal directions, e.g., by asking for repetition of what was stated, as was necessary during this evaluation.
- Have B. B. rehearse learning tasks or assignments and repeat when necessary.
- Help B. B. work more efficiently by reinforcing short, concentrated periods of activity and by progressively increasing the length of these periods.
- Use multimodal presentations that combine auditory/verbal, visual, tactile and/or kinesthetic cues.
- Give directions and instructions in a step-by-step fashion with clearly articulated verbal presentations and sufficient time for processing.
- Supplement lectures with written outlines, handouts, or text containing essential details of the curriculum or assignment.
- Seat B. B. within the classroom in a position that permits easy face-to-face interaction with the teacher and that limits distractions, e.g., a non-window seat, seating away from a distracting child, a study carrel.

A thorough baseline evaluation was accomplished should reevaluation be recommended. The results of this evaluation were communicated to his parents on 00/00/0000 and discussed in great detail along with recommendations for the academic and home environments. Behavioral methods that might prove especially useful were also discussed in detail. If I can answer any further questions, please do not hesitate to contact me at the above phone number.

Ida Sue Baron, Ph.D., ABPP
Board Certified in Clinical Neuropsychology
American Board of Professional Psychology

III

DOMAINS AND TESTS

4

Preliminary Assessment and Classification Scales

While shortened assessment associated with screening instruments or brief tests of specific capabilities is well accepted in psychology, the practice probably has greater demonstrated utility with respect to neuropsychological evaluation of adults than it currently does for children. Of course, there are those who suggest that any neuropsychological evaluation is merely a screening assessment, and to some extent they have a valid point, especially if one compares what we can confidently assess in our relatively brief time with a patient with what still remains perplexing and unknown. Such assessment has both advantages and disadvantages that are worth considering.

PRELIMINARY ASSESSMENT IN CHILD EVALUATION

Neuropsychologists play an important role in the identification of those children at risk for demonstrating future neuropsychological deficit, and in this respect, the notion of screening without an intent to diagnose is considered acceptable (Satz and Fletcher, 1988). Screening may commonly be requested for predicting outcome, although this is made exceptionally difficult in light of widely disparate individual factors and environmental influences and their interaction with developmental factors. Thus, the merit of short screening versus a more comprehensive evaluation that encompasses assessment of a wider range of

cognitive strengths and weaknesses should not be undervalued when used judiciously for reasonable reasons and in appropriate context. In most cases, a comprehensive child evaluation is desirable to better address current concerns. It also provides a database that will enable responsible future reevaluation that can address progression, retrogression, or stalling of the expected developmental trajectory.

Inpatient Screening Assessment

Weaknesses aside, screening does have limited and specific utility in some child evaluation situations. *Inpatient screening* is one circumstance under which screening is often acceptable. A plan for efficient inpatient screening is particularly useful when circumstances outside the examiner's control interfere with the usual control that would be possible for an outpatient evaluation. In the hospital or rehabilitation setting there are often imposed time limitations that shorten the length of time the child will be available for the type of interaction necessary for testing. Interruptions are likely to be frequent in these settings, and the examiner needs to have great flexibility in choosing and administering those tests that will have the greatest utility. Referral for a baseline evaluation to obtain those essential data that will enable current determinations of cognitive status and provide needed data for future comparisons also preempts delaying the evaluation until the child can be more fully evaluated.

Subject-related factors are also influential. The ill, injured, or emotionally distraught child may respond best to a few short tasks, either administered in sequence or dispersed across periods timed to their wellness status. The child's degree of incapacitation may prevent more than a superficial initial screening until they recover more fully.

Screening as a Substitute for Full Evaluation

Screening assessment in child neuropsychology is hotly debated when it is considered to be a *substitute* for a more lengthy and comprehensive evaluation. The substitution of a brief sampling of a range of behaviors for a more thorough investigation has the potential downside that a practitioner will miss highly relevant clinical information. This risk is especially the case when screening depends on only a single instrument sampling a restricted behavioral repertoire (Murphy, 2001). Screening is often considered inappropriate since in most cases the child's diagnosis is already known, and a referral is generated as a request for greater detail about neurocognitive functioning, thus making the referral a request for more, rather than less, information. Some would argue that only with a complete evaluation does a clinician conscientiously examine the extended range of strengths and weaknesses necessary to offer the most appropriate treatment recommendations and intervention strategies. Further, circumstances and qualitative behavioral observations during the actual test session often highlight additional functions a neuropsychologist might wish to explore further to better understand underlying cognitive structure. This exploration may not be possible if only a partial assessment is planned. In general, a screening evaluation is limiting and, therefore, ultimately inconclusive with respect to the full range of etiological factors that may explain the behaviors of concern.

Further complicating matters, there may be external pressures on the neuropsychologist that support considering and proceeding with a screening assessment. These pressures are often generated because of an economic issue or expressed as a preference by a referral source

to which the neuropsychologist is responsible. Such influences must be placed in proper perspective. The neuropsychologist's ethical obligations to the child need to be kept foremost in mind, along with appropriate concern for providing the high quality of service that the child deserves. Such external pressures may present themselves, for example, when a forensic examination is requested, and the referral source requests a screening of particular cognitive functions, although a more thorough evaluation may better address the child's functioning and lead to better identifying the child's full range of neurocognitive strengths and weaknesses. It is also inadvisable to adapt one's typical neuropsychological procedures to include a screening assessment in response to pressures from external oversight parties, such as third party payers, who seek to reduce billable clinical hours and lessen the expense of the more appropriate full evaluation.

Preliminary Screening: Means to an End

There are a number of reasonable reasons to conduct a screening *as a first step* toward a comprehensive and individualized evaluation, as long as one is not totally dependent on the screening instrument, or screening "battery," to the exclusion of relying on one's clinical skills to best evaluate the child. There are various possible screening test choices, and these are often determined by the presumptive diagnosis and reasons for referral. A highly specific test may not be the optimal choice when the intent is to cast a broad net. Therefore, some tests for which successful performance is based on diverse, multiply determined factors may be the most worthwhile screening instruments. A clinician may not know exactly which contributory aspect was impaired at the conclusion of the screening without further evaluation, but the identification of a poor performance yields valuable leads deserving greater attention once the range of variables are considered. These can be analyzed separately after the planned additional testing occurs.

My personal preference is to administer a preliminary screening evaluation at the beginning of a testing session. I consider this "screening-to-be-thorough" a reasonable approach since it does not substitute for a comprehensive evaluation. Thus, *screening* in this discussion refers to a preliminary exploration at the initial stages of a full test session rather than a substitution of a brief battery of tests for a comprehensive evaluation. For instance, while a shorter screening evaluation as the sole evaluation may seem appropriate, given a clearly stated reason for referral, a neuropsychologist must retain some degree of skepticism since there is always the possibility that the presumptive reason for referral that initiated the evaluation is incorrect or incomplete. A shorter preliminary screening directed toward the referral reason may be especially useful in identifying areas of concern and may lead to eventually including critically important data that would be omitted if there were not a more comprehensive follow-up evaluation.

Alternatively, a number of clinical tests can be combined for a productive preliminary screening as preparation for a comprehensive evaluation, when screening is not merely a substitute. The intent of such screening is to prepare to choose the best test instruments—those that will pertain specifically to the individual child—for the remaining testing time. This screening therefore takes place at the start of the testing session, and it must consider the age and capabilities of the child being examined. Such a formal psychometric screening is supplemented with parent questionnaires, rating scales, self-report inventories, a detailed history interview (see Chapter 2), and other information. The sections below provide examples of the approaches taken for a young child, older child, and adolescent.

Preliminary Screening: Exploration with a Young Child

The initial time with a young child is a special circumstance. This is when the examiners' very first actions are crucial to determining whether the child will relax sufficiently to engage actively in the full testing (see Chapter 2 for some suggestions for establishing optimal rapport). One may select nonthreatening screening measures from among the following examples for a young child, especially for one for whom there is limited initial information to direct the evaluation focus (see Table 4–1). Useful introductory tasks often include oral and written alphabet and number sequence production and writing one's name, as well as tests that sample drawing, receptive language, nonverbal reasoning, motor proficiency, attentional capacity, learning and memory, and emotional factors. These may be administered in the order that best suits the child's capabilities, interests, and level of cooperation. Together, they provide both quantitative and qualitative information

Table 4–1. Outline for Preliminary Screening of a Young Child

AUTOMATIC LANGUAGE	Alphabet Production—Oral & Written Number Production—Oral & Written Name Writing
VISUOCONSTUCTION	Beery-Buktenica Test of Visual-Motor Integration Greek cross copy Draw-A-Person; Draw-A-Family
LANGUAGE	Peabody Picture Vocabulary Test-III
REASONING	Raven's Coloured Progressive Matrices
MOTOR	Finger Tapping Test Grooved Pegboard Test
LEARNING & MEMORY	Selective Reminding Test Story Memory Sentence Memory
ATTENTION	Digit Span Block Span Visual Search Cancellation
PROJECTIVE SCREENING	Draw-A-Family Draw-A-Person

that bridge multiple domains, but for convenience, they are assigned here simply on their primary categorization.

Oral and written alphabet, number sequence production, name writing

Oral and written alphabet, number sequence production, and name writing aid in the assessment of the child's proficiency with automatic language sequences through both the oral and written modalities. Oral production provides initial impressions about facility with overlearned sequencing, articulation, voice volume, and prosody. (Some young children will prefer to sing the alphabet.) The examiner examines characteristics of the written formulation, such as size and spatial elements, degree of content elaboration and its sophistication, spelling, grammar, emotional content, the presence of overwriting, indications of erasures, and letter or number reversal or rotation. Handedness, the maturity of the pencil grasp, and any evidence of dyspraxia are also evaluated. Name writing is a useful adjunct measure of fine motor proficiency and overlearned skill.

Drawings

Drawing tests are among the most accepted initial test measures for a young child, as long as the child does not have a motor deficit. The limited emphasis on "talking" and the use of a modality that is much like play combine to make the request for a drawing easily accepted. Drawings provide estimates of visuomotor integration and constructional efficiency, and some can be adapted to serve as a screening for emotional contributions. A standardized test such as the Beery Buktenica Test of Visual Motor Integration (Beery, 1997) or a screening test item such as the Greek-cross copy from the Halstead-Wepman Aphasia Screening Test (Reitan, 1984) are useful. Informal drawings (of a "person" or a "family doing something") can be a stimulus for questioning about the content and relationships among figures. For all drawing tasks one must judge line quality, distortion errors, alignment errors, organization, and style with respect to the child's developmental level. An examiner needs to be alert for perseveration of elements, hemispace omission or distortion, and an inconsistent progression from simple to complex drawing. A distinction needs to be made between errors due to immaturity or delayed development and those that are likely consequent to known or suspected brain dysfunction.

Receptive language

Receptive vocabulary tests, such as the Peabody Picture Vocabulary Test-III (PPVT-III; Dunn and Dunn, 1997), provide information about the child's lexical knowledge and nonverbal comprehension. The PPVT-III can be interpreted as an estimate of verbal IQ that may later be compared with a standardized verbal IQ test result to detect evidence of any receptive, versus expressive, language inconsistency. The picture book presentation is generally quite acceptable to a young child. Importantly for an introductory task, the test provides no basis for the child to judge if his or her responses are right or wrong, thus enabling the examiner to offer unconditional praise for continued cooperation irrespective of the child's accuracy.

Nonverbal reasoning

A test such as the Raven's Coloured Progressive Matrices Test (RCPMT) (Raven, 1965; Raven, Court et al., 1993) is appealing to a young child because it incorporates color and form and demands no verbal response. The RCPMT has three parts that provide clinical information about attention to visual detail, pattern recognition, and nonverbal analysis as well as a summary total score that converts to a percentile ranking.

Motor efficiency

Tests such as the Finger Tapping Test and/or Grooved Pegboard Test provide valuable evidence of differential function between the right and left upper extremities and of the ability to sustain motor responding. These tests are inherently appealing to children without motor deficit. Also, young children are often intrigued by the required stopwatch, which can be used effectively to encourage continued participation on these and other tests.

Learning and memory

Tests of the ability to encode, consolidate, store and retain novel information are multiply determined tests that therefore provide a choice of alternative factors that may be responsible for either good or poor performance. The Verbal Selective Reminding Test is a well-tolerated measure of auditory/verbal learning and memory for unrelated words that requires a relatively brief administration time for the young child while providing numerous indices of function (see Chapter 11).

Attention

Tests requiring visual search cancellation test performance, nonverbal span (block span), and/or auditory number span repetition (digit span forward and digit span backward) provide preliminary indices of the child's capacity for focused or selective attention, working memory, and sustained attention for both the auditory/verbal and nonverbal conditions.

Projective screening for emotional issues

A number of simple tests are useful to begin the examination of the child's mood state and adjustment. For example, the kinetic Draw-A-Family and/or the Draw-A-Person tests elicit additional information beyond that assessed with visuomotor integration tests. Asking the child, "Tell me about the person you drew," or "Tell me what is happening in the family picture," and then also asking for additional detail, such as, "How do you think that makes the child feel?" "What do you think will happen?" and "What will happen next?" elicits a better sense of the child's self-image and perception of family dynamics. Asking for "three wishes" is also a very brief, but sometimes revealing, line of questioning.

The above young-child screening assessment will generally range from 60 to 100 minutes (A summary of selected child and adult tests and their mean approximate time for administration, scoring, interpretation, and reporting was recently published [Lundin and Philippis, 1999]). Together, these tests will screen the young child for attentional aspects, right–left cerebral efficiency, the child's internal dictionary of words, facility with automatic language sequences, visuoconstructional function, visuomotor integration, visuoperceptual and visuospatial ability, nonverbal reasoning capacity, novel verbal learning and memory, and emotional issues. These results should lead to a continued, more focused exploration of cognitive function and provide direction for a rationale of test selection that will balance identifying strengths and weaknesses.

Preliminary Screening: Evaluation for the Older Child

Preliminary screening for an older, school-aged child should take into account her more mature developmental level and sense of what

may be perceived as a threatening task. The same tests administered to a young child will be evaluated for different qualitative features, and a decision made that additional tests may better meet the intent of the preliminary screening. The screening protocol below samples efficiency with oral and written automatic language sequences, auditory and visual attention, right–left cerebral efficiency for motor and sensory tests, verbal fluency, speeded naming, phonological processing, visuoconstruction, visuomotor integration, visuoperception, visuospatial organization, inhibitory capacity, verbal and nonverbal learning and memory, and emotional issues. The following sample measures administered together will range from approximately 100 to 130 minutes (see Table 4–2):

Oral and written alphabet and number sequence production, name writing

These tasks sample behaviors listed above, but are supplemented at these ages with *written paragraph production* to examine written expression proficiency. The child may be asked to respond orally to the paragraph stimulus picture for a gross comparison of written and oral proficiency.

Drawing

As above, a visuomotor test such as the Beery Buktenica Test of Visual Motor Integration (Beery, 1997) and the Greek-cross copy item are useful. In addition, the Draw-A-Clock test (Freedman, Leach et al., 1994; Cohen, Ricci et al., 2000) is an interesting addition for the older child. It provides data leading to conclusions about conceptual difficulty and/or expressive constructional efficiency. The Repeated Patterns Test (Waber and Bernstein, 1994) or other tests requiring production of graphomotor sequences (e.g., ramparts design, alternation of sequences) are also brief but useful measures.

Language

Tests of phonemic and semantic verbal fluency, phonological processing (e.g., Auditory Analysis Test; Rosner and Simon, 1971), and speeded naming (e.g., Rapid Automatized Naming; Denckla and Rudel 1974; Wolf and Biddle 1985) are useful language-screening instruments that have a high probability of detecting developmental delay. Impairment on these tests highlights the need for more

Table 4–2. Outline for Preliminary Screening of a School-Aged Child

AUTOMATIC LANGUAGE	Alphabet Production—Oral & Written Number Production—Oral & Written Name Writing Paragraph Formulation—Oral & Written
VISUOCONSTUCTION	Beery-Buktenica Test of Visual-Motor Integration Greek cross copy Draw-A-Clock Repeated Patterns Test
LANGUAGE	Auditory Analysis Test Verbal Fluency—phonemic & semantic Rapid Automatized Naming
INHIBITORY CAPACITY/EXECUTIVE FUNCTION	Go-No Go Test Stroop Color-Word Test
MOTOR & SENSORY	Finger Tapping Test Grooved Pegboard Test Finger Recognition Fingertip Number (Symbol) Writing Test
LEARNING & MEMORY	Selective Reminding Test Story Memory Sentence Memory Rey-Osterrieth Complex Figure
ATTENTION	Digit Span Block Span Visual Search Cancellation Auditory Consonant Trigrams Test
PROJECTIVE SCREENING	Draw-A-Family Draw-A-Person Children's Depression Inventory

extensive language evaluation, including academic achievement testing, to examine more higher-order abilities such as reading, spelling, writing, and calculation.

Inhibitory capacity

Brief tests, such as one of the existing Stroop Color-Word Test versions or a go-no go test of reciprocal motor actions, are useful for preliminarily examining the inhibitory aspect of executive function, and an older child is well able to take such tests. Later evaluation may need to include additional, more lengthy, measures of inhibitory capacity, across modalities.

Motor and sensory-perceptual efficiency

As noted above, tests comparing the two body sides are especially helpful at any chronological age. For the school-aged child, the Finger Tapping Test and/or Grooved Pegboard Test can be supplemented by finger recognition and/or graphesthesia testing to pro-

vide more extensive information rapidly about differential right-left functioning.

Learning and memory

The ability to encode, consolidate, store, and retain novel auditory/verbal information, for example, with an age-appropriate version of the Verbal Selective Reminding Test, is as useful for the older as it is for the younger child. List learning can be compared with story recall and other verbal learning and memory tasks as part of the more complete evaluation that follows. Assessing learning and recall of novel complex visual information, for example, with the multidimensional Rey-Osterrieth Complex Figure, also provides very interesting information about perceptual ability, organizational style, visuomotor integration, and executive functioning, such as planning ability. The impact in screening of good vs. poor performance is immediately apparent, and the different directions one needs to pursue are often highlighted.

Attention

Verbal and nonverbal attention tests, such as a visual search cancellation, nonverbal span, and auditory number span repetition, produce information about the child's ability to focus attention, selectively attend to information, engage effectively on a working memory task, and sustain attention over time, as noted above. The Auditory Consonant Trigrams Test can be usefully added as an additional screening measure.

Projective evaluation and mood

The Draw-A-Family Test and/or Draw-A-Person Test and a mood questionnaire such as the Children's Depression Inventory (Kovacs, 1992) are brief but revealing measures for school-age children. These can be supplemented later with behavioral questionnaires, personality self-report inventories, or other adaptive behavior measures.

Preliminary Screening: Evaluation for the Adolescent

The adolescent evaluation entails special thoroughness in reviewing the teenager's history prior to direct testing. While many adolescents will accept evaluation as a positive challenge and exert considerable effort, it is also common for them to resent the time needed for a neuropsychological evaluation and to make their displeasure evident. They may be especially reticent about revealing personal details in a history interview. They may also have particular sensitivity to their own self-recognized weaknesses and, therefore, attempt to avoid certain tasks that depend on those abilities or physically or mentally retreat from attempts to assess these weaknesses.

Their unstated objections to evaluation need to be recognized and perhaps elicited in the early discussion preceding the actual test administration. Drawing tests that are often an icebreaker for young children have a different and negative effect on adolescents. Accordingly, I never start with a "childish" Draw-A-Person or any other test or questionnaire that may be perceived as appropriate for a younger child or that might easily reveal sensitive emotional issues. This contrasts with how easily a projective drawing test may be used to introduce the young child to testing.

The importance of knowing the adolescent's history was made quite evident to me when evaluating a female adolescent, with a history of abusing drugs, who was referred because of her poor organizational skill and difficulty following through on academic tasks. She presented as a resentful and sullen young woman. I recognized the need to choose initial tests that would sample domains other than executive function (EF) before asking her to engage in planning or reasoning tests. As a result, motor and sensory-perceptual tests were administered early and were well tolerated (the two sides of the body performed well). List learning was perceived as an acceptable challenge (verbal learning and recall were intact). Spontaneous language was unimpaired. Written paragraph formulation was excellent. Digit span forward and backward were intact (immediate repetition of auditory/verbal stimuli was intact, forward and backward span comparison were as predicted, motivation was maintained). Judgment of line orientation presented no difficulty (visuospatial ability was acceptable, the task suitably nonthreatening). I continued, feeling relatively assured, with each domain sampled, that none was grossly impaired.

Then, came the moment when the first complex problem-solving task was administered, the Wisconsin Card Sorting Test. The cards were arrayed on the table, instructions given, and she attempted the first card, was incorrect, attempted a second card, was incorrect again. She then stood up, stated she would not cooperate further, and left the testing room. Testing was terminated, but by anticipating a negative response to planning and judgment tests, I was able to confirm there were areas of cognitive integrity and no overt lateralized or focal dysfunction related to other cerebral regions that might also have contributed to the concerns expressed in the referral. Not a complete evaluation, but one that was, nonetheless, useful.

POPULATION-SPECIFIC CLASSIFICATION/SCREENING TESTS

No one well-recognized childhood screening instrument currently exists that covers an appropriately extensive range of clinical neuropsychological items, although one is in development (see below). However, there are some individual measures designed for preliminary determination of neurocognitive status for some specific clinical populations familiar to child neuropyschologists. Included among these are the Children's Coma Scale for the severely head-injured child under 36 months old. This scale assesses the best motor response, verbal response (including nonverbalized responses appropriate for a very young child) and eye opening (Hahn, Chyung et al., 1988). Eye opening is rated 4 for spontaneous opening, 3 for nonspecific reaction to speech, 2 for response to painful stimulus, and 1 for no response. Verbal response is rated 5 for smiles, oriented to sound, interacts, and follows objects. A rating of 4 is given for consolable crying, but inappropriate action, 3 for inconsistently consolable, moaning, 2 for inconsolable, restless and irritable, and 1 for no response. Motor response is rated 6 for responds to verbal commands, 5 for localized movement to terminate a painful stimulus, 4 for withdrawal from a painful stimulus, 3 for decorticate posture, 2 for decerebrate posture, and 1 for no response.

The Children's Orientation and Amnesia Test measures the presence and duration of posttraumatic amnesia (Ewing-Cobbs, Levin et al., 1990), and is also of particular value with a traumatic brain-injury population. It was developed with items similar in some respects to its adult counterpart, the Glasgow Coma Scale. Another instance of downward extension from an adult screening measure, the Mini-Mental State (Folstein, Folstein et al., 1975), is a proposed assessment of mental status in children using a Modified Mini-Mental State Examination (Besson and Labbe, 1997).

Rancho Los Amigos Cognitive Scales

While more of a classification scale than a screening instrument, the Rancho Los Amigos Cognitive Scales provide a systematic means for recording consciousness level for traumatic brain injury patients. These scales begin at 6 months old and are applicable throughout

childhood, into adolescence and adulthood. The classification levels are as follows:

Infants, 6 months to 2 years
  Level I: Interacts with Environment
    a. Shows active interest in toys; manipulates or examines them before mouthing or discarding
    b. Watches older children at play; may move toward them purposefully
    c. Initiates social contact with adults; enjoys socializing
    d. Shows active interest in the bottle
    e. Reaches or moves toward a person or object
  Level II: Demonstrates Awareness of Environment
    a. Responds to name
    b. Recognizes mother or other family members
    c. Enjoys imitative vocal play
    d. Giggles or smiles when talked to or played with
    e. Fussing is quieted by soft voice or touch
  Level III: Gives Localized Response to Sensory Stimuli
    a. Blinks when strong light crosses field of vision
    b. Follows moving object passed within visual field
    c. Turns toward or away from loud sound
    d. Gives localized response to painful stimulus
  Level IV: Gives Generalized Response to Sensory Stimuli
    a. Gives generalized startle to loud sound
    b. Responds to repeated auditory stimulation with increased or decreased activity
    c. Gives generalized reflex response to painful stimuli
  Level V: No Response to Stimuli
    a. Complete absence of observable change in behavior to visual, auditory or painful stimuli

Preschool, 2 to 5 Years
  Level I. Oriented to Self and Surroundings
    a. Provides accurate information about self
    b. Knows h/she is away from home
    c. Knows where toys, clothes, etc. are kept
    d. Actively participates in treatment program
    e. Recognizes own room, knows way to bathroom, nursing station, etc.
    f. Is potty trained
    g. Initiates social contact with adult; enjoys socializing
  Level II. Is Responsive to Environment
    a. Follows simple commands
    b. Refuses to follow commands by shaking head or saying "no"

c. Imitates examiner's gestures or facial expressions
d. Responds to name
e. Recognizes mother or other family members
f. Enjoys imitative vocal play

Level III. Gives Localized Response to Sensory Stimuli
a. Blinks when strong light crosses field of vision
b. Follows moving object passed within visual field
c. Turns toward or away from loud sound
d. Gives localized response to painful stimulus

Level IV: Gives Generalized Response to Sensory Stimuli
a. Gives generalized startle to loud sound
b. Responds to repeated auditory stimulation with increased or decreased activity
c. Gives generalized reflex response to painful stimuli

Level V: No Response to Stimuli
a. Complete absence of observable change in behavior to visual, auditory or painful stimuli

School Age, 5 years and Older

Level I. Oriented to Time and Place: Is Recording Ongoing Events
a. Can provide accurate, detailed information
b. Knows way to and from daily activities
c. Knows sequence of daily routine
d. Knows way around unit; recognizes own room
e. Can find own bed; knows where personal belongings are kept
f. Is bowel and bladder trained

Level II. Is Responsive to Environment
a. Follows simple verbal or gestural requests
b. Initiates purposeful activity
c. Actively participates in therapy program
d. Refuses to follow request by shaking head or saying "no"
e. Imitates examiner's gestures or facial expressions

Level III. Gives Localized Response to Sensory Stimuli
a. Blinks when strong light crosses field of vision
b. Follows moving object passed within visual field
c. Turns toward or away from loud sound
d. Gives localized response to painful stimulus

Level IV: Gives Generalized Response to Sensory Stimuli
a. Gives generalized startle to loud sound

b. Responds to repeated auditory stimulation with increased or decreased activity
c. Gives generalized reflex response to painful stimuli

Level V: No Response to Stimuli
a. Complete absence of observable change in behavior to visual, auditory or painful stimuli

THE COMPREHENSIVE NEUROPSYCHOLOGICAL SCREENING INSTRUMENT FOR CHILDREN[1]

The Comprehensive Neuropsychological Screening Instrument for Children (CNSIC) was developed to provide a brief, yet comprehensive, assessment of neurocognitive functioning under standardized conditions for children 6 to 12 years old suspected of having sustained a brain injury. Interest in a more formal screening instrument for psychologists and health professionals led to its development. Empirical data are not yet available to support or refute its usefulness. The authors intended its use for determining whether or not a child has sustained a neurologic insult, the severity of any impairment, whether further evaluation is needed, and how that evaluation should be focused. The CNSIC was designed to obtain quickly a gross measure of potential neurocognitive recovery following a brain injury and a gross profile of impaired and preserved modes of information processing, learning, and communication.

The conceptual model was based on an information-processing model posited by Kaufman (Kaufman, 1996). Following that model, the CNSIC assesses the neurocognitive function of receptive language with two different subtest formats. The first consists of test items presented auditorily and requires expressive language to respond. The second format consists of test items presented visually and requires a motor response. This method of screening neurocognitive functioning was de-

[1]The authors and copyright holders are William J. Ernst, Psy.D., University of Medicine and Dentistry of New Jersey, Robert Wood Johnson Medical School, Cooper Hospital; N. William Walker, Ed.D., James Madison University; and Gary Simpson, M.S., University of Minnesota.

veloped to decrease the likelihood that specific deficits in neurocognitive functions that may not be readily observable or typically assessed by routine mental status examinations would go undetected. Test items considered to be resistant to practice effects according to relevant literature were used as much as possible.

The CNSIC was designed for easy administration to children with suspected or known brain trauma at bedside in acute care or rehabilitation settings. Since these children may have difficulty focusing on testing for a variety of reasons, the subtests and test items that make up the instrument were designed to have a brief administration time (20–30 minutes) and to be easy to administer and score. Consistent with a recognized need, the items and subtests were based on developmental considerations as well as pragmatic issues for children in acute care medical settings. The following neurocognitive functions are assessed: orientation, language, attention, memory, motor control, visuoconstruction, visuoperception, and executive function.

The pediatric brain injury research literature reports that these neurocognitive functions are especially vulnerable (Rosen and Gerring, 1986; Lehr, 1990; Adelson and Kochanek, 1997; Walker, 1997; Taylor, Wade et al., 1999). The CNSIC includes subtests and formats that provide for alternate modes of responding to test items, such as might benefit a child with traumatic brain injury (TBI) or other impairment that restricts usual modes of responding. For example, the Explicit Auditory Memory subtest includes a written response option for children unable to respond verbally and a "head nod" response option for indicating yes or no responses for a nonverbal children.

Test development methods included content validity study, using an expert panel to determine if the prototype subtests assessed the intended neurocognitive functions, to ensure adequate assessment of the construct of neurocognitive functioning in children, to select subtests for the final version, and to revise and improve these selected prototype subtests. Their preliminary pilot testing of the subtests with a small child sample led to further revision and improvement of the prototype subtests selected for the final draft of the CNSIC

prior to normative and validity studies. A second, larger study using 70 non–brain-injured children, 10 per age group, led to further refining of administration and item sequencing. The authors reported that preliminary results support the discriminative robustness of the CNSIC among the targeted age groupings and that more extensive normative and validity studies are in process.

The results of a content validity study and subtest selection procedure using a panel of professional experts resulted in the subtest pool being split into two components: Core and Supplementary Batteries. The *Core Battery* subtests were selected if (*a*) the index of item-objective congruence value was positive and highest for the neurocognitive domain that the subtest was designed to assess, and (*b*) the subtest had the greatest percentage of 1st rankings among the panelists (i.e., assesses most accurately) for the domain that it was designed to assess compared with other subtests in the original pool. Portability also determined the final Core Battery subtests for bedside evaluation, and those items considered unwieldly were omitted or placed on the Supplementary Battery. The Core Battery subtests are listed below with brief descriptions:

Subtest 1: Color Board

Purpose: To assess the child for color blindness.

This subtest consists of a color board with 6 differently colored squares (red, green, yellow, purple, orange, and blue). Squares are ordered in two rows of three, with approximately 3/4 of an inch separating the squares both vertically and horizontally. The examiner points to the squares one at a time in a standardized sequence (left to right/top to bottom) and the child is required to identify the color verbally.

Subtest 2: Orientation

Purpose: To evaluate the child's awareness of self in relation to the environment.

The examiner asks the child 13 questions requiring an oral response. Questions are grouped into three subdomains: orientation to person (items 1–5), place (items 6–9), and, time (items 10–13).

Subtest 3: Receptive Language/Auditory Format

Purpose: To assess the child's receptive language, by having him or her engage in motor sequences in response to verbal commands.

The examiner asks the child to engage in behaviors requiring motor output. The subtest consists of eight questions, the first six requiring single-step motor response, for example, "Stick out your tongue," and the remaining two requiring two-step motor sequences: "First, point to your elbow and then your eye."

Subtest 4: Expressive Language/Naming

Purpose: To assess the child's expressive language with a visual confrontation naming task.

The child is shown colored pictures of common objects (e.g. ear, hand, bird, plane) in succession and asked to identify each of nine stimuli items orally. The first picture (ear) is a teaching item. The correct response is provided if the child responds incorrectly. No further corrections are provided for the timed test items. Points were awarded contingent on both accuracy and speed: 1–10 seconds = 2 points, 11–20 seconds = 1 point, and 20+ seconds = 0 points.

Subtest 5: Short-Term Auditory Attention

Purpose: To assess the child's ability to employ short-term auditory attention and mental flexibility.

The examiner orally presents a series of alternating letters and numbers (e.g., 4-e, 6-b, 1-h) and the child must repeat the identical series or an error is recorded. A practice item is administered, and the correct response provided for any error. The first two items consist of one digit and one letter. For the third item, an additional number is added and subsequent items increase in length. There are 10 items. Testing is discontinued if the child misses two sequences of the same number of letters/numbers.

Subtest 6: Short-Term Auditory Attention and Mental Flexibility

Purpose: To assess the child's working memory and mental flexibility.

The examiner orally presents a series of letters and numbers, arranged in alternating sequence (e.g., 1–a–6–b–2–f). The child must repeat the series backward. A practice item is provided, and the correct response given for an incorrect response. The first two items consist of one digit and one letter. For the third item an additional number is added and subsequent items increase in length. There are 10 items. Testing is discontinued if the child misses two sequences of the same number of letters/numbers.

Subtest 7: Sustained Auditory Attention

Purpose: To assess the child's ability to sustain auditory attention to a target word presented within a word list.

The examiner reads a list of words, and the child is asked to raise a hand each time the target word (e.g., "cat") is read, but he or she should not respond to a non-target word. For teaching, 10 words are read from a sample list at the rate of one every 2 seconds, without emphasis placed on the target word. The child is provided with a standardized correction for mistakes on the sample list. Once task expectations are clear, 40 words are read. No correction occurs during the test. Scores are recorded for both omission and commission errors.

Subtest 8: Sustained Visual Attention

Purpose: To assess the child's ability to sustain visual attention. Additionally, a visual processing speed component is included.

The child is presented with an 8 × 11-inch sheet of paper filled with a variety of geometric shapes. Five different geometric shapes including target triangles are in a sample line of forms at the page top. The examiner demonstrates crossing through a triangle with a pencil mark and asks the child to cross out all of the remaining triangles in the sample. Correction is offered for omissions. The child is then told to work quickly and cross out only target triangles below the line. This subtest is timed. The child indicates when finished, or is stopped at 60 seconds.

Subtest 9: Explicit Auditory Memory/Immediate Trial

Purpose: To assess the child's ability to encode and retrieve from memory a set of 4 words.

The examiner orally presents four words to the child in a standardized sequence. The child must repeat the four words. Credit is awarded if the child responds with the words after this first reading. There is no penalty if the words are not repeated sequentially. A child unable to repeat the four words after the first presentation is provided up to two more list repetitions, but no credit is awarded after the first trial. The subtest is discontinued if the child is unable to repeat the list after the third repetition. The child who successfully repeats words on any trial is instructed to remember the words until asked to repeat them later (Delay Trial).

Subtest 10: Explicit Visual Memory/Immediate Trial

Purpose: To assess the child's ability to encode four ambiguous blots in memory and identify them from an array.

The child is exposed to a picture of a nondescript blot and instructed to look at it carefully. The blot is exposed for 5 seconds, with instruction: "Try to picture it in your mind." After 5 seconds, the blot is removed for 10 seconds. After this delay, an array of blots is presented from which the child is to select the blot previously exposed. The child has 15 seconds to respond. There are four items (blots). Points are awarded for correct responses. Incorrect blot selection leads to demonstration of the correct response, but no points are awarded. The child is then instructed to remember the blots for later identification.

Subtest 11: Visuoconstruction

Purpose: To assess visual reasoning, planning, and construction ability by requiring the child to assemble various geometric shapes.

The child is presented with a variety of geometric shapes, one at a time. Each shape is divided into four component parts. A teaching item (square) is administered first. The examiner models putting the square together. The examiner then scrambles the pieces and asks the child to assemble them. A total of eight geometric shapes are then individually presented. The component parts of each shape are presented in standardized arrays in a horizontal line in front of the child. Timing begins once the child begins to manipulate the pieces and is discontinued once the child completes the item. Points are awarded contingent on accuracy and speed: 1–15 seconds = 2 points, 16–60 seconds = 1 point, and > 60 seconds = 0 points.

Subtest 12: Explicit Auditory Memory/Delay Trial

Purpose: To assess delayed verbal memory ability.

The child is required to recall the four words learned on the Explicit Auditory Memory/Immediate Trial subtest. The first 30 seconds are for free recall of the four words without prompting. The child is then provided with category prompts (semantic cues) for omitted words: "a type of fruit." A multiple-choice, recognition list format is then provided for any words still not recalled. A recognition list consists of three semantically related words: "peach, banana, apple," for the target "banana." The child is awarded 3 points for words recalled during the free recall period, 2 points for words recalled with a category prompt, and 1 point for words recalled during the recognition list condition.

Subtest 13: Explicit Visual Memory/Delay Trial

Purpose: To assess the child's delayed visual memory by evaluating the ability to recognize previously encoded visual stimuli.

The child must identify the four blots previously presented on the Explicit Visual Memory/Immediate Trial subtest. The blots are presented one at a time, embedded in a random array of six shapes. There is a 15-second exposure for each array.

Subtest 14: Executive Functions/ Mental Flexibility Part A

Purpose: To assess flexibility of thinking by requiring the child to switch from one mental set to another.

The child is asked to name as many different animals and foods as he or she can, alternating between categories, such as food, animal, food, etc. Practice with feedback is provided. Once the child has named two series correctly, he or she is directed to stop. The examiner then asks the child to continue to alternate naming as quickly as possible until told to stop. There is a 60-second time limit.

Subtest 15: Executive Functions/ Reasoning Part B

Purpose: To assess the child's verbal problem-solving abilities (reasoning and concept formation).

The examiner requests an oral response to questions: "In what way are a spoon and a fork alike, how are they the same?" The child has 10 seconds to respond to each of 8 questions. Items are scored for accuracy.

Subtest 16: Executive Functions/ Reasoning Part C

Purpose: To assess the child's nonverbal problem-solving abilities (reasoning and concept formation).

The child is presented with sequences of geometric shapes. Subjects are presented with a teaching example and feedback for an incorrect response on the sample only. The sequence at the top of the page shows three shapes and a fourth blank space (for the response). The bottom of the page has four geometric shapes, one of which will complete the sequence correctly. A line separates the two arrays. The child responds by pointing within 10 seconds. Similar items and geometric shapes are used in items 6–8 to elicit stimulus-bound or perseverative responding.

A supplementary battery includes subtests (or subtest formats) that did not meet the core battery selection criteria, but allow for further exploration of suspected areas of deficit and

may provide a more comprehensive assessment. Supplementary subtests include:

Subtest 17: Receptive Language

Purpose: To assess the child's receptive language by requiring naming of two-dimensional drawings of objects.

The child is presented with four different color pictures arranged horizontally. One word is printed in capital letters underneath the four stimuli. There are eight items. The child is provided with the prompt, "Show me the ____," and the examiner reads the target word and gestures to the words under the array of four pictures. The child points to the choice stimulus that matches the word read within 10 seconds.

Subtest 18: Expressive Language

Purpose: To assess the integrity of connections between receptive and expressive language.

The examiner reads individual words and then sentences arranged in a hierarchy, that is, single syllable words early and multisyllabic words later, to the child. Word presentation is followed by sentence items that increase in length and complexity. The child must respond verbatim within 10 seconds. A total of 10 items are administered and scored for accuracy.

Subtest 19: Sustained Auditory Attention and Mental Flexibility

Purpose: To assess the child's ability to sustain auditory attention and inhibit impulsive responses.

The examiner reads a series of words, and the child must raise a hand every time the target word "cat" is read immediately after the word "lamp." A 13-word sample list has 3 target pairs. There is correction if there is no hand raising on the sample. Then the child is read a list of 31 words at the rate of one word/second.

Subtest 20: Motor Control

Purpose: To assess the child's fine motor speed and dexterity.

The child is presented with a board with five bolts secured to it at regularly spaced intervals and provided five nuts with instruction to screw each nut onto a different bolt. The child works from right to left if right-handed or left to right if left-handed. Practice screwing one nut onto a bolt is permitted or an examiner demonstration is allowed. The demonstration nut is then removed from the bolt and the child must screw all five nuts onto separate bolts rapidly without dropping any with the preferred hand. The nut is screwed on to the bolt flush with the board. Once the child is instructed to begin, the number of drops, time to completion, and total number of nuts threaded onto bolts are recorded. The child has 90 seconds to complete the task. The examiner then removes all of the nuts from the bolts, and a trial with the nondominant hand is timed.

CONCLUSION

This chapter has considered a number of alternatives for, or supplements to, a comprehensive evaluation and has noted the development of a soon-to-be published screening test that has inherent interest as a potential instrument for diverse child populations. It will be interesting to see how well other test instruments that are currently used in practice, or are in early stages of development, will fare, and if they are likely to provide a hit when combined together for specific populations. Whether a recombination of developmentally appropriate tests will serve more efficiently as a screening battery remains to be seen.

To date, however, there is no substitute for a well-conceptualized examination that considers all aspects of the child's functioning. My own preference for an initial screening based on the reason for referral remains strong. The discussion in this chapter provides an example of how preliminary information obtained in the first hour of the intended comprehensive evaluation can redirect one's focus and lead to a thorough consideration of the child in the relatively limited time allotted to a formal test session.

REFERENCES

Adelson, P. D., & Kochanek, P. M. (1997). Head injury in children. *Journal of Neurology, 13*, 2–15.

Beery, K. E. (1997). *The Beery-Buktenica Developmental Test of Visual-Motor Integration: Administration, Scoring and Teaching Manual* (4th ed.). Parsippany, NJ: Modern Curriculum Press.

Besson, P. S., & Labbe, E. E. (1997). Use of the Modified Mini-Mental State examination with children. *Journal of Child Neurology, 12*, 455–460.

Cohen, M. J., Ricci, C. A., Kibby, M. Y., & Edmonds, J. E. (2000). Developmental progression of clock face drawing in children. *Child Neuropsychology, 6*, 64–76.

Denckla, M. B., & Rudel, R. (1974). Rapid "automatized" naming of pictured objects, colors, letters and numbers by normal children. *Cortex, 10*, 186–202.

Dunn, L. M., & Dunn, L. M. (1997). *Examiner's manual for the Peabody Picture Vocabulary Test* (3rd ed.) Circle Pines, MN: American Guidance Service.

Ewing-Cobbs, L., Levin, H. S., Fletcher, J., Miner, M., & Eisenberg, H. (1990). The Children's Orientation and Amnesia Test: Relationship to severity of acute head injury and to recovery of memory. *Neurosurgery, 27*, 683–691.

Folstein, M. F., Folstein, S. E., & McHugh, P. R. (1975). Mini-Mental State: A practical method for grading the cognitive state of patients for the clinician. *Journal of Psychiatric Research, 12*, 89–98.

Freedman, M., Leach, L., Kaplan, E., Winocur, G., Shulman, K. I., & Delis, D. (1994). *Clock drawing: A neuropsychological analysis*. New York: Oxford University Press.

Hahn, Y. S., Chyung, C., Barthel, M. J., Bailes, J., Flannery, A., & McLone, D. G. (1988). Head injuries in children under 36 months of age. *Child's Nervous System, 4*, 34–40.

Kaufman, A. S. (1996). *Intelligent testing with the WISC-III*. New York: Wiley.

Kovacs, M. (1992). *Children's Depression Inventory*. North Tonawanda, NY: Multi-Health Systems, Inc.

Lehr, E. (1990). Cognitive aspects. In E. Lehr (Ed.), *Psychological management of traumatic brain injuries in children and adolescents* (pp. 99–132). Rockville, MD: Aspen.

Lundin, K. A., & Philippis, N. A. (1999). Proposed Schedule of Usual and Customary Test Administration Times. *The Clinical Neuropsychologist, 13*, 433–436.

Murphy, K. J. (2001). Is the Bender Gestalt Test an important tool for neuropsychologists? *Journal of the International Neuropsychological Society, 7,* 652–653.

Raven, J. C. (1965). *The Coloured Progressive Matrices.* London, UK: H. K. Lewis.

Raven, J. C., Court, J., & Raven, J. C. (1992). *Raven Manual.* Oxford, UK: Oxford Psychologists Press.

Reitan, R. (1984). *Aphasia and sensory-perceptual deficits in children.* Tucson, Az: Neuropsychology Press.

Rosen, C. D., & Gerring, J. P. (1986). *Head trauma: Educational reintegration.* San Diego, CA: College-Hill.

Rosner, J., & Simon, D. P. (1971). The auditory analysis test: An initial report. *Journal of Learning Disability, 4,* 384–392.

Satz, P., & Fletcher, J. (1988). Early identification of learning disabled children: An old problem revisited. *Journal of Consulting and Clinical Psychology, 56,* 824–829.

Taylor, H. G., Wade, S. L., Yeates, K. O., Drotar, D., Klein, S. K., & Stancin, T. (1999). Influences on first-year recovery from traumatic brain injury in children. *Neuropsychology, 13,* 76–89.

Waber, D. P., & Bernstein, J. H. (1994). Repetitive graphomotor output in learning-disabled and non learning-disabled children: The Repeated Patterns Test. *Developmental Neuropsychology, 10,* 51–65.

Walker, N. W. (1997). *Best practices in assessment and programming for students with traumatic brain injuries.* Raleigh, NC: Public Schools of North Carolina.

Wolf, M., & Biddle, K. R. (1985). *Normative data for RAN and RAS tasks.* Unpublished manuscript, Tufts University, Boston.

5

Intelligence Testing: General Considerations

The existing literature on general intelligence tests is extensive. Entire books, many test manuals, and numerous literature citations are devoted to this topic. It is beyond the scope of this chapter to consider the history of intelligence testing or the history of the development of these tests in substantial detail.

A VERY BRIEF HISTORY OF INTELLIGENCE TESTING

But to appreciate how entrenched intelligence testing is in the psychological community, it is useful to briefly review some major events in it long history. Perceptual and cognitive testing can be traced back to the early to mid-nineteenth century. Landmark dates include 1879, when the first psychology laboratory was founded in Germany by Wilhelm Wundt, and 1888, when J. M. Cattell introduced a psychology testing laboratory in the United States.

Alfred Binet and Théophile Simon developed an intelligence scale in 1905 to assess whether an individual child required academic assistance. Their test resulted in a single mental-age score. Suggesting that intelligence develops with age, they administered their test to a standardization sample of different-aged children to obtain age-appropriate normative data. The Binet-Simon scale was subsequently translated from its original French version into an English test by H. H. Goddard in 1909. A ratio measure was proposed by Wilhelm Stern in 1912 that compared a child's highest achievement or Mental Age (MA) with actual Chronological Age (CA) and thus derived an Intelligence Quotient (IQ), according to the formula $IQ = MA/CA \times 100$. A score of 100 meant MA and CA were equivalent.

Subsequently, a deviation IQ was recommended as an alternative means of reporting results to allow for the limitations of the original calculations that did not account for an individual maturing into adulthood and to reflect the person's relative position among similarly aged individuals (Wechsler, 1949). All Wechsler series IQ tests present summary deviation IQs.

Interest in assessing intelligence of individual adults (16 years and older) led to the development of the Wechsler-Bellevue Intelligence Scale (Wechsler, 1939), to the Wechsler Adult Intelligence Scale in 1955 (Wechsler, 1955), and to subsequent revisions in 1981 and 1997 (Wechsler, 1981; 1997). An instrument for measuring children's intelligence was also developed, the Wechsler Intelligence Scale for Children (WISC; Wechsler, 1949), with subsequent revisions in 1974 and 1991 (Wechsler, 1974; 1991). The WISC rejected the concept of mental age introduced by Binet-Simon as too limiting and introduced the deviation IQ concept of the adult Wechsler test, comparing the child's performance with those in a similar age group but not by comparison with a composite age group.

The deviation IQ is dependent on a normal distribution of test scores, and the child's IQ scores therefore remain constant as the child matures, if no unforseen circumstances occur. Thus, a verbal, performance, or full-scale IQ of 100 always represents a percentile rank of 50 within a comparison group. The Wechsler Preschool and Primary Scales of Intelligence were also developed and revised, but these proved of more questionable value. A third revision is forthcoming, however, that appears to have corrected some of the weaknesses of its predecessor (Wechsler, 2002).

The reader interested in more extensive consideration of the theoretical and practical aspects of intelligence testing will find many excellent resources. These include a discussion of theories of intelligence, including an early idea that general intelligence is an attribute central to all intellectual activity, the influential g (general) factor measured by intelligence test tasks (Spearman 1904; 1923; 1927). As part of his two-factor theory, Charles Spearman proposed an additional number of minor factors, s. The s factor was conceived as specific to a particular test so that performance would depend in part on g but also on the specific capacities inherent to the task: s. In contrast to this theory, a testing battery to assess "primary mental abilities" was developed (Thurstone, 1938) and revised (Thurstone and Thurstone, 1949; 1962) that referred to separable factors of verbal comprehension, word fluency, numerical fluency, spatial visualization, associative memory, perceptual speed, and reasoning. Factor analysis of these abilities resulted in two factors, a verbal-educational factor and a spatial-mechanical factor (Vernon, 1950). It was the Thurstone model that was influential in the development of the current Differential Abilities Scale (DAS) as an alternative means of assessing a child (Elliott, 1990).

Another influential two-factor model emerged in the 1960s, the Theory of Fluid (Gf) and Crystallized (Gc) intelligence (Cattell, 1963; Horn and Cattell, 1966; Horn, 1988), a theory that continues to see application in current psychometric instruments (Flanagan, Mc-

Grew et al., 2000). It has been proposed that fluid intelligence (Gf), or broad reasoning, is used for novel problem solving and procedural knowledge (Caruso and Jacob-Timm, 2001). In contrast to fluid intelligence, crystallized intelligence (Gc) depends on education more than Gf, involves stimuli and concepts available to members of a cultural group, and is related to factual information (Kaufman and Kaufman, 1993).

The Raven's Progressive Matrices Tests (Raven, 1938), Test of Nonverbal Intelligence-3 (Brown, Sherbenou et al., 1997) and Wechsler block design and matrix reasoning subtests are examples of fluid intelligence measures. Such measures were constructed to measure the g factor, or broad construct of general intelligence, of Spearman, as reflected in the capacity to see relations and reason by analogy (Lindgren and Benton, 1980). Examples of measures of crystallized intelligence are tests estimating premorbid IQ by requiring single-word reading, for example, the National Adult Reading Test (NART; Nelson, 1982), and the Wechsler Vocabulary, Similarities, and Information subtests assessing well-learned factual information acquired over time.

Other models were also proposed. A multidimensional Structure of Intellect model of intelligence was proposed by Guilford (Guilford, 1956). A theory of intellectual development from a biological perspective was elucidated by Piaget (Piaget, 1952, 1977). The Das model of simultaneous-sequential processing (Das, Kirby et al., 1975) is the basis for the Das-Naglieri Cognitive Assessment System (Naglieri and Das, 1997). A two-level theory of associative and cognitive abilities, with immediate memory and rote-learning tests falling within the first level; more complex tasks requiring mental functions, such as reasoning and problem solving, in the second level were also proposed (Jensen 1970; 1980).

A model of multiple intelligences has also been offered that rejects the notion of intelligence as a general capacity and takes into account abilities not traditionally represented in intelligence tests, such as musical, bodily-kinesthetic, and personal intelligences (Gardner, 1983), in addition to linguistic, logical-mathematical, and spatial intelligences. The importance of both biological inclination and situational supports for exceptional performance is underscored in the latter model (Gardner, 1995). A triarchic theory of intelligence that conceptualizes intelligence as componential, experiential, and contextual is also proposed (Sternberg, 1982; Sternberg, 1985; Sternberg and Detterman, 1986).

There are many additional references concerning intelligence theories and measurement that might be of interest to the reader. These include a discussion of psychological assessment vs. psychological testing (Matarazzo, 1990), general intelligence tests and their use in child assessment (Kaufman, 1996; Sattler, 2001), standards for educational and psychological tests published by the American Psychological Association (1999), and more complete reviews of the history of intelligence testing (Thorndike, 1997), of the historical bases and development of the Wechsler scales (Boake, 2002), and of the predictive value of IQ (Sternberg, Grigorenko et al., 2001).

COGNITIVE FUNCTION, INTELLIGENCE, AND NEUROLOGICAL INSULT

In earlier years it was believed that the younger the child at the time of neurological insult, the greater the opportunity for recovery to normal afterwards. It is now clearly acknowledged that early brain insult may have more profound consequences on IQ than insult in later childhood (Michaud et al., 1993; Ewing-Cobbs et al., 1994). One focus in child neuropsychology is data collection for outcome study to determine whether a child reaches full recovery or whether intellectual and/or cognitive functioning are compromised as a result of an insult. The interest in determining whether there is recovery to the premorbid intellectual level, or whether a discrepancy from expected cognitive functioning exists as a result of the neurological insult, may be seriously confounded by developmental factors. One possible outcome is that an acquired skill is lost consequent to the insult. For example, a child may stop speaking or experience profound motor dysfunction after normal development.

A second possibility is that there is observable immediate loss of function, but the child regains full mastery with elapsed time, in which case there is presumed to be a full and successful recovery. However, this may not be an accurate conclusion since a third possibility is that there is no loss of function observed, but there is a failure to progress from the time of the neurological insult on, which lasts long after the responsible acute factors have otherwise resolved. As a result, a desired later-onset behavior may fail to appear. This will not be known until the child has matured sufficiently to be expected to demonstrate the behavior. An alternative outcome is that the behavior will emerge, but late or incompletely since the contributory insult occurred at a time in development before the function or behavior was expected to emerge and before it could be assessed.

In such instances, it is only at a later chronological age that the deficit becomes evident. This possibility may be apparent in diverse ways, such as by a delay in the acquisition of developmental milestones in a young child or by demonstration of a learning disability that manifests itself years after the onset and resolution of a neurological condition in a now older child. Another complicating factor is that there rarely are premorbid IQ or other testing data available prior to an insult. Unlike for adults, where estimates may be partly made based on educational and vocational accomplishment, the child presents very much as "blank slate" with respect to how they might have functioned if development had proceeded normally.

PREMORBID IQ ESTIMATION

Examination of the child who experienced early brain insult engenders an interest in estimating premorbid IQ. Most often, baseline data are not available for comparative purposes, and clinicians attempt to make a clinical judgment based on available school and family data for the older child, or family information alone for the very young child, a practice that has its limitations (Redfield, 2001). An inability to estimate IQ may complicate evaluation of the impact of early insult on cognitive function and the determination about whether the child will eventually reach expected premorbid levels over their developmental course. Estimation is considered but one option in gauging the net effect of the neurocognitive disruption.

There are now procedures based on demographic data to supplement the rough clinical assumptions traditionally used (Sellers, Burns et al., 1996). There are also obstacles. Some statistical methods for prediction include such large standard errors of estimation that the formulas have limited applicability to any one individual. Additionally, IQ variations greater than two-thirds of a standard deviation are common over the long-term course of development of normal children.

One of the more interesting recent commentaries on intelligence testing rebuts the recommended use of premorbid IQ estimates as predictors of neuropsychological test performance. These authors redefine the intelligence construct as a composite of neurobehavioral abilities covered in a comprehensive neuropsychological assessment, i.e., including abilities extending beyond those measured by Wechsler IQ tests that include personality, motivational, and other variables assessed by neuropsychologists (Larrabee, 2000). This point of view should have special resonance for child neuropsychologists who are engaged daily in examining the diverse multicomponential contributory factors that may explain behavior, the routine work of neuropsychological investigative efforts. While I strongly endorse this viewpoint, some methods (mentioned below) have been proposed to assist in such calculations.

A variety of options are currently employed to accomplish this estimate of premorbid IQ. The widely used option of estimation based on single word reading of irregular words as available for adults (Nelson, 1982) does not lend itself to child populations. Predicting IQ when parent IQ is known is another method. The formula for this calculation is:

$$(\text{parent IQ} - 100) \times (\text{parent/child correlation}) + 100$$

Information on parent-child IQ correlations are published (Bouchard and McGue, 1981) and an overall correlation of 0.50 between the average of two parents' IQs and a child's IQ was reported. Selected familial IQ correlations from this study are published with associated

standard errors of estimate and confidence limits for estimates based on family members' IQ scores (Redfield, 2001). Therefore, if parent IQ is 99, the calculation is $(99-100) \times (.5) + 100 =$ for a premorbid IQ estimate for a child of 99.5. Since the 0.50 correlation has a standard error of estimate of 12.99, one can then calculate the 95% confidence limits around the child's predicted IQ and determine the magnitude of difference necessary between parent and child IQs to reach significance at $p < .05$. Prediction based on mean parental education was the most powerful demographic predictor of IQ scores in a study of the WISC-III standardization sample children, with ethnic identification explaining an additional 5% of variance (Vanderploeg, Schinka et al., 1998). While a common approach is to consider immediate family members, and despite intelligence being significantly correlated within families, there are limits on the accuracy of IQ estimates based on the abilities of other family members. For the reader wishing to estimate a child's IQ with family IQ, a table of cumulative percentages of expected discrepancies between obtained and predicted IQ for several estimation methods is reported, i.e., one parent's IQ, one sibling's IQ, two parents mean IQ, demographic variables, and previous IQ (Redfield, 2001).

The use of "hold" tests, calculation using parent IQ, and calculation including demographic variables alone or with Wechsler IQ subtest scores, e.g., BEST-3 for adults (information, vocabulary, or picture completion subtests; Vanderploeg, Schinka, et al. 1996) or BEST-2 for children (vocabulary or picture completion subtests; Vanderploeg, Schinka et al., 1998) has also been studied. The notion of using "hold" tests, current tests that are considered more likely to be resistant to the negative cognitive effects of brain injury, has generally not been well supported for premorbid IQ prediction (Vanderploeg, Schinka et al., 1998). While these authors reported that two "hold" measures (information and vocabulary) combined with demographic variables were the best predictors of VIQ and FSIQ, and block design, picture completion, and object assembly, together with demographic variables, were the best predictors of PIQ, their pure demographic-based approach was as equally predictive as the more complicated BEST-2 approach. Importantly, they emphasized that a subtest–demographic formula and BEST-2 approach has limitations once the acute effects of a presumed cerebral insult are past since ongoing cognitive development may fall behind that of the normal peer group, whereas the demographic-based formulas are not subject to such limitations.

Formulas for predicting a child's IQ based on demographic factors alone and on concurrent WISC-III performance are available (Vanderploeg, Schinka et al., 1998). These authors used stepwise multiple regression analyses to determine demographic-based premorbid prediction equations, using the 2123 children from the WISC-III normative sample. They found a correlation of 0.53 with FSIQ, 0.52 with VIQ, and 0.45 with PIQ for the demographic approach. They reported a standard error of estimate of 12.56 for the FSIQ correlation and 95% confidence limits for a demographically predicted IQ of plus or minus 24.6, requiring an IQ difference of 20.7 points for significance at $p < .05$. The Vanderploeg et al. demographic formulas are:

FSIQ = 5.44 (mean parent education)
+ 2.8 (white/non-white)
− 9.01 (black/non-black) + 81.68

VIQ = 5.71 (mean parent education)
+ 4.64 (white/non-white)
− 5.04 (black/non-black) + 79.06

PIQ = 4.18 (mean parent education)
+ 0.26 (white/non-white)
− 11.85 (black/non-black) + 88.09

Parent education refers to the mean of both parents' education level, or a single parent's educational code if only one parent's data are available, and is inserted in the formula as follows: 0 to 8 = 1; 9–11 = 2; 12 = 3; 13–15 = 4; 16+ = 5. Ethnicity codes are white = 1, non-white = 0; and black = 1, nonblack = 0. The 77 children of other ethnic backgrounds in the standardization sample were excluded, and thus, these formulas apply only to white, black, and Hispanic children.

The reader wishing to compare a child's IQ with estimates based on familial IQ or demographic variables is also referred to the appendix in the Redfield article (2001) that lists cumulative percentages of expected discrepancies between obtained and predicted IQ using different estimation methods.

INTELLIGENCE TESTS: SERVICE OR DISSERVICE?

As the brief history above attests, the use of intelligence tests has a long and honored place in child psychology assessment. Many years of their use have resulted in an immensely rich database. These intelligence tests have become a fundamental portion of clinical testing practice and an invariable core in investigative efforts, and a number of distinct advantages are commonly cited, as are some distinct limitations.

Advantages of Intelligence Tests

The long history of intelligence testing in psychology offers the clinician a number of distinct advantages. It is a familiar type of investigation to a broad range of psychologists, allowing for communication across related disciplines or specialties. The ubiquitous IQ test provides the experienced clinician with a well-researched statistical basis for interpretation of individual subtest and factor index scores. Often, a quick appraisal of subtest scaled scores will offer the clinician pertinent cues about potential strengths and weaknesses, despite their consisting of multiple determinants toward successful performance. For example, lowered scores on digit span, coding, and/or picture completion leads a neuropsychologist to consider the relevance of attentional factors. Erratic or fluctuating subtest scores across scales is often characteristic of children with a neurological contribution underlying their behavior. Seemingly intact verbal scores, but a markedly lowered block design subtest scaled score, may lead one to further assess praxis, visuoperceptual, visuospatial, and visual attention components.

Yet, no one subtest score will result in a definitive statement about brain function. In many cases, the IQ subtest scatter is not particularly wide-ranging, and it therefore is less helpful with respect to neuropsychological hypotheses than for establishing where the child falls on the normal bell curve of intelligence for age peers. At a broad level, the obtained IQ(s) on a well-standardized measure will place the child in perspective relative to others of similar chronological age within the general population. Such relative standing has its usefulness, particularly with regard to prediction of academic achievement.

As new intelligence tests are developed and older ones revised, ever more appropriate standardization samples were obtained. More often the most recent U. S. Census survey data have been consulted to apportion the standardization sample representation accordingly. The number of individuals on whom the normative data are collected are generally large and provide a decided advantage for IQ tests in comparison to less well-standardized, specific, individual, neuropsychological tests, which are often based on small regional samples. Several older, and many newer, intelligence tests often have large enough standardization sample size to allow for useful stratification by age, education, and/or gender.

Concomitant with newer test construction and updated revisions, the statistical strengths of many widely used intelligence tests have improved. More sophisticated statistical analyses are published in each test's respective manuals. These allow the clinician to evaluate the appropriateness of the test instrument for the individual child, review improved reliability and validity data, and compare an individual's result with that of the standardization population and subpopulations, including demographic characteristics such as age, educational level, and cultural group. The now more common inclusion of essential base-rate data about frequency of difference between global IQ scores and between IQ index and scaled scores details the prevalence of performance within the general population, that is, the standardization sample.

Therefore, these data tables need to be consulted with respect to identifying the child's performance as within acceptable limits or as significantly different from expectation based on performance of the general population. Intelligence quotient, index, or subtest scaled score discrepancy scores alone do not reveal the clinical significance of the data and should not be interpreted without this additional analysis.

Independent empirical research often soon follows publication of a new test. Such studies, verifying or disconfirming assumptions about underlying factor structure and directing more attention to the potential risks inherent to a test and any biases to interpretation, are enormously valuable and often supportive of the IQ test construction and informative for appropriate interpretive conclusions.

Intelligence tests often consist of multiple parts that are co-normed, allowing the child's performance on one subtest to be compared directly with performance on another. Some of these broad tests also link to other established non-IQ test measures with which they are co-normed. Thus, comparisons within and across measures have a firmer statistical basis and enhanced clinical sensitivity.

Limitations of Intelligence Tests

Despite their prevalence in psychological testing, there are a number of distinct limitations associated with the administration of intelligence tests in child neuropsychological practice. What is pertinent when one wishes to compare a child to age peers is only in small part addressed by an intelligence test, and its use, while often routine, needs to be tempered by recognition of these limitations. Several of these are mentioned below as a personal perspective. Giving full appreciation to the important history and contributions of the intelligence test, my comments below, nonetheless, explain my preference for administering neuropsychological measures and subtests that will contribute maximally to domain-specific understanding of the child's functioning, and for spending as brief a time as possible administering a full intelligence measure.

First, IQ tests can interfere in the sequential hypothesis testing assessment process that enables a clinician to make an educated guess and explore possibilities by choosing tests to confirm or disconfirm these hypotheses. Data obtained from a lengthy IQ test allow for comparisons of a child to his age peer group and across other demographic factors with respect to the potential for intellectual achievement. While the results might offer clues as to how the neuropsychologist should direct an assessment, they often are insufficiently sensitive or specific for neuropsychological dysfunction since the resultant scores and factor indices are multiply determined.

In contrast, an exploratory strategy has often worked well in clinical practice, and it is one I endorse. For this strategy, the referral reason provides useful initial information; the history interview is additive, and the individually determined test selection and administration provides a focus for discovering the child's cognitive strengths and weaknesses. In comparison, the IQ test offers minimal information in this regard. IQ tests require administration of the same subtests irrespective of possible etiology.

Moreover, intelligence tests are not instruments validated with respect to brain function. IQ tests generally do no more than raise a suspicion that must be tested with other measures. Thus, the heavy reliance on IQ and academic achievement tests represents a broad sweep, while neuropsychological evaluation attempts to provide a finer delineation of meaningful elements about how a child perceives, integrates, and expresses information. An emphasis should be placed on examining the child's discrete behavior across a wide variety of domains, especially with tests validated with respect to brain function. Understanding brain function and dysfunction in childhood more likely results when one is grounded in fundamental normal and abnormal child development and can select those tests that will best address the clinical referral questions and respond flexibly to the results of direct interaction with the child and family.

Over years of clinical practice, it has become increasingly evident that intelligence tests are of limited use compared to domain-specific neuropsychological tests for inference about brain function. Recognizing that this criticism can also be directed at many "neuropsychological" test instruments, the problem is especially evident for the IQ test. The relative insensitivity of intelligence tests, and their individual subtests, to brain dysfunction is a deterrent when attempting to choose tests selectively that will elucidate brain function. Intelligence

tests are not "neuropsychological instruments," nor were they constructed for such use. It has been suggested that the insensitivity of global intelligence measures (assessing g) to even mild cognitive impairment, for example, is due to an emphasis on global achievement, rather than specific detail that might be affected in the presence of brain dysfunction (Peavy, Salmon et al., 2001).

Another major disadvantage of standardized intelligence tests is the lengthy time required to administer all their subparts. Since these tests have variable utility in neuropsychological evaluation and contribute minimally to the delineation of cognitive effects of lesions, it is sometimes hard to justify the time spent. Yet, a neuropsychologist finds it obligatory to administer such a general test since school placement decisions generally require it. Federal guidelines as of 2002 continue to endorse a discrepancy model and require that an ability–achievement comparison be made before a child is considered for special education resources. Yet, despite this legal mandate, serious reservations remain about the meaning, purpose, interpretation, and validity of intelligence tests, especially for a child with neuropsychological dysfunction (Fletcher, Francis et al., 1998; Vellutino, Scanlon, et al., 2000).

The reader is referred to an important meta-analysis that addresses the validity of IQ-discrepancy classifications. This study contributed empirical data to the controversy about whether classification of children as learning disabled (LD) are valid if based on such a discrepancy. The study reviewed 320 articles published between 1974 and 1998, focusing on those that described children with reading LD. Without invalidating the concept of LD, the authors concluded that there is minimal support for the validity of classifying children as LD in reading on the basis of the IQ-discrepancy and detailed why they reached this conclusion. Further, diverse policy implications were highlighted. The authors emphasized that the designation of LD failed to take into account the correlation of IQ and achievement, and the regression to the mean that results from this relationship. Since regression to the mean will lead to overidentification of children with higher IQ and underidentification of those with lower IQ, children are sorted by their IQ scores and not by their reading levels. They point out that the discrepancy model favors those with higher IQ scores and that reliance on the IQ-discrepancy classification makes early identification and intervention difficult. They recommend an inclusionary definition and component-based assessment of reading disability. However, beyond this specific subgroup, the article has profound implications for all children with learning disability or low achievement (Stuebing, Fletcher et al., 2002).

Adherence to strict quantitative rules that apply to administration and scoring also hinders detection of subtle but meaningful performance patterns. Documentation of qualitative features of an individual's performance does not regularly occur for most IQ tests. For example, strategic choices, error analysis, and response latency are often not routinely considered. Important behavioral aspects are essentially ignored and make IQ tests limited instruments for the purposes of neurobehavioral assessment.

As a result of these limitations, it is the clinical acumen of the person giving the test that contributes most to detection of those distinctive features associated with brain dysfunction. In the past, good note taking, careful observation of the patient, and testing the limits allowed for more accurate judgments about neuropsychological status. Only recently has this problem begun to be addressed in standardized tests, with less dependence on incidental clinical acumen and more rules for objectifying critical behaviors. Several newer published tests quantify some of the qualitative features that imply neurological compromise, and other tests also utilize scoring procedures that incorporate these features (Kaplan, Fein et al., 1999). Process-oriented modifications of the intelligence tests for children are not in use routinely, and the range of features that would contribute to an expanded knowledge base about a child is often neglected.

While such modifications now appear in some adult intelligence tests, it should be noted that these may add clinical knowledge with the disadvantage of a further lengthened administration time. Such criticism was cited as a limitation of the Wechsler Adult Intelligence Scale—Revised as a Neuropsychological Instrument (WAIS—R NI) (Peavy, Salmon et al., 2001) and may also apply to the WISC-III as a Process Instrument (Kaplan, Fein et al., 1999). Also, these additional scoring instructions often focus on abnormal or worrisome features of the child's performance. They often omit a search for the child's characteristic strengths, and it is these positives that are also central to the child's neuropsychological evaluation.

In addition, the verbal–nonverbal dichotomy on intelligence tests has been misunderstood and misused. It certainly leads inexperienced clinicians to make erroneous conclusions about brain function. Approximately 24% of the WISC-III standardization sample obtained a statistically significant VIQ–PIQ difference (Wechsler, 1991). Yet, frequently, assumptions of right hemisphere dysfunction are made when performance IQ (PIQ) is statistically significantly lower than verbal IQ (VIQ), or of left cerebral hemisphere dysfunction in the presence of a lower VIQ than PIQ. Often, the appropriate table in the IQ test manual has not been consulted to determine whether the difference is also clinically significant, that is, inconsistent with the magnitude of difference found in the normative sample. For example, if one considers the commonly accepted criteria of significant weakness as indicated by a score that falls more than two standard deviations below the mean, one would interpret as clinically significant any performance that falls below the 3rd percentile or below a T score of 30. Further, a lowered PIQ is prevalent in many chronic childhood conditions and not necessarily indicative of lateralized right cerebral dysfunction. The complex nature of the PIQ subtests, and their reliance, in part, on speeded visuomotor function often contributes to a lowered summary PIQ score, but commonly, there is failure to sufficiently consider the diverse potentially responsible subtest features to rightly ascribe etiology.

Another major weakness of IQ tests is that although they are ubiquitous in the lay literature and culture, they are highly subject to misinterpretation, especially by the general public, but also by mental health professionals. This is most evident when a misunderstood IQ or profile analysis influences an academic decision, when data are interpreted out of context, and when IQ results are used in exclusion from other available and relevant data. Too often, assumptions about the meaning of selectively lower or higher subtest scores, along with IQ differences, are interpreted similarly for children as for adults.

For example, The WAIS-III matrix reasoning subtest's moderate association with the Halstead Category Test was reported for English-speaking adults along with a significant relationship between measures of verbal abstract reasoning and fluency and the matrix reasoning subtest. Thus, it is misleading to consider the matrix reasoning task as only a "nonverbal" measure because of the possibility of verbal mediation (Dugbartey, Sanchez et al., 1999). Attempts might even be made to link a specific subtest to a specific brain region or neural network, and data exist suggesting the Wechsler Adult Intelligence Scale picture arrangement subtest is sensitive to frontostriatal dysfunction (McFie and Thompson, 1972; Sullivan, Sagar et al., 1989).

However, to take the next step and say that a low picture arrangement score is evidence proving there is frontostriatal dysfunction would be a naïve response. In a related way, classic teaching in adult neuropsychology taught that a significantly lowered picture arrangement score (compared to all other performance subtest scaled scores) indicated the presence of an anterior right temporal lobe tumor. Yet, such direct test-brain region connectionist teachings are inappropriate for a child, and there is doubt whether such linkage can reliably be made for even an adult, in the absence of additional corroborative data.

Another potential misuse concerns subtest selection for abbreviated testing. For example, some estimate IQ using the vocabulary and block design subtests, since these two subtests' estimate of IQ correlates .90 with full scale IQ based on all subtests (Sattler, 1988). However, a subtest such as block design, which requires visuomotor organization and visuospatial orientation, can be particularly difficult for children with motor impairment, such as Duchenne Muscular Dystrophy (Cotton, Crowe et al., 1998) or hydrocephalus. Impaired upper limb

function is common in children with spina bifida and hydrocephalus (Hetherington and Dennis, 1999).

Finding evidence of motor deficit is not surprising for these children, particularly when visually guided motor movements, such as writing, drawing, and fine motor manipulation of objects, are necessary. Lowered performance IQ relative to verbal IQ might well be a function of the nature of the general intelligence subtests' dependence on such motor coordination and dexterity. The VIQ > PIQ split may therefore be affected by motor, or even noncognitive factors, making discussion of IQ superfluous. This is even more of a concern since the actual deficit might not be known prior to administration, that is, for children whose deficit is as yet undiagnosed. Blind assumption that factor structure is clinically significant is yet another problem. For example, too often the WISC-III Freedom from Distractibility factor is used to justify the presence or absence of an attentional deficit, although the empirical literature does not support such use (Barkley, 1990; Reinecke, Beebe et al., 1999), and alternative explanations for poor performance need to be considered (Wielkiewicz, 1990). The WISC-III index scores have been found to be of questionable value as repeated measures of recovery following traumatic brain injury (Kay and Warschausky, 1999).

Another disadvantage of IQ tests is their failure to contribute to understanding specific underlying reasons for a child's poor performance. For example, an IQ score as a summary score does not reveal the basic processes that contributed to, or negatively impacted, the child's functioning. Basic processes that reveal how knowledge is acquired include, for example, attention and memory (Dennis, Hetherington et al., 1998), component processes of individual IQ subtests, but not definitive markers of such specific impairment in isolation from other data. The movement toward factor interpretation in IQ tests is a more useful direction but still one that provides more general than specific data.

Despite these limitations, an intelligence (IQ) test is routinely administered to a child referred for neuropsychological testing when such evaluation has not been recently obtained. The referral source and the school system often expect its administration. Intelligence tests are often included in evaluations because of Federal legislation mandating their use for ability–achievement discrepancy determination to decide whether a child meets Federal guidelines for access to special education resources. But such use is heavily criticized and is likely to change in favor of domain specific assessment.

An additional problem is that IQ tests are often selected because to do so is a habitual pattern based on years of collective experience. There are clearly times when the intelligence test proves to be a relatively inconsequential part of the evaluation. Depending on the individualized nature of the referral problem, one can envision conducting an excellent, thorough evalaution without an IQ test.

COMMONLY USED INTELLIGENCE TEST MEASURES

Among an ever-enlarging variety of measures of general intelligence are the tests noted below. Several of these, part of the Wechsler series, are presented together. Demographic characteristics for some of these tests are compared in Table 5–1.

Table 5–1. Comparison of Selected Cognitive and Intelligence Tests

	Age Range In Years	Normative Sample Size	Gender No. Male and Female	Race/ Ethnicity According to	Geographic Regions: U.S. Census	Parent Education/ Occupation
BSID-II	1 year to 42 months	1700	Equal	1988 U.S. census	4 regions	Education/ 4 levels
McCarthy	2 : 6 to 8 : 6	1032	Equal	1970 U.S. census		Occupation/ 5 levels
DAS	2 : 6 to 17 : 11	3475	Equal	1988 U.S. census	4 regions	Education/ average of 2 parents
NEPSY	3 to 12	1000	Equal	1995 U.S. census	4 regions	Education/ 3 levels/ average of 2 parents
CAS	5 to 17	2200	Equal	1992 U.S. census	4 regions	Education/ 4 levels; highest used
WISC-III	6 to 16 : 11	2200	Equal	1988 U.S. census	4 regions	Education/ 5 levels
WASI	6 to 89	1100 (100/age 6–16)	Equal 16–74 years; F > M-75–89	1997 U.S. census	4 regions	Education/ 5 levels
KABC	2 : 6 to 12 : 5	2000	Equal	1980 U.S census	4 regions	Education/ 4 levels; highest used
TONI-3	5 to 85	3451 (2118/6–18)	Equal	1990 U.S. census	28 states	Education/ 3 levels
CTONI	6 to 90	2500+	Equal	1997 U.S census	25 states	
WAIS-III	16 to 89	2450	Equal 16–64 years; F > M-65–89	1995 U.S. census	4 regions	Education/ 5 levels

Wechsler Series Intelligence Tests

The *Wechsler Intelligence Scale for Children—Third Edition* (WISC-III) was normed on 2200 children aged 6 years to 16 years, 11 months. The sample included 100 males and 100 females in each of 11 age groups. Race/ethnicity proportion and four geographic regions were based on the 1988 U.S. Census. Five parent educational levels were reported. The WISC-III allows for calculation of verbal IQ, performance IQ, and full-scale IQ, each with a mean of 100 and a standard deviation of 15. There are 13 subtests (10 core, 3 supplemental) that result in scaled scores with a mean of 10 and standard deviation of 3. Four factor-based index scores can be calculated: the Information, Similarities, Vocabulary, and Comprehension subtests for the Verbal Comprehension Index (VCI), the Picture Completion, Picture Arrangement, Block Design, and Object Assembly subtests for the Perceptual Organization Index (POI), the Arithmetic and Digit Span subtests for the Freedom from Distractibility Index (FDI) and the Coding and Symbol Search subtests for the Processing Speed Index (PSI). There is also an optional Mazes subtest.

The WISC-III subtest scaled score descriptive range names, endorsed by psychologists, will vary slightly among different clinicians, and there is probably not much reason to continue their use except that lay individuals are most familiar with these descriptors rather than with standard scores (e.g., z-scores) which are more specific and informative. The following were recommended WISC ranges: 4 and below—mentally retarded or mentally deficient; 5–6, borderline; 7, low average; 8–12, average; 13,

high average; 14–15, superior; 16+, very superior (Sattler, 1988). However, others will refer to 4 and below as "deficient" or "impaired" or use some other term indicating a large deviation from the mean that does not have the stronger negative connotation. Still others who consider scores falling between the 10th and the 90th percentiles as within normal limits will describe 12 as high average, as it translates to a standard score equivalent of 110 and a z score of +0.6 to +0.9. Then, scaled scores of 14 and above are superior or above average, 12–13 are high average, 9–11 are average, 7–8 are low-average, and 6 and lower are below average. It is the latter descriptors that I will use.

Descriptors for IQ scores or standard scores with a mean of 100 and *SD* of 15 are also subject to slightly different descriptors among clinicians. For example, one person may refer to a score of 70 to 79 as borderline while someone else may refer to this range as below average. Or, a score of 69 or lower may be considered intellectually deficient (as in the WISC-III), mentally deficient, or mentally retarded (Sattler, 1988), impaired, or well below average. There is no conclusive labeling, but for those wishing to use a descriptor, a sample proposed classification is presented in Table 5–2. No matter which convention is chosen, the reliability of the score and the standard error of measurement need to be taken into account. Thus, these descriptors will seem appropriate with a very reliable test, but will not necessarily be as useful with an unreliable test that requires a more conservative judgment. Whether the scaled scores are actually based on a normal distribution or a skewed one will also matter. If, for example, z-scores are computed on

Table 5–2. Suggested Descriptors for Full Scale IQs

IQ or Standard Score	Classification	Theoretical Normal Curve
130 and higher	Very Superior	2.2%
120–129	Superior	6.7%
110–119	High Average	16.1%
90–109	Average	50.0%
80–89	Low Average	16.1%
70–79	Below Average	6.7%
69 or lower	Significantly Below Average	2.2%

tests that are not based on a normal distribution, an examiner will not obtain an accurate representation of where the child is in comparison to his/her peers.

Comparisons of the WISC-III data with WISC-R and WAIS-R data have been made, with the result that generational changes in IQ were found, consistent with the Flynn effect (Flynn, 1984; Flynn, 1987). Children administered older versions of tests tend to score better than they do on more recent versions because the norms for earlier versions are only applicable to prior cohorts. The Flynn effect reinforces the importance of comparing a child's performance with current standardization sample data to avoid spurious IQ inflation. Data on 206 children, administered both the WISC-R and WISC-III in counterbalanced order at a median interval of 21 days, found the WISC-R FSIQ to be approximately 5 points higher than the WISC-III FSIQ (108.2 compared to 102,9). Verbal IQ was about 2 points higher, and PIQ about 7 points higher. Another table lists the ranges of expected WISC-III IQ scores for selected WISC-R IQ scores. A sample of 189 16 year olds were administered the WISC-III and WAIS-R at a median interval of 21 days. The WAIS-R FSIQ was about 4 points higher than the WISC-III FSIQ. The WAIS-R VIQ and PIQ scores were approximately 2 and 6 points higher than the WISC-III VIQ and PIQ scores.

The WISC-III is co-normed to the Wechsler Individual Achievement Test measures to enable determination of ability–achievement discrepancy. Data now exist supporting the use of an eight-subtest WISC-III short form (WISC-III SF) that maintains the four-factor structure of the WISC-III (Donders, 2001). It includes administration of the Similarities, Vocabulary, Picture Completion, Block Design, Arithmetic, Digit Span, Coding, and Symbol Search subtests (Donders, 1997). It should be noted that other analyses suggest a five-factor model is a better fit for the WISC-III, with five underlying latent variables identified: Verbal Comprehension, Constructional Praxis, Visual Reasoning, Freedom from Distractibility, and Processing Speed (Burton, Sepehri et al., 2001). A review of the validity of seven WISC-III short forms in a sample of psychiatric inpatients was published (Campbell, 1998).

The WISC-III as a Process Instrument (WISC-III PI; Kaplan, Fein et al., 1999) is a recent addition to this line of tests and is applicable for those 6 to 6 years, 11 months old. It norm references component processes and includes base rate information for some qualitative observations. Building on the WISC-III subtests, this instrument expands coding and arithmetic, adds symbol copy and written arithmetic, includes information and vocabulary multiple-choice stimuli, picture vocabulary and block design multiple-choice stimuli, spatial span, letter span, sentence arrangement cards, and Elithorn mazes.

The newest edition of the Wechsler Preschool and Primary Scale of Intelligence—Third Edition (WPPSI-III; Wechsler, 2002) begins at 2 years, 6 months and extends to 7 years, 3 months. There are 15 subtests, several new to this edition, including receptive language and naming subtests. Different core subtests are now available for the youngest age group and for those children 4 years old and older.

The Wechsler Adult Intelligence Scale—Third Edition (WAIS-III) is normed on 16 to 89 year olds. It allows for calculation of verbal IQ, performance IQ, and full-scale IQ, each with a mean of 100 and a standard deviation of 15. There are 14 subtests that result in scaled scores with a mean of 10 and standard deviation of 3. Four factor-based index scores can be calculated. The Vocabulary, Similarities, and Information subtests comprise the Verbal Comprehension Index (VCI). The Picture Completion, Block Design, and Matrix Reasoning subtests comprise the Perceptual Organization Index (POI). The Arithmetic, Digit Span, and Letter-Number Sequencing subtests comprise the Working Memory Index (WMI). And, the Digit Symbol and Symbol Search subtests comprise the Processing Speed Index (PSI) (Kaufman and Lichtenberger 1999). The WAIS-III was co-normed with the Wechsler Memory Scale—Third Edition. A decision about whether the WISC-III or the Wechsler Adult Intelligence Scale-Third Edition (WAIS-III) should be administered to a 16 year old should be individually determined and might be influenced, for example, by whether reevaluation will be required once the WISC-III normative data are no longer applicable. An American Sign Language translation of the WAIS-III is also available.

The *Wechsler Abbreviated Scale of Intelligence* (WASI; Wechsler, 1999) is normed for those 6 to 89 years old. The normative data is based on 2245 individuals, including 100 at each age level from 6 to 16 years, for a total of 1100 children. Four highly reliable subtests were chosen that each have high loadings (> .70) on *g* (Kaufman, 1996) to maximize the correlation between the WAIS and both the WISC-III FSIQ and WAIS-III FSIQ. The two-subtest form (Vocabulary and Matrix Reasoning) results in a FSIQ, and a four-subtest form (Vocabulary, Similarities, Block Design, and Matrix Reasoning) results in a verbal IQ, performance IQ, and full-scale IQ. WAIS items parallel those of the full Wechsler scale versions, but do differ.

The recommended order of administration is vocabulary, block design, similarities, and matrix reasoning. Only block design has strict time limits, while 30-seconds is recommended as sufficient time for the other subtest items before suggesting the child continue on to the next item. Scores are reported in *T* scores with a mean of 50 and a standard deviation of 10, rather than subtest scaled scores, to extend the range of score points. A table provides data comparing the WASI *T* score to the corresponding subtest scaled scores for the full WISC-III and WAIS-III. A disadvantage of the WASI is its failure to provide some of the clinically useful information obtained with the WISC-III, such as the Processing Speed Index, which has good criterion validity (Donders, 2001).

Cognitive Assessment System

The Cognitive Assessment System (CAS) (Naglieri and Das, 1997) was normed on 2200 children aged 5 years to 17 years, 11 months. The sample included an equal number of males and females in each age group. Race/ethnicity proportion and four geographic regions were based on the 1992 U.S. Census. Parent educational levels were reported. The CAS measures four cognitive processes: planning, attention, simultaneous, and successive (PASS) in children 5 to 17 years, 11 months. These correspond to the three functional units proposed by Luria

(Luria, 1973). Planning represents the third functional unit responsible for forming and carrying out plans and evaluating their efficacy; attention, the first functional unit responsible for cortical tone regulation and focusing attention; and simultaneous and successive, the second functional unit responsible for receiving, integrating, and retaining information.

Simultaneous processing is the mental activity that integrates stimuli into groups and allows for recognition of the interrelated nature of the stimuli while successive processing is the mental activity that integrates stimuli in serial order. The full-scale score includes performance on planning, attention, simultaneous, and successive subtests and has a mean of 100 and a standard deviation of 15. Twelve subtests have a mean of 10 and standard deviation of 3. These subtests comprise the standard battery; there is an 8-subtest basic battery. The planning scale subtests are termed Matching Numbers, Planned Codes, and Planned Connections; the attention scale subtests, Expressive Attention, Number Detection, and Receptive Attention; the simultaneous scale subtests, Nonverbal Matrices, Verbal-Spatial Relations, and Figure Memory; and the successive scale subtests, Word Series, Sentence Repetition, and Speech Rate or Sentence Questions. Reliability and validity data are well documented in the manual.

The Differential Ability Scales

Influenced by the British Abilities Scales (Elliott, Murray et al., 1979), the Differential Ability Scales (DAS; Elliott, 1990) was developed as an alternative test battery for children that provides co-normed data regarding both general cognitive ability (17 subtests) and academic achievement (3 subtests), and it is deservedly gaining wider use. The DAS was normed on 3475 children aged 2 years, 6 months, to 17 years, 11 months. The sample included 175 children for each 6-month age group from 2 years, 6 months to 4 years, 11 months, and 200 per year from 5 years to 17 years, 11 months. There was equal male and female representation for each age group. Race/ethnicity proportion and four geographic regions were based on the 1988 U.S. Census.

Parent education was averaged for two parents or the attainment of a single parent was used. The co-normed academic screener includes word reading, arithmetic, and written spelling, and the manual provides predicted achievement scores based on the General Cognitive Ability composite score (GCA). Overall, the DAS offers flexibility in subtest and item selection to aid differential diagnosis, while IQ estimation is a secondary consideration. The DAS has a hierarchical structure consistent with a cognitive development model. This structure includes subtests as specific ability measures at one level, clusters that include subtests that intercorrelate highly at the next level for children over the age of 3 years, 5 months, and an index of psychometric g at the third level, the GCA. The test utilizes a Rasch model from item-response theory that allows for calculation of difficulty values for each item and estimation of ability values for a person who takes some of the subtest items (Rasch, 1960; 1966). Thus, item difficulty is matched to the child's ability through item selection based on performance of previous item, i.e., adaptive testing, and raw scores are converted to ability scores through the procedure of subtest scaling (Elliott, 1990). The tailoring of item selection based on the child's abilities has the added advantage of introducing more time-efficient sampling than is possible with many general intelligence tests.

The DAS has a preschool level for children 2 years, 6 months to 5 years, 11 months. This level is further subdivided into two levels: lower and upper preschool. In the lower preschool level, those 2 years, 6 months to 3 years 5 months old, the GCA score for conceptual and reasoning ability is computed based on four core subtests (block building, verbal comprehension, picture similarities, naming vocabulary) since there is no evidence for clustering except for g. Two additional diagnostic subtests can be given (digit recall, picture recognition). The GCA for those in the upper preschool level, those 3 years, 6 months to 5 years, 11 months old, is computed based on six core subtests (verbal comprehension, naming vocabulary, picture similarities, pattern construction, copying, and early number concepts), with five additional diagnostic subtests available (block building, matching letter-like forms, digit recall, recall of objects, and picture recognition). The DAS additionally provides two lower level composite scores: cluster scores, for children 3 years, 6 months to 5 years, 11 months old: verbal ability and nonverbal ability. Cluster scores are derived only from core subtests. The DAS is especially advantageous for preschool children and for low-functioning children since it allows for determination of ability structure and calculation of IQ scores below 45. Also, an extended composite based on administration of the preschool subtests can be calculated for lower functioning school-age children.

The school-age level for children aged 6 years to 17 years, 11 months includes six core subtests (word definitions, similarities, matrices, sequential and quantitative reasoning, design recall, pattern construction) and three additional diagnostic subtests (digit recall, recall of objects, speed of information processing). Three cluster scores are computed for these children: verbal ability (word definitions, similarities), nonverbal reasoning ability (matrices, sequential and quantitative reasoning) and spatial ability (recall of designs and pattern construction). The child's scores are compared to same-aged peers from a national normative sample and scale T-scores are combined to produce an overall GCA.

Only two subtests are speeded—speed of information processing and pattern construction. However, an alternative unspeeded administration of the latter is possible, avoiding a penalty for slowed motor performance. Bonus points are earned for rapid response.

Comprehensive Test of Nonverbal Intelligence

The Comprehensive Test of Nonverbal Intelligence (CTONI; Hammill, Pearson et al., 1997) was developed to measure reasoning with figural and symbolic elements that minimize the influences of language, extended education, and acculturation. It is normed on more than 2500 individuals, 6 to 90 years old, from 25 states. Instructions can be administered orally or by pantomime, and examinees need only point to alternative choices. It is intended to be a measure of Gf (Hammill, Pearson et al.,

1997; Lassiter, Harrison et al., 2001). There are six subtests: three geometric (analogies, categories, and sequences) and three pictorial (analogies, categories, and sequences) that together yield a full scale Nonverbal IQ (NIQ).

Two subscale composite scores are obtained—Pictorial NIQ (PNIQ) and Geometric NIQ (GNIQ)—but the interpretation of the difference between these scores is unclear and requires further research. CTONI scores were significantly correlated with WISC-III full-scale IQ ($r = .81$), Test of Nonverbal Intelligence-2 ($r = .82$), and PPVT-R ($r = .74$) scores (Hammill, Pearson et al., 1997). The CTONI PNIQ was strongly correlated with receptive language skills (Gc) and the CTONI GNIQ was strongly related to nonverbal intelligence (Gf) (Lassiter, Harrison et al., 2001). Concurrent validity was evaluated by comparing the CTONI to the Kaufman Adolesent and Adult Intelligence Test (Kaufman and Kaufman, 1993). The authors found CTONI NIQ underestimated general intellectual functioning as measured by the KAIT. They also found that the GNIQ was related to the construct of fluid intelligence, but PNIQ scores measured both fluid and crystallized abilities. Verbal mediation, verbal comprehension, and verbal expression may influence CTONI pictorial subtests, especially analogies, while CTONI GNIQ was associated with nonverbal problem solving. They concluded that the CTONI GNIQ scale was the purest measure of fluid intelligence (Lassiter, Harrison et al., 2001).

Test of Nonverbal Intelligence–3

The Test of Nonverbal Intelligence–3 (TONI-3; Brown, Sherbenou et al., 1997) is a relatively brief, language-free measure of intelligence, aptitude, abstract reasoning, and problem solving for ages 6 to 89. The TONI was first published in 1982 as a nonverbal 50-item test for those 5 to 85 years old (Brown, Sherbenou, & Johnsen, 1982). It was normed on 1,929 individuals in 28 states. It was revised in 1990 and 835 new individuals were added to the original normative data base for a new sample of 2,764. Five items were added to the upper end (Brown, Sherbenou et al., 1990). The current TONI–3 was shortened to 45 items and all new normative data were collected on 3,451 indi-

viduals matched to the 1990 U.S. census results, including 2,118 children between 6 and 18 years. New picture plates were also designed. Bias on the basis of demographic variables and item bias was insignificant. This test should be considered when the child cannot comprehend language well or respond well through verbal expression. It is recommended for screening in the early recovery stages of traumatic brain injury (Farmer and Muhlenbruck, 2000). This test has applicability for a number of profoundly impairing conditions. It may also be useful when English is not the first language. Instructions are pantomimed, and the child responds either by pointing or in response to the examiner's pointing to as many as 45 items arranged in ascending order of difficulty. There are two equivalent forms for test–retest circumstances.

Kaufman Assessment Battery for Children

The Kaufman Assessment Battery for Children (K-ABC; Kaufman and Kaufman, 1983) was normed on 2000 children, aged 2 years, 6 months to 12 years, 5 months. The sample included an equal male and female representation for each of 20 age groups. Race/ethnicity proportion and four geographic regions were based on the 1980 U.S. Census. Four levels of parent education were recorded and the highest parent educational level used. The city, suburb, and rural distribution was based on the 1970 U.S. Census. Educational placement was considered, and 7% of the sample was placed in six categories of special education.

The K-ABC utilizes two component processes according to principal components analysis and principal factor analysis, simultaneous and sequential processing. It is based on Luria's theory of simultaneous and successive information processing. These define intelligence in terms of the child's problem solving and processing styles. Simultaneous processing (seven subtests: Magic Window, Face Recognition, Gestalt Closure, Triangles, Matrix Analogies, Spatial Memory, and Photo series) requires a gestalt integration of stimuli. Sequential processing (three subtests: Hand Movements, Number Recall, Word Order) refers to temporal or serial ordering of stimuli, such as recalling a number sequence or tapping pattern. There are also six achievement subtests: Expressive Vocabulary, Faces and Places, Arithmetic, Riddles, Reading/Decoding, and Reading/Understanding.

To aid in the assessment of cultural or linguistic minorities and handicapped children a nonverbal scale of six subtests was included that involves pantomime presentation of instructions (Anastasi, 1985; Coffman, 1985). The internal factor structure remains similar across cultural groups, e.g. with African children (Boivin, Giordani et al., 1995). Educational placement was included as a stratification variable with six categories represented based on the U. S. Department of Education's 1980 "Condition of Education and State, Regional, and National Summaries of Data" from the 1978 *U. S. Civil Rights Survey of Elementary and Secondary Schools*. The categories were speech-impaired, learning-disabled, mentally retarded, emotionally disturbed, other (e.g., other health impaired), and gifted.

A tetrad short form of the K-ABC includes the subtests Hand Movements (reproducing hand-movement sequences), Word Order (serial recall of words), Triangles (puzzle assembly), and Matrix Analogies (identification of principles of similarity) (Kaufman and Applegate, 1988). This form gives an estimated mental processing composite (MPC). Short-form reliabilities ranged from .90–.93 for 5- to 12-year-old children. Corrected validity coefficients comparing short and long forms range from .87 to .90. Caution has been offered about overstating the neuropsychological implications of this test (Donders, 1992).

Kaufman Adolescent and Adult Intelligence Test

The Kaufman Adolescent and Adult Intelligence Test (KAIT; Kaufman and Kaufman, 1993) was designed to assess the two factors in Cattell and Horn's theory of intelligence, i.e. Gf and Gc, along with the broader g, or general intelligence, that is reflected in a composite IQ The fluid and crystallized IQs from the KAIT were found to be adequate representations of a robust and interpretable factor structure when only the core subtests are administered to young adolescents (Caruso and Jacob-Timm, 2001). Four subtests that combine for fluid IQ are Rebus Learning, Logical

Steps, Mystery Codes, and Memory for Block Designs.

Four subtests that combine for crystallized IQ include Definitions, Auditory Comprehension, Double Meanings, and Famous Faces. Each of the three IQ scores have a mean of 100 and standard deviation of 15. Reliable component analysis (RCA) of the KAIT found the difference between RCA Gf and Gc scores to be more reliable than the difference between equally weighted Crystallized and Fluid IQs. Thus, confidence intervals around the Gf/Gc difference were narrower, and smaller observed differences were necessary for statistical significance (Caruso, 2001b).

The Kaufman Brief Intelligence Test

The Kaufman Brief Intelligence Test (K-BIT; Kaufman and Kaufman, 1983) psychometric intelligence screening test can be administered to children as young as 4 years old. A vocabulary summary score is obtained from performance on Expressive Vocabulary and Definitions subtests, considered a measure of crystallized thinking. Fluid thinking is assessed with a matrices subtest. Together, these subtests can be administered in less than 30 minutes. Vocabulary and matrices combine for an IQ composite score with a mean of 100 and *SD* of 15. The composite correlated .80 with WISC-R FSIQ and .75 with adult WAIS-R FSIQ in a population of 35 normal children (Kaufman and Kaufman, 1990). It is considered useful by some for a number of child and adult clinical populations, including screening early recovery from moderate to severe acquired brain injury (Naugle, Chelune et al., 1993; Donovick, Burright et al., 1996; Farmer and Muhlenbruck, 2000). However, its interchangeable use with the WISC-III, and specifically for those with TBI, is cautioned since the K-BIT overestimated functioning. Correlations ranged from .32 to .79, and standard errors of estimation ranged from 6.87 to 10.39 when the K-BIT was compared to the WISC-III in a TBI population of 47 children.

None of the K-BIT standard scores had a statistically significant relationship with the injury severity measure of coma, but the WISC-III did demonstrate such correlation, with PIQ more strongly related to injury severity than

VIQ. It was postulated that this was due to the K-BIT not emphasizing speeded performance as does the WISC-III performance subtests (Donders, 1995). A measurement error caution with 4-year-olds is that it takes only a difference of one raw item on the K-BIT to generate a difference of a third of a standard deviation (or greater) in the standardized score at many age levels (Jacques Donders, personal communication).

Bayley Scales of Infant Development (2nd ed.)

The Bayley Scales of Infant Development (2nd ed.) (BSID-II) (Bayley 1949; 1993) assesses early cognitive and motor development. It was normed on 1700 children (850 boys and 850 girls) between the ages of 1 month to 42 months, in 17 age groups. There were 50 males and 50 females in each age group. Race/ethnicity proportion and geographic representation were based on the 1988 U.S. Census. Four parent educational levels were recorded. There are three scales: mental scale, motor scale and a 30-item behavior rating scale. A basal level is the level at which five or more items at a given age level are passed. A ceiling level is when three consecutive items are not passed. Two normalized standard scores are derived: a mental development index (MDI) and a psychomotor development index (PDI).

Data are also provided for clinical groups of infants with diagnoses of HIV antibody, prenatal drug exposure, birth asphyxiation, developmental delay, frequent otitis media, autism, and Down syndrome and for those born prematurely. Coefficient alpha reliability, a measure of test internal consistency, is .88 for the MDI and .84 for the PDI. Test–retest after a 6-month interval was .83 for the mental scale and .77 for the motor scale. Concurrent validity data for the MDI was .79 for the McCarthy Scales and .73 for the WPPSI.

Correction for prematurity

Prematurity affects assignment of chronological age and requires special consideration. There are several references that address premature birth (Dorman and Katzir, 1994; Lindsey and Brouwers, 1999) and correction for evaluating cognitive development. Commonly, one stops correcting for prematurity at 24 months old. Some test manuals provide guidance. For example, the Bayley Scales of Infant Development-II manual recommends a "month-by-month" subtraction formula. That is, the examiner should refer to normative data for a chronological age two months earlier than the birth age for a child born two months premature.

There are long-term cognitive effects of low birth weight, that is, up to 2,500 grams (Hack, et al., 1991; Hack, Klein et al., 1995; Picard, Del Dotto et al., 2000), including visuomotor deficit, and effects on language (receptive syntax, verbal reasoning, and receptive phonological awareness), fine motor and tactile abilities, and attention (Taylor, Hack et al., 1995; 1998). The results of a study of children with extremely low birth weight (<1000 grams at birth) supported the idea that magnocellular pathway/dorsal stream dysfunction may underlie problems with visuospatial and visuomotor performance (Downie, 2003). These researchers found that these children experienced difficulties with motion processing and that there was a significant relationship between this ability and performance on the coding and picture arrangement subtests of the Wechsler Intelligence Scale for Children—Third Edition.

Cognitive outcome is not always reported to be one of eventual deficit despite multiple reports of cognitive deficit that are detectable early and may persist into adolescence and adulthood. Premature children of extremely low birth weight without periventricular brain injury during the perinatal period, who were appropriate in size for their gestational age, may function as well as full-term children on tests of reading, spelling, phonological awareness, working memory, and intelligence (Downie, 2003). In another study, children with very low birth weight (VLBW), weighing between 600 and 1250 grams, were evaluated serially at 36, 54, 72, and 96 months of corrected age. They were administered the Peabody Picture Vocabulary Test-Revised (PPVT-R) and age appropriate intelligence tests. Increasing age, residence in a two-parent household, and higher levels of maternal education were significantly associated with higher PPVT-R scores. Early intervention with special services beginning at 36 months old was also found to be helpful. The children of mothers with less than a high school education had greater increases over time compared to those children whose mothers had a high school education or higher educational attainment. Not all VLBW children, however, showed improvement as they matured. Those children with the additional complication of early onset intraventricular hemorrhage and subsequent central nervous system injury had the lowest PPVT-R scores initially and their scores declined over time rather than showing the gains accomplished by the other VLBW children (Ment, 2003). Caution is advised, however, in interpreting results suggesting gain over time too optimistically since impairment of more complex functions than receptive language typically characterize this clinical population (Aylward, 2002), and since a longer follow-up time is necessary to highlight a more complete profile of neurocognitive strengths and weaknesses. Many contributory confounding factors, therefore, make outcome predictions difficult. It is important to consider the full range of factors, inclusive of environmental and biomedical variables (Aylward, 2003).

Mullen Scales of Early Learning

The Mullen Scales of Early Learning (Mullen, 1995) cover a broad early childhood age range, from birth to 68 months. Unlike the Bayley Scales of Infant Development, this test can be administered until the child is nearly old enough for a WISC-III, but alternatively, an examiner might want to transition to the DAS. The Mullen Scales provide estimates of ability within five areas—gross motor skill, fine motor skill, visual reception, receptive language, and expressive language. Thus, more detailed data is generally possible using the Mullen instead of the Bayley scales, both of which have bright and appealing stimulus materials that are appealing to young children. It is often preferred for children who have developmental impairment and for research and clinical studies because of its ability to obtain estimates of more than just broad verbal and motor skill.

McCarthy Scales of Children's Abilities

The McCarthy Scales of Children's Abilities (McCarthy, 1972) includes 18 subtests that yield a General Cognitive Index and scores for verbal, perceptual-performance, quantitative, motor, and memory scales. Ten age groups were defined from 2½ to 8½ years old, spaced at half-year intervals between 2½ and 5½ years. The McCarthy was normed on 1032 children aged 2 years, 6 months to 8 years, 6 months old. There was equal male and female representation for each of 10 age groups. Race/ethnicity was defined as white or nonwhite; Chicanos and Puerto Ricans were classified based on racial background. The four geographic regions were based on the 1970 U.S. Census. Five father's occupation groups were based on a condensation of 10 U.S. Census Bureau groups. Urban-rural residence statistics included 2/3 urban to 1/3 rural, based on 1960 Census data. The test materials are appealing to children, but the considerably older normative data set makes this a limited instrument in comparison to more currently normed measures that were developed for, or extend into, the same age range. Thus, it is no longer advisable to administer the McCarthy Scales of Children's Abilities.

Stanford-Binet Intelligence Scale

The Stanford-Binet Intelligence Scale has a long history in psychology testing (Terman 1916; Terman and Merrill 1937; 1960; 1973), but a history of more limited use in child neuropsychology. This is due, in part, to other tests and measurement techniques for young children providing more salient behavioral and cognitive information. Terman and Merrill published the *Stanford Revision and Extension of the Binet-Simon Intelligence Scale* in 1916. The test is based on a hierarchical model of a general ability factor, *g*, and second-order factors of crystallized abilities, abstract-visual reasoning, and short term memory. The Stanford Binet (4th ed.) (Thorndike, Hagen et al., 1986a; 1986b) replaced the age-scale format with a point-scale format. Limitations continue to be cited, e.g., it can lead to an overestimate of IQ due to scoring procedures that exclude subtests when the raw score is zero (Granau, 2000). The Stanford-Binet-IV was normed on 5013 children between 2 and 18 years old, ranging from 194 in the 18-year age group to 460 in the 5-year age group. The sample was intended to be representative of the 1980 U. S. Census, but required statistical adjustment to correct for too many children with a high socioeconomic status. It groups 15 subtests into four areas: verbal reasoning, abstract/visual reasoning, quantitative reasoning, and short-term memory, but not all subtests are administered at all chronological ages. The Stanford-Binet Intelligence Scales, Fifth Edition (SB5), has been recently published and is normed for those 2 to 85 years old. Five factors are identified: fluid reasoning, knowledge, working memory, visual-spatial processing, and quantitative reasoning. The results lead to a full-scale IQ, verbal IQ and nonverbal IQ, with composite indices also computed.

Leiter International Performance Scales–Revised

Additionally, one might consider the Leiter International Performance Scales—Revised (Roid and Miller, 1997) when English is not the child's first language or for those with impaired hearing, impaired language, cultural deprivation, or autistic-spectrum disorders. The Leiter-Revised normative data extend downward as young as 2 years old.

DEVELOPMENTAL ASSESSMENT IN CHILD NEUROPSYCHOLOGY

The recent emphasis on application of child development principles in developmental assessment in child neuropsychology test development cannot be lauded enough. We have had many years of interpreting test results from measures not developed primarily with developmental considerations in mind. It has been relatively straightforward and easy for someone to take a measure from adult assessment, make a few changes, and then offer it as a measure of child neurodevelopment because it was administered to children and data were collected.

It is apparent that there are enormous weaknesses in the development and application of many of these tests. For example, some items may constrict the range of normal development one wishes to assess. As a result, administration modifications often need to be made outside of the recommended standardized instructions to better evaluate a child. Scoring systems do not always capture the nature of child performance consistent with any theoretical developmental principles. Normative data often are not stratified according to age and education, and gender when important. Thus, the recent emphasis on seriously questioning the applicability of some of our most well-utilized tests for child populations is long overdue. Child neuropsychologists are also critically examining measures and procedures from cognitive and developmental psychology. They are cognizant of the contributions of diverse developmental theorists, whose theories would suggest we should dispense with some of our current tests and explore other means for ecologically valid measurement. The attention that is now being paid to correcting these early neglected aspects in test construction, is more than welcome. It is a huge relief.

The reader should be gratified to know that the developmental focus in testing is becoming even more evident in child neuropsychology in very recent years. Among those following a clear path in these respects are child neuropsychologists Bernstein and Waber, who provided us with a developmental approach to the administration and scoring of the Rey-Osterrieth Complex Figure (Chapter 11), Espy, who is developing a battery of tests appropriate for preschoolers (Chapter 6), and Kerns and colleagues, who are developing novel tests of working memory, inhibition, and spatial perception for young children (Chapters 6 and 10). One relatively recent test battery, the NEPSY, is noted specifically for its reevaluation of how to assess children using Lurian principles and with respect to neurodevelopmental issues.

NEPSY

The NEPSY (Korkman, Kirk et al., 1997) was developed with respect to the flexible model and diagnostic principles of the Russian neuropsychologist Alexandr Luria (Luria, 1973; Korkman, 1999). To its credit, the NEPSY was constructed using a developmental model unlike other multifactorial ability tests such as the WISC-III, which are downward extensions from original adult versions. The NEPSY was originally developed in Finland for young children and was subsequently extended and normed on 1000 English-speaking children, 100 at each age level, from 3 to 12 years. The sample included 50 males and 50 females in each age group. Race/ethnicity proportion and four geographic regions were based on the 1995 U.S. Census. Three parent education levels were recorded and the average of two parents used. There are five broad functional domains: attention/executive function, language, visual-spatial processing, sensorimotor, and memory and learning. Each domain contains core subtests intended as the minimum for administration at each age level, and expanded subtests are available for the language and sensorimotor domains for 3 to 4 years old, and for all domains for those 5 to 12 years old. Administration of the core battery of the NEPSY takes at least 45 minutes for preschoolers and at least one hour for school-aged children. This is a substantial amount of time, especially for the very young child. Thus, as with any test battery, selection of this instrument might mean omission of some other tests that have interest with respect to the emerging profile. The authors recommend inclusion of expanded subtests along with the core subtests when atypical results are found for a core subtest. Selective assessments with subtests from problematic domains are recommended when problems emerge in more than one domain. A full assessment with all subtests is recommended for brain-damaged children or those for whom a complete neuropsychological evaluation is requested. This extends the administration time to approximately one hour for preschoolers and 2 hours for school-aged children.

There are 11 core subtests for those 3 and 4 years old. The language core includes Body Part Naming, Phonological Processing, and Comprehension of Instructions. The visuospatial core includes Design Copying and Block Construction. The attention/executive function core includes Visual Attention and Statue. The sensorimotor core includes Imitating Hand Positions and Visuomotor Precision. The memory and learning core includes Narrative Memory and Sentence Repetition.

There are 14 core subtests for those 5 to 12 years old. The language core includes Comprehension of Instructions, Phonological Processing and Speeded Naming. The visuospatial core includes Arrows and Design Copying. The attention/executive function core includes Auditory Attention/Response Set, Visual Attention, and Tower. The Sensorimotor Core includes Fingertip Tapping, Imitating Hand Positions, and Visuomotor Precision. The memory and learning core includes Memory for Faces, Memory for Names, and Narrative Memory.

The NEPSY has been criticized for conceptually problematic handling of attention and executive functioning for very young ages (Ahmad and Warriner, 2001) and for its psychometric weaknesses, such as placement of subtests within scales that might not be accurate placements and the ease with which a child scores within low-average limits with chance or perseverative responding. It has not gained widespread use in its entirety within the child neuropsychology community; more commonly, individual subtests are selectively administered. In contrast, the battery appears to have generated interest for nonneuropsychologists, who may not fully appreciate its statistical limitations, but find its ease of administration and conceptual packaging as a battery convenient despite their more limited ability to translate data meaningfully within a neuropsychology framework.

CONCLUSION

The progress made over the last three decades in child neuropsychology has been enormous. Our profession has established itself as a recognized clinical specialty and receives deserved lay and professional recognition. Concomitant with the profession's growth, there is a greater depth of understanding about neurodevelopment, an increased emphasis on developmental issues, reduced dependence on adult test instruments for children, new test construction with cognitive development as a primary consideration, establishment of standardized procedures for child assessment, and a full appreciation of the steps one must take to produce a reliable and valid evaluation. All of these contribute immeasurably to the continued growth of child neuropsychology.

Despite these many gains, there are many avenues for future research addressing existent and persisting weaknesses in child neuropsychological testing. There are times when intelligence testing may contribute to those weaknesses. By acknowledging there are limitations, I am not offering potential critics a basis for weakening the profession or diminishing the conclusions neuropsychologists can reach. Weaknesses in test development, normative standards, and clinical application are more than offset for the individual child's evaluation by the responsibly well-trained neuropsychologist's clinical judgment, breadth and depth of knowledge, and experience with normal and abnormal child populations. It is healthy to view our weaknesses along with our strengths, with an eye toward scientific investigation, empirical validation, and evolution of our techniques. It is our duty as psychologists to abide by the ethical and professional guidelines of our profession, including warnings not to overstep the bounds of our competence or provide inappropriate or harmful care.

REFERENCES

Ahmad, S. A., & Warriner, E. M. (2001). Review of the NEPSY: A developmental neuropsychological assessment. *The Clinical Neuropsychologist, 15*, 240–249.

American Educational Research Association. (1999). *Standards for Educational and Psychological Testing.* Washington, D.C.: American Educational Research Association.

Anastasi, A. (1985). Review of Kaufman's Assessment Battery for Children. In *Ninth Mental Measurements Yearbook, Vol. 1* (pp. 769–771).

Aylward, G. P. (2002). Cognitive and neuropsychological outcomes: more than IQ scores. *Mental Retardation and Developmental Disabilities Research Review, 8*, 234–240.

Aylward, G. P. (2003). Cognitive function in preterm infants: no simple answers. *Journal of the American Medical Association, 289*, 752–753.

Barkley, R. A. (1990). *Attention Deficit Hyperactivity Disorder: A Handbook for Diagnosis and Treatment.* New York: Guilford Press.

Bayley, N. (1949). Consistency and variability in the growth of intelligence from birth to eighteen years. *Journal of Genetic Psychology, 75*, 165–196.

Bayley, N. (1993). *Bayley scales of infant development (2nd ed.).* San Antonio, TX: The Psychological Corporation.

Boake, C. (2002). From the Binet-Simon to the Wechsler-Bellevue: Tracing the history of intelligence testing. *Journal of Clinical and Experimental Neuropsychology, 24*, 383–405.

Boivin, M. J., Giordani, B., & Bornefeld, B. (1995). Use of the Tactual Performance Test for cognitive ability testing with African children. *Neuropsychology, 9*, 409–417.

Bouchard, T. J., Jr., & McGue, M. (1981). Familial studies of intelligence: A review. *Science, 212*, 1055–1059.

Brown, L., Sherbenou, R. J., & Johnsen, S. K. (1982). *Test of Nonverbal Intelligence.* San Antonio, TX: Pro-Ed.

Brown, L., Sherbenou, R. J., & Johnsen, S. K. (1990). *Test of Nonverbal Intelligence* (2nd ed.). San Antonio, TX: Pro-Ed.

Brown, L., Sherbenou, R. J., & Johnsen, S. K. (1997). *Test of Nonverbal Intelligence-Third Edition.* San Antonio, TX: The Psychological Corporation.

Burton, D. B., Sepehri, A., Hecht, F., VandenBroek, A., Ryan, J. J., & Drabman, R. (2001). A confirmatory factor analysis of the WISC-III in a clinical sample with cross-validation in the standardization sample. *Child Neuropsychology, 7*, 104–116.

Campbell, J. (1998). Internal and external validity of seven Wechsler Intelligence Scale for Children-Third Edition: Short forms in a sample of psychiatric inpatients. *Psychological Assessment, 10*, 431–434.

Caruso, J. (2001). Increasing the reliability of the fluid/crystallized difference score from the Kaufman Adolescent and Adult Intelligence Test with Reliable Component Analysis. *Assessment, 8*, 155–166.

Caruso, J., & Jacob-Timm, S. (2001). Confirmatory factor analysis of the Kaufman Adolescent and Adult Intelligence Test with young adolescents. *Assessment, 8*, 11–17.

Cattell, R. B. (1963). Theory of fluid and crystallized intelligence. *Journal of Educational Psychology, 54*, 1–22.

Coffman, C. E. (1985). Review of Kaufman's Assessment Battery for Children. In *Ninth Mental Measurements Yearbook*, Vol. 1 (pp. 771–773).

Cotton, S., Crowe, S., & Voudouris, N. (1998). Neuropsychological profile of Duchenne Muscular Dystrophy. *Child Neuropsychology, 4,* 110–117.

Das, J. P., Kirby, J., & Jarman, R. F. (1975). Simultaneous and successive syntheses. *Psychological Bulletin, 82,* 87–103.

Dennis, M., Hetherington, C. R., & Spiegler, B. J. (1998). Memory and attention after childhood brain tumors. *Medical and Pediatric Oncology, Suppl. 1,* 25–33.

Donders, J. (1992). Validity of the Kaufman Assessment Battery for Children when employed with children with traumatic brain injury. *Journal of Clinical Psychology, 48,* 225–230.

Donders, J. (1995). Validity of the Kaufman Brief Intelligence Test (K-BIT) in children with traumatic brain injury. *Assessment, 2,* 219–224.

Donders, J. (1997). A short form of the WISC-III for clinical use. *Assessment, 2,* 219–224.

Donders, J. (2001c). Using a short form of the WISC-III: Sinful or smart? *Child Neuropsychology, 7,* 99–103.

Donovick, P. J., Burright, R. G., Burg, J. S., Davino, S., Gronendyke, J., Klimczak, N., et al. (1996). The K-BIT: A screen for IQ in six diverse populations. *Journal of Clinical Psychology in Medical Settings, 3,* 131–139.

Dorman, C., & Katzir, B. (1994). *Cognitive effects of early brain injury.* Baltimore, MD: Johns Hopkins University Press.

Downie, A. L. S., Jakobson, L. S., Frisk, V,. & Ushycky, I. (2003). Periventricular brain injury, visual motion processing, and reading and spelling abilities in children who were extremely low birthweight. *Journal of the International Neuropsychological Society, 9,* 440–449.

Dugbartey, A. T., Sanchez, P. N., Rosenbaum, J. G., Mahurin, R. K., Davis, J. M., & Townes, B. D. (1999). WAIS-III matrix reasoning test performance in a mixed clinical sample. *The Clinical Neuropsychologist, 13,* 396–404.

Education for All Handicapped Children Act of 1975, 89 Stat. 773.

Elliott, C. D. (1990). *Differential Ability Scales.* San Antonio, TX: The Psychological Corporation.

Elliott, C. D., Murray, D. J., & Pearson, L. S. (1979). *British Abilities Scales.* Windsor, UK: National Foundation for Educational Research.

Ewing-Cobbs, L., Thompson, N. M., Miner, M. E., & Fletcher, J. M. (1994). Gunshot wounds to the brain in children and adolescents: age and neurobehavioral development. *Neurosurgery, 35,* 225–233.

Farmer, J. E., & Muhlenbruck, L. (2000). Pediatric Neuropsychology. In R. G. Frank & T. G. Elliott (Eds.), *Handbook of Rehabilitation Psychology* (pp. 377–397). Washington, D.C.: American Psychological Association.

Flanagan, D. P., McGrew, K. S., & Ortiz, S. O. (2000). *The Wechsler Intelligence Scales and Gf-Gc theory: A contemporary apporach to interpretation.* Boston: Allyn and Bacon.

Fletcher, J. M., Francis, D. J., Shaywitz, S. E., Lyon, G. R., Floorman, B. R., Stuebing, K., et al. (1998). Intelligent testing and the discrepancy model for children with learning disabilities. *Learning disabilities research and practice, 13,* 186–203.

Flynn, J. (1984). The mean IQ of Americans: Massive gains 1932–1978. *Psychological Bulletin, 95,* 29–51.

Flynn, J. (1987). Massive IQ gains in 14 nations: What IQ tests really measure. *Psychological Bulletin, 101,* 171–191.

Gardner, H. (1983). *Frames of Mind: The Theory of Multiple Intelligences.* New York: Basic Books.

Gardner, H. (1995). Why would anyone become an expert? *American Psychologist,* 802–803.

Grunau, R. E., Whitfield, M. F., & Petrie, J. (2000). Predicting IQ of biologically "at risk" children from age 3 to school entry: Sensitivity and specificity of the Stanford-Binet Intelligence Scale IV. *Journal of Developmental and Behavioral Pediatrics, 21,* 401–407.

Guilford, J. P. (1956). The structure of intellect. *Psychological Bulletin, 53,* 267–293.

Hack, M., Breslau, N., Weissman, B., Aram, D., Klein, N. K., & Borowoski, E. (1991). Effect of very low birth weight and subnormal head size on cognitive abilities at school age. *New England Journal of Medicine, 323,* 231–237.

Hack, M., Klein, N. K., & Taylor, H. G. (1995). *Long term developmental outcome of low birth weight infants* (Vol. 5). Los Altos, CA: Packard Foundation.

Hammill, D. D., Pearson, N. A., & Wiederholt, J. L. (1997). *Examiner's Manual. Comprehensive Test of Nonverbal Intelligence.* Austin, TX: Pro-Ed.

Hetherington, R., & Dennis, M. (1999). Motor function profile in children with early onset hydrocephalus. *Developmental Neuropsychology, 15,* 25–51.

Horn, J. L. (1988). Thinking about human abilities. In J. R. Nesselroade & R. B. Cattell (Eds.), *Handbook of multivariate experimental psychology (2nd ed.)* (pp. 645–685). New York: Plenum.

Horn, J. L., & Cattell, R. B. (1966). Refinement and test of the theory of fluid and crystallized general intelligences. *Journal of Educational Psychology, 57,* 253–270.

Individuals with Disabilities Education Act, P.L. 101–476, 104 Stat. 1142.

Jensen, A. R. (1970). Hierarchical theories of mental ability. In W. B. Dockerell (Ed.), *On intelligence: The Toronto symposium on intelligence, 1969.* London: Methuen.

Jensen, A. R. (1980). *Bias in mental testing.* New York: Free Press.

Kaplan, E., Fein, D., Kramer, J., Delis, D., & Morris, R. (1999). *WISC-III as a Process Instrument.* San Antonio, TX: The Psychological Corporation.

Kaufman, A. S. (1996). *Intelligent testing with the WISC-III.* New York: Wiley.

Kaufman, A. S., & Applegate, B. (1988). Short forms of K-ABC Mental Processing and Achievement Scales at age 4 to 12½ years for clinical and screening purposes. *Journal of Clinical and Child Psychology, 17,* 359–369.

Kaufman, A. S., & Kaufman, N. L. (1983). *Kaufman assessment battery for children: Interpretive Manual.* Circle Pines, MN: American Guidance Service.

Kaufman, A. S., & Kaufman, N. L. (1990). *Kaufman Brief Intelligence Test.* Circle Pines, Minnesota: American Guidance Service, Inc.

Kaufman, A. S., & Kaufman, N. L. (1993). *The Kaufman Adolescent and Adult Intelligence Test Manual.* Circle Pines, MN: American Guidance Service.

Kaufman, A. S., & Lichtenberger, E. O. (1999). *Essentials of WAIS-III Assessment.* New York: Wiley.

Kay, J. B., & Warschausky, S. (1999). WISC-III index growth curve characteristics following traumatic brain injury. *Journal of Clinical and Experimental Neuropsychology, 21,* 186–199.

Korkman, M. (1999). Applying Luria's diagnostic principles in the neuropsychological assessment of children. *Neuropsychology Review, 9,* 89–105.

Korkman, M., Kirk, U., & Kemp, S. (1997). *NEPSY: A developmental neuropsychological assessment.* San Antonio: The Pyschological Corporation.

Larrabee, G. J. (2000). Association between IQ and neuropsychological test performance: commentary on Tremont, Hoffman, Scott and Adams (1998). *The Clinical Neuropsychologist, 14,* 139–145.

Lassiter, K. S., Harrison, T. K., Matthews, T. D., & Bell, N. L. (2001). The validity of the Comprehensive Test of Nonverbal Intelligence as a measure of fluid intelligence. *Assessment, 8,* 95–103.

Lindgren, S. D., & Benton, A. (1980). Developmental patterns of visuospatial judgment. *Journal of Pediatric Psychology, 5,* 217–225.

Lindsey, J. C., & Brouwers, P. (1999). Intrapolation and extrapolation of age equivalent scores for the Bayley II: A comparison of two methods of estimation. *Clinical Neuropharmacology, 22,* 44–53.

Luria, A. (1973). *The working brain: An introduction to neuropsychology.* Harmondsworth, UK: Penguin.

Matarazzo, J. D. (1990). Psychological assessment versus psychological testing. *American Psychologist, 45,* 999–1017.

McCarthy, D. (1972). *Manual for the McCarthy Scales of Children's Abilities.* New York: The Psychological Corporation.

McFie, J., & Thompson, J. A. (1972). Picture arrangement: A measure of frontal lobe function? *British Journal of Psychiatry, 121,* 547–552.

Ment, L. R., Vohr, B. R., Allan, W., Katz, K., Schneider, K., Westerveld, M., et al. (2003). Change in cognitive function over time in very low-birth-weight infants. *Journal of the American Medical Association, 289,* 705–711.

Michaud, L. J., Rivara, F. P., Jaffe, K. M., Fay, G., & Dailey, J. L. (1993). Traumatic brain injury as a risk factor for behavioral disorders in children. *Archives of Physical Medicine & Rehabilitation, 74,* 368–375.

Mullen, E. M. (1995). *Mullen Scales of Early Learning.* Los Angeles, CA: Western Psychological Services.

Naglieri, J., & Das, J. P. (1997). *Das-Naglieri: Cognitive assessment system.* Itasca, IL: Riverside.

Naugle, R. I., Chelune, G. J., & Tucker, G. D. (1993). Validity of the Kaufman Brief Intelligence Test. *Psychological Assessment, 5,* 182–186.

Nelson, H. E. (1982). *National adult reading test (NART): Test manual.* Windsor: NFER-Nelson.

Peavy, G. M., Salmon, D. P., Bear, I., Paulsen, J., Cahn, D. A., Hofstetter, C. R., et al. (2001). Detection of mild cognitive deficits in Parkinson's disease patients with the WAIS-R NI. *Journal of the International Neuropsychological Society, 7,* 535–543.

Piaget, J. (1952). *The origins of intelligence in children.* New York: International Universities Press.

Piaget, J. (1977). *The development of thought: Equilibration of cognitive structures.* New York: Viking Press.

Picard, E. M., Del Dotto, J. E., & Breslau, N. (2000). Prematurity and low birthweight. In K. Yeates, M. D. Ris & H. G. Taylor (Eds.), *Pediatric neuropsychology: Research, theory, and practice* (pp. 237–251). New York: The Guilford Press.

Rasch, G. (1960). *Probabilistic models for some intelligence and attainment tests.* Copenhagen: Danish Institute for Educational Research.

Rasch, G. (1966). An item anaysis which takes individual differences into account. *British Journal of Mathematical and Statistical Psychology, 19,* 49–57.

Raven, J. C. (1938). *Progressive Matrices: A perceptual test of intelligence.* London: K. K. Lewis.

Redfield, J. (2001). Familial intelligence as an estimate of expected ability in children. *The Clinical Neuropsychologist, 15,* 446–460.

Reinecke, M. A., Beebe, D. W., & Stein, M. A. (1999). The third factor of the WISC-III: It's (probably) not Freedom from Distractibility. *Journal of the American Academy of Child and Adolescent Psychiatry, 38,* 322–328.

Roid, G. H., & Miller, L. J. (1997). *Leiter Interna-*

tional Performance Scales-Revised. Wood Dale, IL: Stoelting.

Sattler, J. M. (1988). *Assessment of children*, (3rd ed.). San Diego, CA: Author.

Sattler, J. M. (2001). *Assessment of Children: Cognitive Applications*. San Diego, CA: Author.

Sellers, A., Burns, W. J., & Guyrke, J. S. (1996). Prediction of premorbid intellectual functioning of young children using demographic information. *Applied Neuropsychology, 3*, 21–27.

Spearman, C. (1904). "General intelligence," objectively determined and measured. *American Journal of Psychology, 15*, 201–293.

Spearman, C. (1923). *The nature of "intelligence" and the principles of cognition*. London, England: MacMillan.

Spearman, C. (1927). *The abilities of man*. London, England: Macmillan.

Sternberg, R. J. (1985). *Beyond IQ: A triarchic theory of human intelligence*. Cambridge: Cambridge University Press.

Sternberg, R. J. (Ed.). (1982). *Handbook of human intelligence*. New York: Cambridge University Press.

Sternberg, R. J., & Detterman, D. K. (1986). *What is intelligence? Contemporary viewpoints on its nature and definition*. Norwood, NJ: Ablex.

Sternberg, R. J., Grigorenko, E. L., & Bundy, D. A. (2001). The predictive value of IQ. *Merrill-Palmer Quarterly, 47*, 1–41.

Stuebing, K. K., Fletcher, J. M., LeDoux, J. M., Lyon, G. R., Shaywitz, S. E., & Shaywitz, B. A. (2002). Validity of IQ-discrepancy classifications of reading disabilities: A meta-analysis. *American Educational Research Journal, 39*, 469–518.

Sullivan, E. V., Sagar, H. J., Gabrieli, J. D. E., Corkin, S., & Growdon, J. H. (1989). Different cognitive profiles on standard behavioral tests in Parkinson's disease and Alzheimer's disease. *Journal of Clinical and Experimental Neuropsychology, 11*, 799–820.

Taylor, H. G., Hack, M., & Klein, N. K. (1998). Attention deficits in children with <750 gm birth weight. *Child Neuropsychology, 4*, 21–34.

Taylor, H. G., Hack, M., Klein, N. K., & Schatschneider, C. (1995). Achievement in children with birth weights less than 750 grams with normal cognitive abilities: Evidence for specific learning disabilities. *Journal of Pediatric Psychology, 20*, 703–719.

Terman, L. M. (1916). *The measurement of intelligence*. Boston: Houghton Mifflin.

Terman, L. M., & Merrill, M. A. (1937). *Measuring intelligence*. Boston: Houghton Mifflin.

Terman, L. M., & Merrill, M. A. (1960). *Stanford-Binet Intelligence Scale: Manual for the third revision Form L-M*. Boston, MA: Houghton Mifflin.

Terman, L. M., & Merrill, M. A. (1973). *Stanford-Binet Intelligence Scale: Manual for the third revision. Form L-M. 1972 norms edition*. Boston: Houghton Mifflin.

Thorndike, R. (1997). The early history of intelligence testing. In D. P. Flanagan, J. L. Genschaft & P. L. Harrison (Eds.), *Contemporary intellectual assessment: Theories, tests, and issues* (pp. 3—16). New York: Guilford.

Thorndike, R., Hagen, E. P., & Sattler, J. M. (1986a). *Guide for administering and scoring the Stanford-Binet Intelligence Scale* (4th ed.). Chicago, IL: Riverside.

Thorndike, R., Hagen, E. P., & Sattler, J. M. (1986b). *Technical Manual: Stanford-Binet Intelligence Scale* (4th ed.). Chicago, IL: Riverside.

Thurstone, L. L. (1938). *Primary Mental Abilities*. Chicago, IL: University of Chicago Press.

Thurstone, L. L., & Thurstone, T. G. (1949). *Examiner manual for the SRA Primary Mental Abilities Test*. Chicago: Science Research Associates.

Thurstone, L. L., & Thurstone, T. G. (1962). *Primary mental abilities (Rev. ed.)*. Chicago: Science Research Associates.

Vanderploeg, R. D., Schinka, J. A., & Axelrod, B. (1996). Estimation of WAIS-R premorbid intelligence: Current ability and demographic data used in a best performance fashion. *Psychological Assessment, 8* (404–411).

Vanderploeg, R. D., Schinka, J. A., Baum, K. M., Tremont, G., & Mittenberg, W. (1998). WISC-III premorbid prediction strategies: Demongraphic and best performance approaches. *Psychological Assessment, 10*, 277–284.

Vellutino, F. R., Scanlon, D. M., & Lyon, G. R. (2000). Differentiating between difficult-to-remediate and readily remediated poor readers: More evidence against the IQ-achievement discrepancy definition of reading disability. *Journal of Learning Disabilities, 33*, 223–238.

Vernon, P. E. (1950). *The structure of human abilities*. London: Methuen.

Wechsler, D. (1939). *The measurement of adult intelligence*. Baltimore: Williams and Wilkins.

Wechsler, D. (1949). *Manual for the Wechsler Intelligence Scale for Children*. New York: The Psychological Corporation.

Wechsler, D. (1955). *Manual for the Wechsler Adult Intelligence Scale*. New York: The Psychological Corporation.

Wechsler, D. (1974). *The Wechsler Intelligence Scale for Children-Revised*. New York: The Psychological Corporation.

Wechsler, D. (1981). *Wechsler Adult Intelligence Scale-Revised manual.* New York: The Psychological Corporation.

Wechsler, D. (1991). *Wechsler Intelligence Scale for Children—Third Edition.* San Antonio, TX: Psychological Corporation.

Wechsler, D. (1997). *The Wechsler Adult Intelligence Scale-III: Administration and scoring manual.* San Antonio, TX: The Psychological Corporation.

Wechsler, D. (1999). *The Wechsler Abbreviated Scale of Intelligence.* San Antonio, TX: The Psychological Corporation.

Wechsler, D. (2002). *Wechsler Preschool and Primary Scale of Intelligence-Third Edition.* San Antonio, TX: The Psychological Corporation.

Wielkiewicz, R. M. (1990). Interpreting low scores on teh WISC-R third factor: It's more than distractibility. *Journal of Consulting and Clinical Psychology, 2,* 91–97.

6

Executive Function

The construct of executive function (EF) is heterogeneous and includes some very broad, as well as some very specific, behaviors. General terms, such as abstract reasoning, problem solving, and concept formation, are being replaced by more specific terms and operational definitions. Yet, the EF construct remains abstract and open to diverse interpretations, explaining, in part, why sensitive and specific EF tests are not easily developed (Archibald and Kerns, 1999). Executive function has become an umbrella term that encompasses a number of subdomains, some more consistently endorsed than others. These subdomains are derived from empirical studies, such as those that include factor analysis or structural equation modeling to validate the construct, or are labeled based on clinical judgment. Table 6–1 lists some common EF subdomains, but does not include all associated terms. It should also be noted that while a specific EF learning disorder is not described in the *Diagnostic and Statistical Manual of Mental Disorders* (4th ed.) (DSM-IV; American Psychiatric Association, 1994), data supportive of such a disorder is voluminous, and the entity is well recognized. The omission has complicated attempts to provide academic special educational services for children with any form of EF disorder, or EFD, to parallel other DSM-IV learning disability terminology.

There is inconsistency about whether a test is rightly assigned to the EF domain when its multifactorial nature allows for across-domain assignment. Tests of EF tend to be chosen based on face validity (Kafer and Hunter, 1997), although construct validity data do not always support such a decision. EF test construct validity data can easily be compromised because of many alternative versions and varied administration procedures across different studies using "identical" tests. The breadth of functions or behaviors attributed to the EF construct, therefore, often results in overlap with those subsumed under other cognitive domains.

This overlap becomes even more evident in a review of the research literature, including factor analytic studies, and in clinical assessment descriptions based on a focused behavioral sampling. As a result, it becomes apparent that EF cannot always be discretely dissociated from other constructs, such as attention, information processing speed, or memory. Also, it becomes difficult to interpret and generalize research results when the stated definitions overlap semantically, but differ in their theoretical basis. Within this chapter, tests are assigned to the following sections: (*1*) Plan, Organize, Reason, and Shift, (*2*) Working Memory, (*3*) Inhibit, (*4*) Fluency, (*5*) Estimation, (*6*) Questionnaires, and (*7*) Preschool Executive Function Tests.

Importantly, the overlap between certain aspects of EF and other cognitive domains can seriously confound child clinical evaluation conclusions. A practitioner, therefore, needs to consider the particular behavioral demands for success before concluding there is an EF

Table 6–1. Sample Executive Function Subdomains

Set Shifting
Hypothesis Generation
Problem Solving
Concept Formation
Abstract Reasoning
Planning
Organization
Goal Setting
Fluency
Working Memory
Inhibition
Self-monitoring
Initiative
Self-control
Mental Flexibility
Attentional Control
Anticipation
Estimation
Behavioral Regulation
Common Sense
Creativity

deficit. For example, a broad EF deficit might be invoked to explain task difficulty, but since a degree of attentional control is necessary for any successful task performance, the equally plausible alternative hypothesis of specific attentional disorder might be more accurate. A degradation of semantic or phonological memory could explain a semantic or phonemic word fluency deficit (Watson, Balota et al., 2001). Information processing speed might be the component of principal interest for EF tests such as word or design fluency.

Attentional aspects of EF might play a crucial role in the assessment of working memory, while other EF components such as abstraction, problem solving, and planning have only a minimal relationship with memory processes (Vanderploeg, Schinka et al., 1994). Active hypothesis testing during evaluation is essential in order to arrive at the most salient possibility. Thus, those who follow a strict battery approach, with invariant test instruments, might well be at a disadvantage unless their battery is inclusive of all possible cognitive confounds for the particular child being assessed. It is also for this reason that a screening evaluation cannot be considered a complete evaluation, and its limitations in child assessment need to be acknowledged.

Clinicians are acutely aware that patients who exhibit normal performance on an EF measure during testing may be highly dysfunctional in the real-world setting. To borrow an analogy related to electroencephalogram interpretation, referring to its principal usefulness when it is positive, *the absence of EF impairment on neuropsychological testing is not proof of intact EF.* There are varied explanations for a discrepancy between real-world and test-taking behavior. These include failure of the chosen test(s) to assess the requisite capability, scarcity of tests of discrete neuroanatomic regions or neural systems that contribute to the deficit, the child's ability to self-regulate behavior effectively in the artificial testing environment (commonly observed for children with attentional disorder), and selection of tests with poor ecological test validity. Our profession has some distance to travel before these disparities can be sufficiently accounted for.

DEFINITION

Various definitions of EF are proposed, and these often have considerable overlap. There is some consistency in conceptualizing this overarching construct, despite variable assignment of subfunctions within different definitions. A sampling of the range of definitions follows (see Eslinger, 1996, for a review):

Executive function maintains an appropriate set in order to achieve a future goal (Luria, 1973). It is those mechanisms by which performance is optimized in situations requiring the simultaneous operation of a number of different cognitive processes (Baddeley, 1986). It involves strategic planning, impulse control, and organized search as well as flexibility of thought and action (Welsh, Pennington et al., 1991). It requires the ability to plan and sequence complex behaviors, simultaneously attend to multiple sources of information, grasp the gist of a complex situation, resist distraction and interference, inhibit inappropriate responses, and sustain behavior for prolonged periods (Denckla, 1989).

Executive functions are higher functions that integrate others that are more basic, such as perception, attention, and memory. These higher functions include the abilities to anticipate, establish goals, plan, monitor results, and use feedback (Stuss and Benson, 1986; Stuss, 1992). It is conceptualized as regulatory control (Nigg, 2000) and is described as the capacity to engage in independent, purposive, self-serving behavior (Lezak, 1995). Executive functions are conceptualized as a collection of processes that guide, direct, and manage cognitive, emotional, and behavioral functions, especially during active, novel, problem solving (Gioia, Isquith et al., 2000).

My own definition of EF emphasizes the *metacognitive capacities that allow an individual to perceive stimuli from his or her environment, respond adaptively, flexibly change direction, anticipate future goals, consider consequences, and respond in an integrated or common-sense way, utilizing all these capacities to serve a common purposive goal.*

EXECUTIVE FUNCTION SUBDOMAINS

As Table 6–1 indicates, many terms are applicable with an EF framework, and not all overlap with the others. There are important theoretical and clinical distinctions that can be made for each of these subdomains. Two in particular—Inhibit and Working Memory—are given central importance in some theoretical models of EF (Fuster, 1989; Roberts and Pennington, 1996; Barkley, 1997b). The importance of these relatively discrete EF subdomains has been highlighted by others (Tranel, Anderson et al., 1994; Denckla, 1996b) and are discussed briefly below. For the discussion of EF tests and their normative data that follows, tests are subcategorized according to these two major dimensions, when appropriate, while others are listed under more relevant subdomains, when possible.

Inhibition

Because inhibition mediates response selection in planning and problem solving tasks (Levin, Song et al., 2001), it is becoming a focus of even greater attention as investigators attempt to parcel out contributions to effective or impaired inhibitory function. A variety of forms of inhibition are described (Barkley, 1997b; Nigg, 2000), such as cognitive inhibition, interference control, and oculomotor inhibition (Barkley, 1997b; Nigg, 2000), as accumulating evidence suggests that inhibition is not an unitary construct (Kerns, McInerney et al., 2001). Another form, behavioral inhibition, refers to the ability to inhibit a prepotent response and is a form that not only can be directly examined in the clinical setting but is very important to assess.

Examples of clinical measures that assess the ability to inhibit the prepotent response include the many versions of the Stroop Color Word Test (SCWT), the Category Test and its adaptations, the Contingency Naming Test, and go-no go tests of reciprocal motor movements (particularly as reflected by commission errors). It is possible to assess this capacity in even very young children, e.g. with the Shape School test (Espy, 1997; Espy, Kaufmann et al., 2001). Experimental measures of behavioral inhibition are also of great interest, such as the Logan Stop Signal Task (Logan, 1994). All of these tests are discussed below.

Behavioral inhibition constitutes a core deficit in one theoretical model of EF (Barkley 1994; 1997b). In this model, behavioral inhibition refers to *(1)* inhibition of the initial prepotent response to an event, *(2)* stopping an ongoing response or response pattern that permits a delay in the decision to respond or continue stopping, and, *(3)* protecting the delay period and the self-directed responses that occur within it from disruption by competing events and responses. The model claims that behavioral inhibition affects four key executive function processes, identified as self-control of mood, motivation, and arousal; internalization of self-directed speech; working memory; and reconstitution. The latter refers to the ability to break down and then recombine behavior to pursue a goal.

There are substantial data indicating that response inhibition is mediated by frontal cerebral regions (Stuss and Benson, 1986; Mega and Cummings, 1994). Research has demonstrated that inhibitory efficiency is affected by orbitofrontal, inferior frontal, and gyrus rectus lesions (Levin, Song et al., 2001) and that there is involvement of anterior cingulate cortex on inhibition tasks that require conflict monitoring (Bench, Frith et al., 1993) (MacDonald, Cohen et al., 2000). The developmental trajectory on inhibition tasks appears linked to prefrontal maturation (Welsh and Pennington, 1988; Case, 1992; Gerstadt, Hong et al., 1994; Levin, Song et al., 2001). Regions of anterior frontal cortex important for the inhibitory control aspect of executive function continue to develop throughout childhood (Krasnegor, Lyon et al., 1997) and into adolescence (Yakovlev and Lecours, 1967; Eslinger, Biddle et al., 1997). Adult levels of efficiency on EF tasks might be reached in early adolescence (Kolb and Fantie, 1997) or continue until young adulthood (Stuss, 1992).

Importantly, EF impairment in childhood is not necessarily correctly ascribed to anterior, frontal lobe dysfunction as it likely would be for an adult. Because frontal lobe development is actively ongoing in children, unlike in adults, a clinician must consider the possibility that various strategies and/or neural pathways might be operational at different maturational stages. Further, there is evidence that diffuse brain dysfunction can also disrupt EF (Goldberg and Bilder, 1987; Rabbitt, 1998). How well EF data obtained in the testing situation will translate to a child's actual behavior in a real-world setting is not always predictable. Thus, how performance on cognitive measures that depend on inhibitory capacity relate to self-regulation of behavior still remains a subject of conjecture (Levin, Song et al., 2001). Better delineation of the critical regions or neural systems that influence function at different developmental stages is an important area of ongoing research. There is accumulating evidence that children experience inhibitory control impairment and that inhibitory control is dependent on the integrity of the prefrontal cortex but also on the interaction of the prefrontal cortex with other brain regions, including white matter tracts. In one study, the effects on inhibitory control of early damage to white matter tracts consequent to bilateral spastic cerebral palsy was investigated. The clinical group performed more poorly than the control subjects on all inhibitory tasks administered, including the Stroop Color Word Test, a stimulus-response reversal task, and an antisaccade task. These

researchers emphasized that one must control for processing speed when using reaction time as a dependent variable (Christ, White, et al., 2003).

While, in many instances, the EF data come from objective, standardized measures of the ability to inhibit or not inhibit it is often the qualitative observations of the child's performance that will add critical insight into inhibitory strength or weakness. As a result, behavioral observations and error analysis become particularly useful. For example, repetition errors suggest a failure to successfully self-monitor, and perseverative errors further suggest difficulty inhibiting previous response patterns and shifting to a new response set. Subject errors might reveal differences in information processing or explain information decay. The recent interest in quantifying what have traditionally been incidental or qualitative observations holds much promise for clinicians attempting to dissociate component behavioral processes within the EF and other neurocognitive domains. Even in the absence of rules for quantification, our qualitative observations become critical and are valid in formulating hypotheses to be tested in and out of the testing situation.

Working Memory

Working Memory (WM), or primary memory (Baddeley, 1983; 1986), refers to memory for, or information processing of, material or events in a temporary mental workspace, that is, lasting 30 seconds or less. It can be thought of as an on-line information processing and manipulation system (Mesulam, 2000). Two kinds of working memory tasks are distinguished: the generally easier maintenance tasks in which information must be maintained across a delay, and manipulation tasks in which information must be reorganized (Kerns, McInerney et al., 2001). Working memory, or working-with-memory (Moscovitch, 1992), is central to all information processing; it keeps active a limited amount of information within a brief time span and is associated with rapid access and frequent updating. Capacity is limited compared to long-term (secondary) memory but dependent on organization and type of material.

Working memory is working with information in a short-term buffer (Atkinson and

Shiffrin, 1968). It provides the important basis for more complex cognitive functions. For instance, one relies on WM when holding a new telephone number in mind until the person answers, when the number is no longer retained. Working memory can be stressed by adding layers of complexity to the task, such as requiring a longer span (see Chapter 7). Working memory is also associated with rapid forgetting over short intervals when there is interference, and, therefore, it relies on continuous attention (Morris and Baddeley, 1988).

The integrity of prefrontal cortex and its importance for intact WM is receiving wide recognition, particularly with the advances in structural and functional imaging techniques. Adult functional magnetic resonance imaging studies found declining working memory related to functional changes in prefrontal cortex (Jonides, Marshuetz et al., 2000) and that prefrontal cortex is activated during verbal (Awh, Jonides et al., 1996) and nonverbal (Jonides, Smith et al., 1993) working memory tasks (see Cabeza and Nyberg, 2000, for a review). Studies of children have found similar activation in prefrontal cortex in response to working memory tasks and have shown that working memory improves as a function of increasing age, processing speed efficiency (Fry and Hale, 1996), and inhibitory control (Bjorklund and Harnishfeger, 1990). It should be emphasized that localization using EF tests is not well substantiated for children. However, EF tests are valid instruments when the dynamic nature of maturity is appropriately considered and there is recognition that the child's strategic planning may differ in meaningful ways from that demonstrated by an adult. That is, children and adults might both succeed on a task, but the ways in which they accomplish this can be quite different. Therefore, their failures are potentially attributable to different factors as well, and these have implications for structural as well as behavioral etiological considerations.

Working Memory Models

Of the different working memory models that are conceptualized and proposed, one model that has been actively tested and modified accordingly is that of Baddeley and Hitch (1974). Their initial model of WM specified three functional component parts, rather than considering WM merely a unitary short-term store (Atkinson and Shiffrin, 1968). Each component is subject to impairment at any level. The Central Executive System (CES) is at the highest level and has similarity to Norman and Shallice's Supervisory Attentional System (Norman and Shallice, 1986). The CES is responsible for oversight of functions of active short-term memory processes. It has limited-capacity, attentional-control processes responsible for initiating and regulating component mental processes involved with memory. An intact CES is necessary for maintaining information in working (primary) memory, to retrieve information from semantic memory, and to perform divided attention tasks. Two separate storage and retrieval mechanisms controlled by the CES were postulated.

These are the *phonological loop* (originally the articulatory loop), concerned with phonemic auditory processing and a repository for verbal information, and the *visuospatial sketchpad* (originally the visuospatial scratchpad), a repository for visual and spatial information. The phonological loop's two components are the "phonological store," within which traces decay rapidly over about two seconds, and the "articulatory rehearsal system" that is needed to refresh the store so that the rapid decay is delayed. The latter is a process of subvocal articulation that reflects central, but not peripheral (overt articulation), speech control (Baddeley, 2001).

The Baddeley and Hitch model is evolving. Recently, a fourth component was added to the model as an interface between the subsystems and long-term memory, the *episodic buffer* (Baddeley, 2000). The episodic buffer is conceptualized to be a mnemonic storage system for integrated episodes or scenes and a buffer in providing a limited-capacity interface between systems using different codes. It is postulated that multiple information sources are considered simultaneously and that retrieval from the buffer is through conscious awareness. In this new context, the CES is a purely attentional system with a role beyond memory function. The attentional subprocesses of the CES are postulated to be focusing attention, dividing attention, and switching attention.

Since the components of WM are hypothesized to have a limited capacity, the Baddeley

WM model predicts that performance will break down as task demands exceed processing capacity, particularly if the neural resources underlying the CES are compromised. As noted above, demand on the WM system is affected by memory load, or span. For example, an increase in verbal learning test-list length varies the memory load and increases demand on the WM system. Thus, WM may be highly vulnerable to disruption by a variety of neurological conditions or by attentional disorder. Working memory depends on interference control to preclude disruption of WM by ongoing internal and external distracting events and to prevent similarly disrupting influences while motor responding is being guided by WM (Baddeley, 1986; Fuster, 1997; Barkley, Murphy et al., 2001).

Working memory in childhood is receiving enhanced attention (Roberts and Pennington, 1996). Tasks that require the child to solve a problem after a short delay during which he or she must retain information, or track a spatial array over time prior to making a choice decision, would fall within this domain. Treatment considerations are also being addressed. Whether working memory can be trained in 7- to 15-year-old children diagnosed with ADHD was examined in a double blind placebo controlled design. The researchers found that training did enhance performance on the trained working memory task and that motor activity was reduced in the treatment group. They also found that the training generalized to a nontrained visuospatial working memory task, to the Stroop task, and to the Raven's Progressive Matrices nonverbal reasoning task, tasks dependent on working memory and/or inhibition. Similar improvements on cognitive tasks were found for a sample of young adults without ADHD and without a working memory deficit (Klingberg, Forssberg et al., 2002).

Both research and clinical tasks are now available to examine WM in children, with some of the former taken from cognitive psychology research and adapted for clinical neuropsychological use. Examples of instruments that examine WM include the Auditory Consonant Trigram Test (see Chapter 7), a test utilizing the Peterson and Peterson paradigm (Peterson and Peterson, 1959). The Peterson and Peterson paradigm has been shown to be in-

fluenced by the difficulty of the distractor task (Morris and Kopelman, 1986). Of interest as well are the Delayed Alternation Non-Alternation (DANA) task and Self-Ordered Pointing Test (Archibald and Kerns, 1999; see executive function tests for the very young, below), both tasks derived from the experimental literature. A pursuit rotor task and the n-back task are additional examples of experimental WM tasks.

"n-back" Task

The n-back task requires the subject constantly to update information held in working memory (Cohen, Perlstein et al., 1997). This procedure has a history of use in adult research studies. An example of an auditory n-back task is requiring the subject to respond to single letters. In the 0-back condition, the subject presses a key when a specified letter is heard. This is a discrimination condition. In the 1-back condition, the subject presses the key when two identical letters are heard. That is, the letter one-digit back is identical to the current letter. In the 2-back condition, the subject presses the key if the letter two digits back is identical to the target letter. Thus, if the target is "b" and the sequence heard is "b, q, b," the condition for a 2-back is met. In the 3-back, the key is pressed if a letter three back is identical: "b, q, r, b." As the separation increases, the task becomes more difficult.

While not a clinical test, the n-back procedure is nonetheless a task that has clinical and research interest. It should be noted that the Test of Everyday Attention for Children (TEA-Ch) Code Transmission subtest has similarities to the n-back procedure. It requires the child to respond to auditory cues with the number that precedes every presentation of two number 5s on a 13-minute long tape recording. The subtest appears sensitive to both working memory and sustained attention factors (see Chapter 7 for further discussion about the TEA-Ch).

Error analysis is also useful when the task itself might not be interpreted easily as a WM task. For example, omission errors on go-no-go tests might provide additional data concerning WM, as might Wechsler Intelligence Scale for Children-III (WISC-III) digit span backward performance, thereby highlighting the importance of looking at forward span and backward span separately.

EXECUTIVE FUNCTION
AND INTELLIGENCE

There is an important distinction between general intelligence and executive function that often becomes quite apparent with neuropsychological evaluation. EF tests provide data that are substantially different than intelligence test data, although at the lower IQ range the relationship between EF and IQ might be stronger (Duncan, 1995). This has become obvious in numerous studies of lesioned adults, where intelligence data does not contribute substantially to understanding the impact of a lesion on higher cognitive functions (Eslinger and Damasio, 1985; Shallice and Burgess, 1991). It is well recognized by clinicians that success on one does not guarantee success on the other.

Only moderate correlations were found when EF tests were compared to adult IQ tests (Crockett, Bilsker et al., 1986). This dissociation is often clearly apparent in child clinical evaluation as well. While a moderate-to-strong correlation might exist between EF and IQ tests (Welsh, Pennington et al., 1991), differences between tests also become apparent. For example, the Wisconsin Card Sorting Test (WCST) had lower correlation with adult full scale IQ than did the Category Test (Pendleton and Heaton, 1982; Donders and Kirsch, 1991), and the Category Test measured reasoning abilities distinct from Wechsler Adult Intelligence Scale-Revised general intelligence (Johnstone, Holland et al., 1997).

The distinction between EF and intelligence is critically important in clinical interpretation. Since high intelligence is not a guarantee of flexible thinking, an extremely bright individual can demonstrate incapacitating cognitive rigidity and limiting rule-bound behavior contrary to the expectation of others. Similarly, lower intelligence does not dismiss the possibility of good common sense and creativity that lead to effective "overachievement" and an ability to conceptualize beyond the routine.

As stated in an early intelligence test manual, "... intelligence is not always adaptive, nor does it inevitably involve abstract reasoning. Intelligence is multifaceted as well as multidetermined" (Wechsler, 1981, p. 8). There is a need to distinguish for parents and teachers the

difference between intelligence and EF. Toward that end, I find it easier to explain the dissociation between these two constructs with an example. That is, when a child demonstrates a discrepancy between intelligence and EF, I explain how some highly intelligent children can nonetheless be rigid and inflexible in their thinking, unable to demonstrate good common sense or to use their intelligence adaptively.

Yet, I continue to explain, a not-so-bright child by measured IQ score might have especially well-adapted capabilities, and thus succeed or "overachieve" despite formal documentation of more limited intelligence compared to other similarly aged children. When presented with this perspective, many adults recognize the child's characteristic ways of responding, are able to separate these behaviors from their understanding of "intelligence," and are more likely to grasp the importance of discriminating specific strengths from weaknesses. Executive function strengths or weaknesses can impact on declarative learning, but these are dissociable processes (Beebe, Ris et al., 2000).

The relationship of intelligence, gender, and age to scores on EF measures has begun to receive greater attention in children (Welsh and Pennington, 1988; Welsh, Pennington et al., 1991; Grodzinsky and Diamond, 1992; Seidman, Biederman et al., 1997; Seidman, Biederman et al., 2001). In one study, 26 normal children with WISC-III full scale IQs above 130 and 24 normal children with full scale IQs between 110 and 129, were compared, using the WCST and with comparison to the normative sample (Arffa, Lovell et al., 1998). Above average children outperformed average 9–14 year old children on every variable, at every age. While intelligence proved to be a significant qualifier of age trends, gender relationships were nonsignificant in a preliminary analysis.

EXECUTIVE FUNCTION
NEUROANATOMY

It is well recognized from adult studies that lesions in different prefrontal cortical regions in the mature individual result in distinctly different behavioral effects. Dorsolateral prefrontal cortex lesions are associated with cognitive disorders, hypo- or hyperkinesis, impaired temporal integration (Fuster, 1989; Di Stefano, Bachevalier et al., 2000), and impaired planning and response selection in goal-driven behavior (Miller, 2000). Medial prefrontal lesions are associated with disorders of initiation, and individuals with such lesions are likely to be apathetic, less motivated, exhibit inertia, and project flattened affect. Orbitofrontal lesions are associated with a sense of euphoria or mania, uncontained responsiveness to impulses, and the display of behavioral disinhibition (Fuster, 1989; Cummings, 1993). Functional activation study also found an association between the orbitofrontal region and recognition of words that convey mental state (Baron-Cohen, Ring et al., 1994).

The neural substrate underlying EF in childhood is not yet clearly delineated, but there is evidence of frontal and subcortical contributions, as for adults (Cummings, 1993). Data suggest that the functions that best define EF are known to be especially dependent on mature frontal lobes (Luria, 1980; Denckla, 1996b), especially dorsolateral regions (Grattan and Eslinger, 1991), and subcortical (basal ganglia) connections (Denckla, 1989; Eslinger and Grattan, 1993). Documentation of prefrontal activation in infancy using neuroimaging techniques (Chugani, 1987, #1673) supports the results of behavioral & cognitive studies of EF developmental progression over the childhood years. Executive function is considered by some to be a possible behavioral marker of prefrontal functioning from infancy through childhood (Welsh and Pennington, 1988; Pennington, Bennetto et al., 1996). Additional comments regarding EF and neuroanatomy are made below for specific tests or EF subdomains.

EXECUTIVE FUNCTION ASSESSMENT IN CHILDHOOD

The centrality of EF to daily living, coping, interpersonal, academic, and vocational skills underscores the importance of accurate definition and identification in order to remediate or manage executive dysfunction when it oc-

curs. The practical reasons for assessing EF behaviors are significant, and EF tests greatly improve knowledge about a child's characteristic response patterns in a way that traditional intelligence and academic achievement tests cannot. Tests of direct pragmatic or ecologically valid significance are not commonly available, but elements of some EF tests do allow for sharpened clinical judgment about a child's typical behavior.

Communication to parents based on these data underscores the valid and meaningful judgments that can be made about their child after even a single test session. This is especially helpful when there is resistance to the idea that a single assessment session will offer insight, or when assessment is perceived to be of limited utility, encompassing, as it does, the increased structure of one-to-one contact in the artificial testing environment. The translation of behavior and test scores into meaningful judgments about the child's cognitive flexibility, shifting capacity, response to novelty, reaction to routine, or ability to follow multistep instructions helps parents recognize how the behaviors that concern them daily are manifest through formal testing (Baron, Fennell et al., 1995).

Reliable and valid assessment of EF in children is receiving increased and deserved attention as this domain's importance is increasingly appreciated (Denckla, 1994; Anderson, 1998; Archibald and Kerns, 1999; Anderson, Anderson et al., 2001; Espy, Kaufmann et al., 2001). This is particularly relevant for children with neurological problems who are recognized as having EF impairments that interfere with normal maturation, cognition, and academic and social experiences (Fletcher, Ewing-Cobbs et al., 1990; Asarnow, Satz et al., 1991; Mateer and Williams, 1991; Perrott, Taylor et al., 1991; Landry, Jordan et al., 1994). Behavioral disorders are also linked to frontal syndromes. For example, conduct disorder is associated with the pseudopsychopathic syndrome of orbital frontal lesions, Attention Deficit Hyperactivity Disorder (ADHD) is linked to attention disorder and hyperkinesis, autism shares similarities with the apathy syndrome, and Tourette syndrome is analogous to an inhibition deficit (Pennington, 1997).

A wide range of EF measures are available (Pennington, 1997). Among the most useful EF tests are those that best enable the prediction of an individual child's behavior in novel circumstances, in situations of choice and decision making, in planning and reasoning, and in the creative, flexible generation of ideas and concepts. Other tests within the EF domain assess motor function, generative ability, and inhibition and initiation of action. While tests of pragmatic social judgment have yet to be used routinely, tests that require inference and clinical judgment continue to be developed. The thoughtful development of tests based on child development principles, rather than using downward extensions from an adult model, is a particularly appropriate advance.

There has been considerably greater attention directed toward defining, measuring, and interpreting EF in childhood in recent years (Welsh, Pennington et al., 1991; Denckla, 1996; Fletcher, 1996). It is recognized that by adapting tests (Welsh, Pennington et al., 1990) or constructing new tests with developmentally appropriate materials and test stimuli (Archibald and Kerns, 1999), one can successfully evaluate the EF of even very young children (Archibald and Kerns, 1999; Espy, Kaufmann et al., 2001). The focus on EF assessment is increasing in response to the usefulness of the EF construct in understanding the behavioral and academic profiles that present in clinical practice and as recognition increases that early intervention is often a child's best opportunity to ameliorate acquired early-onset and congenital problems.

Executive function has become a focus in studies of children and adolescents with diverse psychological and medical problems. Examples of these include studies of acquired disorder such as traumatic brain injury (Levin, Fletcher, et al., 1996), specific frontal lobe injury (Mateer and Williams, 1991), meningitis (Taylor, Schatschneider et al., 1996), and frontal lobe infarction secondary to sickle cell disease (Watkins, Hewes et al., 1998). Studies of ADHD (Barkley, 1997b), dyslexia (Helland and Asbjørnsen, 2000), and phenylketonuria, a disorder affecting frontal lobe function (Welsh, Pennington et al., 1990; Smith, Klim et al., in press) represent some of the studies of presumed congenital conditions.

The long-existent gap in measurement of EF in adolescents has also begun to narrow. Child neuropsychologists have often been confronted with weak or nonexistent normative data for the adolescent age group, a persisting problem. Yet, progress in considering the special nature of adolescence is increasingly receiving deserved attention (Barr, 2003; Anderson, Anderson et al., 2001).

EXECUTIVE FUNCTION TESTS: PLAN, ORGANIZE, REASON, SHIFT

Category Test and Wisconsin Card Sorting Test

Two tests that received considerable early attention in the child literature were the versions and modifications of the Halstead Category Test (CT; Reitan and Wolfson, 1985) for young children and older children, and the Wisconsin Card Sorting Test (WCST; Heaton, 1981). Both of these generic tests are downward extensions from tests originally developed for adults (Reitan and Davison, 1974) and, therefore, subject to criticism as such. These tests are multifactorial measures that assess more molar abilities such as judgment, reasoning, and hypothesis generation, and are recognized for their elicitation of the ability to initiate and shift. They are ubiquitous in both adult and child neuropsychological practice and are only briefly discussed here. Child normative data are available in published articles and manuals. However, some unpublished meta-normative data are included below, as are Canadian child normative data.

The CT in its different versions and the WCST are not considered interchangeable (Donders and Kirsch, 1991; Beebe, Ris et al., 2000). This is due to their differential requirements: to recall bits of information or respond based on knowledge of a rule or response strategy; to engage in repetition of the stimulus or receive corrective feedback (Donders, 1998a;b). In an adult study, Booklet Category Test (BCT) factor analyses identified perceptual-motor function and nonverbal reasoning factors, while WCST factor analyses resulted in memory and perceptual-motor ability factors. Thus, selective impairment on the BCT might be due to less ability to process novel or complex information, particularly if perceptual-motor or spatial learning is required, while WCST impairment might be due to less ability to recall information. In another study, factor analysis did load the WCST, CT, and Trail Making Test on a distinct factor (Shute and Huertas, 1990). Thus, some clinicians prefer to administer both tests, when EF discrimination is paramount.

Comparison of the CT and WCST tests has also been conducted to determine how interchangeable they are (Pendleton and Heaton, 1982). The two tests did differ in their detection of cerebral dysfunction. Conceptual requirements of the WCST were considered simpler and stimulus attributes more constant than for the CT. The authors concluded that the WCST was more sensitive to frontal than other cerebral lesions and more accurate diagnostically than the CT in their presence. The CT better identified those with focal nonfrontal or diffuse lesions. While the WCST measures perseverative tendencies, the CT was judged the more difficult measure and more sensitive to abstraction and novel concept-formation abilities.

Category Test

Descriptions of constructs assessed by the various CT versions often include concept generation, mental shifting, rule learning, or problem solving in response to external structure. The CT was originally published in 1943 and consisted of 360 figures presented in a rotating-drum apparatus. The test was later shortened to 208 figures and presented in slides on a carousel projector with a button and buzzer/bell apparatus (Reitan, 1955). The Reitan-Indiana Neuropsychological Test Battery Category Test is an 80-item version administered to young children, ages 5 to 8 years old, and the Halstead-Reitan Intermediate Category Test is a 168-item version developed for older children and adolescents, 9 to 15 years old (Knights and Tymchuk, 1968).

There are five subtests for younger and six subtests for older children. The principles underlying the five-subtest version are color recognition, relative amount of a specific color, difference in shape or size, the missing color,

and recall of prior items respectively. The principles underlying the six-subtest version are recognition of Roman numerals, number of stimuli, oddity in left to right serial position, proportion of the whole for two subtests (requiring visuospatial ability and perception of part-whole relationships), and recall of prior items respectively (Donders and Strom, 1995; Donders, 1999). Perseverative responding and response latency patterns of subtest performance also are qualitative features that have clinical importance but are not reflected in published normative data.

The original standard apparatus remains in use, although alternative administration procedures were subsequently developed, including the portable BCT version (DeFilippis & McCampbell, 1979; DeFilippis, McCampbell, & Rogers, 1979) that eliminates the cumbersome standard slide projector apparatus and a computer version of the Intermediate Category Test (Choca, Laatsch et al., 1994). A booklet short form was then developed, the Children's Category Test (CCT; Boll, 1993) for ages 5 to 16 years, 11 months, which is age-normed and co-normed with the California Verbal Learning Test—Children's Version (Delis, Kramer et al., 1994). These different versions have demonstrated equivalence with the original test instrument (McCampbell and DeFilippis, 1979; MacInnes, Forch et al., 1981; Boll, 1993).

The CCT is a booklet version of the Halstead-Reitan Category Test for Children. The normative sample consists of about an equal number of boys and girls at 12 age levels for a total of 920 children representative of the U.S. population for race/ethnicity, parental education, and geographic region. Internal consistency averages about 0.86, and the average standard error of measurement is 3.74 (Boll, 1993). The CCT has adequate internal consistency and concurrent validity (Reeder and Boll, 1992; Donders, 1996). There are two levels: The CCT-Level 1 is appropriate for those 5 to 8 years old, and the CCT-Level 2 is administered to those 9 to 15 years, 11 months old. Despite a single T score resulting from administration of the entire CCT, it was found that the two levels may vary in the constructs measured at each level. Therefore, the subtest error pattern becomes an important clinical consideration, and evidence from other neuropsychological tests supporting presumptive error patterns is valuable (Donders, 1999). A short form scoring procedure for the computer version has been described (Boll, 1993). A CCT computer software version is available, with greater reliability in administration and scoring reported for adults (Fortuny and Heaton, 1996).

The latent structure of the CCT has been examined, using the 920 children from the standardization sample divided into the respective two levels, 320 children, 5 to 8 years old, and 600 children, 9 to 16 years old. Both subgroups had a two-factor solution, although different for each subgroup, and provided support for the notion that this is a multifactorial instrument. For young children, one factor was defined by subtests II and III, i.e., principles of relative amount of a specific color and difference in shape or size. The second was defined by subtests IV and V, i.e., the missing color and recall of prior items respectively, with a moderate loading by subtest III, i.e., difference in shape or size. Subtest I, color recognition, did not load highly on either factor. The factors were moderately correlated ($r = .50$). For older children, high loadings by subtest III, i.e, oddity in left to right serial position, and a moderate loading by subtest VI, i.e., recall of prior items, defined the first factor. The second older children factor had high loadings by subtests IV and V, i.e., proportion of completion of the whole, and a moderate loading by subtest VI, i.e., recall of prior items. Subtests I and II did not load highly, i.e, recognition of Roman numerals and number of stimuli, respectively. The factors were moderately correlated ($r = .55$).

These data suggested it was clinically appropriate to consider the CCT subtest error pattern when 50% or more of the young child's total CCT errors were on subtest IV or when at least 50% of the older child's CCT errors were on subtest III or on subtests IV and V combined (Donders, 1999). These data were consistent with cluster analysis data from the standardization sample for the older children's CCT (Donders, 1998a). In a traumatic head injury (THI) population, a similar two-factor structure emerged that also highlighted the multifactorial nature of the task, suggesting that a summary total error score might be insufficient as a marker for diagnostic utility (Nesbit-Greene and Donders, 2002). Age and IQ need to be considered since a higher full-scale intelligence quotient was associated with fewer errors on the subtests that loaded on these factors, and older children made fewer errors than younger children. Only Factor I (subtests IV, V, and VI) covaried meaningfully with severity of THI.

Differential requirements of the CT and WCST were further examined from a cognitive psychology perspective (Perrine, 1993). The construct of "attribute identification," or the selection of critical features to categorize and encode conceptually in memory, was examined and compared to "rule learning," a more complex cognitive task in concept formation. Only 30% shared variance was found between the CT and WCST. While the tests are related, these data suggested that there are differences attributable to different cognitive processing demands. That is, the WCST depends more on attribute identification and is particularly sensitive to perseverative tendencies, while the CT is more dependent on rule learning and assesses manipulation of higher order concepts.

While the CT and WCST tests are commonly thought to be primarily tests of frontal lobe function in the adult literature (Milner, 1963; Drewe, 1974; Robinson, Heaton et al., 1980), such strict association cannot be made (Anderson, Damasio et al., 1991; Mountain and Snow, 1993; Axelrod, Goldman et al., 1994). In recent years, adult functional neuroimaging studies supported the importance of having intact frontal cortex for performance on such tasks (Berman, Ostrem et al., 1995; Volz, Gaser et al., 1997). The child literature is less clear, with some investigators finding poorer performance in children with frontal dysfunction (Heaton, Chelune et al., 1993; Levin, Song et al., 1997), while others did not find support for this association (Chase-Carmichael, Ris et al., 1999) and questioned their specificity (Anderson, Damasio et al., 1991).

These tests are also useful for documentation of cerebral impairment associated with psychiatric disorders, such as schizophrenia (Kolb and Whishaw, 1983; Crockett, Bilsker et al., 1986), and a study of WCST performance in children and adolescents supported its use in those with learning disability (Snow, 1998).

Developmental trajectories will differ by task (Welsh, Pennington et al., 1991) but EF functions can be documented in the very young child if developmentally appropriate tests are administered. Maturational stages are reported, particularly around 6 years, 10 years and early adolescence (Passler, Isaac et al., 1985; Levin, Culhane et al., 1991; Welsh, Pennington et al., 1991; Anderson, Anderson et al., 1996). Performance on the WCST equivalent to that of an adult was found by 10 years of age (Chelune and Baer, 1986; Welsh, Pennington et al., 1991) and by 11 to 12 years (Rosselli and Ardila, 1993). The greatest increments in EF development occurred between ages 7 and 9 years, and between 11 and 12 years (Anderson, Anderson et al., 1996). Together, these data support neurophysiological evidence of greater anterior cerebral cortex maturation around these ages. Of interest, performance commensurate with normal adults by 10 years was not found in a Taiwanese study using a computerized version of the WCST (Shu, Tien et al., 2000).

There is a higher likelihood that there will be practice effects if one is retested with multifactorial problem solving tests such as the Category Test or WCST, when the test procedures or test stimuli are no longer novel and the patient is more sophisticated in test taking (Dikmen, Heaton et al., 1999). However, in one study using the WCST, variables examined at two test sessions administered 9 months apart to brain-injured and non–brain-injured adults found only a small magnitude of change. The authors concluded that the WCST procedure was stable and suitable for repeat administration (Tate, Perdices et al., 1998). There are no similar data available on repeat administration of the WCST in children.

Older normative data sets (Knights, 1966; Spreen and Gaddes, 1969; Fromm-Auch and Yeudall, 1983) for the original CT apparatus are presented in Table 6–2. The Fromm-Auch and Yeudall data are for thirty-two 15 to 17 year olds and seventy-one 18- to 23 year olds. Their mean scores ranged widely from 16 to 68 and 9 to 106, respectively. These adolescents were part of a larger adult study whose 193 subjects had mean Wechsler IQ scores within high average limits. Disparate normative data sets were combined to obtain meta-norms for the category test.

Table 6–2. Category Test Means and SDs: Three Sources

Age	KNIGHTS DATA[a]		SPREEN & GADDES DATA		FROMM-AUCH & YEUDALL DATA	
	Mean	SD	Mean	SD	Mean	SD
5	25.4	10.0				
6	21.8	10.3				
7	19.6	9.3				
8	15.7	9.0	14.4	7.6		
9	51.3	20.2	59.5	17.7		
10	52.6	21.0	50.0	16.9		
11	49.3	14.2	43.3	18.5		
12	49.6	24.0	36.2	16.5		
13	49.6	19.1	34.6	17.2		
14	35.2	14.5	31.3	11.1		
15			30.6	12.3		
15–17					35.8	16.2
18–23					35.9	21.2

Source: Adapted from Knights (1966), Spreen & Gaddes (1969), and Fromm-Auch & Yeudall (1983), © Swets & Zeitlinger.

Findeis and Weight Meta-Norms

While normative data are available from a number of sources, several of these were combined in 1994 to obtain meta-normative data (Michael K. Findeis and David G. Weight, Brigham Young University, 1994, personal communication) for both the Reitan-Indiana Neuropsychological Test Battery (5 to 8 years old) and the Halstead Neuropsychological Test Battery for Children (9- to 14-years old). Data were collected from 20 articles published between 1965 and 1990 (see Table 6–3) with published statistical properties that allowed for a pooling of normative data for the purpose of creating metameans and standard deviations. Excluded were case studies, preliminary data reports later followed by completed research, reported duplicate results, and research that did not contain means and sample sizes. Scoring ambiguities required the exclusion of the Aphasia Screening Test, the Lateral Dominance Examination, and several of the sensory-perceptual subtests. Metameans were computed by summing the sample group means, weighting by sample size, and dividing by the total number of individuals. The mean of

Table 6–3. Articles Used by Findeis and Weight to Develop Meta-Norms

Boll (1974)
Boll, Berent & Richards (1977)
Boll & Reitan (1972)
Crockett, Klonoff, & Bjerring (1969)
Davis, Adams, Gates, & Cheramie (1989)
Finlayson & Reitan (1976)
Frisch & Handler (1974)
Hughes (1976)
Ingram (1975)
Klonoff & Low (1974)
Maiuro, Townes, Vitaliano, & Trupin, (1984)
Nici & Reitan (1986)
Reitan (1971b)
Reitan (1986)
Reitan (1987)
Sachs, Krall & Drayton (1982)
Selz & Reitan (1979b)
Spreen & Gaddes (1969)
Teeter (1985)
Townes, Trupin, Martin, & Goldstein, (1980).

Source: Unpublished data, courtesy of M. Findeis & D. Weight (1994).

means was represented as $\acute{O}(nx)/\acute{O}(n)$, where x and n are the mean and sample size, respectively. Metastandard deviations were obtained by summing the sum of squares, dividing by the N of the metasample, and extracting the square root. When the sample means are combined into a group mean, the between samples variance is eliminated, leaving only the samples within error variance. The combined average standard deviation was represented as: $\% \ \acute{O}((n)s^2)/\acute{O}(n)$ where n and s are sample size and sample standard deviation squared, respectively.

The final selection included data for 33 subtests and scales from the Indiana-Reitan and Halstead-Reitan test batteries. The total subject size N of 3,225 included 910 males and 805 females (53% of the total N) and 1510 of unspecified gender (47%). Most subjects represented in the normal or control groups were Caucasian, from middle- to upper-middle-class socioeconomic backgrounds, were volunteered by their parents for study, and were identified as being free from any history of neurological abnormalities. The average full-scale IQ was 112.87. The demographic data of the meta-analysis are presented in Table 6–4. These unpublished meta-norms for the CT for children 5 to 14 years old are presented in Table 6–5, along with means and SD for each total age group, i.e. 5 to 8 years old and 9 to 14 years old. Additional meta-normative data from this study are included for the Reitan Indiana Neuropsychological Test Battery Color Form and Progressive Figures Tests and for the Trail Making Test in Chapter 7, for the Speech Sounds Perception Test and Rhythm Test in Chapter 8, for the Finger Tapping Test, Grip Strength Test, and Tactual Performance Test in Chapter 9, for the Matching Figures, Match-

Table 6–4. Findeis & Weight Meta-Normative Study: Demographic Characteristics

Subjects: 3,225 children
Age: 5 to 14 years
Gender: 910 male; 802 female; 1510 unknown (47%)
IQ: average = 112.87
Race: Mostly Caucasian
SES: Mostly middle to upper-middle class
Inclusion criteria: No neurological abnormalities

Table 6–5. Meta-Norms: Category Test Number of Errors

Age	N	Mean	SD
5	216	27.40	9.1
6	202	26.00	12.7
7	244	20.56	8.9
8	221	12.35	6.7
9	129	53.56	17.4
10	216	46.58	18.6
11	213	40.88	16.3
12	226	35.12	16.0
13	112	36.29	16.4
14	114	30.81	12.0
5 to 8	542	16.62	9.8
9 to 14	422	39.0	15.1

Note: Ages 5 to 8 = 80 items; 9 to 14 = 168 items

Source: Unpublished data, courtesy of M. Findeis & D. Weight (1994).

ing V's, Star, Concentric Squares and Matching Pictures tests in Chapter 10, and for the Target Test in Chapter 11.

Wisconsin Card Sorting Test

The Wisconsin Card Sorting Test (WCST) was developed as a measure of "flexibility in thinking" (Berg, 1948). It is widely recognized as a measure of concept generation, cognitive set shifting (Milner, 1963), the ability to inhibit prepotent responses, attribute identification, abstract reasoning, hypothesis testing and problem solving, and sustained attention. Recent factor structure and construct validity studies (Greve, Brooks et al., 1997) generally identified a 3-factor structure. Factor 1 reflects an executive function factor or perseveration component, including primarily response inflexibility as derived from perseverative errors, perseverative responses, and total number of errors scores, and secondarily disrupted problem solving as derived from percent conceptual level responses, number of categories completed, and total number correct scores. Factor 2 reflects an ineffective hypothesis-testing strategy in the absence of perseveration (a concept formation component) and is often absent in high-functioning persons. This factor has high loading for nonperseverative errors and

moderate loadings for percent conceptual level responses, number of categories completed, and total number correct scores. Factor 3, a failure-to-maintain set component, measures the ability to maintain correct responding when the correct sorting principle is determined, with high failure-to-maintain set and fewer number of categories completed scores (Greve, 2001). It has particular interest to clinicians as a test that elicits perseverative responses and failures to maintain mental set in the presence of competing stimuli.

The WCST was standardized for clinical use after years of research application (Heaton, 1981). It is a sensitive clinical and research measure for diverse medical and neuropsychological disorders that affect executive and other cognitive functions and has commonly been interpreted as a measure of frontal lobe function (Robinson, Heaton, et al. 1980). The first study to provide WCST normative data for children and simultaneously examine normal development of the cognitive abilities demanded by this test found that children's performances were indistinguishable from that of adults by the time they reached 10 years (Chelune and Baer, 1986). The demographic data and normative data are provided in Table 6–6 and Table 6–7, respectively, and in an updated manual (Heaton, Chelune et al., 1993). These data corresponded well with those showing that focused attention and inhibition of perseveratory tendencies on tasks adapted from Luria were just about complete by 10 years of age (Passler, Isaac et al., 1985). The WCST measured such "adult-like" constructs by the age of 9 or 10 as response accuracy, failure to self-monitor, and learning (Kizilbash and Donders, 1999). A reduction in perseverative errors on

Table 6–6. Wisconsin Card Sorting Test Demographic Data: Chelune & Baer Study (1986)

Subjects: 105 children in grades 1 through 6
Age: 6 to 12 years
Gender: 53 males; 52 females
IQ: Mean PPVT IQ of 108.3 (13.6)
Handedness: 12 left-handers (11.4%)
Race: Not specified
SES: Not specified
Inclusion Criteria: In a regular class; no exclusion for academic or medical reasons

Table 6–7. Wisconsin Card Sorting Test Means and *SD*s: Chelune & Baer Data

Age	*n*	Categories Achieved	Perseverative Errors	Failures to Maintain Set
6	11	2.73 (2.10)	40.64 (28.03)	1.64 (2.01)
7	14	4.07 (1.94)	25.07 (18.43)	1.93 (1.21)
8	22	4.05 (2.01)	23.18 (13.23)	1.82 (1.26)
9	16	4.81 (1.47)	18.13 (11.55)	1.75 (1.53)
10	20	5.60 (.75)	13.95 (6.50)	1.00 (1.02)
11	12	5.58 (.79)	15.17 (13.49)	1.17 (1.11)
12	10	5.70 (.95)	12.30 (16.94)	.70 (.68)

Source: Chelune & Baer (1986), © Swets & Zeitlinger.

the WCST occured between 7 and 13 years (Chelune and Baer, 1986; Levin, Culhane et al., 1991; Kelly, 2000).

As noted in the Preface, it is inappropriate to rigidly apply lessons learned from adult studies to children. The WCST provides a good example. While studies of adults generally support the idea that the WCST is especially sensitive to frontal lobe dysfunction (Milner, 1963), and positron emission tomography study found the right dorsolateral frontal—subcortical circuit especially critical (Lombardi, Andreason et al., 1999), studies with children provided mixed results. Timing of brain maturation affects when one can presume that a child's frontal lobes, especially the dorsolateral prefrontal areas, are sufficiently mature to be mediating responses to this type of task. These developmental considerations are critical. The ability of the WCST to detect frontal lobe dysfunction is a subject of study in the child literature. For example, in one study, the WCST failed to find more impaired performance in children with frontal lesions than for those with extrafrontal or multifocal/diffuse lesions. Also, lesion lateralization analyses did not find more impairment in left than right lesion groups (Chase-Carmichael, Ris et al., 1999).

A shortened 64-card version, the Wisconsin Card Sorting Test-64 (WCST–64), was published (Kongs, Thompson et al., 2000) and reviewed (Greve, 2001). Normative data are available for those 6 years, 6 months, to 85 years old, with age-corrected norms given for children below age 20. The 3-factor structure described above was reported in the WCST-64

manual for child normative, child lesion, and child diagnostic subsamples. While the WCST-64 appears to be comparable to the WCST (Greve, 2001), and therefore advantageous as a short form, some caution has been advised. Adequate correlation and accuracy scores were obtained for census-based norms for the WCST and WCST-64, but WCST-64 demographically adjusted standardized scores were not comparable to the full WCST scores in adults (Axelrod, 2001). Also, strong practice effects are associated with the WCST, and two evaluations of neurologically normal adult males over 12 months with the WCST-64 found significant improvement on indices of number of categories completed, perseverative errors, percent perseverative errors, and learning-to-learn (Basso, Lowery et al., 2001).

Clinically, the option of the WCST-64 is a positive development. It makes the test all that more appealing for use with the younger children, especially those who may well experience difficulty. The less-prolonged administration means the child has that much less time to experience the complex nature of the task or become frustrated, and the examiner does not lose valuable information inherent to this test. As a result, my concern about administering the standard version to a child with probable EF disorder is better addressed by the ability to tap the same functions under considerably less stressful circumstances. The number of perseverative errors made by 7 to 12-year-old children (*N* of 10 per age level) is reported as part of a larger study of executive function in childhood (Welsh, Pennington et al., 1991).

Table 6–8. Wisconsin Card Sorting Test
Demographic Data: Rosselli and Ardila
Study (1993)

Subjects: 233 children in Colombia, South America
Age: 5 to 12 years
Gender: 119 Males; 114 females
Handedness: 220 right-handed; 13 left-handed
Race: Not specified
Inclusion criteria: No physical handicap

Cross-cultural normative data for the WCST are available for some populations. Developmental norms for 233 5- to 12-year-old Colombian children were reported (Rosselli and Ardila, 1993). The demographic data for this study are presented in Table 6–8. Computerized administration is also possible, and such data were published for a Taiwanese sample of 219 children (Shu et al., 2000). It is of interest that standard vs. computerized WCST administrations were compared in North American and Spanish normal adults and yielded similar results (Artiola i Fortuny and Heaton, 1996). Canadian child normative data are presented below (Paniak, Miller et al., 1996).

A number of alternative test administration strategies exist. For children, both standard or abbreviated administrations are supported by normative data. For the standard administration, four stimulus cards are placed in front of the child, and two sets of 64 response cards become the child's deck. The child must match each consecutive response card to the examiner's stimulus cards according to the principle they devise. The child is told if he or she is right or wrong for each response without being told the active principle. The child is unaware that the sorting principle is changed at a designated time and that he or she must adjust the sorting accordingly. The criterion is six complete correct sorts or until all 128 cards are attempted. For the WCST-64 administration, four stimulus cards are placed in front of the child, and one set of 64 response cards becomes the child's deck. The criterion is six complete correct sorts or termination when all 64 cards are attempted. The shorter WCST-64 has great salience for child assessment and is my preferred administration procedure.

The WCST (Heaton, Chelune et al., 1993) and WCST-64 (Kongs, Thompson et al., 2000)

manuals present specific administration and scoring guidelines. Empiric studies have shown some scores to be more useful than others. Perseverative errors on the WCST, for example, suggest difficulty inhibiting previous response patterns and shifting to a new response set (Anderson, Anderson et al., 2000). The perseveration score is considered especially useful but initially complicated to derive. How to score perseveration is explained both in text (Flashman, Horner et al., 1991) and in a diagrammatic procedure (Berry, 1996), and the WCST manual instructions are further explicated with a computer scoring program (Flashman, Mandir et al., 1991). Computer version scoring systems are available for both the WCST and the WCST-64 (Heaton, 1999; 2000). Repetition errors are one index of the failure to self-monitor well. Field dependency is a related behavior strongly associated with adults who have frontal lobe syndromes. The patient finds it difficult to control behavior and responds to the environmental context or internal associations. For example, when asked to draw a circle, the patient draws a flower and persists in drawing a flower whenever drawing a circle is requested.

Normative data for 685 Canadian children, 9 to 14 years old, were published for the standard 128-card WCST (Paniak, Miller et al., 1996). Demographic data for this study are presented in Table 6–9. Normative data for four selected test scores are presented in Table 6–10 and data for test scores and percentile range on skewed variables of number of categories completed, trials to complete first category, and failure to maintain set in Table 6–11.

Table 6–9. Wisconsin Card Sorting Test
Demographic Data: Paniak Study (1996)

Subjects: 685 children volunteers in Edmonton,
  Alberta, Canada.
Age: 9 to 14 years
Gender: 309 male; 376 female
Handedness: Not specified
Race: Not specified
SES: Not specified
Inclusion criteria: Attending regular classes, not in
  English as a Second Language (ESL) class or a self-
  contained special education class, no history of brain
  disease or injury, no behavior problems for which the
  child was hospitalized

Table 6–10. Wisconsin Card Sorting Test Means and *SDs*: Paniak et al. Data

Age	N	Errors	Perseverative Responses	Nonperseverative Errors	Perseverative Errors
9	80	43.79 (18.04)	26.76 (16.25)	20.34 (10.92)	23.45 (3.08)
10	140	41.44 (19.25)	24.66 (14.64)	19.31 (10.55)	21.94 (11.90)
11	131	38.25 (19.53)	20.64 (12.39)	19.15 (12.41)	18.78 (10.49)
12	123	30.12 (17.50)	17.61 (12.69)	14.30 (9.37)	15.81 (10.52)
13	96	27.95 (15.96)	15.70 (10.66)	13.66 (8.45)	14.29 (9.15)
14	115	24.13 (15.41)	12.89 (8.96)	12.33 (9.40)	11.80 (7.41)

Source: Paniak, Miller, Murphy, Patterson & Keizer (1996)

Table 6–11. Wisconsin Card Sorting Test Scores on Skewed Variables

Age	WCST VARIABLES			
	Percentiles	# Categories	TTF	FMS
9	>16	4–6	10–17	0–2
	11–16	2–3	18–22	3
	6–10	2	23–25	3–4
	2–5	1–2	36–78	4–5
	<1	0–1	79–128	6–21
10	>16	4–6	10–17	0–2
	11–16	2–3	18–21	2–3
	6–10	2	22–37	3
	2–5	2	38–51	4
	<1	0–1	52–128	5–21
11	>16	4–6	10–14	0–1
	11–16	3	15–19	2–3
	6–10	2–3	20–25	3
	2–5	1–2	32–63	3–4
	<1	0–1	64–128	5–21
12	>16	5–6	10–12	0–1
	11–16	4	13–16	2
	6–10	2–4	17–19	2–3
	2–5	2	20–38	3
	<1	0–1	39–128	4–21
13	>16	5–6	10–12	0–1
	11–16	4	13–15	2–3
	6–10	4	16–22	3
	2–5	3–4	23–31	3–5
	<1	0–2	32–128	6–21
14	>16	6	10–15	0–1
	11–16	4–5	16–18	1–2
	6–10	4	19–21	2
	2–5	3–4	22–39	3–4
	<1	0–3	40–128	4–21

Note: TTF = Trials to Complete First Category; FMS = Failure to Maintain Set
Source: Paniak et al. (1996)

Contingency Naming Test

The Contingency Naming Test (CNT) (Taylor, 1987, #725) was modeled after the Stroop Color Word Test (SCWT; Stroop, 1935) and is a measure of the ability to inhibit, but also to switch, mental set. It relies on color and shape stimuli and is distinguished from other similar Stroop-like tasks because it makes no demands on literacy and word knowledge. The CNT assesses rapid memory retrieval abilities (Taylor, Albo et al., 1987), reactive flexibility, and name retrieval speed in school-aged children (Anderson, Anderson et al., 2000) and is sensitive to brain injury sequelae in childhood (Taylor, Albo et al., 1987; Taylor, Schatschneider et al., 1991). These functions are believed to be mediated in humans through a frontal-striatal network that includes the prefrontal cortex and the basal ganglia (Eslinger and Grattan, 1993).

The CNT and its easily specified shift component appears to be superior to the WCST as a measure of shifting (Fletcher, 1998). Factor analysis also found the CNT loading on a speculative factor of response speed or psychomotor efficiency (Taylor, Schatschneider et al., 1996), along with the paper and pencil WISC-R coding subtest and a paper-and-pencil visual search test. It was included in studies of a number of clinical populations, including bacterial meningitis (Taylor, Barry et al., 1993; Taylor, Schatschneider et al., 1996; Taylor, Schatschneider et al., 2000; Grimwood, Anderson et al., 2000), acute lymphocytic leukemia (Taylor, Albo et al., 1987), and low birth weight (Taylor, Hack et al., 1995; 1998). Data suggest that the reactive flexibility inherent to success on this task is mediated by a frontal-striatal network, implicating the prefrontal region and the basal ganglia (Eslinger and Grattan, 1993). Of related interest, the striatal contribution to category learning was investigated in Parkinson's disease patients, and results reinforced the notion that there are multiple categorization systems likely mediated by different neural networks. The striatum was implicated in the learning of complex nonverbalizable nonlinear categorization rules but did not appear involved in learning simple linear categorization rules. These rules were learned by amnesic patients and therefore did not ap-

pear to involve declarative memory systems (Maddox and Filoteo, 2001).

The CNT requires the child to name a series of colored shapes by their color or shape, according to a specified naming rule. Each shape contains a smaller inside shape. Sometimes the inside and outside shapes are the same, and sometimes they are different. For simple rules, the child names the color or shape of each design while ignoring the other dimension. Part 1 requires the child to name only the colors; for Part 2 the child names only the outside shapes. For complex rules, the child names the color or shape contingent on other dimensions. For example, the child might need to name a color when the primary shape matches the smaller shape within it, and name the primary shape when this is not the case. Thus, Part 3 has the contingency that requires the child to name the color if the outside and inside shapes match, and to name the outside shape if the two shapes do not match. For Part 4, the child applies the same naming rule as in Part 3, but when a backward arrow appears over the stimuli, the child responds to a reverse contingency, e.g., name the color, not the shape (Taylor, Schatschneider et al., 1996). A learning phase begins each part. The child is given up to five trials to learn the rule. The criterion is errorless performance on one trial or completion of the five training trials. Part 4 might be omitted for young children. In this case, the test can be scored for naming time for Parts 1 and 2 (name retrieval speed) and for error rate increase in Part 3, compared to Parts 1 and 2 (mental set shifting).

Preliminary normative data with a maximum of 24 children per age group (H. G. Taylor 1987, personal communication; see Table 6–12) are supplemented by more recent data obtained on a sample of Australian children (Anderson, Anderson et al., 2000). Demographic data are presented in Table 6–13. The developmental normative data for errors are presented in Table 6–14, for self-correction in Table 6–15, for self-regulation in Table 6–16, and for age group and gender on time and efficiency variables in Table 7–17.

Strong age effects for accuracy and speed were found, with substantial improvement noted between 7 and 9 years old and less pro-

Table 6–12. Contingency Naming Test Means and *SD*s: Taylor Data

	Age	N	Mean	SD
Self-corrections	6.0–7.5	6	7.00	3.84
plus errors:	7.6–8.11	11	3.63	3.77
Parts 1 and 2	9.0–10.11	25	2.32	2.54
	11.0–12.11	24	1.87	1.54
	13.0–14.11	18	1.50	1.54
	15.0–16.11	13	1.69	1.65
Self-corrections	6.0–7.5	5	34.00	16.80
plus errors:	7.6–8.11	11	24.72	11.48
Parts 3 and 4	9.0–0.11	24	12.66	8.31
	11.0–12.11	24	12.95	8.34
	13.0–14.11	18	7.88	5.33
	15.0–16.11	13	7.46	5.07
Time: A	6.0–7.5	6	75.16	21.38
Parts 1 and 2	7.6–8.11	11	58.81	13.11
	9.0–10.11	25	47.08	9.47
	11.0–12.11	24	41.04	9.01
	13.0–14.11	18	34.61	5.05
	15.0–16.11	13	32.69	5.83
Time: B	6.0–7.5	5	193.00	43.07
Parts 3 and 4	7.6–8.11	11	148.63	28.47
	9.0–10.11	24	132.08	26.90
	11.0–12.11	24	117.54	21.25
	13.0–14.11	18	95.77	18.70
	15.0–16.11	13	105.33	31.20

Source: Courtesy of H. G. Taylor, personal communication.

nounced gains at older ages along with steady speed increments across all ages, particularly for those 7 and 11 to 13 years old (Anderson, Anderson et al., 2000). These authors also reported on another study, establishing validity data. The latter study included clinical populations of children with phenylketonuria (PKU), bacterial meningitis (BM), and acute lymphoblastic leukemia (ALL) and found that these groups differed from a clinical control group of

79 healthy children, supporting the CNT as a test sensitive to cognitive impairment.

The PKU and ALL groups were slower and less accurate than the control group, and the BM group made more errors than controls on two-dimensional shifting. Comparisons of the clinical groups found the PKU group slower than ALL and BM on trials 3 and 4 (requiring shifting), the ALL group making the most errors and the least self-corrections, and the BM group doing well on trials 1 to 3, but not on trial 4. Also, for adolescents, trials 1 and 2 (naming) were sensitive to deficits in speed of name retrieval and shifting tasks identified group differences in both accuracy and speed (Anderson, Anderson et al., 2000).

Table 6–13. Contingency Naming Test Demographic Data: Australian Sample

Subjects: 381 children in Australia
Gender: 189 male; 192 female
Age: 7.0 to 15 years
IQ: range = 101.7 to 110.3; average = 106.3
Race: Not reported
SES: Mainly low to middle SES (34% low, 49% middle, 17% upper SES)
Exclusion criteria: IQ below 80

Source: Anerson, Anderson, Northam, & Taylor (2000)

Concept Generation Test

Concept generation and sorting behavior in very young children have long been difficult to partition out from other contributory functions inherent in most of the commonly used tasks

Table 6–14. Contingency Naming Test—Errors: Anderson et al. Data

Age (years)	7	8	9	10	11	12	13	14	15
N	22	34	26	49	59	60	50	37	44
Trial 1									
1 or more errors (%)	27	15	4	4	14	7	8	5	7
3 or more errors (%)	14	0	0	0	0	0	0	0	0
No. errors (90th percentile)	2.9	1.0	0	0	1.0	0	0	0	0
Trial 2									
1 or more errors (%)	14	17	12	8	9	12	4	3	7
3 or more errors (%)	5	6	0	0	0	0	0	0	0
No. errors (90th percentile)	1.0	1.0	1.0	0	0	1.0	0	0	0
Trial 3									
1 or more errors (%)	64	44	35	33	39	38	36	30	33
3 or more errors (%)	27	9	4	8	10	7	6	3	9
No. errors (90th percentile)	8.8	2.0	1.0	2.0	2.1	2.0	2.0	1.2	2.6
Trial 4									
1 or more errors (%)	90	85	69	76	69	73	74	57	70
3 or more errors (%)	75	52	27	41	33	37	26	14	19
No. errors (90th percentile)	17.6	9.6	5.9	6.0	6.0	6.0	4.99	3.2	4.6
Total									
1 or more errors (%)	95	91	77	84	81	83	80	76	84
3 or more errors (%)	73	62	42	47	42	45	42	19	36
No. errors (90th percentile)	26.1	12.0	6.6	8.0	7.1	7.9	6.9	4.0	6.0

Source: Anderson, Anderson, Northam and Taylor, personal communication (2002), updating Anderson, Anderson et al. (2000).

Table 6–15. Contingency Naming Test—Self-Corrections: Anderson et al. Data

Age (years)	7	8	9	10	11	12	13	14	15
N	22	34	26	49	59	60	50	37	44
Trial 1									
1 or more self-corrections (%)	50	35	27	37	49	40	22	24	27
No. self-corrections (90th percentile)	1.9	2.0	2.0	2.0	2.0	1.9	1.9	1.0	1.0
Trial 2									
1 or more self-corrections (%)	59	56	54	37	41	30	36	22	32
No. self-corrections (90th percentile)	2.9	2.0	2.3	2.0	2.0	1.0	1.9	1.0	1.6
Trial 3									
1 or more self-corrections (%)	59	82	85	71	59	67	72	54	67
No. self-corrections (90th percentile)	5.7	4.0	4.6	4.0	4.1	2.9	3.0	2.2	3.0
Trial 4									
1 or more self-corrections (%)	80	61	81	71	77	68	80	70	70
No. self-corrections (90th percentile)	4.9	4.0	4.3	4.0	5.0	3.0	3.0	3.2	3.0
Total									
1 or more self-corrections (%)	95	94	92	94	93	92	94	78	95
No. self-corrections (90th percentile)	13.5	10.2	10.5	11.0	10.0	6.9	7.0	6.2	7.0

Source: Anderson, Anderson, Northam and Taylor, personal communication (2002), updating Anderson, Anderson et al. (2000) published data.

Table 6–16. Contingency Naming Test—Self-Regulation: Anderson et al. Data

Age (years)	7	8	9	10	11	12	13	14	15
N	22	34	26	49	59	60	50	37	44
Trial 1									
Self-regulation score (median)	1	0	0	0	1	0	0	0	0
Self-regulation (90th percentile)	6.8	3.0	2.0	2.0	3.0	2.0	2.0	2.0	2.0
Trial 2									
Self-regulation score (median)	1	1	1	0	0	0	0	0	0
Self-regulation (90th percentile)	4.8	3.6	3.3	2.0	2.0	2.0	2.0	1.0	2.0
Trial 3									
Self-regulation score (median)	3	3	3	2	2	2	2	2	2
Self-regulation (90th percentile)	18.9	8.0	6.3	7.0	7.0	5.0	6.0	6.0	6.0
Trial 4									
Self-regulation score (median)	15.5	8	5	5	5	5	4.5	3	4
Self-regulation (90th percentile)	36.2	20.6	13.2	13.0	13.1	13.9	10.8	8.4	10.0
Total									
Self-regulation score (median)	28.5	15	9.5	8	9.5	9	8	5	7
Self-regulation (90th percentile)	55.9	32.2	17.3	21.0	23.1	20.9	17.0	11.2	16.6

Source: Anderson, Anderson, Northam and Taylor, personal communication (2002), updating Anderson, Anderson et al. (2000) published data.

that purport to measure these functions. For example, the Raven's Progressive Matrices Tests depend on visual perception, the WCST depends on recall, and the CNT depends on naming skill. Efforts are being made in a number of laboratories to address these executive functions more specifically. Among the tests that have been developed or adapted for young children is the Concept Generation Test for Children (CGT-C; Jacobs, Anderson et al., 2001), which was adapted from an adult version (Levine, Stuss et al., 1995) to attempt these finer delineations of cognitive processes. The original adult task incorporates three conditions, with successively increasing structure. The individual sorts six black-and-white diagrams, which each contain the name of an animal and a figure, according to a common feature. The requirement is that each group contains three items. Six predetermined groupings include animal habitat, animal domestication, direction of lines, location of writing, inside shape, and size of the inside shape.

The adaptation for children required a change to concepts more familiar to young children, i.e., animals, colors, shapes. The child must sort six stimulus cards with both pictorial and verbal information. There are seven predetermined conceptual groupings: animal habitat, color of the card outline, card shape, direction of lines, animal size, writing size (capital or lower case), and location of writing on the card. The three performance levels provide increased levels of structure: free generation, identification of the category constructed by the examiner, and cued generation when the rule was provided.

The CGT-C was administered to 105 children (47 males, 58 females) aged 7 to 15 years, 9 months old, with no history of neurologic or psychiatric disorder, from metropolitan Australian primary and secondary schools (see Table 6–18). They were in mainstream educational placements, and English was the first language. Three age groups were constructed to reflect anatomical growth spurts in the frontal lobes: 7.0 to 8.1 years (Group 1), 9.0 to 11.11 years (Group 2), and 12.0 to 15.11 years (Group 3). Data from this study suggested that there may be an important spurt in conceptual reasoning skills around 9 to 10 years of age. No significant group differences were found for either gender or IQ. The expected developmental trends of more efficient strategizing

Table 6-17. Contingency Naming Test Means and SDs for Age Group and Gender for Time and Efficiency

Age	TRIAL 1		TRIAL 2		TRIAL 3		TRIAL 4		TOTAL	
	Time M(SD)	Efficiency M(SD)	Time M(SD)	Efficiency M(SD)	Time M(SD)	Efficiency M(SD)	Time M(SD)	Efficiency M(SD)	Time M(SD)	Efficiency M(SD)
7 yr (n = 22)	28.9(6.3)	3.2(1.1)	44.2(14.2)	2.4(0.8)	77.8(16.8)	0.9(0.4)	91.3(19.3)	0.5(0.3)	241.8(28.5)	0.2(0.1)
Male (n = 7)	29.1(6.0)	3.0(1.0)	48.7(19.4)	2.2(1.1)	85.0(24.2)	0.7(0.3)	88.2(15.1)	0.4(0.1)	254.2(27.9)	0.1(0.1)
Female (n = 15)	28.8(6.7)	3.4(1.2)	42.1(11.2)	2.5(0.7)	74.4(11.7)	1.1(0.4)	92.3(20.9)	0.5(0.3)	237.6(28.4)	0.2(0.1)
8 yr (n = 34)	24.8(5.2)	4.0(1.0)	37.8(13.3)	2.7(1.0)	65.1(13.0)	1.3(0.4)	80.2(19.7)	0.7(0.3)	205.0(31.4)	0.2(0.1)
Male (n = 18)	25.6(5.8)	3.8(1.0)	40.9(15.4)	2.5(1.0)	65.9(12.6)	1.4(0.4)	80.8(19.5)	0.8(0.3)	208.2(28.4)	0.2(0.1)
Female (n = 16)	23.9(4.6)	4.2(0.9)	34.3(9.9)	3.0(1.0)	64.3(13.7)	1.3(0.4)	79.6(20.6)	0.7(0.3)	202.1(34.7)	0.2(0.1)
9 yr (n = 26)	21.7(4.2)	4.7(1.0)	28.3(8.0)	3.7(1.0)	57.3(11.2)	1.6(0.5)	75.2(13.8)	1.0(0.4)	182.6(28.2)	0.4(0.2)
Male (n = 15)	22.9(4.2)	4.5(0.8)	30.7(8.6)	3.3(0.8)	58.3(11.2)	1.5(0.4)	74.7(15.0)	1.0(0.4)	186.5(29.4)	0.3(0.1)
Female (n = 11)	20.4(4.0)	5.0(1.1)	25.0(5.8)	4.1(1.1)	56.0(11.6)	1.7(0.6)	76.0(12.6)	0.9(0.5)	177.2(26.9)	0.4(0.2)
10 yr (n = 49)	20.7(3.9)	5.0(1.0)	27.1(6.8)	3.8(1.0)	52.9(11.2)	1.7(0.5)	74.8(18.6)	0.9(0.5)	175.5(31.4)	0.4(0.2)
Male (n = 21)	21.4(3.4)	4.8(0.8)	29.6(7.9)	3.5(1.0)	53.3(11.4)	1.7(0.5)	75.9(18.4)	0.9(0.5)	180.1(29.8)	0.3(0.2)
Female (n = 28)	20.1(4.2)	5.1(1.1)	25.2(5.2)	4.1(0.9)	52.7(11.3)	1.8(0.6)	74.0(19.0)	1.0(0.4)	172.0(32.6)	0.4(0.2)
11 yr (n = 59)	19.5(4.0)	5.1(1.1)	24.0(5.2)	4.2(1.0)	50.7(11.9)	1.8(0.6)	72.7(20.8)	1.0(0.5)	166.8(36.4)	0.4(0.2)
Male (n = 29)	20.4(4.3)	4.8(1.1)	24.0(6.0)	4.3(1.1)	51.1(12.2)	1.8(0.6)	72.6(23.0)	1.1(0.5)	168.2(39.6)	0.4(0.2)
Female (n = 30)	18.5(3.5)	5.4(1.0)	24.0(4.5)	4.2(0.9)	50.4(11.9)	1.7(0.6)	72.7(18.7)	1.0(0.5)	165.3(33.4)	0.4(0.2)
12 yr (n = 60)	18.4(3.3)	5.5(1.1)	22.6(6.4)	4.5(1.1)	47.3(10.5)	1.9(0.6)	65.6(15.3)	1.1(0.5)	153.8(29.0)	0.4(0.2)
Male (n = 30)	18.9(3.6)	5.5(0.9)	24.8(8.0)	4.1(1.1)	48.2(12.3)	2.0(0.6)	63.6(14.7)	1.1(0.5)	155.5(32.9)	0.4(0.2)
Female (n = 30)	17.9(2.9)	5.5(1.2)	20.4(3.0)	4.9(0.9)	46.3(8.5)	1.9(0.7)	67.5(15.8)	1.0(0.5)	152.1(24.9)	0.4(0.2)
13 yr (n = 50)	16.5(4.6)	6.2(1.4)	20.9(5.4)	5.0(1.2)	44.6(11.0)	2.1(0.7)	61.3(16.2)	1.2(0.6)	143.3(32.9)	0.5(0.2)
Male (n = 28)	17.8(5.6)	5.8(1.5)	21.9(5.8)	4.8(1.1)	46.2(10.8)	2.0(0.6)	63.2(16.4)	1.2(0.6)	149.0(34.4)	0.5(0.2)
Female (n = 22)	15.0(2.2)	6.7(1.1)	19.8(4.7)	5.1(1.3)	42.6(11.2)	2.2(0.8)	58.8(16.0)	1.3(0.6)	136.1(30.0)	0.5(0.2)
14 yr (n = 37)	16.8(3.2)	6.0(1.1)	21.4(6.0)	4.9(1.0)	41.9(7.4)	2.2(0.5)	58.9(12.2)	1.4(0.5)	139.1(22.0)	0.5(0.2)
Male (n = 21)	17.8(3.4)	5.6(1.1)	22.0(3.9)	4.7(0.8)	44.1(7.4)	2.1(0.5)	60.9(12.9)	1.3(0.4)	144.8(19.9)	0.5(0.2)
Female (n = 16)	15.6(2.6)	6.6(1.0)	20.7(8.0)	5.1(1.2)	39.0(6.4)	2.4(0.5)	56.4(11.2)	1.4(0.5)	131.6(22.9)	0.5(0.2)
15 yr (n = 44)	15.9(2.8)	6.3(1.1)	18.6(3.9)	5.4(1.0)	41.3(12.3)	2.3(0.7)	57.2(20.1)	1.4(0.6)	133.4(34.3)	0.5(0.2)
Male (n = 20)	16.8(3.0)	5.8(1.1)	19.6(3.9)	5.2(0.9)	45.6(15.7)	2.1(0.8)	59.9(26.6)	1.3(0.6)	143.2(45.2)	0.4(0.2)
Female (n = 24)	15.2(2.4)	6.7(1.0)	17.8(3.8)	5.6(0.9)	38.1(7.9)	2.4(0.7)	55.1(13.1)	1.4(0.6)	126.1(21.5)	0.6(0.2)
Total (n = 381)	19.6(5.3)	5.3(1.4)	25.6(10.1)	4.2(1.3)	51.0(14.8)	1.8(0.7)	69.0(19.7)	1.1(0.5)	164.5(41.3)	0.4(0.2)
Male (n = 189)	20.2(5.2)	5.1(1.3)	26.8(11.0)	4.1(1.3)	52.0(15.1)	1.8(0.6)	68.7(19.8)	1.1(0.5)	166.5(40.8)	0.4(0.2)
Female (n = 192)	18.9(5.3)	5.5(1.5)	24.4(9.0)	4.4(1.3)	50.1(14.5)	1.9(0.7)	69.2(19.6)	1.1(0.5)	162.5(41.8)	0.4(0.2)

Source: Anderson, Anderson, Northam and Taylor, personal communication (2002), updating Anderson, Anderson et al. (2000) published data.

Table 6–18. Concept Generation Test Demographic Characteristics: Jacobs et al. Study (2001)

Subjects: 105 Australian children.
Age: 7 to 15 years
Gender: 58 male; 47 female
Handedness: Not specified
Race: Not specified
SES: Not specified
Inclusion criteria: No history of neurologic or psychiatric disorder; mainstream educational placement; English as the first language.

and higher scores for the older age children were found. This result has significant implications for this test's potential to discriminate performances of younger and older children and, therefore, its usefulness in monitoring recovery from childhood neurologic insult. The CGT-C normative data are presented in Table 6–19, by age group.

A similar task that has only two conditions is now part of the Delis-Kaplan Executive Function System (Delis, Kaplan et al., 2001). This sorting test has applicable normative data, beginning at 8 years old. The same stimuli are used for adults and children. The child must sort six cards in as many ways as possible, placing three cards in each of two groups for each trial. There are three possible verbal sorts (semantic category, mode of transport, and linguistic structure) and five perceptual sorts

(based on aspects of dimension, form, and appearance). Condition 1 is free sorting. Sorting time is recorded. For Condition 2, sort recognition, the child must determine the concepts used by the examiner who sorts the cards into two groups of three cards each on eight trials.

Tower of Hanoi

The Tower of Hanoi (TOH) is a three-disk or four-disk transfer task (Simon, 1975) that is considered a test of working memory, planning, rule application, and behavioral inhibition. The task requires the child to place five disks of different size onto one of three equally sized posts from a prearranged configuration. The largest disk must be on the bottom, and the blocks decrease consecutively in size until the smallest is on top. The rules allow for movement of only one disk at a time, and a bigger disk cannot be placed on top of smaller disk. There are computerized and noncomputerized versions of the TOH. One computerized version for adults was developed for the U. S. Military Personnel Assessment Battery (Reeves, Kane et al., 1994), and another computerized version was used with children 4 to 8 years old (Luciana and Nelson, 1998). However, preliminary data suggested a standard apparatus version was easier for children (Bishop, Aamodt-Leeper et al., 2001).

Developmental data are reported in a study using the TOH and other tests, conducted on 100 normal preschool children without learn-

Table 6–19. Summary Scores for Concept Generation Test

	SUMMARY SCORES FOR CGT-C: MEAN (SD)		
	Group 1	Group 2	Group 3
No. correct free sorts generated	2.4 (1.2)	3.7 (1.7)	5.5 (1.0)
Score for free generation	4.8 (2.8)	7.6 (3.3)	11.1 (2.1)
No. repetitions	0.3 (0.8)	00 (00)	00 (00)
No. of cue trials administered	3.7 (1.8)	2.5 (1.8)	1.4 (0.9)
Strategic Scores for CGT-C across age groups			
Proportion correct sorts: free generation	33.2 (16.5)	51.6 (25.8)	70.8 (19.7)
Proportion correct sorts: identification	19.7 (2.7)	34.7 (37.4)	37.6 (43.7)
Proportion correct sorts: cued	80.7 (27.3)	100 (00)	100 (00)
Proportion: children repeating sorts	5%	00	00
Proportion: children making rule breaks	2.6%	00	00

Source: Adapted from Jacobs et al. (2001).

ing disabilities (LD), intellectual or sensory handicap, or emotional problems from schools in a large metropolitan area. The sample included 10 children at each age level from 3 to 12 years old with equal male and female representation (Welsh, 1991; Welsh, Pennington et al., 1991). In another study, the relationship between the TOH and a modified version, the NEPSY Tower, was examined. The data revealed a strong relationship between raw scores for the two tasks, but limited correlation when tower raw scores were converted to standardized scores (Gioia, Isquith et al., 1999). Also, intellectual level appears influential. Those with lowered general intelligence experienced difficulty on the TOH (Borys, Spitz et al., 1982).

Because grading TOH item difficulty proved to be an obstacle, an adapted and simpler version was developed, the Tower of London (TOL), which uses colored balls and posts of different lengths (Shallice, 1982). Intercorrelation between the TOH and TOL tasks was somewhat low ($r = 0.37$) (Humes, Welsh et al., 1997). Some studies have investigated reliability. Test–retest reliability over only a 25-minute time interval using a noncomputerized TOH task with young children was $r = 0.72$ (Gnys and Willis, 1991). However, test–retest reliability improved for children 10 to 14 years old, retested one week after initial testing (Aman, Roberts et al., 1998). For a modified TOH task scored for accuracy, not time, test–retest reliability for 45 children between 7 and 10 tested after a 30 to 40 day interval was lower, $r = 0.528$ for raw scores and $r = 0.508$ for age-adjusted z-scores. Test–retest reliabilities were not significantly different for younger and older children (Bishop, Aamodt-Leeper et al., 2001).

Due to their low reliability, it was suggested that tower tasks might not be useful clinical tests of EF for an individual child (Bishop, Aamodt-Leeper et al., 2001), despite their intrinsic interest in experimental group studies of frontal lobe function and planning ability. The literature reports an association between TOH or TOL performance and adult frontal lobe function (Owen, Downes et al., 1990; Goel and Grafman, 1995). There is evidence on positron emission tomography (PET) imaging in normal adults of specifically activated dorsolateral prefrontal cortex during TOL test performance (Baker, Rogers et al., 1996) and of left frontal cortical activation using single photon emission computerized tomograph study (SPECT; Morris, Ahmed et al., 1993). Such specific correlation is not made for children, given their prefrontal circuitry immaturity (Nelson, 1995; Luciana and Nelson, 1998), and the continued maturation of prefrontal regions into adolescence and young adulthood (Huttenlocher, 1994). Of particular interest to child clinicians is the conclusion of one child tower study that "factors other than regional brain development may exert so powerful an influence on performance of executive function tasks that they swamp any variation due to individual differences in underlying neurology" (Bishop, Aamodt-Leeper et al., 2001, p. 555).

Tower of London

The Tower of London test (TOL) was originally designed for adults (Shallice, 1982), and was later successfully adapted for children in a variety of forms. The TOL is typically considered a test of planning ability that is also useful in the assessment of working memory, the ability to engage in anticipatory planning, and the ability to inhibit responding. It had a low correlation with receptive vocabulary, but a moderate correlation with other EF tasks (Krikorian, Bartok et al., 1994; Anderson, Anderson et al., 1996). However, some adult studies found the TOL failed to discriminate between patient and control groups (Ponsford and Kinsella, 1992; Cockburn, 1995), and that the construct of planning/problem solving was not reliably or validly measured by the test (Kafer and Hunter, 1997). In contrast, a study with children aged 7 to 15 supported the idea of a separable planning component and of the sensitivity of the TOL to maturational change (Levin, Culhane et al., 1991). Importantly, more recent data suggest that it might not be possible to assume that the TOL measures the same functions in children as it does for adults (Baker, Segalowitz et al., 2001).

Two complementary developmental normative data studies with different scoring rules are published for the Shallice TOL test. One

Table 6–20. Tower of London: Anderson et al. Study (1996)

Subjects: 376 children in Australia; age group N ranges from 18 to 30/cell for males, 24 to 33/cell for females; and 51 to 59 for Total n.

Gender: 180 male; 196 female

Age: 7.0 to 13.11 years

Race: Not reported

SES: Mean in 4 range (1 = high; 7 = low) on Daniel's Scale of Occupational Prestige

Inclusion/Exclusion Criteria: English first language; educated in English speaking school; no history of neurological deficit, LD, or special educational assistance

Table 6–22. Tower of London Planning Time Means and SDs

Age	Mean (SD) (in seconds)
7	65.9 (16.0)
8	57.1 (22.7)
9	55.6 (18.4)
10	59.6 (30.0)
11	43.9 (15.4)
12	48.8 (18.7)
13	52.9 (28.7)
ALL	54.7 (23.0)

Source: Anderson, Anderson, and Lajoie (1996). © Swets & Zeitlinger.

study's procedure rewarded rapid performance with bonus points and imposed a time limit for each trial (Anderson, Anderson et al., 1996). This procedure used a weighted performance time score and deducted the number of failed attempts. A maximum of 60 seconds was allowed. Normative data are presented for children 7 to 13 years, 11 months old. The demographic data for this study are presented in Table 6–20. The normative data for raw score means and standard deviations are presented in Table 6–21. The normative data for planning time means and standard deviations are presented in Table 6–22. A computerized version was published (Davis and Keller, 1998).

The other developmental scoring procedure rewarded performance accuracy but not speed (Krikorian, Bartok et al., 1994). The authors used the problems from Shallice's original study (Shallice, 1982). They found a linear increase in performance with advancing age.

Table 6–21. Tower of London Raw Score Means and SDs

Age	Mean (SD)
7	59.7 (10.0)
8	64.1 (9.8)
9	70.0 (9.8)
10	71.8 (9.0)
11	73.2 (9.1)
12	77.2 (9.0)
13	78.7 (7.3)
ALL	71.1 (11.0)

Source: Anderson, Anderson, and Lajoie (1996), © Swets & Zeitlinger.

Children aged 12 to 14 years old had performance statistically equivalent to a young adult group. Thus, by the sixth to eighth grade, they performed as well as 74 subjects with a mean age of 21 years. They made the qualification that their population was middle-class, intact cognitively, and therefore not representative of the general population. The authors recommended comparison of TOL performance with Porteus Maze test performance to distinguish types of planning impairments and found a moderate correlation between these two measures, but not full overlap. They attributed this to the TOL attention component and its requirement for retaining a sequence of moves, while the Porteus Maze test requires a planned action in response to a set, externally represented, configuration (Krikorian, Bartok et al., 1994).

The instructions for the Krikorian et al. study are:

"I want you to arrange the balls on thee pegs to match the picture." After successful matching, "I will be showing you some more pictures and asking you to match them by rearranging the balls on the pegs. I'm also going to tell you to do it in a certain number of moves. I may say make it look like the picture in two, three, four, or five moves. A move means taking a ball from a peg and placing it on another peg. You cannot pick up a ball and hold it while you move another, and you cannot move two balls at the same time. As you can see, the pegs are different sizes; this one holds zero or one ball, this one up to two, and this one up to three balls." Examiner positions balls in starting arrangement. "We will start every problem from this arrangement. This will be the start position for each problem." First problem presented. "Now, make it look like this in two moves."

Three trials are allowed for each problem. A score of three points for successful solution on the first trial, two points for success on the second trial, one point for success on the third trial, or zero points for no success is assigned for each problem. The maximum score is 3 points for each of 12 trials, for a total of 36 points. Scoring for latency/planning or execution time is possible, but normative data are not provided for these indices. This study's demographic data are presented in Table 6–23. The normative data for 205 children aged 7 to 13 years old, in grades 1 to 8, are presented in Table 6–24.

A comparison of these two scoring methods found that the scoring method influenced conclusions regarding developmental trends (Baker, Segalowitz et al., 2001), such that holding the administration procedure constant but using different scoring systems resulted in the potential for different developmental hypotheses. The subjects were 112 Canadian children and 48 undergraduates from 18 to 23 years old who were not identified as gifted, learning disabled, ADHD, traumatic brain-injured, or having a psychiatric or neurologic disorder. The authors used both scoring methods and found different developmental trajectories for each method. Scoring for accuracy showed continued development into adulthood. Scoring for speed showed an asymptote by 13 years old. Correlations between the two systems were significant for age, with a reliable drop in the

Table 6–23. Tower of London Demographic Data: Krikorian et al. Study (1994)

Subjects: 205 1st through 8th grade children in suburban Cincinnati, OH
Age: 7 to 13 years; grade cell N ranges from 24 to 31.
Gender: 87 male; 118 female
Handedness: Not specified
Race: Not specified
SES: Middle class; rating of 3.3 (.66) on 5-point Hollingshead index
Inclusion: No children with learning, ADHD, or behavioral problems

Table 6–24. Means and *SD*s for Tower of London Performance by Grade

Grade	n	Mean (SD)
1	24	27.8 (3.7)
2	25	29.0 (2.6)
3	24	30.3 (2.7)
4	24	30.4 (2.9)
5	24	30.5 (2.8)
6	26	31.8 (2.9)
7	27	31.6 (2.3)
8	31	32.5 (1.9)

Source: Krikorian, Bartok & Gay (1994), © Swets & Zeitlinger.

correlation coefficient with increased age. In a French TOL study of 214 children and 17 young adults between 7 and 17+ years, the data found that "planification" develops and refines until 16 years old (Lussier, Guerin et al., 1998). Thus, caution must be taken in interpreting data within a developmental model in exclusion of consideration of the methodology.

Tower of London–Drexel University

A third procedure is available commercially for children: the Tower of London—Drexel University (Culbertson and Zillmer, 2000). This 10-item version allows only one trial per item so that the final score does not reflect number of trials to solution. It has a higher ceiling than the TOL. There is one form for children 7 to 15 years old and another for those 16 and older. It includes two tower sets, each with three differently sized pegs and three differently colored beads. One set is for the child, and the other for the examiner, for demonstration, and as a model for the 10 test items that range from three to seven moves. The child must copy the examiner's model in as few moves as possible, moving one bead at a time. Each item is timed, with a maximum 2-minute time limit per item. There are seven measurement variables: total moves, total correct, time violations, rule violations, initiation time, execution time and total problem-solving time.

NEPSY Tower

The NEPSY tower subtest (Korkman, Kirk et al., 1997) is another modification of the TOL

(Shallice, 1982). The NEPSY Tower subtest is a 20-problem version with a maximum of seven moves (Korkman, Kirk et al., 1997), in which the child of 5 to 12 years is encouraged to work quickly. This contrasts with the planning and open number of moves allowed by other tower tasks, e.g., the TOH, Delis-Kaplan Executive Function System (D-KEFS) Tower, and TOL (Welsh, Pennington et al., 1991; Delis, Kaplan et al., 2001). The NEPSY tower requires the child to produce a response that reproduces an existing model presented in a stimulus book within a specified number of moves and does not evaluate the child's efficiency in reaching the target. The NEPSY tower relies on a total-outcome subtest score, not a process score such as number of trials to solution, as described in other methods (Levin, Culhane et al., 1991).

Unlike the TOL, the NEPSY tower includes items that require identical initial moves since all items begin with the balls on the pegs in a standard starting position. In contrast, the TOL varies the initial moves. As a result, the TOL appears to elicit response inhibition and flexible planning to a greater extent than the NEPSY tower. The NEPSY tower is criticized for its insensitivity to the purported executive function it is intended to measure, along with other executive function subtests of this battery, and for its lack of construct validity, i.e., its inability to discriminate among clinical populations. Several explanations are proposed, including that of dampened variance in raw scores, further restricted when raw scores are converted to standard scores (Gioia, Isquith et al., 1999).

In their study comparing the NEPSY tower subtest with the three-ring Tower of Hanoi (TOH3; Welsh, Pennington et al., 1991) for 38 children, aged 6 to 12 years old, there was a significant correlation between NEPSY tower and TOH3 raw scores. This disappeared when NEPSY tower standard scores were compared to TOH3 raw scores and when NEPSY tower standard scores were compared to TOH3 standard scores (Gioia, Isquith et al., 1999). Such data suggest that the NEPSY norms potentially reduce the variance and sensitivity of the task. The authors further noted the high correlation of the NEPSY tower with general intellectual function and the significant correlation of the TOH with performance IQ, but not verbal IQ, consistent with prior report (Gioia, 1993). As a result of such preliminary data, along with clinical observation of decreased sensitivity of the NEPSY tower subtest and concern that it merely reflects maturation effects, it appears that those wishing to use a tower test should consider one of the other available options. Further, greater clinically significant score differences are apparent for groups of children with global impairment since the NEPSY attention/executive function domain has a strong correlation with general intellectual function (Gioia, Isquith et al., 1999).

The apparatus consists of three posts of different length and three colored balls. The child changes the pattern from the starting pattern to the presented pattern following five rules: (1) only one ball is moved at a time; (2) only one ball is allowed in the child's hands at a time; (3) the balls cannot be placed on the table while the child uses only one hand, (4) only one ball is placed on the small stick, two balls on the middle stick, and three balls on the tallest stick, and, (5), the new pattern must be made in a specified number of moves. After a sample item, the test begins with the examiner saying, "I have a series of patterns just like that last one that I want you to copy." Timing begins when the stimulus card is placed before the child. For the sample item and all 12 test items the examiner says, "I want you to copy this pattern using only N moves." The easiest pattern involves two moves, and the hardest requires five moves. Scoring is for number of trials, latency to first move, solution time, and number of problems solved on the first try.

Table 6–25. Delis-Kaplan Executive Function System Demographic Data

Subjects: 700 children 8 to 15 years, 175 aged 16 to 19 years
Age: 8 to adult
Gender: Roughly equal proportion male and female
Race: Stratified for 2000 U.S. Census
Education: 5 major educational groups according to 2000 U.S. Census
SES: Not available
Exclusion criteria: Any medical or psychiatric symptom or condition

The Delis-Kaplan Executive Function System Tower Test

A tower task is included in the Delis-Kaplan Executive Function System (D-KEFS) (Delis, Kaplan et al., 2001), a compilation of executive function measures that allow for comparability determination since all subtests are normed on the same national standardization sample (see Table 6–25). The sample is nationally representative of age, gender, race/ethnicity, education, and geographic region based on the 2000 U. S. Census. Child norms begin at age 8 years and continue into adulthood. As for the TOL, the D-KEFS Tower Test requires forward planning of a sequence of steps as the child tries to move a pattern of beads efficiently from a start configuration to a goal configuration to match a target pattern. Difficulty level rises by increasing the minimum number of moves necessary to achieve the goal configuration.

Porteus Maze Test

Maze learning performance has a long history in cognitive psychology (Milner, 1965). The Porteus Maze Test (PMT); Porteus, 1924; 1950; 1959) and Vineland Revision Form (Porteus, 1965) were developed in 1914 as a measure of planning and as a screening for intellectual efficiency. Besides the Vineland Revision, there are the more difficult extension series, and supplemental series, which can be used for retesting. Early studies suggested that maze performance was indicative of ability to adapt, plan, anticipate and use practical knowledge and measured something different than intelligence tests for the psychosurgery population (Riddle and Roberts, 1978). The PMT was included in studies of children with ADHD (Homatidis and Konstantareas, 1981; Kuehne, Kehle et al., 1987; Grodzinsky and Diamond, 1992) and was chosen for studies where a "culture-free" measure of nonverbal motor reasoning skill, not strongly influenced by educational level, was desired. However, cultural influences are complex, and face validity may be misleading. Studies comparing children of European descent and children from other cultural contexts reinforce the notion that these tests may not be nearly as culturally fair as first believed.

Standard procedure requires an individual at least 3 years old to draw a line from a starting point to the end goal on a set of increasingly more difficult mazes, with no imposed time limits, beginning with Maze V (Porteus, 1965). The child is instructed not to enter a dead end, draw through walls represented by solid lines, cut corners, or lift the pencil. An error results in immediate termination and presentation of another trial. Contemporary performance standards were introduced for children in grades 1 to 8, and a young adult group, using the Vineland Revision form (Krikorian and Bartok, 1998). Maze learning improved with age, but plateaued at 12 to 14 years. However, strong ceiling effects were not found in a traumatic brain injury study comparing children with frontal or extrafrontal lesions using extended range maze stimuli (Levin, Song et al. 2001). The child demographic data for the normative study are presented in Table 6–26 and the means and standard deviations for the PMT are presented in Table 6–27.

The Cronbach coefficient alpha value of .81 indicated the PMT had moderately high internal consistency. Greater efficiency with increasing age was found, and there was evidence of performance plateaus at Grades 1 and 2, 4 through 8, and for young adults. Similar to maturational data for another nonverbal planning task, the TOL, (Krikorian, Bartok et al., 1994), a ceiling on PMT performance was reached at about 13 years. A small gender difference was found, favoring males, consistent with evidence that males perform spatial tasks better than females. These data also found that IQ did not contribute appreciably to PMT performance.

This instrument was found to be sensitive to TBI severity and volume of circumscribed prefrontal (inferior frontal and orbitofrontal) le-

Table 6–26. Demographic Data: Krikorian & Bartok Study (1998)

Subjects: 246 children from suburban Cincinnati, OH
Gender: No. of males and females not reported
Age: 7 to 13 years
Race: Not reported
SES: 3.2 on Hollingshead scale of social position
Inclusion: No gross, debilitating cognitive, or mental disorder

Table 6–27. Porteus Maze Test Means and Standard Deviations

Grade	N	Mean	SD
1	26	10.6	2.7
2	27	11.8	3.4
3	24	13.8	2.4
4	24	14.0	2.0
5	26	14.7	2.0
6	47	14.6	2.1
7	32	14.9	2.0
8	40	15.4	1.8

Source: Adapted from Krikorian and Bartok (1998).

sions (Levin, Song et al., 2001) in children studied at least three years post-injury. In this study, the investigators also recorded "planning time," that is, the time spent looking at the maze before beginning to draw, with 30 seconds maximum given before they were prompted to start drawing. This was recorded, along with number of trials required to complete each level, total solution time, and number of errors. In addition, the motor speed factor was considered separately from the cognitive demands. The three most difficult mazes successfully completed by the child were presented again, so that the child could rapidly trace the existing path. The total time was the motor speed component score. Motor speed did not explain the TBI severity effect.

EXECUTIVE FUNCTION TESTS: INHIBITION

Stroop Color-Word Test

The Stroop Color Word Test (SCWT) is a brief measure of selective or focused attention (Lowe and Mitterer, 1982), the ability to shift from one perceptual set to another as test requirements change, and the ability to inhibit responding. It provides insight into the ability to concentrate and resist distraction (Lezak, 1995). The Stroop procedure requires the individual to inhibit a prepotent well-learned verbal response when faced with a novel one. Specifically, the child must inhibit an automatized reading response and produce a competing color-naming response. The EF character-

istics of cognitive flexibility and mental set shifting in response to environmental stimuli also affect performance, as do visual competence, color blindness (Lezak, 1995), and the capacity to focus and sustain attention (Johnston and Venables, 1982).

The SCWT is based on the Stroop Effect (Stroop, 1935), the difficulty experienced when attempting to eliminate meaningful but conflicting information from a task, even when that information is irrelevant to the task (Mesulam, 1985). This work was itself based on earlier psychological studies of normal subjects that found the time to read color name words was less than the time needed to name actual colors, even after practice (Cattell, 1886; Brown, 1915). The Stroop Effect is an example of automatic, uncontrolled word reading, along with the ability to control or inhibit reading (Rafal and Henik, 1994). By obtaining reading and color-naming, speeded performances on the Stroop Test prior to the target interference condition, the interference condition result can be interpreted with respect to selective attention and response inhibition. The reader is referred to Henik (1996) for discussion and recommendations on following Stroop's logic to benefit from the paradigm and effect bearing his name.

The Stroop has a long history in psychology (MacLeod, 1991). Studies of adults with brain damage support the neuropsychological use of the Stroop procedure (Nehemkis and Lewinsohn, 1972; Golden, 1976; Dodrill, 1978), although construct validity is confounded by multiple demands inherent in the task, such as response inhibition, response shifting, sustaining attention, selective visual attention reading level, and naming ability. Left-frontal brain-damaged subjects had greater difficulty than subjects with lesions in other cerebral locations (Perret, 1974), hypothesized due to inhibition of a verbal automatic response. However, later study found a right prefrontal lesion location had greater influence on number of errors during the interference condition than did a left prefrontal location (Vendrell, Jungue, et al., 1995).

Human functional activation study found evidence of orbitofrontal and ventral frontal activation for response inhibition tasks such as the Stroop (Bench, Frith et al., 1993). Also, functional imaging studies, using a Stroop paradigm for emotional and nonemotional words, found activation in a region of the anterior cingulate cortex (ACC) (Whalen, Bush et al., 1998), an area that mediates the monitoring of conflict during information processing and influences arousal and effort over time. Activation of the left anterior cingulate cortex, the supplementary motor cortex, thalamus and the cerebellum was found in a positron emission tomography (PET) study of young adults. The authors emphasized that the activation, while in the frontal lobe, was not prefrontal (Ravnkilde, Videbech et al., 2002). They contrasted these data with verbal fluency data that appeared to be more specific for prefrontal function.

In another functional neuroimaging study of healthy adults, the left inferior precentral sulcus appeared to be a central brain structure mediating the interference effect associated with the Stroop paradigm. This region was significantly activated during the incongruent color words condition along with significant deactivations in the rostral portion of the ACC and posterior cingulate gyrus. These results were interpreted as likely related to the mediation of competing articulatory demands during the interference condition. The proximity of the inferior precentral sulcus to the left inferior frontal gyrus and its role in speech production suggested to these researchers that the Stroop effect may be mediated by increased response competition associated with subvocal articulatory processes (Mead, Mayer et al., 2002). Overall, demonstration of activation of the ACC has been inconsistent and methodological factors appear responsible for this inconsistency. Thus, the role of the ACC remains under investigation.

Developmental data indicate that while reading does not interfere in color naming for first graders, it does interfere for second and third graders (Comalli, Wapner et al., 1962; Schiller, 1966). A robust Stroop effect noticeable in the early school grades, reaches its highest level around Grades 2 to 3, commensurate with increased reading skill. The SCWT was administered to high-achieving and low-achieving Indian second and third graders in schools teaching the tribal language Oriya or English. The high-achiever children read words and colors faster than the low-achiever subjects. The high-achiever girls, third graders, and children in English schools had greater cognitive interference between color naming and word reading than their counterparts, suggesting interference differences were due to higher verbal ability and/or bilingual competency (Dash and Dash, 1987).

Comparison of Stroop Test performances of 10- to 15-year-old, mentally retarded and normal children found the retarded children naming colors faster than reading words and showing relatively less of an interference effect. They functioned like normal first graders. Reading speed and interference measures appeared to reflect stable individual differences likely related to learning differences (Das, 1969). When retarded children were compared by mental age level, word-reading and color-naming speeds increased with increasing age, as did the interference effect. Compared to normal children of equivalent mental age, they were slower in changing from a direct to a verbal mode as evidenced by color-naming speed and interference (Das, 1970)

Clinical interpretive guidelines indicate that children with reading problems can present with diminished color-word-reading scores, but normal color naming and color naming under the interference condition (Golden, 1978). Therefore, good interference performance might indicate good ability to inhibit automatic response tendencies and lead to a prediction of an association between the interference score and other response inhibition tasks. Or, good interference performance might indicate lack of an interference effect for the individual and no such prediction (Cox, Chee et al., 1997). In the latter study, the impact on the interference effect when reading is not automatized (i.e., for poor readers) was examined. Reading proficiency affected the construct validity of the SCWT interference score. The validity of the Stroop interference score as a measure of the ability to inhibit an automatic response pattern was supported.

Significant correlation was found between inhibition of the automatized reading response and the inhibition of a preponderant motor response, when reading automaticity was operationally defined as a single-word reading score equal to or higher than estimated full scale IQ. Caution has been offered about inferring an ability to inhibit automatized behavior based on the Stroop interference score if phonological decoding skills and strength of single-word reading in relation to overall ability level are not known (Cox, Chee et al., 1997). Increased inhibitory control is reflected in greater Stroop Test gains between the ages 7 to 13 (Kelly, 2000).

Research on the Stroop procedure with adults has found acceptable reliability and validity (MacLeod, 1991). Test–retest reliability was .90, .83, and .91, respectively, for each of the three parts (word reading, color naming, color-word interference) when there was a 1-month interval between tests (Spreen and Strauss, 1998). Besides age effects noted above, gender effects in favor of females are reported for color and word trials, but not always for the interference trial (Stroop, 1935; Perriti, 1971; Golden, 1974). Ethnic or cultural normative data are limited. In one study of adults 19 and older, a modified Stroop (Comalli, Wapner et al., 1962), which was further modified to present color naming before word reading, was used. Modification was made to check for color blindness, stuttering, or dysnomia, and to increase the likelihood that a priming effect would be exerted by reading words just before the interference trial. Using a modification of the Comalli version, the normative data for 42 subjects found African American

women outperformed men (Strickland, D'Elia et al., 1997), as has been previously documented. Besides time-to-completion, data were also provided for number of errors and number of near misses.

Normative data for a SCWT in Spanish were published (Armengol, 2002) for 349 Mexican children aged 6 to 12 years old, in first through sixth grade (see Table 6–28 for these demographic data). Normative data were presented in separate tables for either the 170 children in public or 179 children in private school (see Table 6–29 and Table 6–30, respectively).

Modifications of the SCWT for deaf adults are also reported (Wolff, Radecke et al., 1989). In one child study, there were no significant differences between deaf and hearing children on the SCWT when they were of similar age, the deaf having no difficulty compared to the hearing on this attention task. A greater interference in the SCWT task for younger deaf and hearing groups than for older groups was reported, leading to a recommendation for norms based on developmental age (Ojile, Das et al., 1993).

Adult studies find interference performance declines through the adult years (Cohn, Dustman et al., 1984; Uttl and Graf, 1997), possibly increasing again around age 60 (MacLeod, 1991). Some adult investigations of task dependence on language supported the idea that different orthographies activate different processing strategies but this was later contradicted in a meta-analysis (Chen, 1999; Lee and Chan,

Table 6–28. Stroop Color Word Test: Mexican Children

	Male/ Female		Father's Education[a]	Mother's Education	Age: Years & Months	K-BIT Matrices
Private School $N = 179129.82$	91/88	M	5.85	5.37	9.9	103
		SD	1.39	1.43	1.88	12
Public School $N = 170$	85/85	M	2.64	2.28	9.5	90
		SD	1.84	1.61	1.99	14
t values, Private Public			$t = 16.15$ $p < .001$°°	$t = 16.76$ $p < .001$°°	$t = 1.803$ $p = 0.07$	$t = 9.68$ $p < .001$°°

Source: Armengol (2002), © Swets & Zeitlinger.

[a]Measures by degree or partial degree attained: 1 = elementary, 2 = junior high, 3 = partial senior high, 4 = senior high, 5 = partial college/associate's degree, 6 = baccalaureate, 7 = post-baccalaureate.

Table 6–29. Means and Standard Deviations for Stroop Variables–Public School

Age	N	Statistic	TIME TO COMPLETION (SEC.)				UNCORRECTED ERRORS			CORRECTED ERRORS			TVIP[1]	K-BIT[2]
			Color	Word	Inter	Diff	Color	Word	Interf	Color	Word	Interf		
6	9	Mean	143.22	138.6	220.6	77.33	1.22	1.89	5.67	1.77	1.89	5.67	116.88	95.67
		SD	45.63	46.85	53.93	54.85	1.48	1.62	3.39	3.39	1.62	3.39	11.03	16.38
7	27	Mean	128.26	111.0	244.2	115.9	1.26	0.33	2.63	3.0	0.78	6.77	114.15	92.00
		SD	21.74	58.47	58.85	50.89	1.26	0.87	2.42	2.75	0.97	4.6	11.24	11.37
8	22	Mean	125.82	87.18	228.0	102.2	1.05	4.54	2.86	2.68	1.0	7.05	115.05	93.77
		SD	23.23	17.68	50.32	43.39	1.58	0.21	3.15	2.32	1.83	4.81	15.28	10.68
9	30	Mean	118.57	80.43	216.7	98.13	1.0	0.17	3.07	1.7	0.20	4.4	113.23	89.57
		SD	25.75	15.73	61.57	48.31	1.55	0.53	4.17	1.39	0.48	2.66	17.25	11.14
10	25	Mean	100.72	68.28	178.4	77.72	1.16	0.00	3.52	1.36	0.16	3.6	111.44	84.84
		SD	17.39	13.22	37.64	33.13	1.75	0.00	5.65	1.35	0.47	3.19	13.99	14.72
11	33	Mean	91.97	59.21	164.5	72.55	0.97	0.12	13.79	1.52	.242	4.27	107.21	86.52
		SD	16.12	11.32	40.45	31.74	1.19	0.42	3.71	1.33	0.50	5.62	18.55	11.76
12	12	Mean	93.0	60.75	175.8	82.83	1.50	0.25	4.5	0.58	0.00	2.0	111.83	79.67
		SD	17.86	10.76	52.01	41.90	1.51	0.62	4.48	0.99	0.00	2.17	13.09	14.94

Source: Armengol (2002), © Swets & Zeitlinger.

[1]Test de Vocabulario en Imágenes Peabody, Scaled Scores

[2]Kaufman Brief Intelligence Test, Scaled Scores

Table 6–30. Means and Standard Deviations for Stroop Variables–Private School

Age	N	Statistic	SECONDS TO COMPLETION				UNCORRECTED ERRORS			CORRECTED ERRORS			TVIP[1]	K-BIT[2]
			Color	Word	Inter	Diff	Color	Word	Interf	Color	Word	Interf		
6	5	Mean	138.4	83.2	267.6	129.2	1.6	0.40	13.8	3.6	0.20	3.8	132.2	103
		SD	31.90	15.12	92.88	100.3	1.7	0.89	17.8	1.82	0.45	2.68	11.17	9.7
7	26	Mean	126.3	82.8	241.9	114.2	0.85	0.40	0.20	2.27	0.805	6.4	126.8	100.4
		SD	28.44	16.34	65.00	55.1	1.0	1.30	0.58	1.59	1.08	3.57	13.54	9.5
8	33	Mean	125.9	70.3	210.5	103.9	2.09	3.0	0.21	.42	0.39	4.27	125.9	102.6
		SD	25.39	16.01	61.04	50.16	2.20	0.93	0.48	.71	0.79	3.97	8.94	12.2
9	30	Mean	99.7	61.5	182.7	83.2	0.57	2.0	0.00	1.46	0.20	3.6	129.5	108.2
		SD	13.96	9.49	39.10	34.50	0.68	0.48	0.00	1.66	0.48	3.10	11.23	13.1
10	25	Mean	93.6	57.4	184.8	91.2	0.83	2	0.17	1.83	0.21	4.33	130.2	100.2
		SD	20.77	9.46	47.55	34.51	1.05	0.60	0.20	1.20	0.51	3.28	9.63	10.7
11	30	Mean	136.6	53.2	140.6	58.7	0.30	2.0	0.00	1.27	2.0	4.67	136.6	102.6
		SD	11.96	8.54	19.2	16.78	0.59	0.61	0.00	1.18	0.61	3.49	8.94	13.2
12	30	Mean	74.8	48.3	125.9	51.13	0.5	2.0	0.00	1.3	0.20	2.7	129.2	104.7
		SD	14.25	8.92	24.90	21.60	0.73	0.48	0.00	1.24	0.48	2.17	10.52	12.2

Source: Armengol (2002), © Swets & Zeitlinger.

[1]Test de Vocabulario en Imagenes Peabody, Scaled Scores

[2]Matrices Subtest of the Kaufman Brief Intelligence Test, Scaled Scores

2000). These recent investigations found no significant difference in the Stroop effect for Chinese and English orthographies and no gender difference (Lee and Chan, 2000).

A modification was also developed that better differentiated between TBI and control groups than did other Stroop versions (Bohnen, Jolles et al., 1992). The authors used a four-color, 100-items-per-page, version of the Stroop, published in the Netherlands, that measures the speed at which the 100 items are read. In this more complex task that better detected the subtle disturbances of mild TBI, 20 items on the third part, the interference trial, were randomly selected and had rectangles drawn around the words. This page constituted a fourth trial. The subject read the word name of the items in rectangles while responding with the color ink of those words not in rectangles. This procedure is incorporated in the D-KEFS Color Word Interference Test. Given the limited, and older, available child normative data, it remains to be determined whether the D-KEFS version will exceed the standard SCWT in usefulness for children.

Versions of the Stroop Procedure

Stroop versions differ by colors presented, type and arrangement of stimuli, order of presentation, or tasks. A considerable variety of administration procedures and methodologies exist (Jensen and Rohrer, 1966), although only one version had associated child normative data available until very recently (Golden, 1978). Although it is expected with traditional measures that reading is a requirement for Stroop administration (Cox, Chee et al., 1997), modified versions relying on color and form are reported for very young children (Arochova, 1971; Butollo, Bauer et al., 1971; Archibald and Kerns, 1999).

Several examples of the more common versions are provided below:

Original Stroop Version
A five-color version with three tasks—reading words, naming color patches, reading color names—printed in nonmatching colored inks (Stroop, 1935).

Golden version
The Stroop Color Word Test (SCWT; Golden 1976; 1978) is a three-color version (blue, green, red). There are three 100-item pages, one each for three 45-second trials of word reading of black typed words, color naming of "XXXX" in randomized color sequences, and color naming when the words are printed in nonmatching colored ink: the word "red" is printed in green ink, and the correct response is "green." One reads down columns of stimuli on each trial. If the last column is completed before the 45-second time limit elapses, the subject starts over until the time limit is completed. Four scores are obtained—the number of items read correctly for each of the three trials and an interference score, which should be calculated (Golden, undated manuscript): INT = Age Corrected CW observed–CW predicted. The formula for CW predicted = C × W/C + W. Thus, the INT score is calculated by the formula: $I = CW - (C \times W)/(C + W))$. The interference effect is considered the indicator of selective attention.

Age corrections for raw scores obtained for each of the three 45-second trials of the Golden version are presented in Table 6–31 for children aged 7 to 16 years. The age-corrected scores are then used to obtain the *T*-scores for each of the three tasks, and also for the difference score between predicted and obtained interference scores. These data are presented in Table 6–32.

Table 6–31. Stroop Age Corrections for Children

Age Group	Word	Color	Color-Word
7	52	40	26
8	46	36	24
9	41	29	20
10	34	24	16
11	26	16	11
12	15	10	7
13	10	7	5
14	5	0	2
15	3	0	0
16	0	0	0

Source: Golden (1978); Reprinted with permission of The Stoelting Corporation.

Table 6–32. T Scores for Stroop Color-Word Test—Age-Corrected Raw Scores

T-score	Word	Color	Color-Word	Interference
80	168	125	75	30
78	164	122	73	28
76	160	119	71	26
74	156	116	69	24
72	152	113	67	22
70	148	110	65	20
68	144	107	63	18
66	140	104	61	16
64	136	101	59	14
62	132	98	57	12
60	128	95	55	10
58	124	92	53	8
56	120	89	51	6
54	116	86	49	4
52	112	83	47	2
50	108	80	45	0
48	104	77	43	−2
48	100	74	41	−4
44	96	71	39	−6
42	92	68	37	−8
40	88	65	35	−10
38	84	62	33	−12
36	80	59	31	−14
34	76	56	29	−16
32	72	53	27	−18
30	68	50	25	−20
28	64	47	23	−22
26	60	44	21	−24
24	56	41	19	−26
22	52	38	17	−28
20	48	35	15	−30

Source: Golden (1978); Reprinted with permission of The Stoelting Corporation.

Regard version

The Stroop Color Word Test—Victoria version (Regard 1981a; 1981b): This is a four-color version (blue, green, red, and yellow) with six rows of four items. Part D consists of color dots. Part W is common words unrelated to color. Part C is color words. Each color is used six times, appearing only once in a row. The requirement is to name colors of printed stimuli, disregarding verbal content.

Comalli version

In the Comalli version (Comalli, Wapner et al., 1962) there are three stimulus cards, each with 100 items arranged in 10 rows of 10 items per row. A row of practice items is provided at the top of the card. Card 1 requires reading color words (red, blue, green) printed in black ink. Card 2 requires naming colored rectangles. Card 3 has words printed in incongruous ink, and the subject must name the ink color. The subject reads from left to right and completes all 100 items for each of the three parts. A time-to-completion score is recorded for each part. A Comalli-Kaplan modification presents the colored rectangles first, then the word-reading trial, and finally the incongruous ink-word trial, with errors recorded (Armengol, 2002).

Dodrill version

In this 176-item, four-color version (red, orange, green, blue), a difference score is obtained using two tasks, the color and color-word tasks (Dodrill, 1978). The length of the trials presumably allows for demonstration of cognitive slowing over the extended trials.

Trenerry version

The Stroop Neuropsychological Screening Test (SNST; Trenerry, Crosson et al., 1989). This 112-item version was developed to address methodological problems of other versions, that is, the direction the subject must read (rows or columns) and syllable length of color name, which affects speed and score. There are two tasks: color naming and color-word reading for words with nonmatching ink color. Form C consists of 112 color names for four colors (red, green, blue, tan) arranged in four columns. Normative data begin at 18 years old.

Some SCWT variations are subtests within larger batteries. For example, a Stroop-like task in the Das Naglieri Cognitive Assessment System (CAS; Nagleri and Das, 1997) is the Expressive Attention subtest. It requires size responses to animal pictures for those 5 to 7 years old; 8- to 17-year-old children respond to colors and color words.

The NEPSY Auditory Attention and Response subtest requires response to a tape recording of words, with colors interspersed among noncolor words. A conflicting instruction is part of the Auditory Response Set that follows the Auditory Attention task. Three specific colors require three different responses.

When the child hears the first color, a square of the second color must be immediately put in a box. When the second color is heard, the square of the first color is placed in the box. When the third color is heard, a square of the same color is put in the box. The subtest is scored for time and accuracy.

The Test of Everyday Attention for Children (TEA-Ch) Opposite Worlds subtest also requires inhibition of a prepotent response (see Chapter 7). The D-KEFS Color Word Interference Test is a version of the SCWT that, in addition to word reading, color naming, and an interference trial, has a shift-condition fourth trial, as recommended by Bohnen and colleagues (1992) (see Executive Function Tests: Inhibition).

Other modifications include individual tests specifically designed for children, such as the Day-Night Stroop (Gerstadt, Hong et al., 1994). The Day-Night Stroop test was used in a study of verbal inhibition in childhood (Passler, Isaac et al., 1985) and requires inhibition and switching in order to respond to a light-colored card as "night" and to a dark-colored card as "day." The test is not recommended for children under 6 years old who are unable to inhibit and switch simultaneously. Dramatic improvement in test performance on an adapted version that incorporated color was found between 5 and 6 years of age (Diamond, 1991). The task was subsequently adapted due to anticipated ceiling effects at about 7 years old with the Day-Night Stroop with explicit stimulus-verbal response associations using moon and sun pictures on black and white cards, respectively (Gerstadt, Hong et al. 1994), the Sun-Moon Stroop (Archibald and Kerns, 1999) (see below).

There is also an Auditory Stroop Test (Jerger, Martin et al., 1988) and The Fruit Stroop test (Santostefano, 1988) (see below). The latter auditory version of the SCWT was administered to 3- to 6-year-olds. This reaction time task required the children to respond quickly and accurately to words spoken by male or female voices. The child was instructed to ignore what was said and push the "mommy" button if mommy were talking or the "daddy" button if daddy were talking. Reaction time increased with conflict between semantic and auditory dimensions and decreased relative to a neutral condition, with congruence between the two dimensions (Jerger, Martin et al., 1988).

Sun-Moon and Fruit Stroop Tests

The Archibald and Kerns modifications to the Stroop test deemphasized the reading skill required for other Stroop versions (Archibald and Kerns, 1999). The Sun-Moon Stroop used colored pictures of suns and moons, arranged pseudorandomly. The child had to first rapidly respond "sun" to sun pictures and "moon" to moon pictures for 45 seconds, stopping the progression across the row and stating the correction when an error was made. For the second trial, the child had to say "moon" to sun pictures and "sun" to moon pictures. The Interference score was calculated by the formula: (No. of items correct on part 2—No. of items correct on part 1)/(No. of items correct on part 1).

The Fruit Stroop task modification of the Fruit Distraction Task (Santostefano, 1988) had four pages. On page 1 the child had 45 seconds to rapidly name colored rectangles (blue, green, yellow, red). On page 2 the child rapidly names the color of appropriately colored fruits. On page 3 the child rapidly names the colors that the fruits should be now that they are colorless. On page 4 the child rapidly names the color the fruit should be for incorrectly colored fruits. The predicted score was calculated according to the formula: (No. items correct page 1 × No. items correct page 3)/No. items page 1 + page 3). The predicted score is subtracted from the actual score to obtain the summary Interference score. A negative value indicates more interference.

The resulting Sun-Moon Stroop and Fruit Stroop were administered and compared to results on the Golden Stroop version. The normative data for all three Stroop tasks are presented later in this chapter in Table 6–63.

There are also other adapted versions of the Stroop Test. One version employs words with emotional significance. This Emotional Stroop Test is a cognitive method utilized in clinical and diagnostic psychiatry since the emotional salience of words causes interference in color naming in various populations. Possibly, these emotional interferences arise from attentional disturbances. Color word methodology appears

Table 6–33. Matching Familiar Figures Test Normative Data

Age	N	RESPONSE TIME		NO. ERRORS	
		Mean	SD	Mean	SD
7	10	27.3	30.3	12.6	6.43
8	10	18.9	17.4	11.8	5.73
9	10	22.5	16.1	11.0	6.77
10	10	39.3	27.2	6.30	4.37
11	10	35.5	20.0	4.20	3.36
12	10	34.7	16.3	4.10	2.13

Source: Welsh et al. (1991), courtesy of Lawrence Erlbaum Associates.

relatively unaffected by motivational biases and can be used to distinguish between genuine and fictitious psychological disorders (Greco, 1993). A Food Stroop test and parallel, alternate version Shape Stroop test have been used in investigation of psychopathology in eating disorders (Kay, Ben-Tovim et al., 1992).

Matching Familiar Figures Test

The Matching Familiar Figures Test (MFFT; Kagan, Rosman et al., 1964; Kagan, 1966; Arizmendi, Paulsen et al., 1981) is a measure of impulsivity, appropriate for children or adults. The child must find an identical match for a stimulus from one of six similar pictures. There are six items for 6- to 12-year-olds and eight for those 13 years old and older. The test is scored for number correct and response time. Rapid responding will likely result in more errors (Arizmendi, Paulsen et al., 1981). A speed–accuracy trade-off is evident when impulsive responding produces more errors. The test also taps inhibition and strategic search. Commission errors were of interest in a study of 6-year-old children with behavioral issues, who made significantly more errors than the control children (Mariani and Barkley, 1997). The MFFT appears useful in documenting a fast, but inaccurate, response strategy in ADHD children (Barkley, 1991; DuPaul, Anastopoulos et al., 1992). Internal consistency for response time was 0.89 and 0.62 for errors (Welsh, Pennington et al., 1991). Normative data for children 7 to 12 years old are presented in Table 6–33. Adult level performance was achieved by age 10.

Go-No Go Tasks

Go-no go tasks are considered measures of the ability to inhibit (inability reflected in commission errors), but it has also been suggested that omission errors might reflect attention and concentration factors underlying effortful cognitive processes and therefore, they may correlate with working memory measures (Archibald and Kerns, 1999). Early correlation of go-no go task performance with frontal systems brain function (Drewe, 1975) is reinforced by recent functional human neuroimaging data linking frontal systems function to go-no go performance (Kawashima, Satoh et al., 1996; Rolls, 1996), especially orbitofrontal cortex (Fuster, 1989; Casey, Trainor et al., 1997). It is just this type of information about behavior that one needs to inquire about in history taking, since assessment of the orbitofrontal region is not specifically test-linked in the clinical setting and depends on more than a suggestive test result. Thus, the convergence of test results suggesting more anterior cerebral dysfunction with behavioral descriptions compatible with what is known about orbitofrontal dysfunction (or mesial frontal or dorsal lateral prefrontal dysfunction) is required to feel more confident about making such an informed suggestion.

A variety of go-no go tasks are used in research or clinical practice. A reciprocal motor movements task (Christensen, 1975; Luria, 1980) is one commonly used screening measure. For the contrasting motor program part of this screening test, the child is instructed to tap twice if the examiner taps once, and to tap once if the examiner taps twice. Data suggest that this is under a child's control by age 6 (Becker, Isaac et al. 1987; Diamond, 1991). For the next part of the go-no go task, the child is instructed to tap twice if the examiner taps once, but to do nothing if the examiner taps twice. In this latter step, the examiner looks to see if the finger moves when the child should be inhibiting the action. One procedure I follow is to administer the "one tap" four times before tapping twice for the first time, and then to randomly intersperse one and two taps until confident that the child is performing without error.

Two response inhibition tasks were employed to assess motor response inhibition in a study of children with ADHD, and two additional tasks assessed motor persistence (Mostofsky, Russell et al., 2001). For the Contralateral Motor Response Task the child placed both hands on a table, and the examiner touched one hand, instructing the child to raise the opposite hand quickly and then place it back on the table. After eyes-open practice, 48 trials were randomly administered (24 for each hand), with the eyes closed, at a rate of one per second. Same-side errors were recorded. A Conflicting Motor Response Task that was part of an earlier study or ADHD (Shue and Douglas, 1992) was also use in this child study. The child placed both hands on a table. The examiner's instructions were, "If I show you my finger, you show me your fist. If I show you my fist, you show me your finger." There were 2 practice trials and 48 trials at a rate of one per second, with the child responding using the dominant hand. Echopraxic errors were recorded.

The two motor impersistence tasks were the NEPSY Statue Test and a lateral eye gaze persistence task. The NEPSY Statue Test requires the child to stand still in a designated position while the examiner provides occasional distracters. Errors involving the child's response to these distracters are recorded. The lateral eye gaze persistence task requires the child to sustain looking at an eraser tip held 45 degrees from the plane between the examiner and child's midline. The eraser tip is held in the contralateral visual field, and the child needs to sustain looking for 20 seconds. If the child

does not sustain looking for 20 seconds, the task is repeated, and the time score for each trial is added. If sustained for 20 seconds, the trial is not repeated, and the subject is automatically given a score of 40. Two trials in each direction allow for scoring mean time for right gaze, left gaze, and total mean time.

A motor impersistence subtest is included as part of the Benton Laboratory of Neuropsychology Tests (Benton, Sivan et al., 1994). There are eight tests that require maintenance of a movement or posture: keeping eyes closed, tongue protrusion while blindfolded and with eyes open, fixating gaze in lateral visual fields, keeping one's mouth open, maintaining central fixation during visual fields confrontation testing, head turning during sensory testing, and saying "ah."

Other examples of go-no go tasks include the Archibald and Kerns go-no go task (Archibald and Kerns, 1999, #934) modified from another task (LaPierre, Braun et al., 1995) to develop a more challenging task for a wider developmental spectrum. The task requires the child to respond rapidly by pressing a computer keyboard space bar to 1 per second flashes appearing in 60 white squares in pseudorandom locations against a blue background. These trials were not scored, but established the needed learned "prepotent" response. The scoreable trials were three parts of 50 trials each, for a total of 150 trials. In the first part, the child had to respond rapidly to white crosses, but not respond to the learned prepotent response—white squares. In the second part, the child responded to squares. The child again responded to crosses in the third part. Commission and omission errors were scored as responses to a no-go response and no response to a go response, respectively. Summary scores for each error type were added across all three parts. Normative data for this go-no go task are presented later in this chapter in Table 6–63.

Stop Signal Task

The stop signal task is a choice reaction time experimental task that presents a classic paradigm for behavioral inhibition (Logan, 1994). The child must respond to a visual stimulus and voluntarily inhibit his or her response on an infrequent presentation of an auditory stop signal (Logan and Cowan 1984; Logan, Cowan et al., 1984). The ability to stop, to inhibit the prepotent response, is an internally generated and automatic process that is constant across strategies or tasks (Logan, 1981). The stop signal reaction time (SSRT) is the primary outcome measure, a measure of the speed of the inhibitory process (Kooijmans, Scheres et al., 2000). Difficulty can be adjusted by varying the interval between stimulus presentation and stop signal presentation. This paradigm is evident in the requirements of the Walk, Don't Walk subtest of the TEA-Ch.

The test was administered along with the Stroop test and TOL test in studies of inhibitory deficits in reading-disabled children (van der Schoot, Licht et al., 2000) and in children with DSM-IV diagnoses of ADHD (Pliszka, Borcherding et al., 1997) and DSM-IV ADHD-Combined type (Nigg, 1999). It was used in studies of impulsivity and inhibitory control in normally developing children and in those with childhood psychopathology, including ADHD, conduct disorder, learning disorder, and emotional disorder (Schachar and Logan, 1990). These studies supported its use as a measure of inhibitory control. Its validity as a measure of response inhibition was also supported by a study of the effects of methylphenidate for hyperactive children (Tannock, Schachar et al., 1989) and in a study investigating whether motivational factors (reward) influence the stopping performance in ADHD and TBI children (Konrad, Gauggel et al., 2000).

The latter study presumed different inhibitory control mechanisms underlying each clinical population: a motivational/energetic model for ADHD children that depends on the state of the child and allocation of energy, and a primary response inhibition deficit as part of general impairment in executive functions secondary to structural brain damage for TBI children. They found that ADHD children brought their performance level up to that of normal controls under reward contingencies, but rewards were less effective for brain-injured children. The Logan stop-signal paradigm was also incorporated in a study of response

inhibition and measures of psychopathology in which the authors found externalizing behavior was positively related to response inhibition, and symptoms of ADHD were better predictors of inhibitory functioning than aggressive behavior-disorder symptoms (Kooijmans, Scheres et al., 2000). A meta-analysis of studies utilizing the task has been published (Oosterlaan, Logan et al., 1998).

EXECUTIVE FUNCTION TESTS: FLUENCY

Verbal Fluency Tests

Verbal fluency tests are known by a number of terms, e.g., controlled oral word association (COWA), FAS Test, controlled word association (CWA), verbal word generation, word fluency, word retrieval, phonemic fluency or rapid verbal naming. Included are tests of *letter fluency,* which test the ability to generate words in response to a letter cue, and of *semantic fluency,* which test the ability to produce words in response to a category cue. Verbal fluency tests may be verbal or require a written response.

Verbal fluency tests involve speeded lexical production, promote automatic lexical access, and reflect efficient lexical organization (Dunn, Gomes et al., 1996). Two components of verbal fluency tests are (1), the linguistic component associated with left cerebral hemisphere function and (2) an ideational component associated with frontal lobe function. Performance is not independent of intelligence or vocabulary (Tager-Flusberg, 1985) or of attention. There is also a working memory component since the child must retrieve new words while remembering previously retrieved words to avoid perseverative responding (Watson, Balota et al., 2001). The ability to self-monitor, initiate, and shift characterizes performance on such tasks. Inhibition of rule-breaks is required, making it more a test of EF (Mahone, Cirino et al., 2002).

It is also of interest when a child provides a burst of responses initially, but then tapers off dramatically. Such responding is contrasted with the typical pattern of a greater number of errors in the first 15 to 20 seconds, followed by fewer responses, and then continued responding, but relatively few responses at the end of the time interval. To better assess this production pattern, I routinely record responses indicating either 20-second-interval responses or, following procedure associated with newer child normative data for verbal fluency, responses within each 15-second interval.

Adult studies found fluency influenced by age, intelligence, or gender, with older, higher IQ, and female superiority evident (Parkin and Lawrence, 1994; Spreen and Strauss, 1998). Semantic fluency is correlated higher with dysfunction of posterior cerebral regions, and letter fluency is correlated higher with more anterior cerebral region dysfunction in adult studies. Task difficulty level varies between letter and semantic fluency. Letter verbal fluency is considered more difficult for children than semantic fluency and assesses a linguistic ability that is minimally related to word knowledge (vocabulary) or verbal memory (Halperin, Healey et al., 1989). While word retrieval efficiency increases with age (Cohen, Morgan et al., 1999), it remains a question as to when adult response levels are reached. Some suggest that adult levels are reached around age 10 (Regard, Strauss et al., 1982), while others postulate continued development into adolescence (Welsh, Pennington et al., 1991).

Since the frontal lobes and a key relay zone of the hippocampal formation continue to develop into adolescence (Benes, Turtle et al., 1994), it has been suggested that some cognitive abilities, such as verbal fluency, continue to develop into adolescence as well. Thus, it may be that verbal fluency is more sensitive to neurodevelopment (Cohen, Morgan et al., 1999). An association of fluency tasks with frontal lobe efficiency has been consistently reported in adults (Borkowski, Benton et al., 1967; Jones-Gotman and Milner, 1977; Butler, Rorsman et al., 1993; Tucha, Smely et al., 1999). These studies particularly implicate anterior, left prefrontal regions (Milner, 1964; Pendleton, Heaton et al., 1982; Elfgren and Risberg, 1998), and activation was also found in supplementary motor cortex, anterior cingulate cortex, and the cerebellum (Ravnkilde, Videbech et al., 2002). How well verbal and nonverbal fluency correlates with focal or lateralized cerebral lesions is of continued inter-

est to researchers. Impaired performance in the presence of left frontal lobe lesions was reported early (Perret, 1974; Jones-Gotman and Milner, 1977; Tucha, Smely et al., 1999) and supported by recent neuroimaging studies (Parks, Lowenstein et al., 1988; Frith, Friston et al., 1991). However, the dissociation is not entirely discrete. Some studies show reduced verbal fluency with right frontal lesions (Miller, 1984; Tucha, Smely et al., 1999; Butler, Rorsman et al., 1993) and reduced verbal and nonverbal fluency in left-sided compared to right-sided lesion patients (Butler, Rorsman et al., 1993). The temporal lobes are also associated with verbal fluency function. Decreased verbal fluency is reported after either left or right temporal lobectomy (Loring, Meador et al., 1994), further supporting the idea of a relevant contribution to such ability from either cerebral hemisphere. Yet, fluency impairment after frontal lesions in adults often appears greater than after temporal lesions (Crowe, 1992), emphasizing the relative importance of anterior cerebral regions. Also, evidence of greater nonverbal fluency impairment with right frontal lesions has not always been found, arguing against a hypothesis of a clean, double dissociation between verbal and nonverbal fluency and frontal lesion side (Tucha, Smely et al., 1999).

Clustering and Switching

Semantic clustering is a strategy adults with well-developed EF use to group rote information in conceptually meaningful clusters during memory encoding (Beebe, Ris et al., 2000). The ability to cluster semantically appears to follow a developmental trajectory from childhood to adult maturation, reaching adult levels in the second decade of life (Bjorklund and Douglas, 1997). While children begin to adopt such strategies early, in response to explicit instruction before they are able to self-impose a strategy (Cox and Waters, 1986), it is not advisable to interpret a young child's clustering scores in the same way one evaluates an adult's clustering score (Cowan, 1997), for example, on the California Verbal Learning Test (CVLT).

A study of the tendency of adult subjects to switch spontaneously between subcategories on semantic verbal fluency testing has demonstrated that those with frontal lobe lesions are less likely to switch (Troyer, Moscovitch et al., 1998). The importance of distinguishing between endogenous (spontaneous) and exogenous (external) directed switching has been recommended since these might be differentially sensitive to frontal lobe damage, that is, switching following endogenous cueing may be impaired following focal frontal lesions, while switching in response to exogenous cueing may remain intact (Baldo, Shimamura et al., 2001). Adult studies have also found spontaneous strategy use is impaired in frontal lobe lesion patients. Thus, adults failed to cluster target words when attempting free recall. Their impaired spontaneous semantic clustering contrasted with more intact function when explicitly directed to employ semantic categories (Gershberg and Shimamura, 1995).

Qualitative inspection of aspects of letter and semantic fluency tests is also helpful, and guidelines have been reported for quantifying such qualitative features. For example, clustering and switching are easily observed and scored, and both are needed for optimal test performance. Scoring guidelines have been published (Troyer, Moscovitch et al., 1997; 1998). (On semantic fluency tests, *clustering* refers to generation of two or three consecutive words with a shared meaning or the generation of contiguous words within subcategories; *switching* to the ability to shift from one subcategory to another.) Scoring examples of clustering on a semantic fluency test would be two or three successive words in the same semantic subcategory.

On letter fluency tests, clustering is scored by reference to the sequence of words and might include *(a)* words beginning with the same two letters, *(b)* words in which the vowel changes (e.g., rate, rote) or *(c)* homophones— words with the same sound but different spelling. Letter fluency scoring requires data about word production, semantic clusters (above three sequences), phonemic clusters, and related words. Switching is scored by the formula "WP-RW + No. Clusters = No. Switches," where WP = word production and RW = related words. It is noted that the D-KEFS quantifies several qualitative aspects of

fluency (Delis, Kaplan et al., 2001), including naming errors, reading errors, inhibition errors, and inhibition/switching errors.

Switching on letter-cued word generation tasks was associated with frontal function and clustering with temporal lobe function in the adult literature (Rich, Troyer et al., 1999). Examination of clustering and switching has recently been considered in childhood and adolescence (Roncadin and Rich, 2002; Caroline Roncadin, Jill Bee Rich, Janice Johnson, and Marcia Barnes, 2002, personal communication). The later maturation of frontal than temporal brain regions and the continuation of frontal lobe myelinization into adolescence or young adulthood has led investigators to consider differential observations of clustering and switching by using verbal fluency tests. The expectation was that clustering would plateau earlier than switching (Roncadin and Rich, 2002).

Letter (FAS) and semantic (animals) fluency tests were administered to 96 children and adolescents between 6 and 17 years of age (4 boys and 4 girls per age) who were native English speakers, had no history of neurological or developmental disorders, and had an IQ in the broad normal range (79–128). Using the detailed scoring protocol of Troyer and colleagues (Troyer, Moscovitch et al., 1997), three scores were separately calculated for letter and for semantic fluency: total correct (number of correct words generated), clustering (mean number of words per subcategory), and switching (number of switches between subcategories). Means and standard deviations by age are presented in Table 6–34. Clustering and switching showed different developmental trajectories as predicted.

While age correlated strongly with total words generated and number of switches in both the letter and semantic conditions, mean cluster score was unrelated to age for either condition. Consistent with their prediction, clustering appeared to plateau early in development, with adult levels in clustering (Troyer, 2000) demonstrated by children as young as 6 years of age. These data therefore suggested that developmental gains in clustering occur in the preschool years. In contrast to clustering, switching developed over a more protracted

Table 6–34. Means (Standard Deviations) for Fluency Measures by Chronological Age

Age	n	PHONEMIC FLUENCY			SEMANTIC FLUENCY		
		Total Correct	Clustering	Switching	Total Correct	Clustering	Switching
6	8	7.75 (4.27)	0.18 (0.23)	5.38 (2.56)	9.75 (2.87)	0.90 (0.66)	6.00 (1.69)
7	8	16.63 (4.81)	0.33 (0.18)	10.88 (3.98)	11.50 (2.39)	1.24 (0.61)	6.00 (2.20)
8	8	17.00 (6.95)	0.24 (0.17)	12.38 (5.90)	12.50 (3.96)	1.24 (0.46)	6.25 (2.19)
9	8	21.63 (8.47)	0.30 (0.20)	14.63 (5.93)	12.13 (4.22)	1.22 (0.82)	6.50 (2.73)
10	8	28.63 (8.80)	0.41 (0.13)	19.00 (7.31)	14.63 (3.74)	1.33 (0.86)	7.50 (2.39)
11	8	29.38 (6.95)	0.27 (0.15)	21.75 (5.23)	15.63 (1.77)	1.16 (0.51)	8.00 (1.51)
12	8	29.63 (8.19)	0.35 (0.22)	20.38 (7.84)	12.75 (2.25)	0.92 (0.67)	8.00 (3.07)
13	8	33.88 (10.80)	0.28 (0.10)	25.13 (8.10)	15.13 (2.03)	1.19 (0.42)	8.00 (1.77)
14	8	32.50 (7.98)	0.33 (0.11)	22.63 (4.98)	16.13 (3.52)	1.29 (0.62)	8.38 (4.07)
15	8	27.75 (8.12)	0.31 (0.20)	19.00 (5.13)	17.50 (5.58)	1.38 (1.04)	8.25 (3.06)
16	8	37.13 (11.01)	0.34 (0.14)	26.25 (9.68)	19.25 (4.68)	1.42 (0.77)	8.63 (1.69)
17	8	38.88 (10.06)	0.31 (0.11)	28.13 (9.78)	19.13 (3.00)	1.17 (0.61)	10.13 (3.80)

Source: Courtesy of Caroline Roncadin, Jill B. Rich, Janice M. Johnson, and Marcia A. Barnes (2002), personal communication.

period, not reaching maturity until adolescence. When clustering was not used, as was the case in letter fluency in typically developing children, then "total correct" and "switching" become almost the same score.

These data appeared consistent with the adult literature, where switching appears to depend on the frontal system and clustering on posterior, temporal regions. The investigators suggested that switching might be less useful for assessing letter fluency performance in children than in adults. They further suggested that adjunct scoring of clustering and switching may improve the diagnostic utility of verbal fluency tests with atypically developing children and adolescents.

Verbal Fluency for Letters

Various letter generation tests are essentially identical to one another in procedure, but the specific data obtained may differ. For example, some word-generation measures assess verbal production, while others assess written production. For some, the score is the total of multiple trials, while others rely on a single trial. Normative data have been reported for letters of progressively increasing associative value, e.g., C, F, L, along with recommendation of the alternates P, R, W (Benton and Hamsher, 1976).

For some letter fluency tests, the letters and their presentation sequence were determined by each letter's verbal productivity and English-language frequency of occurrence. One test version (FAS) elicits responses for three letters that have been determined to fall within the easy difficulty range: F, A, S. Another version (CFL) requires responses to C, F, L (or the P, R, W alternative—PRW), in which one letter of the three falls within a moderately difficult range: L and R (Borkowski, Benton et al., 1967). Despite three easy letters for the FAS form, and two easy and one hard letter for CFL, investigation of the comparability of FAS and CFL found equivalence of the two forms across settings and diagnostic groups, with correlations ranging from .87 to .94 (Lacy, Gore Jr. et al., 1996). Normative data for PRW are not available, but correlation of the PRW with CFL for 54 normal subjects (counterbalanced order) was a moderately strong .82. A comparison of mean scores for the CFL and PRW forms found the means to be nonsignficantly different (Benton, Hamsher et al., 1994).

The question sometimes arises about whether normative data obtained for FAS or CFL are equivalent. The comparability of FAS and CFL was investigated, and it was concluded that the two forms are essentially equivalent. A correlation between CFL and FAS of between .87 and .94, which surpassed the CFL and PRW correlation, was found in a clinical sample of 287 adults. These data suggest that CFL and FAS forms can be used interchangeably and as alternate forms (Lacy, Gore Jr. et al., 1996). A similar study with children has not been reported.

Verbal Fluency: Letter F

Word retrieval data for a single letter, F, has been reported, along with additional data for design fluency, animal naming, block design, and vocabulary scores from a normative study on eighty 6- to 13-year-old Canadian children by four grade levels (Regard, Strauss et al., 1982). These demographic data for both males and females in first, third, fifth and seventh grade are presented in Table 6–49 and the normative data are presented in Table 6–50, along with five-point design fluency (see Design Fluency Tests, below), animal fluency, and block design and vocabulary raw score data.

NEPSY Verbal Fluency

The NEPSY Verbal Fluency subtest requires the child aged 3 to 6 years old to generate words in response to two semantic cues (animals, and things you can eat or drink). Unlike other such tests, the examiner is allowed to probe for response within any 15-second segment of the 60-second trial. A child aged 7 to 12 must generate words in response to the two above-noted semantic cues and two phonemic (the letters S and F) letter cues (Korkman, Kirk et al., 1997). Probes are also allowed for these children. The NEPSY standard scoring procedure combines all trials to obtain one total score. Supplemental scoring data for considering these two tasks separately are provided. An

examiner will likely want to consult these supplemental data, given the interesting dissociation that results and that may have relevant clinical meaning. It should be noted, however, that discrete norms for both letter and semantic tests are discussed later in this chapter, and these may offer the examiner a better appreciation of the child's competence with each type of word-generation task.

Verbal Fluency: Letters F, A, S

The FAS Test is part of the Neurosensory Center Comprehensive Examination for Aphasia (NCCEA; Spreen and Benton, 1977). Child normative data were published for kindergarten through sixth grade (ages 6 to 12 years) (Benton and Hamsher, 1976; Schum, Sivan et al., 1989; Benton, Hamsher et al., 1994). Early normative data for children aged 6 to 13 were published (Gaddes and Crockett, 1975) (see Table 6–35). Data were also published for oral and written FAS production that included 15 to 20 year olds ($N = 62$) along with adults (Yeudall et al., 1986) (see Table 6–36). Retest reliability ranges from .67 to .88 (Spreen and Strauss, 1998). Normative data for 14-year-olds were omitted.

Three 60-second trials are given for the three letter word retrieval task—one trial each for the letter F, A, and S. The examiner says,

"I am going to say a letter of the alphabet and I want you to say as quickly as you can all the words you can think of that begin with that letter. For instance, if I say "B" you might say "bad, battle, bed . . ." or other words like that. I do not want you to use words

Table 6–35. Normative Data for FAS Word Generation

Age	FEMALES			MALES			TOTAL		
	n	Mean	SD	n	Mean	SD	n	Mean	SD
6	30	4.6	5.0	22	4.1	4.1	52	4.4	4.6
7	24	16.0	7.3	27	14.1	6.5	51	15.0	6.9
8	23	23.1	5.7	25	22.5	7.7	48	22.8	6.8
9	30	25.0	7.3	23	22.6	6.4	53	24.0	6.9
10	25	27.4	7.1	25	23.8	8.2	50	25.6	7.8
11	22	31.1	6.8	22	28.2	8.1	44	29.7	7.6
12	13	32.0	6.8	13	29.4	8.1	26	30.7	7.4
13	12	37.3	5.8	17	28.8	8.3	29	32.3	8.4

Source: Adapted from Gaddes and Crockett (1975).

Table 6–36. Oral and Written FAS Normative Data for 15–20-Year-Old Males and Females

	Mean	SD
Males		
Oral		
F	13.82	4.36
A	12.48	3.87
S	15.87	4.52
Total FAS	42.17	6.82
Written		
F	13.85	3.65
A	12.06	3.24
S	14.81	3.34
Total FAS	40.72	6.14
Females		
Oral		
F	13.60	4.29
A	11.93	3.82
S	15.93	4.31
Total FAS	41.46	6.71
Written		
F	14.40	3.97
A	13.00	3.15
S	15.88	3.27
Total FAS	42.75	6.33

Source: Adapted from Yeudall et al. (1986)

that are proper names, such as the names of people or places, so you would not say words such as "Boston, Bob, or Buick." Also, do not use the same word again with a different ending, such as "eat" and "eating." Do you have any questions? (pause) Okay, begin when I say the letter. The first letter is "F." Go ahead."

Timing begins immediately. The number of correct words for all three trials is the total score. Incidentally, intrusion and perseverative errors should be recorded for their qualitative value. An intrusion error is a word that is not appropriate for the target stimulus, such as saying "circular" when generating words for the letter S. A perseveration error is a repetition of a word already stated. Perseverative errors raise concern about the ability to maintain words in the brief short-term buffer, also referred to as working memory (see above).

Yeudall and colleagues (1986) have provided data on adolescents with relatively high education levels (see Table 6–36). It should be noted that those with education levels below grade

12 achieved about four to five words less on the sum total score. FAS, semantic generation, and set shifting fluency trials are part of the D-KEFS (Delis, Kaplan et al., 2001).

Verbal Fluency: Letters C, F, and L

The Controlled Oral Word Association Test (COWAT) version using letters C, F, and L was introduced in the Multilingual Aphasia Examination (MAE) (Benton and Hamsher, 1976; Schum, Sivan et al., 1989; Benton, Hamsher et al., 1994). The procedure is identical to that described above for the FAS test, i.e., three 60-second trials are given for each of the letters C, F, and L (or the alternates P, R, and W). Normative data for 6- to 12-year-old children, in kindergarten through sixth grade, are presented in Table 6–37. Percentiles by grade are presented in Table 6–38.

More recent investigation expanded the MAE child normative data to include seventh and eighth graders, children aged 13 and 14 years old (Steven Zorich and Kerry Hamsher, unpublished data, 2002, personal communication). Interpretation of these data should be qualified by the fact that these data were being prepared for a doctoral dissertation committee when submitted for this book. Subjects of average verbal ability were included, as assessed with the Peabody Picture Vocabulary Test-3 (PPVT-3). Children with PPVT-3 Scores between 80 and 120 were accepted, with the seventh grade mean = 102.06 (11.21) and eighth grade mean = 106.85 (8.66). The 32 seventh and 33 eighth graders children were from a small midwestern town in the United States and were tested in the summer follow-

Table 6–37. MAE Normative Data for CFL Generation

Age	Grade	Mean	SD
6.3	K	9.1	5.2
7.3	1	14.4	4.6
8.2	2	17.6	6.2
9.3	3	22.7	6.5
10.2	4	26.7	7.4
11.3	5	24.2	6.9
12.3	6	25.8	5.0

Source: Benton, Hamsher, and Sivan (1994); Schum, Sivan and Benton (1989); © Swets & Zeitlinger.

Table 6–38. MAE Controlled Oral Word Association—Percentiles for Children by Grade

Score	K	1st	2nd	3rd	4th	5th	6th	Score
40					99	99		40
38				99	95	95	95	38
36				97	85	90	90	36
34				96	80	85	85	34
32			99	90	75	80	80	32
30			95	87	65	75	75	30
28			92	80	60	70	70	28
26		99	90	70	55	60	55	26
24		97	85	60	45	40	45	24
22		95	80	50	35	30	30	22
20	99	90	65	40	30	25	20	20
18	95	80	55	30	25	20	10	18
16	85	60	40	20	15	15	5	16
14	80	40	30	10	5	5	1	14
12	70	35	20	5	1	1		12
10	55	20	15					10
8	45	10	5					8
6	35	5	1					6
4	20	1						4
2	10							2
1	5							1

Source: Benton, Hamsher, & Sivan (1994); Schum, Sivan & Benton (1989); © Swets & Zeitlinger Publishers.

ing their seventh and eighth grade school year, respectively. An independent samples T-test on the mean PPVT-3 scores was calculated: $t = -1.923$, $df = 58.34$, sig. (two-tailed) = 0.059.

There was approximately equal male and female representation, the majority was Caucasian, and the town's mean socioeconomic status was lower-middle class (S. Zorich, 2002, personal communication). The means and standard deviations by grade for CFL word generation by these children are presented in Table 6–39.

Adolescent data for 100 high school athletes were reported for COWAT performance across

Table 6–39. MAE Normative Data for CFL Generation: 7th and 8th graders

Age	N	Grade	Mean	S. D.
13	32	7	25.97	8.04
14	33	8	28.24	6.47

Source: Unpublished data, courtesy of Steven Zorich and Kerry Hamsher.

two sessions separated by approximately 60 days, along with data on selected WAIS-III subtest scores, the Trail Making Test, and the Hopkins Verbal Learning Test (Barr, 2003). The demographic data for this study are presented in Table 7–14. The complete data sets are presented in Tables 11–18, 11–19, and 11–20, and include a table of adjusted reliable change indices calculated for 90%, 80%, and 70% confidence intervals along with percent of sample with scores falling below the lower limit. The results are presented with a caution about interpreting test data from high-school athletes, raise question about test–retest reliability, and suggest that separate norms for males and females are warranted.

Verbal Fluency: Letters C, P, B, and R

A study of word retrieval in response to four letters (C, P, B, and R), and for 30-second trials, was reported for 6- to 12-year-old children (Cohen, Morgan et al., 1999). As with the above letter fluency tasks, no proper names or plural forms of previously verbalized responses are scored. A four-letter paradigm was suggested to enable qualitative discriminations related to EF and word retrieval. The 30-second limit resulted from the observation that children, especially young children, exhaust their retrieval at around 15 to 20 seconds (Morris Cohen, 2002, personal communication). Whether this procedure meets its intended goals without eliminating valuable data remains to be determined empirically. The choice of a more traditional procedure of three letters for 60-second trials currently provides more substantial normative data. The demographic data for this study are presented in Table 6–40, and the normative data in Table 6–41.

Verbal Fluency for Category: Semantic Fluency

Semantic fluency, or word generation in response to a category cue, is believed to develop more rapidly than letter fluency since the latter depends on maturation of spelling ability. Prototypical response norms for category word generation tests are available (Uyeda and Mandler, 1980). One can consider the quality of the response along with intrusion and perseveration errors as characteristic features of the child's performance that might distinguish between normal and abnormal response patterns.

Animal Fluency

Word retrieval data for the category Animals was reported along with additional data for design fluency, letter F fluency, block design, and vocabulary raw scores in a normative study on 6- to 13-year-old Canadian children by four grade levels (Regard, Strauss et al., 1982). These data are presented in Table 6–50.

Table 6–40. Demographic Data for CPBR Word Generation: Cohen et al. Study (1999)

Subjects: 130 children
Gender: 64 male; 66 female
Age: 6 to 12 years
Race: 84.6% Caucasian; 15.4% African American
SES: N/A
Inclusion Criteria: Normal intelligence (Otis-Lennon standard score ≥85
Mean = 106.28 ± 10.92), grade level reading, no behavior problems, no academic retention

Table 6–41. Means and SD for CPBR Word Generation

Age	N	Mean	SD
6.0–6.11	19	15.53	4.99
7.0–7.11	19	19.47	5.61
8.0–8.11	18	23.67	6.82
9.0–9.11	17	23.76	3.58
10.0–10.11	19	26.63	4.81
11.11–11.11	19	28.32	5.43
12.0–12.11	19	30.42	5.81

Source: Cohen et al. (1999), © Swets & Zeitlinger.

McCarthy Scales of Children's Abilities Category Fluency

The McCarthy Scales of Children's Abilities (McCarthy, 1972) includes a semantic fluency subtest requiring a verbal response to category cues. These 1972 normative data for a standardization sample of 1032 children include sample sizes ranging from 100 to 106 for each age level, i.e., 10 age groups spaced at half-year intervals between 2½ and 5½ years and at yearly intervals until 8½ years. The child is required to name things to eat, animals, things to wear, and things to ride. The score is the total number of words generated for all four categories, with a 20-second time limit per trial. Table 6–42 provides these older normative data from 1972.

A comparatively small number of children were assessed with the McCarthy word fluency subtest as part of a study of prefrontal function in children (Welsh, Pennington, et al., 1991), with the age range extended to 12 years. The mean total raw scores and SDs by age for number of words generated for all four categories (things to eat, animals, things to wear, and things to ride) in a 40-second time limit per trial, instead of the 20-second McCarthy time limit, are presented in Table 6–42.

Multilingual Aphasia Examination: Semantic Fluency

Category fluency data for adolescents generating words in response to animals, fruits, or vegetables, and a combined score, are now available for a limited size age sampling. The Multilingual Aphasia Examination (MAE) Semantic Fluency norms were expanded to in-

Table 6–42. Means and *SD*s for Two Category Fluency Test Versions

Age	40-SECOND TRIALS[1]			20-SECOND TRIALS[2]		
	N	Mean	SD	N	Mean	SD
2				102	2.5	2.7
3	10	12.7	4.60	104	4.7	3.6
3.5				100	6.2	3.8
4	10	16.6	6.29	102	9.1	4.3
4.5				104	11.1	5.2
5	10	19.5	5.72	102	12.9	4.8
5.5				104	14.8	5.3
6	10	28.7	4.76	104	18.4	4.3
7	10	29.6	6.80	104	21.5	5.5
8	10	33.4	9.32	106	23.5	5.3
9	10	35.0	5.23			
10	10	39.0	8.93			
11	10	45.1	6.59			
12	10	54.9	9.79			

Source: [1]Welsh et al. (1991), courtesy of Lawrence Erlbaum Associates. [2]Adapted from Table 17, McCarthy Scales of Children's Abilities Manual (1972).

clude 65 seventh and eighth graders (S. Zorich and K. Hamsher, 2002, personal communication) (see C, F, L above for demographic data). These data supplement the original data for first to sixth graders and are presented in Table 6–43.

A number of larger test batteries also include semantic fluency subtests. For example, the Clinical Evaluation of Language Fundamentals (3rd ed.) (CELF-3) provides normative data for word generation to two categories, plus occupation names (Semel, Wiig et al., 1995). Normative data are provided for total number of responses for all three categories and 60-second trials.

First Name Fluency

The use of first name fluency tests was stimulated by the interest in developing a control task with fewer organizational and phonological demands than the more commonly used letter and semantic word retrieval tests. It was used to discriminate an initiation problem from more linguistic or semantic aspects of word generation. That is, better first name than letter or category fluency suggests initiation problems are not the most likely explanation for poor performance. Whereas, if first name fluency is poor, along with letter or category fluency, then initiation problems need to be strongly considered as do possible linguistic or semantic difficulty.

A study of 73 public school children was the first to present first name fluency norms, and these results were compared with those of 146 children referred for learning difficulties (see Table 6–44 and Table 6–45) (Harris, Marcus et al., 1999). A standard 60-second trial was given.

Table 6–43. MAE Normative Data for Animals, Fruits, Vegetables, and Total Generation: 7th and 8th graders

Age	N	Grade	ANIMALS		FRUITS		VEGETABLES		TOTAL	
			Mean	S. D.	Mean	S. D.	Mean	S. D.	Mean	S. D.
13	32	7	18.9	3.6	10.5	2.8	7.3	2.6	36.7	7.1
14	33	8	18.3	3.5	11.15	2.9	8.4	2.2	37.96	6.8

Source: Unpublished data courtesy of Steven Zorich and Kerry Hamsher.

Table 6–44. First Name Fluency Test: Controls: Harris et al. Study (1999)

Subjects: 73 children
Gender: 38 male; 35 female
Age: 7 to 10 years; Mean = 110 months, $SD = 12.5$
Race: Not reported
SES: Mostly middle class families
Inclusion Criteria: No known learning or medical problems

The results presented in Table 6–46 indicate that referred learning disabled (LD) children generated fewer first names than controls, girls generated more names than boys for each group, and there was clear improvement with increasing age.

Naming of Animals, Foods, and Words Beginning with "SH"

A developmental naming study of normal children aged 6 to 12, 111 boys and 130 girls, (Halperin, Healey et al., 1989) consisted of three standard 1-minute trials. The child had to name animals, then food, and then words beginning with the sound "sh" (the sound is said, not the letters). Normative data are presented in Table 6–47. In one study, a decrement score was calculated for each subject, subtracting the number of words generated during the latter half of the test from words generated in the first half and dividing by the total number of generated words (Lockwood, Marcotte et al., 2001).

Written Fluency Test

Thurstone Word Fluency Test

The Thurstone Word Fluency Test (TWFT) requires written production of words under

Table 6–45. First Name Fluency Test: Learning-Disabled Children: Harris et al. Study (1999)

Subjects: 219 children; 146 referred for learning problems
Gender: Referred: 92 male; 54 female
Age: 7 to 10 years; Mean = 110 months, $SD = 12.1$
Race: Not reported
SES: Mostly middle class families
Inclusion Criteria: Referred for learning difficulties and participation in a larger study

timed conditions (Thurstone and Thurstone, 1938; 1949; 1962). It was adapted to assess spontaneity of language in brain-injured individuals (Milner, 1964; Ramier and Hécaen, 1970). The task gives subjects 5 minutes to generate words beginning with "S" and then 4 minutes to produce four-letter words beginning with "C." The test was considered useful in detecting the presence or absence of focal or diffuse brain damage, but not useful in lateralizing a lesion. It was affected more by frontal than by nonfrontal, left hemisphere than right hemisphere, and left frontal than right frontal lesions in an adult study (Pendleton, Heaton et al., 1982). Child normative data (Kolb and Whishaw, 1985) are presented in Table 6–48. Qualitative features to look for include rule breaking, such as producing "C" words greater than four letters, and quality of written production.

Design Fluency Tests

Design fluency tests are considered analogous to verbal fluency tests and potential measures of right frontal cerebral function (Lee, Strauss et al., 1997). However, these tests are likely to be sensitive to brain dysfunction in other locations, and poor design generation cannot be interpreted as specific evidence of such focal dysfunction. Like verbal fluency tests, design fluency tests tap the EF subdomains of initiate, shift, self-regulate, and self-monitor. One contrast between verbal and design fluency is that the former require strategic generation of stored words, while the designs of the latter are not stored in memory.

Design fluency tasks typically require rapid generation of nonrepresentational designs, although at least one version has no time constraints—graphic pattern generation (Glosser and Goodglass, 1990). Some versions are "fixed" with restriction to a specific number of lines (e.g., four) and include a free condition (Jones-Gotman and Milner, 1977). Others only require unrestricted or free drawings, and some restrict generation to printed configurations of dots (Regard, Strauss et al., 1982; Ruff, 1988; Delis, Kaplan et al., 2001). These might vary dot positions or include interference stimuli (Ruff, 1988).

Early studies employing design fluency often depended on investigators' subjective scor-

Table 6–46. First Name Fluency Means (*SD*) and *N*s for Control and Learning-Disabled (LD) Children

| Age | CONTROLS | | REFERRED LD | |
	Male	Female	Male	Female
7	11.2 (2.9)	14.8 (5.1)	9.13 (2.8)	11.4 (2.8)
	N = 5	N = 5	N = 15	N = 10
8	13.8 (5.8)	16.9 (5.1)	12.1 (3.5)	15.67 (5.8)
	N = 11	N = 14	N = 20	N = 12
9	17.0 (5.9)	20.22 (8.7)	14.78 (4.4)	18.61 (7.0)
	N = 10	N = 9	N = 31	N = 18
10	18.25 (5.9)	25.86 (5.2)	15.23 (4.4)	20.6 (5.4)
	N = 12	N = 7	N = 26	N = 14

Source: Harris et al. (1999).

ing judgments, while later test development resulted in a structured procedure that enhanced reliability and ease of administration, with persons 16 years old and older (Evans, Ruff et al., 1985; Ruff, Light et al., 1987; Vik and Ruff, 1988). Perseverative and nonperseverative errors are considered indicative of a failure to self-regulate or self-monitor. Qualitative observations should at least include notation about perseveration, rule breaking, and line quality, as well as total generated correct output. Some investigators quantified one or more of these observations. For example, perseverative errors on the Five-point Test were useful in distinguishing right frontal from nonfrontal adult patients, while left frontal patients had the second highest perseverative error scores, but did not differ significantly from other clinical groups (Lee, Strauss et al., 1997).

Early studies found right frontal and right frontocentral patients tended to perform worse than left frontal patients on design fluency (Jones-Gotman and Milner, 1977), but later studies suggested the characteristic distinction between left frontal mediation of verbal fluency and right frontal mediation of design fluency was less clear than originally thought. Specifically, more recent studies have suggested there is a contribution to design fluency from both right and left frontal regions (Glosser and Goodglass, 1990).

In another study, a prominent contribution of the left hemisphere was suggested, since left frontal lobe tumor patients had both poorer verbal and nonverbal fluency than right frontal lobe tumor patients (Butler, Rorsman et al., 1993). Further, results of a regional cerebral blood flow study found that design fluency activated the frontal lobes bilaterally (Elfgren and Risberg, 1998). Only recently have both design and verbal fluency been studied in adults with focal frontal lesions and compared

Table 6–47. Normative Data for Naming of Animals, Foods, and Words Beginning with "sh"

| Age | ANIMALS | | | FOODS | | | "SH WORDS" | | | TOTAL FLUENCY | | |
	N	M	SD	N	M	SD	N	M	SD	N	M	SD
6	34	10.74	2.4	34	9.74	3.3	34	4.24	1.6	34	24.71	5.9
7	40	12.43	2.9	40	11.88	2.7	40	5.53	1.6	40	29.83	5.5
8	32	12.31	2.7	36	11.11	3.4	38	5.21	2.1	31	28.45	6.4
9	38	13.76	3.7	37	14.05	3.9	44	5.95	2.4	36	33.33	7.7
10	22	14.27	3.7	29	13.97	2.2	38	6.00	2.0	21	34.48	6.3
11	28	15.50	3.8	30	14.80	4.6	36	6.28	2.4	27	36.78	8.0
12	10	18.90	6.2	10	17.70	4.0	10	6.10	1.8	10	42.70	9.7

Source: Halperin et al. (1989), © Swets & Zeitlinger.

Table 6–48. Written Fluency Normative Data

	TOTAL			MALE			FEMALE		
Age	N	M	SD	N	M	SD	N	M	SD
6	80	9.28	4.47	40	8.70	4.33	40	9.85	4.58
7	133	15.87	8.22	61	14.26	8.00	72	17.22	8.20
8	197	21.52	9.29	112	19.85	8.05	85	23.72	10.34
9	208	25.93	10.18	118	24.03	10.01	90	28.41	9.93
10	189	29.98	11.92	103	27.32	11.39	86	33.16	11.83
11	146	37.08	11.98	71	35.01	13.07	75	39.03	10.57
12	140	40.58	13.00	56	34.61	10.61	84	44.52	12.98
13	167	45.07	14.10	91	39.81	12.26	76	51.37	13.65
14	175	48.46	14.72	90	44.52	14.08	85	52.64	14.30
15	120	47.35	15.22	69	44.23	15.88	51	51.57	13.28
16	69	48.28	13.69	41	44.76	14.56	28	53.43	10.54
17	79	49.65	17.51	42	46.12	16.83	37	53.65	17.63
18	30	61.47	15.29	12	57.33	5.42	18	64.22	14.98

Source: Adapted from Kolb and Whishaw (1985).

to an age- and education-matched control group. Of interest was the finding that, whereas left frontal patients performed worse than right frontal patients on verbal fluency, as expected, the two groups had comparable design fluency performance (Baldo, Shimamura et al., 2001), suggesting design fluency is somewhat dependent on bilateral anterior cerebral regions.

Age can have an impact on design fluency performance. Normative studies found that the number of generated figures increased with age, peaked between ages 16 and 24, remained constant between 25 and 55, and then declined. Although age effects for normal subjects are reported, they did not occur in a clinical sample of adults with a history of unilateral cerebrovascular accident (Glosser and Goodglass, 1990).

Motor speed did not appear to correlate significantly with performance, performance IQ had a moderate correlation with performance, and verbal fluency and Ruff Figural Fluency Test (RFFT) correlation lacked significance for both adults and children (Ruff, Light et al., 1987). The RFFT appears to be sensitive to discriminating between moderate and severe head-injury patients (Ruff, Evans et al., 1986).

Five-Point Test

The Five-point Test (Regard, Strauss et al., 1982) is a timed figural fluency test. The adult version has 40 dot matrices within rectangles arranged in 5 columns and 8 rows, and originally allowed 5 minutes, although some report a 3-minute time limit, comparable to common verbal fluency time limits. In an adult study, patients with frontal lobe dysfunction had a higher percentage of perseverative errors than nonfrontal neurological or psychiatric patients, and there was higher classification accuracy for right frontal impaired patients. These data were interpreted as support for the Five-point Test's sensitivity to frontal brain dysfunction (Lee, Strauss et al., 1997).

The child version consists of a sheet of paper on which the 40 4 × 3 cm rectangles with a fixed pattern of five symmetrically placed dots as placed on dice are printed. After two samples are shown, the child has 5 minutes to produce as many different, unique designs as possible by connecting the dots with one or more straight lines. A warning is given the first time he or she makes either of two error types: drawing a line that does not connect dots and/or repeating a design. The responses can be scored for total number of figures, number of perseverative designs, number of rotated figures, number of figures using added dots, number of self-corrections, and percent correct. Data for number of figures produced, number of rotated figures, and number of self-corrections are presented in Table 6–50. There were no significant effects for number of repeated designs, number of figures using added dots, or percent correct.

Table 6–49. Five-point Test Demographic Data: Regard et al. Study (1982)

Subjects: 80 children in public school in Victoria, Canada
Gender: 40 male, 40 female (10 each in each grade: 1, 3, 5 and 7)
Age: Mean age 6.3 in Grade 1, 8.4 in Grade 3, 10.6 in Grade 5 and 12.4 in Grade 7
Handedness: All right-handed
Inclusion/Exclusion criteria: No failed grade, no psychiatric or neurological disorders

The design fluency test was only moderately correlated with intelligence, as assessed with WISC-R block design and vocabulary scores. Normal children produced unique designs that increased in number linearly up to approximately age 10 years, when performance became comparable to that of normal adults; only 10- and 12-year-olds self-monitored productions; and early male > female gender differences in performance disappeared by adolescence (Regard, Strauss et al., 1982). The demographic data for this sample is presented in Table 6–49, a sample of 80 normal, right-handed, 6- to 13-year-olds in four grades. The mean age was 6.3 years for those in grade 1, 8.4 years for grade 3, 10.6 years for grade 5, and 12.4 years for grade 7. The results provided the normative data for mean number of figures, number of rotated figures, and number of self-corrections listed in Table 6–50.

In another study, the original 5-minute version and a 3-minute version were administered to 30 children aged 11 years, 9 months to 14 years, 8 months (Mean = 13.0 years), in grades 6, 7, and 8 (Risser and Andrikopoulos, 1996). The two versions were equivalent, and the neurologically normal adolescents performed at the level of neurologically normal adults. For the 3-minute version, adolescents averaged 29.5 unique designs (*SD* = 7.77). They made on average 1.27 perseverative errors (*SD* = 1.76). For the 5-minute version, adolescents averaged 42.6 unique designs (*SD* = 11.45). They averaged 2.57 perseverative errors (*SD* = 2.97). Age and gender did not affect performance.

NEPSY design fluency modification

The NEPSY battery (Korkman, Kirk et al., 1997) includes a 35-item modification of the Five-point Test as a design fluency subtest for 5- to 12-year-olds. Instead of the original 5-minute time limit, there is a 60-second time limit for each of two parts, a structured array of dots for the first part, and a random array of dots for the second. NEPSY design fluency normative data are available, based on 800 children since the normative sample is comprised of 100 children at each age level.

Ruff Figural Fluency Test

The Five-point Test was adapted to construct the Ruff Figural Fluency Test (RFFT) (Ruff, Light et al., 1987), a measure that consists of five pages or parts, 35 squares to a page, and 5 black dots arranged within each square. Parts I, II, and III have the same dot arrangement, but distractors are superimposed on Parts II and III. Parts IV and V have no distractors, and the dot arrangement is less symmetrical. Normative data are provided for the summary total score and error ratio, but not for the individual subtests, for those in grades 1 to 8, and also aged 16 and older.

The RFFT instructions for children ask them to view a pattern of dots and then connect two or more dots, using straight lines, to make a design or picture. They are instructed to work quickly and make sure each picture drawn is different from the others. Each of five parts is preceded by three sample items. There is a 60-second time limit per part.

Recognizing the importance of determining whether a child's strategy is similar to that of the adult, qualitative aspects of figural fluency have been examined in addition to the usual quantitative variables of number of designs generated and number of perseverative responses. *Rotation strategy* has been defined as "either the entire figure is systematically rotated or some portion of the figure is rotated while the rest of the figure remains fixed." *Quantitative strategy* was determined if the "basic figure remains constant while a single line is systematically added to or removed from each successive figure in the strategy" (Vik and Ruff, 1988, p. 66). Design complexity, defined as the number of lines used for each design, was also measured to determine whether young children draw random figures that require more time to complete than drawings by older children. Also, a slight but nonsignificant learning effect has been seen to take place over

Table 6–50. Five-point Test Means and SDs by Grade and Gender

| | | FIVE-POINT TEST | | | | | | F TEST | | | | | | | | | | |
| | | FIGURES | | ROTATED FIGURES | | SELF-CORRECTIONS | | WORDS | | NON-WORDS | | ANIMAL NAMING | | BLOCK DESIGN | | VOCABULARY | |
Grade/Sex	N	M	SD	M	SD	M	SD	M	SD	M	SD	M	SD	M	SD	M	SD
1	20	22.48	12.56	5.90	3.89	0.10	0.31	5.80	2.65	0.20	0.52	10.05	3.25	15.15	5.86	17.05	5.72
Girls	10	20.46	12.46	6.30	4.76	0.10	0.32	6.60	2.80	0.10	0.32	9.10	3.31	13.20	5.69	16.0	3.37
Boys	10	24.50	12.96	5.50	2.99	0.10	0.32	4.90	2.33	0.30	0.67	11.00	3.06	17.10	5.63	18.10	7.43
3	20	30.10	9.92	10.90	4.34	0.05	0.22	8.45	3.30	0.00	0.00	13.40	3.00	28.60	8.46	27.40	5.30
Girls	10	27.10	7.52	11.70	4.57	0.00	0.00	8.00	2.26	0.00	0.00	13.70	2.83	28.30	9.75	28.20	5.51
Boys	10	33.10	11.46	10.10	4.18	0.10	0.32	8.90	4.18	0.00	0.00	13.10	3.28	28.90	7.46	26.60	5.23
5	20	37.35	8.99	13.25	5.82	0.50	0.69	10.20	3.07	0.00	0.00	15.70	4.02	29.15	11.05	34.55	6.17
Girls	10	36.40	7.63	11.00	3.92	0.40	0.52	10.30	2.79	0.00	0.00	14.60	4.27	27.40	9.41	34.40	5.93
Boys	10	38.30	10.50	15.50	16.70	0.60	0.84	10.10	3.48	0.00	0.00	16.70	3.65	30.90	12.74	34.70	6.72
7	20	44.00	8.71	18.60	6.79	0.35	0.67	10.90	3.27	0.00	0.00	15.70	3.69	40.90	12.45	36.75	5.68
Girls	10	45.00	9.09	17.50	7.43	0.20	0.42	12.00	3.27	0.00	0.00	16.00	2.54	43.00	14.91	37.00	4.90
Boys	10	43.00	8.68	19.70	6.27	0.50	0.00	9.70	2.98	0.00	0.00	15.40	4.70	38.80	9.76	36.50	6.64

Source: Regard, M., Strauss, E. & Knapp. P. Children's production on verbal and non-verbal fluency tasks. *Perceptual and Motor Skills,* 1982, 55, 839-844. © Perceptual and Motor Skills 1982.

the five parts, but the number of strategies generated has tended to be negatively affected, once the dot matrix becomes more random, as it is in Parts IV and V.

It was found that older children (Grades 5 to 8) made more mean total and unique figures than younger children (Grades 1 to 4) and that older children employed more strategies and produced a greater number of figures in a strategy than younger children. Children in Grades 1 to 4 rarely used strategies; strategy use began to appear more consistently around fifth grade, at about 11 to 12 years old, but was not applied by all older children. Perseverations, error ratio (perseverations/unique figures), and average line number were not significantly different between grades. Intelligence was correlated significantly with strategy use in Grades 5 to 8, a higher IQ associated with strategy use (Vik and Ruff, 1988).

The subjects' demographic data are described in Table 6–51. It should be noted that mean Expressive One Word Picture Vocabulary Test IQ scores for Grades 1 to 2, 3 to 4, and 5 to 6 was over 120 (within superior limits), while the mean score for Grades 7 and 8 was 105 (within average limits). Normative data by grade and RFFT part are presented in Table 6–52.

Delis-Kaplan Executive Function System— Design Fluency

The Delis-Kaplan Executive Function Scale (D-KEFS) Design Fluency Test rules require the child aged 8 or older to complete three conditions (Delis, Kaplan et al., 2001). The general rules are that the child must use only four straight lines, each line must start at a dot and end at a dot, and each line must touch at least one other line at a dot. On Condition 1, the child is required to generate novel designs connecting filled dots on the answer sheet. On

Table 6–51. Figure Fluency Test Demographic Data: Vik and Ruff Study (1988)

Subjects: 87 children
Gender: Not reported
Age: 6.4 to 14.6 years
Race: Not reported
Intelligence: Estimated with Expressive One Word Picture
    Vocabulary Test; ranged from 79 to 145
SES: Not reported; attending public and private schools

Table 6–52. Figural Fluency Test Mean Scores

Grades	RFFT PART				
	I	II	III	IV	V
1 and 2	7.21	8.26	8.84	9.32	8.84
3 and 4	9.14	9.86	9.89	10.57	10.93
5 and 6	12.39	13.35	13.26	14.04	14.70
7 and 8	14.44	16.00	16.31	16.13	17.25

Source: Vik & Ruff (1988), Courtesy of Lawrence Erlbaum Associates.

Condition 2, the child generates designs connecting only empty dots. Condition 3 requires the child to switch between filled and empty dots. Each condition is 60 seconds long, and the primary measure is the total number of correct designs. There are procedures for quantifying several additional aspects of design fluency, set loss errors, repetition errors, total number of attempted designs, and design accuracy percentage.

EXECUTIVE FUNCTION TESTS: ESTIMATION

Biber Cognitive Estimation Test

Cognitive estimation refers to when an individual provides an answer to a question based on his or her best judgment since the necessary or relevant knowledge is not known (Shallice and Evans, 1978). The mental operations involved in estimation are similar to those deficient in the presence of brain injury and ADHD. Estimation skill requires inhibition of impulsive responding as well as appropriate judgment. Thus, it may be that this type of test has greater ecological validity than other tests in assessing executive functions, although this remains to be examined. The Biber Cognitive Estimation Test (BCET) was developed to establish quantitative rather than subjective judgments of normality for items in several content areas. A broad definition of the normal range was reached through a large participant sample. The final version consists of 20 items (see Table 6–53), 5 each in the categories of time/age, quantity, weight, and distance/length) (Fein, Gleeson et al., 1998). Participants' an-

Table 6–53. Biber Cognitive Estimation Test Questions

1. How many seeds are there in a watermelon?
2. How much does a telephone weigh?
3. How many sticks of spaghetti are there in a one pound package?
4. What is the distance an adult can walk in an afternoon?
5. How high off a trampoline can a person jump?
6. How long does it take a builder to construct an average-sized house?
7. How much do a dozen, medium-sized apples weigh?
8. How far could a horse pull a farm cart in one hour?
9. How many brushings can someone get from a large tube of toothpaste?
10. How many potato chips are there in a 40-cent, one-ounce bag?
11. How long would it take an adult to handwrite a one-page letter?
12. What is the age of the oldest living person in the United States today?
13. How long is a tablespoon?
14. How much does a folding chair weigh?
15. How long does it take to iron a shirt?
16. How long is a giraffe's neck?
17. How many slices of bread are there in a one-pound loaf?
18. How much does a pair of men's shoes weigh?
19. How much does the fattest man in the United States weigh?
20. How long does it take for fresh milk to go sour in the refrigerator?

Source: D. Fein, M. Gleeson, S. Bullard, R. Mapou, & E. Kaplan (1998).

swers to each question were scored on a 0–2 point scale, based on answers given by a large sample of normal adults. These ranges are reported by Fein and colleagues (1998) and are presented in Table 6–54. Scores that fell within the response range of 95% of the normal sample received a score of 1. Scores that fell between the 25th and 75th percentile of the adult distribution received a score of 2.

Data were obtained for a cognitive estima-

Table 6–54. Item Characteristics from the BCET Adult Normative Sample

Item	Category	Units	Mean	SD	Normative Range	25–75% Range
1	Quantity	Seeds	218.1	194.8	25–1000	80–300
2	Weight	Pounds	2.7	2.0	0.3–10	1–3
3	Quantity	Sticks	186.6	129.7	35–600	85–250
4	Distance/Length	Miles	12.8	6.9	1–35	8–17.5
5	Distance/Length	Feet	9.4	4.9	2–20	4.5–15
6	Time/age	Months	3.2	2.1	.25–10	1.25–4
7	Weight	Pounds	4.3	2.3	1–13	2.5–5
8	Distance/Length	Miles	5.7	3.8	1–20	2.5–8
9	Quantity	Brushings	99.0	82.2	20–500	45–100
10	Quantity	Chips	30.6	19.8	7–100	16–40
11	Time/age	Minutes	15.8	9.1	3–45	9–20
12	Time/age	Years	111.7	5.6	102–127	105–114
13	Distance/Length	Inches	5.9	2.1	1–12	4–7
14	Weight	Pounds	5.6	4.0	0.5–20	2.3–7
15	Time/age	Minutes	8.0	4.6	2–20	4–10
16	Distance/Length	Feet	7.0	3.3	1–16.4	4–8
17	Quantity	Slices	21.2	5.5	10–35	17–25
18	Weight	Pounds	2.3	1.3	0.375–8	1–3
19	Weight	Pounds	687.0	260.9	210–1500	478–830
20	Time/age	Days	11.2	4.9	3–30	6–14

Source: Courtesy of the authors, Fein et. al. (1998).

tion test administered to 315 school aged children aged 5 to 16 years old, in Kindergarten through 11th grade in four northeastern U.S. public school systems. Socioeconomic status ranged from lower-middle to upper-middle class. The 30-item, WISC-III Information subtest was also administered. The construct of cognitive estimation was found to be reliable, and a positive developmental trend was noted on inspection of the trajectories for each domain. Performance plateaued at about 9 years old. Age, intelligence, and fund of knowledge correlated with overall test performance. There were no gender effects. The resulting normative data are presented in Table 6–55.

Time Estimation

Time estimation has a long history in psychological research but has received even greater interest recently as investigators attempt to support or refute the hypothesis that children with ADHD should manifest time sense impairment due to working memory impairment (Barkley, 1997a). A test of this theory with 6- to 13-year-old children with ADHD and a matched control group found those with ADHD performed significantly below controls on measures of inhibition, attention, and time reproduction, but not differently than controls on working memory tasks (Kerns, McInerney

et al., 2001). There is also interest in better understanding the time perception paradigms that elicit the most difficulty (West, Douglas et al., 2000). Time perception has been assessed in children using estimation, production, or reproduction methods (see Zakay, 1990, for a review). *Estimation* tasks require a verbal report of the length of a sample duration. *Production* tasks involve producing a time duration in some way to match the duration length indicated. This could be accomplished by drumming the fingers for the specified length of time, for example. Time *reproduction* tasks require manual replication of a demonstrated time duration, e.g., 15 seconds of finger drumming. Time reproduction tasks are considered the most effortful WM tasks since the specific time duration to be replicated must he held in mind and used as a template for motor duplication (Barkley, Murphy et al., 2001). Poor motor inhibition is also associated with these time sense deficits. This is especially true with time reproduction paradigms, in which those who are less inhibited make more underreproductions than those who are more inhibited (Barkley, Murphy et al., 2001). A computer-administered test of time perception is the Timetest, with four subtests: a visual subtest without distractors, a visual subtest with distractors, an auditory subtest without distractors, and an auditory subtest with distractors (Barkley, 1998).

Table 6–55. Means (Standard Deviations) of Cognitive Estimation Scores by Age

Domains	5	6	7	8	9	10	11	12	13	14	15	16	Means
							AGE						
Quantity (0–10)	2.93_a	$3.88_{a,b}$	$4.74_{b,c}$	$5.82_{c,d}$	$6.96_{d,e}$	$6.71_{d,e}$	$6.68_{d,e}$	$6.83_{d,e}$	7.45_e	$7.04_{d,e}$	$6.45_{d,e}$	$7.07_{d,e}$	6.33
	(1.82)	(1.50)	(1.73)	(1.77)	(1.64)	(1.45)	(1.38)	(1.20)	(1.30)	(1.15)	(1.84)	(1.58)	(1.89)
Time (0–10)	1.29_a	2.25_a	3.84_b	$4.96_{b,c}$	$5.96_{c,d}$	$5.93_{c,d}$	6.60_d	$6.34_{c,d}$	$6.36_{c,d}$	7.00_d	6.87_d	7.18_d	5.79
	(1.73)	(1.39)	(1.80)	(1.71)	(1.64)	(1.77)	(1.44)	(1.56)	(1.81)	(1.41)	(1.59)	(1.28)	(2.21)
Weight (0–10)	3.00_a	$3.69_{a,b}$	$4.32_{a,b,c}$	$5.50_{b,c,d}$	6.30_d	6.56_d	6.36_d	$6.00_{c,d}$	6.50_d	6.22_d	6.87_d	6.66_d	5.96
	(2.15)	(1.85)	(2.16)	(1.95)	(2.16)	(2.12)	(2.25)	(2.04)	(1.79)	(1.93)	(1.61)	(1.84)	(2.21)
Distance (0–10)	2.14_a	$3.44_{a,b}$	$4.74_{b,c}$	$6.21_{c,d}$	6.70_d	$6.27_{c,d}$	$6.08_{c,d}$	6.66_d	6.77_d	6.87_d	7.16_d	7.30_d	6.21
	(2.51)	(2.39)	(1.73)	(1.42)	(1.29)	(1.36)	(1.58)	(2.02)	(1.48)	(1.58)	(1.46)	(1.61)	(2.07)
Composite (0–10)	2.34_a	3.31_a	4.41_b	5.63_c	$6.48_{c,d}$	$6.37_{c,d}$	$6.43_{c,d}$	$6.46_{c,d}$	6.77_d	6.78_d	6.84_d	7.05_d	6.07
	(1.34)	(1.26)	(1.21)	(1.05)	(0.91)	(0.93)	(1.07)	(1.36)	(0.94)	(0.84)	(0.94)	(0.81)	(1.59)
N	14	16	19	28	23	41	25	29	22	23	31	44	

Note. Cells within a row that have a common subscript are not significantly different from each other.

Source: Courtesy of Brian Harel, unpublished master's thesis (Deborah A. Fein, Brian T. Harel, Antonius Cillessen, Edith Kaplan, Mary Kay Gleeson, Robb Mapou, Alyson Aviv, Sarah E. Bullard).

MATRICES

A number of matrices tests of nonverbal reasoning are available for children and adolescents. Some versions are subtests within larger batteries, such as the WAIS-III matrix reasoning for those 16 years old and older, nonverbal matrices in the CAS for 5 to 17 year olds, the matrices subtest of the DAS for 5 to 17 year olds, and a subtest within the Kaufman Brief Intelligence Test (K-BIT). The Raven's Coloured Progressive Matrices and Raven's Standard Progressive Matrices Tests are individual tests with a long history of clinical use.

Raven's Progressive Matrices Tests

The Ravens Coloured Progressive Matrices Test (Raven, 1965) is a nonverbal visuospatial reasoning test requiring attention to visual detail (Part A), pattern matching (Part AB), and the ability to analyze and reason about nonverbal stimuli (Part B). Normative data are available for children aged 11 years old or younger, with data extrapolated down to age 3½. Its association with right anterior cerebral impairment in clinical evaluation received neuroimaging support since the right dorsolateral prefrontal cortex was activated during Raven's test performance (Prabhakaran, Smith et al., 1997). While considered to be a more culturally fair instrument for the evaluation of cognitive ability than many other tests, it, like many cognitive measures, is negatively affected by lowered socioeconomic status (SES) (Raven, Court et al., 1992). There are three parts, each with 12 items, allowing for a maximum score of 36 (Raven, Summers et al., 1986).

The Raven's Standard Matrices Test is similarly an untimed test that requires pattern recognition and analogy to choose among a multiple-choice array of six to eight possibilities for the correct answer for a series of black-and-white designs that have a portion missing. There are five parts, A, B, C, D, and E, each with 12 items. There is also a short version with six items from each part. The answers depend on appreciating spatial, design, or numerical relationships for pattern matching or completion. Normative data for British children 8 to 13 and 13 and older are published in the 1977 manual, along with normative data on 3464 Irish children aged 5 to 11 years old (Raven, Court et al., 1977).

TESTS ELICITING PERSEVERATION

Perseveration refers to an abnormal continuation of behavior in the absence of the appropriate stimulus, or the immediate recurrence of a previous response to a later stimulus. It is not modality specific, but rather, is observed across modalities, such as the verbal perseveration in speech or graphomotor perseveration in design copying. Perseveration is closely associated with frontal lobe damage in adults (Kolb and Whishaw, 1990), but occurs with damage to other brain regions or when there is frontal system pathway disruption. While not unique to frontal lobe dysfunction, it is often more pervasive in the presence of such disruption while nonfrontal lesions may be associated with less severe perseveration that is restricted to domains related to the specific compromised regions. It has been proposed that clinical features of prefrontal syndromes do not necessarily imply there is selective structural or biochemical damage to the prefrontal cortex and that a structurally diffuse central nervous system (CNS) disease may masquerade as a selective frontal lobe disease (Goldberg, 1986).

Perseveration is also observed in non–CNS-diagnosed individuals, including some patients with psychiatric disorders such as schizophrenia. In a study of perseverative tendencies of dementia patients, it was concluded that perseverative behavior is hierarchically arranged in terms of specific levels of cognitive complexity, with an overall pattern of cognitive deficits associated with each dementia type (Lamar, Podell et al., 1997). A 3-factor model was found with perseveration related to semantic knowledge, motor functioning, or an intermediary factor (Lamar, Podell et al., 1997). The authors postulated that some perseverations are due to impaired complex cognitive functioning, while others are secondary to a breakdown of more elementary cognitive functions.

Perseveration is conceptualized in various ways. The Supervisory Attention System (SAS) model (Norman and Shallice, 1986) explains perseveration and other attentional problems by frontal-lobe-damaged patients as resulting from an impaired SAS, which leads to action being captured by the immediate environmental stimuli (Shallice, 1982). In another description, three types of perseverative behavior were each associated with a specific neuroanatomic substrate (Sandson and Albert, 1984). One, *continuous perseveration,* refers to the inappropriate prolongation of a behavior without interruption as seen in graphomotor disturbances. This was associated with subcortical pathology, that is, basal ganglia damage. A second, *recurrent perseveration,* refers to a repetition of a previous response to a subsequent stimulus, caused by faulty memory function. It is seen, for example, in Alzheimer's dementia and aphasic disturbances of the posterior left hemisphere. The third, *stuck-in-set perseveration,* refers to the inability to switch mental set from one mode of output to another and is uniquely associated with frontal lobe pathology. This taxonomy was compared with that of Goldberg and Tucker (Goldberg and Tucker, 1979; Goldberg, 1986). Overlap was found, such that continuous perseveration was compatible with the latter's *hyperkinesia-like motor perseveration,* recurrent perseveration was viewed by the latter as able to be split into two subtypes: *perseveration of features* and *perseveration of elements,* and stuck-in set perseveration matched with *perseveration of activities.*

Intrusion errors are considered a form of perseverative error. Specifically, they refer to a delayed repetition of a previous response after intervening stimuli. A number of child neuropsychological tests allow for scoring of intrusion errors, and only a few provide normative data for these errors, e.g., intrusion errors committed on the 12-word Selective Reminding Test (SRT) as a measure of EF (Vellutino and Scanlon, 1985). The WCST perseverative error and perseverative responses scores are valuable indices of mental shifting capacity. The adult literature suggests that intrusion and false positive errors are related to temporal lobe impairment, with or without frontal lobe dysfunction (Crosson, Sartor et al., 1993).

In addition to qualitative observations of perseveration, some cognitive tasks specifically elicit such responding more easily than other tasks. The Repeated Patterns Test and the Graphical Sequences Test are two such tests that are brief, easily accepted by children without graphomotor problems, and worthwhile including in testing sessions that are specifically concerned with evaluating EF as well as when more information is needed about handwriting and visuomotor integrative capacity.

Repeated Patterns Test

The Repeated Patterns Test (RPT) is a modification (Waber and Bernstein, 1994) of the Rhythmic Writing subtest of the Purdue Perceptual-Motor Inventory (Roach and Kephart, 1966) and Kephart designs. The RPT is a brief test used to assess prevalence and severity of graphomotor output problems. The ability to distinguish between motor and linguistic demands in the presence of written language disorder makes this test a potentially valuable additional screening instrument for LD children. Graphomotor output is evaluated independently since there are no linguistic demands like spelling or letter formation. The test therefore differs from other visuomotor integration and dexterity tests in its direct applicability to handwriting, assessing the ability to control and sustain repetitive or sequential movement or to routinize a motor program.

The instructions are: "For each of these patterns, I would like you to continue the pattern across the page until I tell you to stop." Five sequences are presented on a single sheet of paper. The child places a pen at the end of each printed pattern until a "go" signal is given. No explicit indication is given that speed is a goal. There is a time limit of 15 seconds for each pattern.

The production is scored for quality of patterns and number of repetitions. For the quality score, responses are compared to exemplars (Waber and Bernstein, 1994), and each pattern production is ranked from 1 for poor, 3 for average, to 5 for excellent. A "goodness judgment" is made, and a numeric value of 1 to 5 assigned for each pattern. The sum of the 5 ratings is a global score, QSUM. The number of repetitions score is based on single units for each of the five patterns.

A normative sample based on results of a group administration only to right-handed school children (105 male, 103 female), not identified as learning disabled, is also available. The author found a main effect for sex, girls exceeding boys, on the quality scores but not on the number of repetitions scores. These data are presented by trial in Table 6–56.

Groups of learning disabled children, controls, and a smaller subset of children post

Table 6–56. RPT Means & *SDs* of Quality and Number of Repetitions by Age and Gender

Age		N	FEMALES Quality M (SD)	# Reps M (SD)	N	MALES Quality M (SD)	# Reps M (SD)
8		18			17		
	Trial 1		4.39 (0.61)	5.94 (1.76)		3.59 (0.87)	7.12 (1.76)
	Trial 2		3.94 (0.454)	13.06 (4.08)		3.53 (0.62)	14.24 (5.65)
	Trial 3		3.44 (0.78)	8.28 (2.52)		3.12 (0.86)	10.82 (3.50)
	Trial 4		3.61 (1.04)	2.56 (0.86)		3.00 (1.12)	3.00 (1.46)
	Trial 5		2.83 (0.99)	3.44 (1.15)		2.71 (1.05)	3.41 (1.77)
9		17			14		
	Trial 1		4.24 (0.66)	7.18 (1.42)		3.57 (0.65)	7.43 (2.10)
	Trial 2		4.35 (0.61)	18.47 (5.65)		3.93 (0.47)	16.21 (5.82)
	Trial 3		3.76 (0.83)	12.24 (3.54)		3.36 (0.84)	12.21 (4.54)
	Trial 4		3.65 (0.70)	4.88 (0.70)		3.21 (0.97)	4.50 (1.65)
	Trial 5		2.71 (1.05)	4.59 (1.62)		3.21 (1.12)	4.57 (1.79)
10		7			15		
	Trial 1		4.57 (0.53)	7.00 (1.00)		3.80 (0.86)	6.93 (2.12)
	Trial 2		4.43 (0.53)	17.71 (3.53)		4.30 (0.82)	15.00 (5.22)
	Trial 3		3.86 (0.38)	11.14 (3.53)		3.8 (1.26)	12.20 (3.36)
	Trial 4		4.43 (0.79)	5.14 (1.57)		3.3 (1.03)	4.20 (1.42)
	Trial 5		3.00 (1.41)	4.57 (2.57)		2.67 (0.98)	4.67 (1.27)
11		18			14		
	Trial 1		4.44 (0.70)	7.06 (1.70)		4.43 (0.51)	7.43 (1.50)
	Trial 2		4.50 (0.62)	15.17 (4.40)		4.14 (0.95)	15.93 (4.87)
	Trial 3		4.06 (1.00)	12.44 (2.83)		3.86 (0.53)	12.21 (2.97)
	Trial 4		4.06 (0.87)	4.39 (1.42)		4.07 (0.92)	4.79 (0.70)
	Trial 5		3.78 (0.94)	4.72 (1.93)		3.64 (1.08)	5.07 (1.44)
12		16			18		
	Trial 1		4.44 (0.73)	7.37 (1.54)		4.22 (0.88)	6.89 (1.53)
	Trial 2		4.50 (0.52)	15.87 (2.70)		4.17 (0.79)	15.22 (4.47)
	Trial 3		4.25 (0.58)	12.00 (3.10)		3.78 (0.88)	11.78 (2.62)
	Trial 4		4.19 (0.91)	4.75 (0.68)		4.06 (0.54)	5.00 (1.37)
	Trial 5		3.87 (1.02)	6.12 (2.55)		3.78 (0.94)	5.00 (1.85)
13		17			15		
	Trial 1		4.53 (0.80)	7.12 (1.50)		4.53 (0.74)	6.07 (1.53)
	Trial 2		4.53 (0.51)	16.47 (4.53)		4.47 (0.52)	15.73 (3.10)
	Trial 3		4.12 (0.78)	12.06 (2.82)		4.20 (0.56)	12.4 (3.02)
	Trial 4		4.41 (0.62)	4.53 (1.01)		4.27 (0.80)	4.73 (1.03)
	Trial 5		3.88 (0.86)	5.53 (1.59)		4.20 (0.94)	6.00 (1.69)
14		10			12		
	Trial 1		4.60 (0.52)	7.30 (1.25)		4.67 (0.49)	6.67 (1.07)
	Trial 2		4.70 (0.48)	17.40 (4.84)		4.50 (0.52)	16.17 (3.13)
	Trial 3		4.50 (0.53)	13.50 (2.01)		3.92 (1.08)	13.25 (1.62)
	Trial 4		4.40 (0.97)	5.20 (0.92)		3.92 (1.08)	4.58 (1.50)
	Trial 5		3.80 (0.92)	6.30 (1.42)		4.00 (1.85)	5.67 (1.50)

Source: Courtesy of Deborah Waber, personal communication.

Table 6–57. Demographic Data for Learning Disabled Subjects: Waber and Bernstein Study (1994)

Learning Disability Subjects: 174 children in Boston, Massachusetts, area
Age: 8 to 14 years; majority between 8 and 11 years
Gender: 127 male, 47 female
Handedness: 18% left handed
Race: Not specified
Inclusion criteria: Estimated IQ at least 85

Table 6–59. Demographic Data for Acute Lymphoblastic Leukemia Subjects: Waber and Bernstein Study (1994)

Acute Lymphoblastic Leukemia Subjects: 51 children in the Boston area
Age: 8 to 14 years
Gender: 29 male, 22 female
Handedness: Not specified
Race: Not specified
Inclusion criteria: Received CNS treatment for Acute Lymphoblastic Leukemia

central nervous system treatment for acute lymphoblastic leukemia (ALL) were studied (Waber and Bernstein 1994) and their demographic data are presented in Table 6–57, Table 6–58, and Table 6–59. The control data for QSUM are presented in Table 6–60, and data for the LD subjects are presented in Table 6–61. A subsequent study of children with attentional problems but without learning disability also supported the reliability and validity of this instrument (Marcotte and Stern, 1997).

A procedure has been outlined for obtaining a speed score, the number of times a unit is repeated in the 15-second time interval, and an objective score (Waber and Bernstein, 1994). For the latter, coding of two specific pattern features can be made: motor control and motor programming. Motor control was evaluated by size and deviation from the horizontal. Calculation rules for height (H) and width (W) scores are given along with summary categorical variable scores of 0, 1, or 2 for each. The sum of H + W becomes the MOT-CON variable, summarized as 0 (sum of zero), 1 (sum of one or two), and 2 (sum of three or greater). Deviation is scored only if the entire form is

outside guidelines. The motor programming score refers to output errors programming direction and shape, and samples are provided. Errors are scored for any error in item repetition for each design. Each design then receives a score of 0 for no errors, or 1 for one or more errors. Alternation errors, scored for only designs 4 and 5, are subtracted from the speed score (total number of repetitions) for an error score that is collapsed into a categorical score of 0 (no errors), 1 (3 or more errors) or 2 (3 or more errors).

Graphical Sequences Test

The Graphical Sequences Test (GST) (Goldberg and Tucker, 1979; Bilder and Goldberg, 1987; Jaeger, Goldberg et al., 1986) is a motor regulation and sequencing task. It was derived from the Graphomotor Sequences Test in the Luria Neuropsychological Investigation (Christensen, 1979), and is now part of the Execu-

Table 6–58. Demographic Data for Control Subjects: Waber and Bernstein Study (1994)

Control Subjects: 229 children in Boston, Massachusetts, area
Age: 8 to 14 years
Gender: 122 male, 108 female°
Handedness: 10% left handed
Race: Not specified
Inclusion criteria: Suburban children without learning disability

°Table sum differs by 1 with text sum.

Table 6–60. Repeated Patterns Test Means & SDs of QSUM by Age and Gender for the Control Group

Age	FEMALE			MALE		
	N	Mean	SD	N	Mean	SD
8	18	18.22	2.96	18	16.11	2.67
9	19	18.57	2.36	16	17.56	2.68
10	7	20.28	1.79	16	17.87	3.84
11	21	21.00	2.68	20	19.65	3.08
12	16	21.25	1.80	19	19.89	2.97
13	17	21.47	2.42	19	21.63	2.24
14	10	22.00	2.16	14	20.85	2.17

Source: Waber & Bernstein (1994); courtesy of Lawrence Erlbaum Associates.

Table 6–61. Repeated Patterns Test Means & SDs of QSUM by Age and Gender for the Learning Disability Group

Age	FEMALE			MALE		
	N	Mean	SD	N	Mean	SD
8	13	12.00	3.71	32	10.75	3.49
9	10	14.60	1.71	16	13.31	4.58
10	5	11.00	2.28	27	14.11	3.67
11	7	17.71	3.68	18	16.50	3.79
12	2	20.50	4.95	11	16.36	2.20
13	8	17.62	5.44	13	17.23	4.06
14	2	23.50	0.70	10	16.20	3.76

Source: Waber & Bernstein (1994); courtesy of Lawrence Erlbaum Associates.

tive Control Battery (Goldberg, Podell et al., 2000) along with three additional tests—the Competing Programs Test, Manual Postures Test, and Motor Sequences Test. The GST requires the individual to draw simple shapes or write the name of these shapes, numbers, or well-learned objects. It has proved useful in eliciting perseverative responding in a dementia study (Lamar, Podell et al., 1997). Only recently, have child data been collected and analyzed (Kenneth Podell, 2002, personal communication).

Alternating Sequences Tests

The ramparts design is a single line of alternating elements. It requires the subject to copy the design while it is left in view. The examiner then can observe whether the child can maintain the alternating set, whether perseverative responding emerges, and whether he can sustain responding in order to produce a sequence as long as the stimulus. When the stimulus drawing is positioned at the top of the answer page, the *closing-in phenomenon* might be observed that is associated with anterior cerebral dysfunction. Closing-in is a phenomenon in which an individual seems pulled toward a stimulus, that is, the individual may draw the design overlapping with or too close to the original stimulus (Loring, 1999).

I may also ask an older child or adolescent to write a connected sequence of alternating "m"s and "n"s (lower case) across the page. The

child is instructed to keep the pencil on the paper. Both of these tests may evoke perseverative responding. One has to be careful about interpreting errors on the m–n repetition task for a child who is too young to carry out the task successfully or whose handwriting problems are especially prominent. One may ask a younger child to print "X" and "O" in alternation.

EXECUTIVE FUNCTION TESTS FOR THE VERY YOUNG

There is limited availability of discrete EF tests for the very young child, even within the context of those standardized test batteries now available for young children. Importantly, as our knowledge of EF capacities in the very young child grows, there is also an accompanying interest in and development of a wider variety of EF test instruments and of empirical validation of these measures. Currently, these often have limited ecological validity data to support their use. One line of research is concerned with measurement of "basic" EF, those simple tasks that are less likely to require nonexecutive cognitive abilities (Archibald and Kerns, 1999). These authors chose to investigate the self-ordered pointing and delayed alternation/non-alternation (DANA) tasks, heavily dependent on working memory, and go-no go, Sun-Moon Stroop, and Fruit Stroop tests, tasks dependent on ability to inhibit. They published normative data for 89 Canadian children (see Table 6–62 for demographic data and Table 6–63 for the normative data).

Table 6–62. Demographic Data: Archibald and Kerns Study (1999)

Subjects: 89 children in Victoria, Canada
Gender: 38 male; 51 female
Age: 7 to 12 years; Mean = 10.03 years, SD = 1.72, Range = 6.9–12.91
Intelligence: Mean = 109.76, SD = 10.49, Range = 88–144
Race: Not reported
SES: Not reported
Inclusion Criteria: No neurological, psychiatric, developmental or learning difficulties

Table 6–63. Means (*SD*) for Four Executive Function Measures

Working Memory	Age	SOP-Err	DA-Err	DNA-Err	G-NG/O
	7	18.07 (6.64)	1.40 (2.47)	4.67 (5.67)	2.46 (2.18)
	8	16.41 (6.65)	4.00 (5.83)	2.75 (1.21)	1.89 (1.45)
	9	13.92 (3.57)	3.42 (3.34)	3.42 (1.93)	1.11 (1.27)
	10	12.72 (4.44)	3.65 (6.52)	13.00 (1.95)	0.74 (0.96)
	11	11.88 (4.16)	0.71 (1.25)	1.71 (0.76)	0.14 (0.38)
	12	12.00 (3.20)	2.73 (4.56)	2.07 (1.03)	0.20 (0.56)
Inhibitory Capacity	Age	G-NG/CO	Fruit	Golden	SunMo
	7	11.15 (4.16)	2.16 (4.18)	−7.67 (6.69)	−0.3046 (0.1115)
	8	8.11 (2.89)	4.43 (4.70)	−4.50 (4.26)	−0.2651 (0.0981)
	9	6.11 (3.02)	5.47 (5.77)	−6.56 (5.90)	−0.2806 (0.0912)
	10	5.35 (4.04)	8.64 (7.03)	−0.1544 (5.46)	−0.1714 (0.1128)
	11	3.86 (2.19)	10.58 (5.72)	2.82 (5.14)	−0.1183 (0.1695)
	12	4.27 (3.84)	15.52 (5.84)	3.37 (4.63)	−0.1584 (0.0795)

Note; SOP = Self-ordered Pointing; DA = Delayed Alternation; DNA = Delayed Non-alternation; GNG = Go/NoGo; Fruit = Fruit Stroop Interference; Golden = Golden Stroop Interference; SunMo = Sun Moon Stroop Interference; Err = errors; O = Omissions; Com = Commissions

Source: Archibald and Kerns (1999), © Swets & Zeitlinger.

Self-Ordered Pointing Test

The Self-Ordered Pointing Test (SOPT; Kates and Moscovitch, 1989), based on earlier work (Petrides and Milner, 1982), is primarily a measure of working memory due to its requirement that the child make a response, retain knowledge of that response, and self-monitor performance over trials. In terms of the working memory dichotomy between maintenance and manipulation, the SOPT is a maintenance task (Kerns, McInerney et al., 2001). It has been used in adult studies (Shimamura and Jurica, 1994; Bryan and Luszcz, 2001) as well as developmental child studies (Shue and Douglas,

1992; Archibald and Kerns, 1999). A normal adult positron emission tomography scanning study confirmed an association with frontal lobe function (Petrides, Alivisatos et al., 1993).

The SOP task was modified for school-aged children by using a booklet format with representational drawings of common, familiar objects, requiring a pointing rather than a verbal response, and using multiple subtests of increasing difficulty to improve sensitivity and appropriateness (Archibald and Kerns, 1999). The booklet consisted of 36 pages and four sections. Each page had a set of 6, 8, 10, or 12 line drawings of objects arranged in a matrix. The same pictures were printed on each page of a section, but in different spatial locations. The child was required to select a different picture on each page and the aim was to reach the end of a set without repeating a choice. Each section was presented three times, and the child had to begin with a different object than was selected first on a prior trial. The summary score is the total number of errors, summed across the sections. Normative data for this task are presented in Table 6–63.

Delayed Alternation/Nonalternation

Delayed alternation/nonalternation (DANA) is a spatial working memory computerized task. It was adapted as a child's "sports game" by Archibald and Kerns, from an existing task (Patriot, Verin et al., 1996). The child is required at each beep to press one of two keys, which will throw a basketball at the bottom of the computer screen into either of two basketball hoops at the top of the screen. A correct response results in the baskets disappearing and the word WIN appearing with the sound of cheering. An incorrect response receives no reinforcement.

The next trial begins 15 seconds later. A delayed alternation condition requires the child to alternate responses (win-shift), while the delayed nonalternation condition requires the child not to alternate between baskets (win-stay). The extended delay modification places demands on working memory and challenges older children. A summary score for each condition is the number of errors before reaching a criterion of 10 consecutive correct trials; the failure criterion is 80 trials. Final scores are the total number of errors for each condition. Normative data for this task are presented in Table 6–63. It was suggested that the skills required for DANA may asymptote around 7 to 8 years old (Levin, Culhane et al., 1991; Archibald and Kerns, 1999).

Espy Preschool Executive Function Battery

A battery of tests for preschool children 2 to 5 years of age is also in development that considers the more limited verbal repertoire, manual skill, and attention span of the very young

child (Espy, 1997; Espy, Kaufmann et al., 2001). For example, a colorful storybook presentation and easy-to-hold rubber stamp are effectively used to translate the Trail Making Test for this age group. The test is entitled Trails-P (Espy, 2002). A description of Trails-P and the instructions, along with preliminary normative data, follow. Other tests in development include Shape School (Espy, 1997), A-not-B (Espy, Kaufmann et al., 2001), Spatial Reversal, and Color Reversal. These tests are discussed here as a battery, although the reader will recognize that subtests might be divided between Chapter 7, and its discussion of working memory tasks, and this chapter on executive function. Another test in development by Espy and colleagues is the Continuous Recognition Test–Pre-memory measure (see Chapter 11).

Trails-P

Trails-P includes four conditions, or trials. In Condition A, the child is given an inked stamp with a easy-gripping handle and instructed to stamp dog pictures in order of size, starting with the "baby," through to the "daddy." In Condition B, pictures of like-sized bones are introduced, and the child must match the dogs with their appropriate-sized bone. In Condition C, the child must stamp the dogs in size order, but ignore the bones. In Condition D, pictures of cats are introduced as distractors, and the child must once again alternate between dogs and bones in size order. Performance is scored both for time to completion, including correction, as for the Trail Making Test, and for number of errors. In an initial study of 20 preschool children, there were 11 girls and 9 boys with a mean age of 4.3 years ($SD = 1.03$, range 2.9–5.9 years) (Espy, Cwik et al., 2002). Latency to complete the four conditions was stable: Mean time for Condition A was 35.6 seconds, Condition B, 35.1 seconds, Condition C, 31.7 seconds, and Condition D, 35.1 seconds. The children made more errors on Conditions C ($\bar{X} = 2.9$) and D ($\bar{X} = 2.7$) than on Conditions A ($\bar{X} = 1.8$) and B ($\bar{X} = 1.6$). Reliability and discriminant validity studies are yet to be conducted. Preliminary normative data for 44 children are presented in Table 6–64. The instructions are:

Table 6–64. Trails-P Preliminary Normative Data Means (*SD*)

Age Group		Control (Dogs)	Switch (Dogs & Bones)	Inhibit (Dogs, Ignore Bones)	Switch & Inhibit (Dogs & Bones, Ignore Cats)
3-year-olds	Mean				
M age = 3.36	Latency	43.56 sec	37.38 sec	41.56 sec	47.44 sec
(*SD* = .48)	(*SD*)	(20.91)	(15.67)	(18.64)	(25.16)
7 females	Mean Errors	2.44	1.63	2.63	1.44
9 males	(*SD*)	(2.45)	(2.16)	(1.67)	(1.68)
4-year-olds	Mean				
M age = 4.50	Latency	30.86 sec	29.93 sec	23.86 sec	28.79 sec
(*SD* = .33)	(*SD*)	(9.99)	(19.33)	(7.51)	(14.97)
6 females	Mean Errors	1.64	1.14	2.07	2.00
8 males	(*SD*)	(1.69)	(1.29)	(2.30)	(2.83)
5-year-olds	Mean				
M age = 5.60	Latency	16.71 sec	19.21 sec	18.21 sec	17.43 sec
(*SD* = .40)	(*SD*)	(11.78)	(12.10)	(12.34)	(10.01)
9 females	Mean Errors	0.79	0.57	0.57	0.29
5 males	(*SD*)	(1.72)	(0.76)	(0.65)	(0.47)

Source: Espy, Cwik, Senn, & Polcari (2002)

Race *n* = 28 Caucasian (68%), 13 nonwhite, 3 nonreporting.

The child is presented with pages of colorful dog characters in a storybook and told (for Condition A), "Here is a family of doggies. The littlest one is the baby dog, then the sister dog, then the brother dog. The mommy dog is here, and the biggest dog, the daddy dog, is right here. This dog family lives in this house." Adequate understanding of the differently sized dogs is then confirmed by saying, "Can you show me the little baby dog?" "The sister dog is the next biggest, where is she?" "Then comes the brother dog. Where is that brother dog?" The mommy dog is the next biggest dog, can you show me where she is?" and "Finally, the daddy is the biggest dog—where is he?" These instructions and questions are repeated until the child understands and answers correctly each time. The examiner says for the next picture, "The dog family loves to play outside. Here is the baby and sister playing soccer. The daddy and brother dogs are playing catch with a ball. The mommy dog is chewing on a shoe." For the next picture, the examiner says, "Now it is time for the dogs to come home. To get them home here, you have to stamp each doggie in order, from littlest to biggest, with this marker. Start with the little baby dog, then sister, brother, mommy dog, and finally, the big daddy dog and then get them home by mark-ing the home. Try and go as fast as you can without making any mistakes. Do you understand? Go!" Any time the child makes an error, the examiner returns the child to the last correctly stamped dog and tells the child to "Stamp the next biggest doggie."

The examiner marks the order of stamps on the sheet when the child is finished, turns to the next picture, and says (for Condition B), "Okay, now the doggies are home. They are hungry. Doggies like to eat bones. Here are some bones. Guess what, the little bones are for the baby dog, the next biggest bones are for the sister dog, and the biggest bones are for the brother dog." Turning to the next picture: "Now look at this picture. Here is the baby dog. Which bones are baby's? Stamp them. Here is sister dog. Which bones are sister's? Stamp them. Here is brother dog. Which big bones are brother's? Stamp them too." Turning to the next picture, "Now you are going to feed the doggies. To feed them, you have to stamp each doggie and then their bones with this marker in order. Start with the little baby dog, stamp baby, then find baby's bones, and stamp them to feed him. Then stamp sister and sister's bones to feed her, and then big brother and big brother's bones to feed him. Try and go as fast as you can with-out making any mistakes. Do you understand? Go!"

If the child errs, the child is returned to the last correctly stamped stimulus and told, "Stamp the next doggie, stamp the (e.g., sister) doggie's bones." Errors are marked in order at the conclusion.

The next picture is presented (Condition C) and the examiner says, "Yum, Yum, that was good! Now they are all full and ready to go to bed. They have eaten all the bones they can, and they don't want any more. But look! There are too many bones. This time, get the dogs home without eating any bones. To get them home here, you have to stamp each doggie in order, from littlest to biggest, with this marker. Start with the little baby dog, then sister, brother, mommy dog, and finally, the big daddy dog and then get them home by marking the home. Don't stamp any of the bones, remember they aren't hungry anymore. Try and go as fast as you can without making any mistakes. Do you understand? Go!" If an error is made, the child is returned to the last correctly stamped dog and told, "Stamp the next biggest doggie." The order of stamps is marked at the end. For the next picture, the examiner says, "All of the doggies are asleep in their house," and then for the next, "Here is the sun, it is a new day."

For the final picture (Condition D), the examiner says, "The doggies are hungry! They are ready to eat breakfast. But look, the cats are trying to eat their bones. Oh no! To let them eat, you have to stamp each doggy and then their bones with this marker in order. Start with the little baby dog, stamp baby, then find baby's bones, and stamp them. Then stamp sister and sister's bones, and then big brother and big brother's bones. Don't stamp a cat. If you do, the cat gets the bones. Try and go as fast as you can without making any mistakes. Do you understand? Go!" If errors are made, the examiner corrects the child by returning the child to the last correctly stamped stimulus and saying, "Stamp the next doggie, stamp the (e.g., sister) doggie's bones." Errors are marked in order at the conclusion.

Shape School

The Shape School test is a measure of inhibition and switching appropriate for the very young child (Espy, 1997) that uses a colorful storybook format. Early research data suggest it is sensitive to maturation. Importantly, it was designed to separate the inhibition and switching processes. The initial publication reported data on 70 Caucasian children from middle- and upper-middle income families who were born full term and had unremarkable developmental courses (Espy, 1997). Additional data were collected for a total N of 144 children (73 boys, 71 girls), including 22 nonwhite ethnic minority Black, Hispanic, and Asian children, and these data (Kimberly Espy, 2002, personal communication) are presented in Tables 6–37–6–40.

The Shape School has four conditions: Control (baseline naming), Inhibit, Switch, and Both (Inhibit and Switch). For the Control condition, the child views a picture of a schoolyard with a colored circle and square figures. (The color represents the pupil's name.) The child must then look at a picture of the pupils lined up to enter school from the yard. The child's task is to rapidly name the pupils in order without error: "red, blue, green . . . ."

In the Inhibit condition, figures have either happy or frustrated facial expressions, indicating their readiness for lunch. The child must name the pupils (colors) ready for lunch (the happy figures) and leave frustrated pupils unnamed. Stimuli naming was nearly perfect at all ages for the Control and Inhibit conditions, but speed decreased with age (see Tables 6–37–6–38). Inhibition improved greatly between 3 and 4 years (Espy, 1997).

In general, the Shape School appears sensitive to age-related changes in executive skill efficiency as young as 32 months old in Caucasian middle- and upper-middle family-income strata (Espy, 1997) and when a small subset of non-Caucasian children were included in data analyses (Kimberly Espy, 2002, personal communication).

Children over 48 months old are administered the Switch and Both conditions that employ shape as well as color. For Switch, another classroom picture is presented in which some pupils wear hats, and their name is their shape. All pupils have neutral facial expressions. The child is told that the pupils are going to storytime, and they must be named, i.e., color if hatless or shape if with hat. The ability to switch improved from 4 to 5 years (Espy, 1997).

In the Both condition, a picture of pupils with happy and frustrated faces, and with and without hats, is presented. The child is told that not all pupils are ready for art, and the child must name the happy-faced pupils who are

Table 6–65. Shape School Baseline Naming Control Condition Data

Age	N; Girls/Boy	CORRECT Mean	SD	TIME Mean	SD	EFFICIENCY Mean	SD
2.0–2.11	18; 10G/8B	14.67	0.84	44.77	17.26	0.37	0.12
3.0–3.5	20; 6G/14 B	14.25	1.33	47.75	32.00	0.37	0.14
3.6–3.11	29; 17G/12B	14.89	0.56	33.52	17.62	0.54	0.23
4.0–4.5	33; 18G/15B	14.36	2.00	28.30	13.29	0.62	0.28
4.6–4.11	18; 9G/9B	14.89	0.32	27.06	10.39	0.64	0.27
5.0–5.11	26; 11G/15B	14.88	0.43	23.15	10.27	0.74	0.25

Source: Espy (personal communication).

ready (i.e., by color or shape) and not name those who look frustrated. This condition proved too difficult for children younger than 5 (Espy, 1997). Preliminary normative data are presented in Table 6–65, Table 6–66, Table 6–67, and Table 6–68.

A-not-B

A-not-B is a Piagetian task that has been used in studies of prefrontal cortex lesioned rhesus monkeys (Diamond and Goldman-Rakic, 1989) and humans. Young children's ability to perform an A-not-B task suggests structures are in place that facilitate sensory encoding of the relevant object and that the child can demonstrate knowledge of the context with which to respond (Luciana and Nelson, 1998). The subject observes an object being hidden in one of two positions and is allowed to reach for the object after a specified delay. The object is placed in position A until the subject reaches consistently for it there, and then the object placement is switched to position B. To answer correctly, the subject must recall the position,

inhibit habitual behavior, and shift response set (Anderson, Anderson et al., 2000). Perseverative error on this task is the continued reaching to position A despite the change to position B. It has been speculated that delayed response might depend especially on the sulcus principalis, a subregion of the dorsolateral prefrontal cortex (Diamond, 1991).

QUESTIONNAIRE

Behavior Rating Inventory of Executive Function

The Behavior Rating Inventory of Executive Function (BRIEF; Gioia, Isquith et al., 2000) (see Baron, 2000, for a review) is a parent and teacher questionnaire that provides normative data for children aged 5 to 18 years. Normative data are based on ratings from 1419 parent respondents and 720 teacher respondents from urban, suburban, and rural school areas in Maryland, reflecting the 1999 U. S. Census demographic variables of gender, socioeco-

Table 6–66. Shape School Inhibition Condition Data

Age	N; Girls/Boy	CORRECT Mean	SD	TIME Mean	SD	EFFICIENCY Mean	SD
2.0–2.11	14; 8G/6B	13.21	2.26	81.69	31.22	0.19	0.09
3.0–3.5	15; 3G/12B	12.80	2.59	87.13	82.28	0.25	0.19
3.6–3.11	25; 15G/10B	13.96	1.95	36.04	17.40	0.48	0.23
4.0–4.5	30; 15G/15B	14.13	1.25	28.34	9.91	0.56	0.20
4.6–4.11	18; 9G/9B	14.22	1.70	23.94	10.32	0.70	0.29
5.0–5.11	25; 11G/14B	14.60	0.91	23.04	10.90	0.76	0.30

Source: Espy (personal communication).

Table 6–67. Shape School Switch Condition Data

Age	N; Girls/Boy	CORRECT		TIME		EFFICIENCY	
		Mean	SD	Mean	SD	Mean	SD
4.0–4.5	25; 12G/13B	12.04	3.48	48.72	15.26	0.26	0.09
4.6–4.11	18; 9G/9B	12.77	2.26	48.16	12.21	0.28	0.08
5.0–5.11	23; 10G/13B	13.22	3.06	36.26	9.32	0.39	0.14

Source: Espy (personal communication).

nomic status, ethnicity, age, and geographical population density (See Table 6–69). The BRIEF includes an 86-question Parent Form, a Parent Form Scoring Summary, an 86-question Teacher Form and a Teacher Form Scoring Summary. The answer sheets use a 3-point scale (Never, Sometimes, Often) for respondents with at least a fifth-grade education. Two validity scales intended to detect bias are included, a Negativity Scale (Acceptable, Elevated or Highly Elevated) and an Inconsistency Scale (Acceptable, Questionable or Inconsistent).

Each questionnaire form takes approximately 10 to 15 minutes to complete. Raw scores are translated to T scores by hand or with the assistance of a computer-scoring program that also provides interpretive information. T scores are derived for each scale relative to the normative sample. The manual includes tables of T scores, percentile ranks, and 90% confidence interval values for each scale by gender for four age groupings: 5 to 7 years, 8 to 10 years, 11 to 13 years, and 14 to 18 years. The demographic characteristics for both the parent and teacher questionnaires are presented in Table 6–69. Parent educational level, socioeconomic status, and ethnic group status were considered. Equivalence was found

between mothers' and fathers' responses, and it was determined that the findings were not biased by a teacher's length of time knowing the student.

The BRIEF Self-Report version with 135 items was developed for those 11 to 22 years old and at least a fourth-grade reading level (Guy, Gioia et al., 1998). Support for the ecological validity of the BRIEF for adolescents has begun to be reported (Turkstra and Kuegeler, 2001; Zabel, Verda et al., 2002). A preschool version is also in development (Gioia, Espy et al., 2002; Isquith, Gioia et al., 2002). The authors report only a small correlation between BRIEF scores and IQ (Gioia, Isquith et al., 2000).

Eight subdomains of executive function were identified by principal components analysis. The Inhibit, Shift, and Emotional Control subdomains compose an additional broader composite Behavioral Regulation Index (BRI). The subdomains Initiate, Working Memory, Plan/Organize, Organization of Materials, and Monitor provide a composite Metacognition Index (MI). The BRI and MI are then combined for an overall Global Executive Composite (GEC). Base rate data are provided for both the parent and teacher normative sample to aid determination about whether a statisti-

Table 6–68. Shape School "Both" Condition Data

Age	N; Girls/Boy	CORRECT		TIME		EFFICIENCY	
		Mean	SD	Mean	SD	Mean	SD
4.0–4.5	24; 12G/12B	12.04	2.85	59.59	32.14	0.28	0.18
4.6–4.11	16; 7G/9B	12.31	2.65	45.06	18.47	0.31	0.13
5.0–5.11	24; 11G/13B	12.71	3.26	37.50	19.46	0.41	0.19

Source: Espy (personal communication).

Table 6–69. Demographic Data for the Behavior Rating Inventory of Executive Function

Parent Forms: 1419 children from Maryland
Gender of Child: 604 males and 815 females
Teacher Forms: 720 children from Maryland public and private schools
Gender of Child: 317 males and 463 females
Geographic Distribution: urban (26.5%), suburban (59%) and rural (14.5%)
Age: 5 to 18 years
Race: Actual and census-weighted ethnicity reported for White, African American, Hispanic, Asian/Pacific Islander, and Native American/Eskimo
SES: Hollingshead (1975) scores: 3.12 for Parent form; 2.89 for Teacher form
Inclusion criteria: No special education history or psychotropic medication usage; no more than 10% of questionnaire items with missing responses

Source: Gioia et al. (2000).

cally significant BRI-MI difference allows for interpretation of the GEC score as a summary measure of executive dysfunction. It is noted that behavioral regulation should be examined initially since it underlies metacognitive problem solving. Maximum likelihood confirmatory factor analysis compared four alternative factor models of children's EF with a revised nine-scale BRIEF that separated the Monitor scale into two components, self-monitor and task monitor. A 3-factor model emerged as the best fit: Behavior Regulation (Inhibit and Self-Monitor scales), Emotional Regulation (Emotional Control and Shift scales), and a Metacognition factor (Working Memory, Initiate, Plan/Organize, Organization of Materials, Task-Monitor scales) (Gioia, Isquith et al., 2002).

The Cronbach α coefficient measure of internal consistency ranged from .80–.98 for parent and teacher form and clinical and normative samples. Parent-teacher interrater agreement was only moderate but was indicated to be consistent with expectation for different environmental settings, $r = .32$ (range: .15–.50). The authors discuss two of the lowered correlations, Initiate and Organization of Materials with respect to the environment differences between home and school. Test–retest reliability correlation across clinical scales for a Parent Form normative subsample was $r = .81$ (range: .76–.85) for an average interval of two weeks. BRI, MCI, GEC retest correlations were .84, .88, .86 respectively. Parent form clinical subsample correlation was $r = .79$ (range: .72–.84), with BRI, MCI, GEC retest correlations of .80, .83, .81, respectively, for a mean interval of 3 weeks. Teacher form normative subsample correlation was $r = .87$ (range: .83–92), and BRI, MCI, GEC retest correlations were .92, .90, .91 respectively, with a mean interval of 3.5 weeks. Test–retest T score differences showed T score stability over a 2 to 3 week interval, supporting use of the BRIEF for repeat administration (Baron, 2000, p. 236–237).

Convergent and discriminant validity data correlations with the ADHD-Rating Scale-IV (DuPaul, Power et al., 1998), Child Behavior Checklist (Achenbach, 1991a), Behavior Assessment for Children (Conners, 1989; Reynolds and Kamphaus, 1992), and Teacher's Report Form (Achenbach, 1991b) found the BRIEF adding substantially different information. Correlation between the BRIEF and ADHD-IV found a relationship of the MCI scale to inattention, and of the BRI scale to impulsivity and hyperactivity, that is, inattentive-type children tend to have an elevated Metacognitive profile and a relatively lower Behavioral Regulation profile. It was useful when diagnostic group membership was examined using logistic regression analyses.

Children with ADHD-Inattentive (ADHD-I) or ADHD-Combined (ADHD-C) diagnoses received significantly higher ratings from parents and teachers than control children on the WM scale, but the WM scale did not distinguish between ADHD-I and ADHD-C. The Inhibit scale analyses were useful in distinguishing children with ADHD-C from ADHD-I or controls (Gioia, Isquith et al., 2000). Preliminary data were reported in the manual on studies of Pervasive Developmental Disorder, Tourette syndrome, high-functioning autism, low birth weight, reading disorder, traumatic brain injury, phenylketonuria, frontal lobe lesions and mental retardation. An investigation of executive function profiles for acquired and developmental disorders—ADHD-I, ADHD-C, TBI-Moderate, TBI-Severe, Reading Disability (RD), and Autistic Spectrum Disorders (ASD)—compared children in these six clinical groups to 208 children from the normative sample matched for age, sex, ethnicity, and socioeconomic status (Gioia, Isquith et al., 2002).

Of special interest, the children with ADHD (both types) and ASD exhibited greater difficulty than children with RD or severe TBI, and these had greater difficulty than children with moderate TBI. ADHD-I and RD groups had greater difficulty with metacognitive aspects of EF, and the problems exhibited by the ADHD-I were more severe than for the RD group. ADHD-C had more difficulty than ADHD-I with inhibition and emotional control, and the most profound difficulty in most metacognition and behavioral regulation domains, excepting shifting set. As expected, the ASD group had greater difficulty with flexibility than ADHD-C and more difficulty shifting than all other groups. The authors emphasize the importance of using this instrument in context with other measures, as it is not a diagnostic instrument, and evaluating domain-specific aspects of behavior to understand fully the significance of the obtained findings about self-regulated problem solving and social functioning. A computerized scoring program is available to support interpretation and suggest recommendations.

CONCLUSION

The extraordinarily wide variety of tests highlighted in this chapter underscores the enormous interest in the EF cognitive domain. The trend from consideration of EF as a unitary dimension to one that is fractionated and crosses modalities is evident. This chapter's arbitrary division into sections, those of planning, organizing, reasoning, shifting, working memory, inhibition, fluency, and estimation, not only serves to provide structure for discussion but points out the multiple influential components within EF tests that require careful clinical and experimental examination. It is exciting that some of the newest tests are being developed with developmental issues given priority. Their eventual impact in child evaluation remains to be seen, but there appears to be encouraging progress in child neuropsychological knowledge. These tests should focus attention on the dynamic changes that characterize development and the importance of ap-

preciating the child's developmental level before one makes conclusions about cognitive status.

REFERENCES

Achenbach, T. M. (1991a). *Manual for Child Behavior Checklist 4–18 and 1991 Profile*. Burlington, VT: University of Vermont, Department of Psychiatry.

Achenbach, T. M. (1991b). *Manual for the Teacher Report Form and 1991 profile*. Burlington: VT: University of Vermont, Department of Psychiatry.

Aman, C. J., Roberts, R. J., Jr., & Pennington, B. F. (1998). A neuropsychological examination of the underlying deficit in attention deficit hyperactivity disorder: Frontal lobe versus parietal lobe theories. *Developmental Psychology, 34,* 956–969.

American Psychiatric Association. (1994). *Diagnostic and statistical manual of mental disorders,* Fourth edition. Washington, DC: American Psychiatric Association.

Anderson, P., Anderson, V., & Lajoie, G. (1996). The Tower of London Test: Validation and standardization for pediatric populations. *The Clinical Neuropsychologist, 10,* 54–65.

Anderson, P., Anderson, V., Northam, E., & Taylor, H. G. (2000). Standardization of the Contingency Naming Test (CNT) for school-aged children: A measure of reactive flexibility. *Clinical Neuropsychological Asessment, 1,* 247–273.

Anderson, S. W., Damasio, H., Jones, R. D., & Tranel, D. (1991). Wisconsin Card Sorting Test performance as a measure of frontal lobe damage. *Journal of Clinical and Experimental Neuropsychology, 13,* 909–922.

Anderson, V. (1998). Assessing executive functions in children: Biological, psychological, and developmental considerations. *Neuropsychological Rehabilitation, 8,* 319–349.

Anderson, V., Anderson, P., Northam, E., Jacobs, R., & Catroppa, C. (2001). Development of executive functions through late childhood and adolescence in an Australian sample. *Developmental Neuropsychology, 20,* 385–406.

Archibald, S., & Kerns, K. A. (1999). Identification and description of new tests of executive functioning in children. *Child Neuropsychology, 5,*(2) 115–129.

Arffa, S., Lovell, M., Podell, K., & Goldberg, E. (1998). Wisconsin Card Sorting Test performance in above average and superior school children: Relationship to intelligence and age. *Archives of Clinical Neuropsychology, 13,* 713–720.

Arizmendi, T., Paulsen, K., & Domino, G. (1981). The Matching Familiar Figures Test—A primary, secondary, and tertiary Evaluation. *Journal of Clinical Psychology, 37*, 812–818.

Armengol, C. C. (2002). Stroop Test in Spanish: Children's norms. *The Clinical Neuropsychologist, 16*, 67–80.

Arochova, O. (1971). The use of a modified Stroop Test in pre-school children. *Psychologia a Patopsychologia Dietata, 6*, 261–266.

Artiola i Fortuny, L., & Heaton, R. K. (1996). Standard versus computerized administration of the Wisconsin Card Sorting Test. *The Clinical Neuropsychologist, 10* (419–424).

Asarnow, R. F., Satz, P., Light, R., Lewis, R., & Neumann, E. (1991). Behavior problems and adaptive functioning children with mild and severe closed head injury. *Journal of Pediatric Psychology, 16*, 543–555.

Atkinson, R. C., & Shiffrin, R. M. (1968). Human Memory: A proposed system and its control processes. In K. W. Spence (Ed.), *The psychology of learning and motivation: Advances in research and theory* (pp. 89–195). New York: Academic Press.

Awh, E., Jonides, J. J., Smith, E. E., Schumacher, E. H., Koeppe, R. A., & Katz, S. (1996). Dissociation of storage and rehearsal in verbal working memory: Evidence from positron emission tomography. *Psychological Science, 7*, 25–31.

Axelrod, B. N. (2001). Comparability of norms for the 64-card and full WCST. [abstract] *The Clinical Neuropsychologist, 15*, 269.

Axelrod, B. N., Goldman, R. S., Tompkins, L. M., & Jiron, C. C. (1994). Poor differential performance on the Wisconsin Card Sorting Test in schizophrenia, mood disorder, and traumatic brain injury. *Neuropsychiatry, Neuropsychology, and Behavioral Neurology, 7*, 20–24.

Baddeley, A. D. (1983). Working memory. *Philosophical Transcripts of the Royal Society of London, 302*, 311–324.

Baddeley, A. D. (1986). *Working Memory*. New York: Oxford University Press.

Baddeley, A. D. (2000). The episodic buffer: A new component of working memory? *Trends in Cognitive Science, 4*, 417–423.

Baddeley, A. D. (2001). Is working memory still working. *American Psychologist, 56*, 851–864.

Baddeley, A. D., & Hitch, G. J. (1974). Working memory. In G. H. Bower (Ed.), *The Psychology of Learning and Motivation Volume VIII* (pp. 47–88). New York: Academic Press.

Baker, K., Segalowitz, S. J., & Ferlisi, M.-C. (2001). The effect of differing scoring methods for the Tower of London task on developmental patterns of performance. *The Clinical Neuropsychologist, 15*, 309–313.

Baker, S. C., Rogers, R. D., Owen, A. M., Frith, C. D., Dolan, R. J., Frackowiak, R. S., et al. (1996). Neural systems engaged by planning: A PET study of the Tower of London task. *Neuropsychologia, 34*, 515–526.

Baldo, J. V., Shimamura, A. P., Delis, D., Kramer, J., & Kaplan, E. (2001). Verbal and design fluency in patients with frontal lobe lesions. *Journal of the International Neuropsychological Society, 7*, 586–596.

Barkley, R. A. (1991). The ecological validity of laboratory and analogue assessment methods of ADHD symptoms. *Journal of Abnormal Child Psychology, 19*, 149–178.

Barkley, R. A. (1994). Impaired delayed responding: A unified theory of attention deficit disorder. In D. K. Routh (Ed.), *Disruptive behavior disorders in childhood* (pp. 11–57). New York: Plenum.

Barkley, R. A. (1997a). *ADHD and the nature of self-control*. New York: Guilford.

Barkley, R. A. (1997b). Behavioral inhibition, sustained attention, and executive functions: Constructing a unifying theory of ADHD. *Psychological Bulletin, 121*, 65–94.

Barkley, R. A. (1998). Time perception application (version 1.0) [computer software]. *University of Massachusetts Medical Center: Chesapeake Technology.*

Barkley, R. A., Murphy, K. R., & Bush, T. (2001). Time perception and reproduction in young adults with attention deficit hyperactivity disorder. *Neuropsychology, 15*(3), 351–360.

Baron, I. S. (2000). Test review: Behavior Rating Inventory of Executive Function. *Child Neuropsychology, 6*, 235–238.

Baron, I. S., Fennell, E. B., & Voeller, K. K. S. (1995). *Pediatric Neuropsychology in the Medical Setting*. New York: Oxford University Press.

Baron-Cohen, S., Ring, H., Moriarty, J., Schmitz, B., Costa, D., & Ell, P. (1994). Recognition of mental state terms: Cinical findings in children with autism and a functional neuroimaging study of normal adults *British Journal of Psychiatry, 165*, 640–649.

Barr, W. B. (2003). Neuropsychological testing of high school athletes: Preliminary norms and test-retest indices. *Archives of Clinical Neuropsychology, 18*, 91–101.

Basso, M. R., Lowery, N., Ghormley, C., & Bornstein, R. A. (2001). Practice effects on the Wisconsin Card Sorting Test-64 card version across 12 months. *The Clinical Neuropsychologist, 15*, 471–478.

Becker, M., Isaac, W., & Hynd, G. W. (1987). Neuropsychological development of nonverbal behaviors attributed to "Frontal Lobe" functioning. *Developmental Neuropsychology, 3,* 275–298.

Beebe, D. W., Ris, M. D., & Dietrich, K. N. (2000). The relationship between CVLT-C process scores and measures of executive functioning: Lack of support among community-dwelling adolescents. *Journal of Clinical and Experimental Neuropsychology, 22,* 779–792.

Bench, C. J., Frith, C. D., Grasby, P. M., Friston, K. J., Paulesu, E., Frackowiak, R. S., et al. (1993). Investigations of the functional anatomy of attention using the Stroop test. *Neuropsychologia, 31,* 907–922.

Benes, F. M., Turtle, M., Khan, Y., et al. (1994). Myelination of a key relay zone in the hippocampal formation occurs in the human brain during childhood, adolescence, and adulthood. *Archives of General Psychiatry, 51,* 477–484.

Benton, A. L. & Hamsher, K. (1976). *Multilingual Aphasia Examination.* Iowa City: University of Iowa.

Benton, A. L., Hamsher, K. & Sivan, A. B. (1994). *Multilingual Aphasia Examination: Manual of instructions* (3rd ed.). Iowa City: AJA Associates, Inc.

Benton, A. L., Sivan, A. B., Hamsher, K., Varney, N. R., & Spreen, O. (1994). *Contributions to neuropsychological assessment.* (2nd ed.) A clinical manual. New York: Oxford University Press.

Berg, E. A. (1948). A simple objective technique for measuring flexibiity in thinking. *Journal of General Psychology, 39,* 15–22.

Berman, K. F., Ostrem, J. L., Randolph, C., Gold, J., Goldberg, T. E., Coppola, R., et al. (1995). Physiological activation of a cortical network during performance on the Wisconsin Card Sorting Test: A positron emission tomography study. *Neuropsychologia, 33,* 1027–1046.

Berry, S. (1996). Diagrammatic procedure for scoring the Wisconsin Card Sorting Test. *The Clinical Neuropsychologist, 10,* 117–121.

Bilder, R. M., & Goldberg, E. (1987). Motor perseverations in schizophrenia. *Archives of Clinical Neuropsychology, 2,* 195–214.

Bishop, D. V. M., Aamodt-Leeper, G., Creswell, C., McGurk, R., & Skuse, D. H. (2001). Individual differences in cognitive planning on the Tower of Hanoi task: Neuropsychological maturity or measurement error? *Journal of Child Psychology and Psychiatry, 42,* 551–556.

Bjorklund, D. F., & Douglas, R. N. (1997). The development of memory strategies. In N. C. Cowan & C. Hulme (Eds.), *The development of memory in childhood* (pp. 201–246). Hove East Sussex, UK: Psychology Press.

Bjorklund, D. F., & Harnishfeger, K. K. (1990). The resources construct in cognitive development: Diverse sources of evidence and a theory of inefficient inhibition. *Developmental Review, 10,* 48–71.

Bohnen, N., Jolles, J., & Twijnstra, A. (1992). Modification of the Stroop Color Word Test improves differentiation between patients with mild head injury and matched controls. *The Clinical Neuropsychologist, 6,* 178–184.

Boll, T. (1974). Behavioral correlates of cerebral damage in children aged 9 through 14. In R. M. Reitan & L. A. Davison (Eds.), *Clinical Neuropsychology: Current Status and Application.* New York: John Wiley & Sons.

Boll, T. (1993). *Children's Category Test.* San Antonio, TX: The Psychological Corporation.

Boll, T., Berent, S., & Richards, H. (1977). Tactile-perceptual functioning as a factor in general psychological abilities. *Perceptual and Motor Skills, 44,* 535–539.

Boll, T., & Reitan, R. (1972). Motor and tactile-perceptual deficits in brain-damaged children. *Perceptual and Motor Skills, 34,* 343–350.

Borkowski, J., Benton, A., & Spreen, O. (1967). Word fluency and brain damage. *Neuropsychologia, 5,* 135–140.

Borys, S. V., Spitz, H., & Dorans, B. A. (1982). Tower of Hanoi performance of retarded young adults and non-retarded children as a function of solution length and goal state. *Journal of Experimental Child Psychology, 33,* 87–110.

Brown, W. (1915). Practice in associating color names with colors. *The Psychological Review, 22,* 45–55.

Bryan, J., & Luszcz, M. A. (2001). Adult age difference in self-ordered pointing task performance: Contributions from working memory, executive function, and speed of information processing. *Journal of Clinical and Experimental Neuropsychology, 23,* 608–619.

Butler, R. W., Rorsman, I., Hill, J. M., & Tuma, R. (1993). The effects of frontal brain impairment on fluency: Simple and complex paradigms. *Neuropsychology, 7,* 519–529.

Butollo, W. H., Bauer, B., & Riedl, H. (1971). The equivalence to the Stroop Test for the preschool age? An experimental investigation of interference tendency and its development in young children. *Zeitschrift fuer Entwicklungspsychologie und Paedagogische Psychologie, 3,* 181–194.

Cabeza, R., & Nyberg, L. (2000). Imaging cognition: II. An empirical review of 275 PET and fMRI studies. *Journal of Cognitive Neuroscience, 12,* 1–47.

Case, R. (1992). The role of the frontal lobes in the

regulation of cognitive development. *Brain and Cognition, 20,* 51–73.

Casey, B. J., Trainor, R. J., Orendi, J. L., Schubert, A. B., Nystrom, L. E., Giedd, J. N., et al. (1997). A developmental functional MRI study of prefrontal activation during performance of go-no-go task. *Journal of Cognitive Neuroscience, 9,* 835–847.

Cattell, J. M. (1886). The time it takes to see and name objects. *Mind, ii,* 63–65.

Chase-Carmichael, C. A., Ris, M. D., Weber, A. M., & Schefft, B. K. (1999). The neurological validity of the Wisconsin Card Sorting Test with a pediatric population. *The Clinical Neuropsychologist, 13*(4), 405–413.

Chelune, G. J., & Baer, R. A. (1986). Developmental norms for the Wisconsin Card Sorting Test. *Journal of Clinical and Experimental Neuropsychology, 8,* 219–228.

Chen, H. C. (1999). Comparing intralingual Stroop interference in Chinese and English: A meta-analysis. *Proceedings of the 40th Annual Meeting of the Psychonomic Society, 4,* 69.

Choca, J., Laatsch, L., Garside, D., & Amemann, C. (1994). *The Computer Category Test.* Toronto: Multi-Health Systems.

Christ, S. E., White, D. A., Brunstrom, J. E., & Abrams, R. A. (2003). Inhibitory control following perinatal brain injury. *Neuropsychology, 17,* 171–178.

Christensen, A.-L. (1975). *Luria's Neuropsychological Investigation.* New York: Spectrum Publications, Inc.

Christensen, A.-L. (1979). *Luria's Neuropsychological Investigation,* (2nd Ed.) Copenhagen: Munksgaard.

Cockburn, J. (1995). Performance on the Tower of London test after severe head injury. *Journal of the International Neuropsychological Society, 1,* 537–544.

Cohen, J., Perlstein, W., Braver, T., Nystrom, L., Noll, D., & Jonides, J. J. (1997). Temporal dynamics of brain activation during a working memory task. *Nature, 386,* 604–608.

Cohen, M. J., Morgan, A. M., Vaughn, M., Riccio, C. A., & Hall, J. (1999). Verbal fluency in children: Developmental issues and differential validity in distinguishing children with Attention-Deficit Hyperactivity Disorder and two subtypes of dyslexia. *Archives of Clinical Neuropsychology, 14*(5), 433–443.

Cohn, N. B., Dustman, R. E., & Bradford, D. C. (1984). Age-related decrements in Stroop Color Test performance. *Journal of Clinical Psychology, 40*(5), 1244–1250.

Comalli, P. E., Jr., Wapner, S., & Werner, H. (1962). Interference effects of Stroop color-word test in childhood, adulthood, and aging. *Journal of Genetic Psychology, 100,* 47–53.

Conners, C. K. (1989). *Manual for Conners' Rating Scales.* North Tonawanda, NY: Multi-Health Systems.

Cowan, N. C., & Hulme, C. (1997). *The development of memory in childhood.* Hove East Sussex, UK: Psychology Press.

Cox, C. S., Chee, E., Chase, G. A., Baumgardner, T. L., Schuerholz, L. J., Reader, M. J., et al. (1997). Reading proficiency affects the construct validity of the Stroop Test interference score. *The Clinical Neuropsychologist, 11,* 105–110.

Cox, D., & Waters, H. S. (1986). Sex differences in the use of organizational strategies: A developmental analysis. *Journal of Experimental Child Psychology, 41,* 18–37.

Crockett, D., Bilsker, D., Hurwitz, T., & Kozak, J. (1986). Clinical utility of three measures of frontal lobe dysfunction in neuropsychiatric samples. *International Journal of Neuroscience, 30,* 241–248.

Crockett, D., Klonoff, H., & Bjerring, J. (1969). Factor analysis of neuropsychological tests. *Perceptual and Motor Skills, 29,* 791–802.

Crosson, B., Sartor, K. J., Jenny, A. B., Nabors, N. A., & Moberg, P. J. (1993). Increased intrusions during verbal recall in traumatic and non-traumatic lesions of the temporal lobe. *Neuropsychology, 7,* 193–208.

Crowe, S. (1992). Dissociation of two frontal lobe syndromes by a test of verbal fluency. *Journal of Clinical and Experimental Neuropsychology, 14,* 327–339.

Culbertson, W. C., & Zillmer, E. A. (2000). *Tower of London-Drexel University.* Chicago, IL: Multi-Health Systems, Inc.

Cummings, J. L. (1993). Frontal-subcortical circuits in human behavior. *Neurological Review, 50,* 873–879.

Das, J. P. (1969). Development of verbal abilities in retarded and normal children as measured by the Stroop Test. *British Journal of Social and Clinical Psychology, 8,* 59–66.

Das, J. P. (1970). Changes in Stroop-Test responses as a function of mental age. *British Journal of Social and Clinical Psychology, 9,* 68–73.

Dash, J., & Dash, A. S. (1987). Studies on the Stroop Test: I. School, grade, sex and achievement differences. *Indian Journal of Behaviour, 11,* 8–11.

Davis, H. P., & Keller, F. R. (1998). *Colorado Assessment Tests (v 1.1).* Colorado Springs, CO: Author.

Davis, R., Adams, R., Gates, D., & Cheramie, G. (1989). Screening for learning disabilities: A neuropsychological approach. *Journal of Clinical Psychology, 45,* 423–428.

DeFilippis, N. A., & McCampbell, E. (1979). *Manual for the Booklet Category Test: Research and clinical form.* Odessa, FL: Psychological Assessment Resources, Inc.

DeFilippis, N. A., McCampbell, E., & Rogers, P. (1979). Development of a booklet form of the Category Test: Normative and validity data. *Journal of Clinical Neuropsychology, 1,* 339–342.

Delis, D., Kaplan, E., & Kramer, J. (2001). *Delis-Kaplan Executive Function System.* San Antonio, TX: The Psychological Corporation.

Delis, D., Kramer, J. H., Kaplan, E., & Ober, B. A. (1994). *California Verbal Learning Test-Children's Version.* San Antonio, TX: Psychological Corporation.

Denckla, M. B. (1989). Executive function, the overlap zone between attention deficit hyperactivity disorder and learning disabilities. *International Pediatrics, 4,* 155–160.

Denckla, M. B. (1994). Measurement of executive dysfunction. In G. R. Lyon (Ed.), *Frames of reference for the assessment of learning disabilities: New views on measurement issues* (pp. 117–142). Baltimore, MD: Paul Brookes.

Denckla, M. B. (1996b). A theory and model of executive function: A neuropsychological perspective. In G. R. Lyon & N. A. Krasnegor (Eds.), *Attention, memory, and executive function* (pp. 263–278). Baltimore: Paul H. Brookes.

Diamond, A. (1991). Guidelines for the study of brain-behavior relationships during development. In H. Levin, H. Eisenberg & A. Benton (Eds.), *Frontal lobe function and dysfunction* (pp. 339–378). New York: Oxford University Press.

Diamond, A., & Goldman-Rakic, P. S. (1989). Comparison of human infants and rhesus monkeys on Piaget's AB task: Evidence for dependence on dorsolateral prefrontal cortex. *Experimental Brain Research, 74,* 24–40.

Dikmen, S., Heaton , R. K., Grant, I., & Temkin, N. R. (1999). Test-retest reliability and practice effects of Expanded Halstead-Reitan Neuropsychological Test Battery. *Journal of the International Neuropsychological Society, 5,* 346–356.

Di Stefano, G., Bachevalier, J., Levin, H. S., Song, J., Scheibel, R. S., & Fletcher, J. (2000). Volume of focal brain lesions and hippocampal formation in relation to memory function after closed head injury in children. *Journal of Neurology, Neurosurgery and Psychiatry, 69,* 210–216.

Dodrill, C. B. (1978). A neuropsychological battery for epilepsy. *Epilepsia, 19,* 611–623.

Donders, J. (1996). Validity of short forms of the Intermediate Halstead Category Test in children with traumatic brain injury. *Archives of Clinical Neuropsychology, 11,* 131–137.

Donders, J. (1998a). Cluster subtypes in the Children's Category Test standardization sample. *Child Neuropsychology, 4,* 178–186.

Donders, J. (1998b). Performance discrepancies between the Children's Category Test (CCT) and the California Verbal Learning Test-Children's version (CVLT-C) in the standardization sample. *Journal of the International Neuropsychological Society, 4,* 242–246.

Donders, J. (1999). Latent structure of the Children's Category Test at two age levels in the standardization sample. *Journal of Clinical and Experimental Neuropsychology, 21,* 279–282.

Donders, J., & Kirsch, N. (1991). Nature and implications of selective impairment on the Booklet Category Test and Wisconsin Card Sorting Test. *The Clinical Neuropsychologist, 5,* 78–82.

Donders, J., & Strom, D. (1995). Factor and cluster analysis of the Intermediate Halstead Category Test. *Child Neuropsychology, 1,* 19–25.

Drewe, E. A. (1974). The effect of type and area of brain lesion on Wisconsin Card Sorting Test performance. *Cortex, 10,* 159–170.

Drewe, E. A. (1975). Go-no go learning after frontal lobe lesions in humans. *Cortex, 11,* 8–16.

Duncan, J. (1995). Attention, intelligence, and the frontal lobes. In M. Gazzaniga (Ed.), *The cognitive neurosciences* (pp. 721–733). Cambridge, MA: MIT Press.

Dunn, M., Gomes, H., & Sebastian, M. (1996). Prototypicality of responses of autistic, language disordered, and normal children in a word fluency task. *Child Neuropsychology, 2,* 99–108.

DuPaul, G. J., Anastopoulos, A. D., Shelton, T. L., Guevremont, D. C., & Metevia, L. (1992). Multimethod assessment of attention deficit hyperactivity disorder: The diagnostic utility of clinic-based tests. *Journal of Clinical Child Psychology, 21,* 394–402.

DuPaul, G. J., Power, T. J., Anastopoulos, A. D., & Reid, R. (1998). *ADHD Rating Scale-IV.* New York: Guilford Press.

Elfgren, C., & Risberg, J. (1998). Lateralized blood flow increases during fluency tasks: Influence of cognitive strategy. *Neuropsychologia, 36,* 505–512.

Eslinger, P. J. (1996). Conceptualizing, describing, and measuring components of executive function. In G. R. Lyon & N. A. Krasnegor (Eds.), *Attention, Memory, and Executive Function* (pp. 367–395). Baltimore, MD: Paul H. Brookes.

Eslinger, P. J., Biddle, K. R., & Grattan, L. M. (1997). Cognitive and social development in children with prefrontal cortex lesions. In N. A. Krasnegor, G. R. Lyon & P. S. Goldman-Rakic (Eds.), *Development of the prefrontal cortex: Evolution, neurobiology, and behavior* (pp. 295–335). Baltimore, MD.: Paul H. Brookes.

Eslinger, P. J., & Damasio, A. R. (1985). Severe disturbance of higher cognition after bilateral frontal lobe ablation: Patient EVR. *Neurology, 35,* 1731–1741.

Eslinger, P. J., & Grattan, L. M. (1993). Frontal lobe and frontal-striatal substrates for different forms of human cognitive flexibility. *Neuropsychologia, 31,* 17–28.

Espy, K. A. (1997). The Shape School: Assessing executive function in preschool children. *Developmental Neuropsychology, 13,* 495–499.

Espy, K. A., Cwik, M. F., Senn, T. E., & Polcari, J. (2002). *Assessing executive functions in preschoolers: Trails P.* Poster presented at the Annual Meeting of the American Psychological Association, Chicago, IL.

Espy, K. A., Kaufmann, P., Glisky, M., & McDiarmid, M. D. (2001). New procedures to assess executive functions in preschool children. *The Clinical Neuropsychologist, 15,* 46–58.

Evans, R., Ruff, R., & Gualtieri, C. (1985). Verbal fluency and figural fluency in bright children. *Perceptual and Motor Skills, 61,* 699–709.

Fein, D., Gleeson, M. K., Bullard, S., Mapou, R., & Kaplan, E. (1998). *The Biber Cognitive Estimation Test.* Paper presented at the Poster presented at the 26th Annual Meeting of the International Neuropsychological Society, Honolulu, Hawaii.

Findeis, M. K., & Weight, D. G. (1994). *Meta-norms for Indiana-Reitan Neuropsychological Test Battery and Halstead-Reitan Neuropsychologial Test Battery for Children, ages 5–14.* Unpublished manuscript.

Finlayson, M. A., & Reitan, R. M. (1976). Handedness in relation to measures of motor and tactile perceptual functions in normal children. *Perceptual and Motor Skills, 43,* 475–481.

Flashman, L. A., Horner, M. D., & Freides, D. (1991). Note on scoring perseveration on the Wisconsin Card Sorting Test. *The Clinical Neuropsychologist, 5,* 190–194.

Flashman, L. A., Mandir, A. S., Horner, M. D., & Friedes, D. (1991). Increasing interscorer reliability on the Wisconsin Card Sorting Test (WCST) using classified scoring rules. *Journal of Clinical and Experimental Neuropsychology, 13,* 431.

Fletcher, J. (1996). Executive functions in children: Introduction to the special series. *Developmental Neuropsychology, 12,* 1–3.

Fletcher, J. (1998). Attention in children: Conceptual and methodological issues. *Child Neuropsychology, 4,* 81–86.

Fletcher, J., Ewing-Cobbs, L., Miner, M. E., Levin, H. S., & Eisenberg, H. M. (1990). Behavioral changes after closed head injury in children. *Journal of Consulting and Clinical Psychology, 58,* 93–98.

Fortuny, L. A., & Heaton , R. K. (1996). Standard versus computerized administration of the Wisconsin Card Sorting Test. *The Clinical Neuropsychologist, 10,* 419–424.

Frisch, G., & Handler, L. A. (1974). A neuropsychological investigation of "functional disorders of speech articulation. *Journal of Speech and Hearing Research, 17,* 432–445.

Frith, C. D., Friston, K. J., Liddle, P. F., & Frackowiak, R. S. (1991). A PET study of word finding. *Neuropsychologia, 2,* 1137–1148.

Fromm-Auch, D., & Yeudall, L. T. (1983). Normative data for the Halstead-Reitan Neuropsychological Tests. *Journal of Clinical Neuropsychology, 5,* 221–238.

Fry, A. F., & Hale, S. (1996). Processing speed, working memory, and fluid intelligence: Evidence for a developmental cascade. *Psychological Science, 7,* 237–241.

Fuster, J. M. (1989). *The prefrontal cortex: Anatomy, physiology and neuropsychology of the frontal lobe* (2nd ed.). New York: Raven Press.

Fuster, J. M. (1997). *The prefrontal cortex: Anatomy, physiology and neuropsychology of the frontal lobe* (3rd ed.). New York: Lippincott Williams Wilkins.

Gaddes, W. H., and Crockett, D. J. (1975). The Spreen-Benton aphasia tests: Normative data as a measure of normal language development. *Brain and Language, 2,* 257–280.

Gershberg, F., & Shimamura, A. P. (1995). Impaired use of organizational strategies in free recall following frontal lobe damage. *Neuropsychologia, 13,* 1305–1333.

Gerstadt, C. L., Hong, Y. J., & Diamond, A. (1994). The relationship between cognition and action: Performance of children $3^{1}/_{2}$ to 7 years on a Stroop-like day-night test. *Cognition, 53,* 129–153.

Gioia, G. A. (1993). The Tower of Hanoi task and developmental executive dysfunction. *Journal of Clinical and Experimental Neuropsychology, 15,* 88.

Gioia, G., Espy, K., & Isquith, P. (2002). Executive function in preschool children: Examination through everyday behavior. *[abstract] Journal of the International Neuropsychological Society, 8,* 164.

Gioia, G. A., Isquith, P. K., Guy, S. C., & Kenworthy, L. (2000). *Behavior Rating Inventory of Executive Function.* Odessa, FL: Psychological Assessment Resources, Inc.

Gioia, G. A., Isquith, P. K., Hoffhines, V., & Guy, S. C. (1999). Examining the clinical utility of the

NEPSY Tower: A tale of two towers. *[abstract] Journal of the International Neuropsychological Society, 5,* 117.

Gioia, G., Isquith, P. K., Kenworthy, L., & Barton, R. M. (2002). Profiles of everyday executive function in acquired and developmental disorders. *Child Neuropsychology, 8,* 121–137.

Gioia, G., Isquith, P. K., Retzlaff, P., & Espy, K. (2002). Confirmatory factor analysis of the Behavior Rating Inventory of Exectuive Function (BRIEF) in a clinical sample. *Child Neuropsychology, 4,* 249–257.

Glosser, G., & Goodglass, H. (1990). Disorders in executive control functions among aphasic and other brain-damaged patients. *Journal of Clinical and Experimental Neuropsychology, 12,* 485–501.

Gnys, J. A., & Willis, W. G. (1991). Validation of executive function tasks with young children. *Developmental Neuropsychology, 7,* 487–501.

Goel, V., & Grafman, J. (1995). Are the frontal lobes implicated in "planning" functions? Interpreting data from the Tower of Hanoi. *Neuropsychologia, 33,* 623–642.

Goldberg, E. (1986). Varieties of perseveration: A comparison of two taxonomies. *Journal of Clinical and Experimental Neuropsychology, 8,* 710–726.

Goldberg, E., & Bilder, R. M. (1987). The frontal lobes and hierarchical organization of cognitive control. In E. Perecman (Ed.), *The frontal lobes revisited* (pp. 155–159). New York: IRBN.

Goldberg, E., Podell, K., Bilder, R. M., & Jaeger, J. (2000). *The Executive Control Battery.* Melbourne, Australia: Psych Press.

Goldberg, E., & Tucker, D. (1979). Motor perseveration and long-term memory for visual forms. *Journal of Clinical Neuropsychology, 1,* 273–288.

Golden, C. J. (1974). Sex differences in performance on the Stroop color and word test. *Perceptual and Motor Skills, 39,* 1067–1070.

Golden, C. J. (1976). Identification of brain disorders by the Stroop color and word test. *Journal of Clinical Psychology, 32,* 654–658.

Golden, C. J. (1978). *Stroop Color and Word Test: Manual for clinical and experimental uses.* Chicago: Stoetling.

Grattan, L. M., & Eslinger, P. J. (1991). Frontal lobe damage in children and adults: A comparative review. *Developmental Neuropsychology, 7,* 283–326.

Greco, E. (1993). The Emotional Stroop Test: A review of the literature. *Psichiatria e Psicoterapia Analitica, 12,* 219–223.

Greve, K. W. (2001). The WCST-64: A standardized short-form of the Wisconsin Card Sorting Test. *The Clinical Neuropsychologist, 15,* 228–234.

Greve, K. W., Brooks, J., Crouch, J., Williams, M., & Rice, W. (1997). Factorial structure of the Wis-consin Card Sorting Test. *British Journal of Clinical Psychology, 36,* 283–285.

Grimwood, K., Anderson, P., Anderson, V., Tan, L., & Nolan, T. (2000). Twelve-year outcomes following bacterial meningitis: Further evidence for persisting effects. *Archives of Disease in Childhood, 83,* 111–116.

Grodzinsky, G., & Diamond, R. (1992). Frontal lobe functioning in boys with Attention-Deficit Hyperactivity Disorder. *Developmental Neuropsychology, 8,* 427–445.

Guy, S., Gioia, G. A., & Isquith, P. K. (1998). *Behavior Rating Inventory of Executive Function, Adolescent Self-Report Form (BRIEF-SR).* Unpublished manuscript.

Halperin, J. M., Healey, J. M., Zeitchik, E., Ludman, W. L., & Weinstein, L. (1989). Developmental aspects of linguistic and mnestic abilities in normal children. *Journal of Clinical and Experimental Neuropsychology, 11,* 518–528.

Harris, N. S., Marcus, D. J., Rancier, S. A., & Weiler, M. D. (1999). First name fluency in learning disabled children vs. controls [Abstract]. *The Clinical Neuropsychologist, 13,* 226.

Heaton, R. K. (1981). *Wisconsin Card Sorting Test manual.* Odessa, FL: Psychological Assessment Resources, Inc.

Heaton, R. K. (1999). *Wisconsin Card Sorting Test: Computer version for Windows-Research edition.* Odessa, FL: Psychological Assessment Resources.

Heaton, R. K. (2000). *WCST-64: Computer Version 3 for Windows-Research Edition.* Odessa, Fl: Psychological Assessment Resources.

Heaton, R. K., Chelune, G. J., Talley, J. L., Kay, G., & Curtiss, G. (1993). *Wisconsin Card Sorting Test. Manual.* Odessa, FL: Psychological Assessment Resources.

Helland, T., & Asbjørnsen, A. (2000). Executive functions in dyslexia. *Child Neuropsychology, 6,* 37–48.

Henik, A. (1996). Paying attention to the Stroop Effect? *Journal of the International Neuropsychological Society, 2,* 467–470.

Homatidis, S., & Konstantareas, M. M. (1981). Assessment of hyperactivity: Isolating measures of high discriminant ability. *Journal of Consulting and Clinical Psychology, 47,* 533–541.

Hughes, H. (1976). Norms Developed. *Journal of Pediatric Psychology, 1,* 11–15.

Humes, G. E., Welsh, M. C., Retzlaff, P., & Cookson, N. (1997). Towers of Hanoi and London: Reliability of two executive function tasks. *Assessment, 4,* 249–257.

Huttenlocher, P. R. (1994). Synaptogenesis, synapse elimination, and neural plasticity in human cerebral cortex. In C. A. Nelson (Ed.), *Threats to optimal development: Integrating biological, psy-*

chological, and social risk factors (pp. 35–54). Hillsdale, NJ: Lawrence Erlbaum Associates.

Ingram, D. (1975). Motor Asymmetries in young children. *Neuropsychologia, 13,* 95–102.

Isquith, P., Gioia, G., & Espy, K. (2002). Development of the Behavior Rating Inventory of Executive Function—Preschool Version. [abstract] *Journal of the International Neuropsychological Society,* 8, 303.

Jacobs, R., Anderson, V., & Harvey, A. S. (2001). Concept Generation Test: A measure of conceptual reasoning skills in children: Examination of developmental trends. *Clinical Neuropsychological Assessment, 2,* 101–117.

Jensen, A. R., & Rohrer, W. D., Jr. (1966). The Stroop color-word test: A review. *Acta Psychologica, 25,* 36–93.

Jerger, S., Martin, R. C., & Pirozzolo, F. J. (1988). A developmental study of the auditory Stroop effect. *Brain and Language, 35,* 86–104.

Johnston, A., & Venables, P. H. (1982). Specificity of attention in the Stroop test: An EP study. *Biological Psychology, 15,* 75–83.

Johnstone, B., Holland, D., & Hewett, J. E. (1997). The construct validity of the Category Test: Is it a measure of reasoning or intelligence? *Psychological Assessment, 9,* 28–33.

Jones-Gotman, M., & Milner, B. (1977). Design fluency: The intervention of nonsense drawings after focal cortical lesions. *Neuropsychologia, 15,* 653–674.

Jonides, J. J., Marshuetz, C., Smith, E. E., Reuter-Lorenz, P. A., Koeppe, R. A., & Hartley, A. (2000). Age differences in behavior and PET activation reveal differences in interference resolution in verbal working memory. *Journal of Cognitive Neuroscience, 12,* 188–196.

Jonides, J. J., Smith, E. E., Koeppe, R. A., Awh, E., Minoshima, S., & Mintun, M. A. (1993). Spatial working memory in humans as revealed by PET. *Nature, 363,* 623–625.

Kafer, K. L., & Hunter, M. (1997). On testing the face validity of planning/problem-solving tasks in a normal population. *Journal of the International Neuropsychological Society, 3,* 108–119.

Kagan, J. (1966). Reflection-impulsivity: The generality and dynamics of conceptual tempo. *Journal of Abnormal Psychology, 71,* 17–24.

Kagan, J., Rosman, B. L., Day, L., Albert, J., & Phillips, W. (1964). Information processing in the child: Significance of analytic and reflective attitudes. *Psychological Monographs, 78,* Whole No. 578.

Kates, M., & Moscovitch, M. (1989). *Development of frontal-lobe functioning in children: The ability to order information in time.* Unpublished manuscript.

Kawashima, R., Satoh, K., Itoh, H., Yanagisawa, T., & Fukuda, H. (1996). Functional anatomy of go/no go discrimination and response selection: A PET study in man. *Brain Research, 728,* 79–89.

Kay, W. M., Ben-Tovim, D. I., Jones, S., & Bachok, N. (1992). Repeated administration of the adapted Stroop Test: Feasibility for longitudinal study of psychopathology in eating disorders. *International Journal of Eating Disorders, 12*(1), 103–105.

Kelly, T. (2000). The development of executive function in school-aged children. *Clinical Neuropsychological Asessment, 1,* 38–55.

Kerns, K. A., McInerney, R. J., & Wilde, N. J. (2001). Time reproduction, working memory, and behavioral inhibition in children with ADHD. *Child Neuropsychology, 7,* 21–31.

Kizilbash, A., & Donders, J. (1999). Latent structure of the Wisconsin Card Sorting Test after pediatric traumatic head injury. *Child Neuropsychology, 5*(4), 224–229.

Klingberg, T., Forssberg, H., & Westerberg, H. (2002). Training of working memory in children with ADHD. *Journal of Clinical and Experimental Neuropsychology, 24,* 781–791.

Klonoff, H., & Low, M. (1974). Disordered brain function in young children and early adolescents: Neuropsychological and electroencephalographic correlates. In R. M. Reitan & L. A. Davison (Eds.), *Clinical Neuropsychology: Current Status and Applications* (pp. 121–178). New York: John Wiley and Sons.

Knights, R. M. (1966). *Normative data on tests evaluating brain damage in children 5–14 years of age. Research Bulletin No 20.* London, Ontario: Department of Psychology, University of Western Ontario.

Knights, R. M., & Tymchuk, A. J. (1968). An evaluation of the Halstead-Reitan Category Tests for children. *Cortex, 4,* 403–414.

Kolb, B., & Fantie, B. (1997). Development of the child's brain and behaviour. In C. R. Reynolds & E. Fletcher-Janzen (Eds.), *Handbook of clinical child neuropsychology* (pp. 17–41). New York: Plenum Press.

Kolb, B., & Whishaw, I. Q. (1983). Performance of schizophrenic patients on tests sensitive to left or right frontal, temporal, or parietal function in neurological patients. *Journal of Nervous and Mental Disease, 171,* 435–443.

Kolb, B., & Whishaw, I. Q. (1985). *Fundamentals of Human Neuropsychology* (2nd ed.). New York: W. H. Freeman.

Kolb, B., & Whishaw, I. Q. (1990). *Fundamentals of human neuropsychology* (3rd ed.). New York: W. H. Freeman.

Kongs, S. K., Thompson, L. L., Iverson, G. L., & Heaton, R. K. (2000). *WCST-64: Wisconsin Card*

Sorting Test-64 Card Version Professional Manual. Odessa, Fl: Psychological Assessment Resources.

Konrad, K., Gauggel, S., Manz, A., & Schöll, M. (2000). Lack of inhibition: A motivational deficit in children with Attention Deficit/Hyperactivity Disorder and children with traumatic brain injury. *Child Neuropsychology, 6,* 286–296.

Kooijmans, R., Scheres, A., & Oosterlaan, J. (2000). Response inhibition and measures of psychopathology: A dimensional analysis. *Child Neuropsychology, 6,* 175–184.

Korkman, M., Kirk, U., & Kemp, S. (1997). *NEPSY: A developmental neuropsychological assessment.* San Antonio: The Pyschologica Corporation.

Krasnegor, N. A., Lyon, G. R., & Goldman-Rakic, P. S. (Eds.). (1997). *Development of the prefrontal cortex: Evolution, neurobiology, and behavior.* Baltimore: Paul H. Brookes.

Krikorian, R., & Bartok, J. (1998). Developmental data for the Porteus Maze Test. *The Clinical Neuropsychologist, 12,* 305–310.

Krikorian, R., Bartok, J., & Gay, N. (1994). Tower of London procedure: A standard method and developmental data. *Journal of Clinical and Experimental Neuropsychology, 16,* 840–850.

Kuehne, C., Kehle, T. H., & McMahon, W. (1987). Differences between children with attention deficit disorder, children with specific learning disabilities, and normal children. *Journal of School Psychology, 25,* 161–166.

Lacy, M. A., Gore Jr., P. A., Pliskin, N., Henry, G. K., Heilbronner, R. L., & Hamer, D. P. (1996). Verbal fluency task equivalence. *The Clinical Neuropsychologist, 10,* 305–308.

Lamar, M., Podell, K., Carew, T. G., Cloud, B. S., Resh, R., Kennedy, C., et al. (1997). Perseverative behavior in Alzheimer's disease and subcortical ischemic vascular dementia. *Neuropsychology, 11,* 523–534.

Landry, S. H., Jordan, T., & Fletcher, J. (1994). Developmental outcomes for children with spina bifida and hydrocephalus. In M. G. Tramontana & S. R. Hooper (Eds.), *Advances in child neuropsychology,* Vol. 2 (pp. 85–118). New York: Springer-Verlag.

LaPierre, D., Braun, C. J., & Hodgins, S. (1995). Ventral frontal deficits in psychopathy: Neuropsychological test findings. *Neuropsychologia, 33,* 139–151.

Lee, G. P., Strauss, E., Loring, D. W., McCloskey, L., Haworth, J. M., & Lehman, R. A. W. (1997). Sensitivity of figural fluency on the Five-Point Test to focal neurological dysfunction. *The Clinical Neuropsychologist, 11,* 59–68.

Lee, T. M. C., & Chan, C. C. H. (2000). Stroop Interference in Chinese and English. *Journal of Clinical and Experimental Neuropsychology, 22,* 465–471.

Levin, H. S., Culhane, K. A., Hartmann, J., Evankovich, K., Mattson, A. J., Harward, H., et al. (1991). Developmental changes in performance on tests of purported frontal lobe functioning. *Developmental Neuropsychology, 7,* 377–395.

Levin, H. S., Fletcher, J. M., Kufera, J. A., Harward, H., Lilly, M. A., Mendelsohn, D., Bruce, D., & Eisenberg, H. M. (1996). Dimensions of cognition measured by the Tower of London and other cognitive tasks in head-injured children and adolescents. *Developmental Neuropsychology, 12,* 17–34.

Levin, H. S., Song, J., Ewing-Cobbs, L., & Roberson, G. (2001). Porteus maze performance following traumatic brain injury in children. *Neuropsychology, 15,* 557–567.

Levin, H. S., Song, J., Scheibel, R. S., Fletcher, J., Harward, H., Lilly, M., et al. (1997). Concept formation and problem-solving following closed head injury in children. *Journal of the International Neuropsychological Society, 3,* 598–607.

Levine B., Stuss, D. T., & Milberg, W. P. (1995). Concept generation: Validation of a test of executive functioning in a normal aging population. *Journal of Clinical and Experimental Neuropsychology, 17,* 740–758.

Lezak, M. (1995). *Neuropsychological Assessment, 3rd Edition.* New York: Oxford University Press.

Lockwood, K. A., Marcotte, A. C., & Stern, C. (2001). Differentiation of Attention-Deficit/Hyperacitivy Disorder Subtypes: Application of a neuropsychological model of attention. *Journal of Clinical and Experimental Neuropsychology, 23,* 317–330.

Logan, G. D. (1981). Attention, automaticity, and the ability to stop a speeded choice response. In J. B. Long & A. Baddeley (Eds.), *Attention and Performance IX* (pp. 205–222). New York: Erlbaum.

Logan, G. D. (1994). On the ability to inhibit thought and action: A user's guide to the stop signal paradigm. In D. Dagenbach & T. H. Carr (Eds.), *Inhibitory processes in attention, memory, and language* (pp. 189–239). San Diego, CA: Academic Pres.

Logan, G. D., & Cowan, W. B. (1984). On the ability to inhibit thought and action: A theory of an act of control. *Psychological Review, 91*(295–327).

Logan, G. D., Cowan, W. B., & Davis, K. A. (1984). On the ability to inhibit simple and choice reaction time responses: A model and a method. *Journal of Experimental Psychology: Human Perception and Performance, 10,* 276–291.

Lombardi, W. J., Andreason, P. J., Sirocco, K. Y., Rio, D. E., Gross, R. E., Umhau, J. C., et al. (1999). Wisconsin Card Sorting Test performance following head injury: Dorsolateral frontal-striatal circuit activity predicts perseveration. *Journal of Clinical and Experimental Neuropsychology, 21,* 2–16.

Loring, D. (Ed.). (1999). *INS dictionary of neuropsychology.* New York: Oxford University Press.

Loring, D. W., Meador, K. J., & Lee, G. P. (1994). Effects of temporal lobectomy on generative fluency and other language functions. *Archives of Clinical Neuropsychology, 9,* 229–238.

Lowe, D. G., & Mitterer, J. O. (1982). Selective and divided attention in a Stroop task. *Canadian Journal of Psychology, 36,* 684–700.

Luciana, M., & Nelson, C. A. (1998). The functional emergence of prefrontally-guided working memory systems in four- to eight-year-old children. *Neuropsychologia, 36,* 273–293.

Luria, A. (1973). *The working brain: An introduction to neuropsychology.* Harmondsworth, UK: Penguin.

Luria, A. (1980). *Higher cortical functions in man (2nd ed.).* New York: Basic Books.

Lussier, F., Guerin, F., Dufresne, A., & Lassonde, M. (1998). Etude normative developpementale des fonctions executives: La tour de Londres. *Approche Neuropsychologique des Apprentissages Chez L'Enfant, 10*(2 [47]), 42–52.

MacDonald, A. W., Cohen, J. D., Stenger, V. A., & Carter, C. S. (2000 (June9)). Dissociating the role of the dorsolateral prefrontal and anterior cingulate cortex in cognitive control. *Science, 288,* 1835–1838.

MacInnes, W. D., Forch, J. R., & Golden, C. J. (1981). A cross-validation of a booklet form of the Category Test. *Clinical Neuropsychology, 3,* 3–5.

MacLeod, C. M. (1991). Half a century of research on the Stroop effect: An integrative review. *Psychological Bulletin, 109,* 163–203.

Maddox, W. T., & Filoteo, J. V. (2001). Striatal contributions to categorization learning: Quantitative modeling of simple linear and complex nonlinear rule learning in patients with Parkinson's disease. *Journal of the International Neuropsychological Society, 7,* 710–727.

Mahone, E. M., Cirino, P. T., Cutting, L. E., Cerrone, P. M., Hagelthorn, K. M., Hiemenz, J. R., et al. (2002). Validity of the Behavior Rating Inventory of Executive Function in children with ADHD and/or Tourette syndrome. *Archives of Clinical Neuropsychology, 17,* 643–662.

Maiuro, R., Townes, B. D., Vitaliano, P., & Trupin, E. (1984). Age norms for the Reitan-Indiana Neuropsychological Test Battery for Children. In R. A. Glow (Ed.), *Advances in the Behavioral Measurement of Children, Volume 1* (pp. 159–173).

Marcotte, A. C., & Stern, C. (1997). Qualitative analysis of graphomotor output in children with attentional disorders. *Child Neuropsychology, 3,* 147–153.

Mariani, M. A., & Barkley, R. A. (1997). Neuropsychological and academic functioning in preschool boys with attention deficit hyperactivity disorder. *Developmental Neuropsychology, 13,* 111–129.

Mateer, C., & Williams, D. (1991). Effects of frontal lobe injury in childhood. *Developmental Neuropsychology, 7,* 359–376.

McCampbell, E., & DeFilippis, N. A. (1979). The development of a booklet form of the Category Test. *Clinical Neuropsychology, 1,* 33–35.

McCarthy, D. (1972). *Manual for the McCarthy Scales of Children's Abilities.* New York: The Psychological Corporation.

Mead, L. A., Mayer, A. R., Bobholz, J. A., Woodley, S. J., Cunningham, J. M., Hammeke, T. A., et al. (2002). Neural basis of the Stroop interference task: Response competition or selective attention. *Journal of the International Neuropsychological Society, 8,* 735–742.

Mega, M. S., & Cummings, J. L. (1994). Frontal-subcortical circuits and neuropsychiatric disorders. *Journal of Neuropsychiatry and Clinical Neurosciences, 6,* 358–370.

Mesulam, M.-M. (1985). *Principles of behavioral neurology.* Philadelphia: F. A. Davis Co.

Mesulam, M.-M. (2000). *Principles of behavioral and cognitive neurology.* New York: Oxford University Press.

Miller, E. (1984). Verbal fluency as a function of a measure of verbal intelligence and in relation to different types of cerebral pathology. *British Journal of Clinical Psychology, 23,* 53–57.

Miller, E. K. (2000). The prefrontal cortex and cognitive control. *Nature Reviews, 1,* 59–65.

Milner, B. (1963). Effects of different brain lesions on card sorting. *Archives of Neurology, 9,* 90–100.

Milner, B. (1964). Some effects of frontal lobectomy in man. In J. M. Warren & K. Akert (Eds.), *The frontal granular cortex and behavior* (pp. 313–331). New York: McGraw-HIll.

Milner, B. (1965). Visually-guided maze learning in man: Effects of bilateral hippocampal, bilateral frontal, and unilateral cerebral lesions. *Neuropsychologia, 3,* 317–338.

Morris, R. G., Ahmed, S., Syed, G. M., & Toone, B. K. (1993). Neural correlates of planning ability: Frontal lobe activation during the Tower of London test. *Neuropsychologia, 31,* 1367–1378.

Morris, R. G., & Baddeley, A. D. (1988). Primary and working memory functioning in Alzheimer-type dementia. *Journal of Clinical and Experimental Neuropsychology, 10,* 279–296.

Morris, R. G., & Kopelman, M. D. (1986). The memory deficits in Alzheimer-type dementia: A review. *Quarterly Journal of Experimental Psychology, 38A,* 575–602.

Moscovitch, M. (1992). Memory and working-with-memory: A component process model based on modules and central systems. *Journal of Cognitive Neuroscience, 4,* 257–267.

Mostofsky, S. H., Russell, E., Kofman, O., Carr, J., & Denckla, M. B. (2001). Deficits in motor response inhibition and motor persistence in ADHD. *Journal of the International Neuropsychological Society, 7,* 208.

Mountain, M. A., & Snow, W. G. (1993). Wisconsin Card Sorting Test as a measure of frontal pathology: A review. *The Clinical Neuropsychologist, 7,* 108–118.

Naglieri, J., & Das, J. P. (1997). *Das-Naglieri: Cognitive assessment system.* Itasca, IL: Riverside.

Nehemkis, A. M., & Lewinsohn, P. M. (1972). Effects of left and right cerebral lesions on the naming process. *Perceptual and Motor Skills, 35,* 787–798.

Nelson, C. A. (1995). The ontogeny of human memory: A cognitive neuroscience perspective. *Developmental Psychology, 31,* 723–738.

Nesbit-Greene, K., & Donders, J. (2002). Latent structure of the Children's Category Test after pediatric traumatic head injury. *Journal of Clinical and Experimental Neuropsychology, 24,* 194–199.

Nici, J., & Reitan, R. M. (1986). Patterns of neuropsychological ability in brain-disordered versus normal children. *Journal of Consulting and Clinical Psychology, 54,* 542–545.

Nigg, J. T. (1999). The ADHD response-inhibition deficit as measured by the Stop Task: Replication with DSM-IV combined type, extension, and qualification. *Journal of Abnormal Child Psychology, 27,* 393–402.

Nigg, J. T. (2000). On inhibition/disinhibition in developmental psychopathology: Views from cognitive and personality psychology and a working inhibition taxonomy. *Psychological Bulletin, 126,* 220–246.

Norman, D. A., & Shallice, T. (1986). Attention to action: Willed and automatic control of behaviour. In R. J. Davidson, G. E. Schwarts & D. Shapiro (Eds.), *Consciousness and self-regulation: Advances in research and theory* (Vol. 4, pp. 1–18). New York: Plenum.

Ojile, E., Das, J. P., & Mishra, R. K. (1993). Comparison of deaf and hearing children on measures of selective attention in two age groups. *The Clinical Neuropsychologist, 7,* 136–144.

Oosterlaan, J., Logan, G. D., & Sergeant, J. (1998). Response inhibition in ADHD, CD, comorbid ADHD+CD, anxious and normal children: A meta-analysis of studies with the stop task. *Journal of Child Pschology and Psychiatry, 39,* 411–425.

Owen, A. M., Downes, J. J., Sahakian, B. J., Polkey, C. E., & Robbins, T. W. (1990). Planning and spatial working memory deficits following frontal lobe lesions in man. *Neuropsychologia, 28,* 1021–1034.

Paniak, C. E., Miller, H. B., Murphy, D., Patterson, L., & Keizer, J. (1996). Canadian Developmental Norms for 9 to 14 year-olds on the Wisconsin Card Sorting Test. *Canadian Journal of Rehabilitation, 9*(4), 233–237.

Parkin, A., & Lawrence, A. (1994). A dissociation in the relation between memory tasks and frontal lobe tests in the normal elderly. *Neuropsychologia, 12,* 1523–1532.

Parks, R. W., Lowenstein, D. A., Dodrill, K. L., Barker, W. W., Yoshii, F., Chang, J. Y., et al. (1988). Cerebral metabolic effects of a verbal fluency test: A PET scan study. *Journal of Clinical and Experimental Neuropsychology, 10,* 565–575.

Passler, M., Isaac, W., & Hynd, G. W. (1985). Neuropsychological development of behavior attributed to frontal lobe functioning in children. *Developmental Neuropsychology, 4,* 349–370.

Patriot, A., Verin, M., Pillon, B., Teixeira-Ferreira, C., Agid, Y., & Dubois, B. (1996). Delayed response tasks in basal ganglia lesions in man: Further evidence for a striato-frontal cooperation in behavioral adaptation. *Neuropsychologia, 34,* 709–721.

Pendleton, M. G., & Heaton, R. K. (1982). A comparison of the Wisconsin Card Sorting Test and the Category Test. *Journal of Clinical Psychology, 38,* 392–396.

Pendleton, M. G., Heaton, R. K., Lehman, R. A., & Hulihan, D. (1982). Diagnostic utility of the Thurstone Word Fluency Test in neuropsychological evaluations. *Journal of Clinical Neuropsychology, 4,* 307–317.

Pennington, B. F. (1997). Dimensions of executive functions in normal and abnormal development. In N. A. Krasnegor, G. R. Lyon & P. S. Goldman-Rakic (Eds.), *Development of the prefrontal cortex: Evolution, neurobiology and behavior* (pp. 265–281). Baltimore, MD: Paul H. Brookes.

Pennington, B. F., Bennetto, L., McAleer, O., & Roberts, R. J. (1996). Executive functions and working memory: Theoretical and measurement issues. In G. R. Lyon & N. A. Krasnegor (Eds.), *Attention, Memory, and Executive Function* (pp. 327–348). Baltimore: Paul H. Brookes Publishing Co.

Perret, E. (1974). The left frontal lobe of man and the suppression of habitual responses in verbal categorical behavior. *Neuropsychologia, 12,* 323–330.

Perrine, K. (1993). Differential aspects of conceptual processing in the Category Test and Wisconsin Card Sorting Test. *Journal of Clinical and Experimental Neuropsychology, 15,* 461–473.

Perriti, P. (1971). Effects of non-competitive, competitive instructions and sex on performance in color word interference task. *Journal of Psychology, 79,* 67–70.

Perrott, S. B., Taylor, H. G., & Montes, J. L. (1991). Neuropsychological sequelae, family stress, and environmental adaptation following pediatric head injury. *Developmental Neuropsychology, 7,* 69–86.

Peterson, L. R., & Peterson, M. J. (1959). Short-term retention of individual verbal items. *Journal of Experimental Psychology, 58,* 193–198.

Petrides, M., Alivisatos, B., Evans, A., & Meyer, E. (1993). Dissociation of human mid-dorsolateral from posterior dorsolateral frontal cortex in memory processing. *Society for Neuroscience Abstracts, 90* (873–877).

Petrides, M., & Milner, B. (1982). Deficits on subject ordered tasks after frontal and temporal lobe lesions in man. *Neuropsychologia, 20,* 263–274.

Pliszka, S. R., Borcherding, S. H., Spratley, K., Leon, S., & Irick, S. (1997). Measuring inhibitory control in children. *Developmental and Behavioral Pediatrics, 18,* 254–259.

Ponsford, J., & Kinsella, G. (1992). Attentional deficits following closed head injury. *Journal of Clinical and Experimental Neuropsychology, 14,* 822–838.

Porteus, S. D. (1924). *Guide to Porteus Maze Test.* Vineland, NJ: The Training School.

Porteus, S. D. (1950). *The Porteus Maze Test and intelligence.* Palo Alto, CA: Pacific Books.

Porteus, S. D. (1959). *The maze test and clinical psychology.* Palo Alto, CA: Pacific Books.

Porteus, S. D. (1965). *Porteus Maze Test: Fifty years' application.* New York: The Psychological Corporation.

Prabhakaran, V., Smith, J. A. L., Desmond, J. E., Glover, G. H., & Gabrieli, J. D. E. (1997). Neural substrates of fluid reasoning: An fMRI study of neocortical activation during performance of Raven's Progressive Matrices Test. *Cognitive Psychology, 33,* 43–63.

Rabbitt, P. (1998). *Methodology of frontal and executive function.* London: Psychology Press.

Rafal, R., & Henik, A. (1994). The neurology of inhibition: Integrating controlled and automatic processes. In D. Dagenbach & T. H. Carr (Eds.), *Inhibitory processes in attention, memory, and language.* San Diego: Academic Press.

Ramier, A.-M., & Hécaen, H. (1970). Role respectif des atteintes frontales et de la lateralisation lésionnelle dans les deficitsde la "fluence verbale". *Revue de Neurologie, 123,* 17–22.

Raven, J. C. (1965). *Guide to using the Coloured Progressive Matrices.* London, UK: H. K. Lewis.

Raven, J. C., Court, J., & Raven, J. C. (1977). *Manual for Raven's Progressive Matrices and Vocabulary Scores. Section 3. Standard Progressive Matrices.* London: H. K. Lewis & Co.

Raven, J. C., Court, J., & Raven, J. C. (1992). *Manual for Raven's Progressive Matrices & Vocabulary Scores.* Oxford, UK: Oxford Psychologists Press.

Raven, J. C., Summers, B., & Birchfield, M. (1986). *Manual for Raven's Progressive Matrices and vocabulary scales. Research Supplement 3: A compendium of North American normative and validity studies.* London: H. K. Lewis.

Ravnkilde, B., Videbech, P., Rosenberg, R., Gjedde, A., & Gade, A. (2002). Putative tests of frontal lobe function: A PET-Study of brain activation during Stroop's test and verbal fluency. *Journal of Clinical and Experimental Neuropsychology, 24,* 534–547.

Reeder, K. P., & Boll, T. (1992). A shortened intermediate version of the Halstead Category Test. *Archives of Clinical Neuropsychology, 7,* 53–62.

Reeves, D., Kane, R., & Winter, K. (1994). *Automated neuropsychological assessment metrics: Test administrator's guide.* Washington, DC: Office of Military Performance Aassessment Technology, Division of Neuropsychiatry, Walter Reed Army Institute of Research.

Regard, M. (1981a). *Cognitive rigidity and flexibility: A neuropsychological study.* Unpublished manuscript, Victoria, British Columbia.

Regard, M. (1981b). The left frontal lobe of man and the suppression of habitual responses in verbal categorical behavior. *Neuropsychologia, 12,* 323–330.

Regard, M., Strauss, E., & Knapp, P. (1982). Children's production on verbal and non-verbal fluency tasks. *Perceptual and Motor Skills, 55,* 839–844.

Reitan, R. (1955). An investigation of the validity of Halstead's measures ob biological intelligence. *Archives of Neurology and Psychiatry, 73,* 28–35.

Reitan, R. (1971). Sensorimotor functions in brain-damaged and normal children of early school age. *Perceptual and Motor Skills, 33,* 655–664.

Reitan, R. M. (1986). *Trail-Making Test: Manual for administration and scoring.* Tucson: AZ: Neuropsychology Press.

Reitan, R., & Davison, L. (1974). *Clinical neuropsychology: Current status and applications.* New York: Hemisphere.

Reitan, R., & Wolfson, D. (1985). *The Halstead-Reitan Neuropsychological Test Battery.* Tucson, AZ: Neuropsychological Press.

Reitan, R. M. (1987). *Neuropsychological Evaluation of Children.* Tucson, AZ: Neuropsychology Press.

Reynolds, C. R., & Kamphaus, R. W. (1992). *Behavior Assessment System for Children.* Circle Pines, MN: American Guidance Service.

Rich, J. B., Troyer, A. K., Bylsma, F. W., & Brandt, J. (1999). Longitudinal analysis of phonemic clustering and switching during word-list generation in Huntington's disease. *Neuropsychology, 13,* 525–531.

Riddle, M., & Roberts, A. (1978). Psychosurgery and the Porteus Maze Tests: Review and reanalysis of data. *Archives of General Psychiatry, 35,* 493–497.

Risser, A. H., & Andrikopoulos, J. (1996). *Regard's Five-Point Test: Adolescent cohort stability.* Paper presented at the 24th Annual International Neuropsychological Society Conference, Chicago.

Roach, E. G., & Kephart, N. C. (1966). *The Purdue perceptual-motor survey.* Columbus, OH: Merrill.

Roberts, R. J., & Pennington, B. F. (1996). An interactive framework for examining prefrontal cognitive processes. *Developmental Neuropsychology, 12,* 105–126.

Robinson, A. L., Heaton, R. K., Lehman, R. A. W., & Stilson, D. W. (1980). The utility of the Wisconsin Card Sorting Test in detecting and localizing frontal lobe lesions. *Journal of Consulting and Clinical Psychology, 48,* 605–614.

Rolls, E. T. (1996). The orbitofrontal cortex. *Philosophical Transactions of the Royal Society of London, 351,* 1433–1443.

Roncadin, C., & Rich, J. B. (2002). Clustering and switching on verbal fluency tasks in childhood and adolescence. *Journal of the International Neuropsychological Society, 8,* 206.

Rosselli, M., & Ardila, A. (1993). Developmental norms for the Wisconsin Card Sorting Test in 5- to 12-year-old children. *The Clinical Neuropsychologist, 7,* 145–154.

Ruff, R. M. (1988). *Ruff Figural Fluency Test: Professional Manual.* Odessa, FL: Psychological Assessment Resources, Inc.

Ruff, R. M., Evans, R., & Marshall, L. (1986). Impaired verbal and figural fluency after head injury. *Archives of Clinical Neuropsychology, 1,* 87–106.

Ruff, R. M., Light, R., & Evans, R. (1987). The Ruff Figural Fluency Test: A normative study with adults. *Developmental Neuropsychology, 3,* 37–51.

Sachs, H., Krall, V., & Drayton, M. A. (1982). Neuropsychological assessment after lead poisoning without encephalopathy. *Perceptual and Motor Skills, 54,* 1283–1288.

Sandson, J., & Albert, M. L. (1984). Varieties of perseveration. *Neuropsychologia, 22,* 715–732.

Santostefano, S. (1988). *Cognitive Control Battery.* Los Angeles, CA: Western Psychological Services.

Schachar, R. J., & Logan, G. D. (1990). Impulsivity and inhibitory control in normal development and childhood psychopathology. *Developmental Psychology, 26,* 710–720.

Schiller, P. H. (1966). Developmental study of color-word interference. *Journal of Experimental Psychology, 72,* 105–108.

Schum, R. L., Sivan, A. B., & Benton, A. (1989). Multilingual Aphasia Examination: Norms for Children. *The Clinical Neuropsychologist, 3,* 375–383.

Seidman, L. J., Biederman, J., Faraone, S. V., Weber, W., Mennin, D., & Jones, J. (1997). A pilot study of neuropsychological function in girls with ADHD. *Journal of the American Academy of Child and Adolescent Psychiatry, 36,* 366–373.

Seidman, L. J., Biederman, J., Monuteaux, M. C., Doyle, A. E., & Faraone, S. V. (2001). Learning disabilities and executive dysfunction in boys with Attention-Deficit/Hyperactivity Disorder. *Neuropsychology, 15,* 544–556.

Selz, M., & Reitan, R. M. (1979). Neuropsychological test performance of normal, learning-disabled, and brain-damaged older children. *Journal of Nervous and Mental Disease, 167,* 298–302.

Semel, E., Wiig, E. H., & Secord, W. (1995). *Clinical Evaluation of Language Fundamentals-Third Edition.* San Antonio, TX: The Psychological Corporation.

Shallice, T. (1982). Specific impairments of planning. *Philosophical Transactions of the Royal Society of London, 298,* 199–209.

Shallice, T., & Burgess, P. (1991). Deficits in strategy application following frontal lobe damage in man. *Brain, 114,* 727–741.

Shallice, T., & Evans, M. (1978). The involvement of the frontal lobes in cognitive estimation. *Cortex, 14,* 294–303.

Shimamura, A. P., & Jurica, P. J. (1994). Memory interference effects and aging: Findings from a test of frontal lobe dysfunction. *Neuropsychology, 8,* 408–412.

Shu, B.-C., Tien, A. Y., Lung, F.-W., & Chang, Y.-Y. (2000). Norms for the Wisconsin Card Sorting Test in 6- to 11-year old children in Taiwan. *The Clinical Neuropsychologist, 14,* 275–286.

Shue, K. L., & Douglas, V. I. (1992). Attention deficit hyperactivity disorder and the frontal lobe syndrome. *Brain and Cognition, 20,* 104–124.

Shute, G. E., & Huertas, V. (1990). Developmental variability in frontal lobe function. *Developmental Neuropsychology, 6,* 1–11.

Simon, H. A. (1975). The functional equivalence of problem solving skills. *Cognitive Psychology, 7,* 268–288.

Smith, M. L., Klim, P., & Hanley, W. B. (in press). Executive function in school-aged children with Phenylketonuria. *Journal of Developmental and Physical Disabilities.*

Snow, J. H. (1998). Developmental patterns and use of the Wisconsin Card Sorting Test for children and adolescents with learning disabilities. *Child Neuropsychology, 4,* 89–97.

Spreen, O., & Benton, A. (1977). *Neurosensory centre comprehensive examination for aphasia. Manual of instructions.* Victoria, B.C.: University of Victoria.

Spreen, O., & Gaddes, W. H. (1969). Developmental Norms for 15 neuropsychological tests age 6 to 15. *Cortex, 5,* 171–191.

Spreen, O., & Strauss, E. (1998). *A compendium of neuropsychological tests: Adminstration, norms, and commentary* (2nd ed.). New York: Oxford University Press.

Strickland, T. L., D'Elia, L., James, R., & Stein, R. (1997). Stroop color-word performance of African Americans. *The Clinical Neuropsychologist, 11,* 87–90.

Stroop, J. R. (1935). Studies of interference in serial verbal reactions. *Journal of Experimental Psychology, 18,* 643–662.

Stuss, D. T. (1992). Biological and psychological development of executive functions. *Brain and Cognition, 20,* 8–23.

Stuss, D. T., & Benson, D. F. (1986). *The frontal lobes.* New York: Raven Press.

Tager-Flusberg, H. (1985). The conceptual basis for referential word meaning in children with autism. *Child Development, 56,* 1167–1178.

Tannock, R., Schachar, R. J., Carr, R. P., Chajczyk, D., & Logan, G. D. (1989). Effects of methylphenidate on inhibitory control in hyperactive children. *Journal of Abnormal Child Psychology, 17,* 473–491.

Tate, R. L., Perdices, M., & Maggiotto, S. (1998). Stability of the Wisconsin Card Sorting Test and the determination of reliability of change in scores. *The Clinical Neuropsychologist, 12,* 348–357.

Taylor, H. G., Albo, V., Phebus, C., Sachs, B., & Bierl, P. (1987). Postirradiation treatment outcomes for children with acute lymphoblastic leukemia: Clarification of risks. *Journal of Pediatric Psychology, 12,* 395–411.

Taylor, H. G., Barry, C. T., & Schatschneider, C. (1993). School-age consequences of Haemophilus influenzae Type b meningitis. *Journal of Clinical Child Psychology, 22,* 196–206.

Taylor, H. G., Hack, M., & Klein, N. K. (1998). Attention deficits in children with <750 gm birth weight. *Child Neuropsychology, 4,* 21–34.

Taylor, H. G., Hack, M., Klein, N. K., & Schatschneider, C. (1995). Achievement in children with birth weights less than 750 grams with normal cognitive abilities: Evidence for specific learning disabilities. *Journal of Pediatric Psychology, 20,* 703–719.

Taylor, H. G., Schatschneider, C., & Minich, N. (2000). Longitudinal outcomes of *Haemophilus influenzae* meningitis in school-age children. *Neuropsychology, 14,* 509–518.

Taylor, H. G., Schatschneider, C., Petrill, S., Barry, C. T., & Owens, C. (1996). Executive dysfunction in children with early brain disease: Outcomes post Haemophilus Influenzae Meningitis. *Developmental Neuropsychology, 12,* 35–51.

Taylor, H. G., Schatschneider, C., & Rich, D. (1991). Sequelae of Haemophilus Influenzae meningitis: Implications for the study of brain disease and development. In M. Tramontana & S. Hooper (Eds.), *Advances in Child Neuropsychology* (Vol. 1, pp. 50–108). New York: Springer-Verlag.

Teeter, P. A. (1985). Neurodevelopmental investigation of academic achievement: A report of years 1 and 2 of a longitudinal study. *Journal of Consulting and Clinical Psychology, 53,* 709–717.

Thurstone, L. L., & Thurstone, T. G. (1949). *Examiner manual for the SRA Primary Mental Abilities Test.* Chicago: Science Research Associates.

Thurstone, L. L., & Thurstone, T. G. (1962). *Primary mental abilities (Rev. ed.).* Chicago: Science Research Associates.

Townes, B., Trupin, E., Martin, D., & Goldstein, D. (1980). Neuropsychological correlates of academic success among elementary school children. *Journal of Consulting and Clinical Psychology, 48,* 675–684.

Tranel, D., Anderson, S. W., & Benton, A. (1994). Development of the concept of "executive function" and its relationship to the frontal lobes. In F. Boller & J. Grafman (Eds.), *Handbook of Neuropsychology,* Vol. 9 (pp. 125–148): Amsterdam: Elsevier.

Trenerry, M. R., Crosson, B. A., DeBoe, J., & Leber, W. R. (1989). *Stroop Neuropsychological Screening Test.* Odessa, FL: Psychological Assessment Resources.

Troyer, A. K. (2000). Normative data for clustering and switching on verbal fluency tasks. *Journal of Clinical and Experimental Neuropsychology, 22,* 370–378.

Troyer, A. K., Moscovitch, M., & Winocur, G. (1997). Clustering and switching as two components of verbal fluency: Evidence from younger and older healthy adults. *Neuropsychology, 11,* 138–146.

Troyer, A. K., Moscovitch, M., Winocur, G., Alexander, M., & Stuss, D. T. (1998). Clustering and switching on verbal fluency: The effects of focal frontal- and temporal-lobe lesions. *Neuropsychologia, 36,* 499–504.

Tucha, O., Smely, C., & Lange, K. W. (1999). Verbal and figural fluency in patients with mass lesions of the left or right frontal lobes. *Journal of*

Clinical and Experimental Neuropsychology, 21, 229–236.

Turkstra, L., & Kuegeler, E. (2001). Executive function and conversational fluency in adolescents. [abstract] *Journal of the International Neuropsychological Society, 7,* 218–219.

Uttl, B., & Graf, P. (1997). Color-Word Stroop test performance across the adult life span. *Journal of Clinical and Experimental Neuropsychology, 19,* 405–420.

Uyeda, K., & Mandler, G. (1980). Prototypicality norms for 28 semantic categories. *Behavior Research Methods and Instrumentation, 12,* 587–595.

van der Schoot, M., Licht, R., Horsley, T. M., & Sergeant, J. (2000). Inhibitory deficits in reading disability depend on subtype: Guessers but not Spellers. *Child Neuropsychology, 6,* 297–312.

Vanderploeg, R. D., Schinka, J. A., & Retzlaff, P. (1994). Relationships between measures of auditory learning and executive functioning. *Journal of Clinical & Experimental Neuropsychology, 16,* 243–252.

Vellutino, F. R., & Scanlon, D. M. (1985). Free recall of concrete and abstract words in poor and normal readers. *Journal of Experimental Child Psychology, 39,* 363–380.

Vendrell, P., Junque, C., Pujol, J., Jurado, M. A., Molet, J., & Grafman, J. (1995). The role of prefrontal regions in the Stroop task. *Neuropsychologia, 33,* 341–352.

Vik, P., & Ruff, R. R. (1988). Children's figural fluency performance: Development of strategy use. *Developmental Neuropsychology, 4,* 63–74.

Volz, H. P., Gaser, G., Hager, F., Rzanny, R., Mentzel, H. J., Kreitschmann-Andermahr, I., et al. (1997). Brain activation during cognitive stimulation with the Wisconsin Card Sorting Test: A functional MRI study on healthy volunteers and schizophrenics. *Psychiatry Research: Neuroimaging Section, 75,* 145–157.

Waber, D. P., & Bernstein, J. H. (1994). Repetitive graphomotor output in learning-disabled and non learning-disabled children: The Repeated Patterns Test. *Developmental Neuropsychology, 10,* 51–65.

Watkins, K. E., Hewes, D. K. M., Connelly, A., Kendall, B. E., Kingsley, D. P. E., Evans, J. E. P., et al. (1998). Cognitive deficits associated with frontal-lobe infarction in children with sickle cell disease. *Developmental Medicine and Child Neurology, 40,* 536–543.

Watson, J. M., Balota, D. A., & Sergent-Marshall, S. D. (2001). Semantic, phonological, and hybrid veridical and false memories in healthy older adults and in individuals with dementia of the Alzheimer type. *Neuropsychology, 15,* 254–267.

Wechsler, D. (1981). *Wechsler Adult Intelligence Scale-Revised manual.* New York: The Psychological Corporation.

Welsh, M. C. (1991). Rule-guided behavior and self-monitoring on the Tower of Hanoi disk-transfer task. *Cognitive Development, 6,* 59–76.

Welsh, M. C., & Pennington, B. F. (1988). Assessing frontal lobe functioning in children: Views from developmental psychology. *Developmental Neuropsychology, 4,* 199–230.

Welsh, M. C., Pennington, B. F., & Groisser, D. B. (1991). A normative-developmental study of executive function: A window on prefrontal function in children. *Developmental Neuropsychology, 7,* 131–149.

Welsh, M. C., Pennington, B. F., Ozonoff, S., Rouse, B., & McCabe, E. R. B. (1990). Neuropsychology of early-treated phenylketonuria: Specific executive function deficits. *Child Development, 61,* 1697–1713.

West, J., Douglas, G., Houghton, S., Lawrence, V., Whiting, K., & Glasgow, K. (2000). Time perception in boys with attention-deficit/hyperactivity disorder according to time duration, distration and mode of presentation. *Child Neuropsychology, 6,* 241–250.

Whalen, P. J., Bush, G., McNally, R. J., Wilhelm, S., McInerney, S. C., Jenike, M. A., et al. (1998). The emotional counting Stroop paradigm: A functional magnetic resonance imaging probe of the anterior cingulate cortex affective division. *Biological Psychiatry, 44,* 1219–1228.

Wolff, A. B., Radecke, D. D., Kammerer, B. L., & Gardner, J. K. (1989). Adaptation of the Stroop Color and Word Test for use with deaf adults. *The Clinical Neuropsychologist, 3,* 369–374.

Yakovlev, P. I., & Lecours, A. R. (1967). The myelogenetic cycles of regional maturation of the brain. In A. Minkiniwski (Ed.), *Regional development of the brain in early life* (pp. 3–70). Oxford, UK: Blackwell.

Yeudall, L. T., Fromm, D., Reddon, J.R., and Stefanyk, W.O. (1986). Normative data stratified by age and sex for 12 neuropsychological tests. *Journal of Clinical Psychology, 42,* 918–946.

Zabel, A. T., Verda, M., Kinsman, S., & Mahone, E. M. (2002). Parent and self-report Behavior Rating Inventory of Executive Function (BRIEF) in adolescents with myelomeningocele. [abstract] *Journal of the International Neuropsychological Society, 8,* 297.

Zakay, D. (1990). The evasive art of subjective time measurement: Some methodological dilemmas. In R. A. Block (Ed.), *Cognitive models of psychological time* (pp. 59–84). Hillsdale, NJ: Erlbaum.

7

Attention

Attention is an inherent function in any cognitive performance, yet it is not a unitary function (Denckla, 1989). While the capacity to focus available attentional resources is important, not all simple or even complex tasks are necessarily heavily dependent on this capacity (Baddeley, 2001). Intact arousal, orientation, concentration, span of apprehension, perseverance, and vigilance are desirable, while distractibility, impersistence, poor inhibition, neglect, and confusion characterize some of the problematic aspects (Mesulam, 1985; Denckla, 1989). It is helpful to assess routinely whether there is poor arousal or poor modulation of the individual's information-processing state that would suggest disruption of the ascending reticular activating system in brain stem and midbrain regions or whether the child is poorly oriented or some form of inattention contributes to compromised overall performance (Mesulam, 1985).

For example, it appears that the ability to orient attention develops gradually, with internally driven ability to scan the environment actively established by 5 or 6 years of age, the ability to focus attention expected to be established by 7, and sustained attention developing into adolescence (Helland and Asbjørnsen, 2000). A neurology perspective allows us to consider whether motivational aspects of attention that depend on the limbic system and cingulate cortex, sensory-representational aspects of attention dependent on posterior parietal cortex, or motor exploratory portions of the attention network that depend on frontal cortical regions can be distinguished (Denckla, 1989). It is even more desirable if this can be accomplished with partitioning of functional attention subsystems that lead to better diagnostic differentiation and to specific and effective intervention strategies.

In clinical neuropsychology practice, attention is a process or domain that is assessed as one component contributing to the child's overall neurocognitive competence. Attention is not mediated by a single brain region or by the brain as a whole, but instead is carried out by discrete anatomical networks, within which specific computations are assigned to different brain areas (Posner and Peterson, 1990; Fernandez-Duque and Posner, 2001). Variability of attention is expected in the course of any evaluation and its presence alone does not justify a disorder determination. Other explanations should therefore be considered.

Attention will fluctuate in response to many factors, including motivation, self-esteem, anxiety, mood, and lingering effects of a mild illness. Test order needs to be considered as tests administered later in a test session might be more poorly responded to than those administered earlier. For example, sequential administration of multiple measures tapping a particularly weak domain may result in poor performance on the later tests, when tests that tap the child's strengths were not interspersed to provide a break and sense of success. Fatigue affects performance (Stuss, Stethem et al., 1989). Task sensitivity and test challenge may affect results, that is, a more sensitive test may prove more difficult for a child with a particular impairment. The modality—verbal mediation, spatial integration, or tactile/kinesthetic manipulation—needed for successful performance may be influential. Further, no pure test of attention exists to aid in definitive determination about whether the degree of attentional problem noted exceeds that appropriately attributed to normal variability.

The most common disorder of attention in childhood is Attention Deficit Hyperactivity Disorder (ADHD). As defined by the *Diagnostic and Statistical Manual of Mental Disorders* (4th ed.) (DSM-IV; American Psychiatric Association, 1994) ADHD is characterized by a core disorder of inattention, impulsivity, and/or hyperactivity. It is estimated that as many as 20% of U.S. children manifest ADHD symptoms (Barkley, 1990). While specific evidence of a distinct neurobehavioral profile sufficient to meet ADHD DSM-IV diagnostic criteria may be apparent on evaluation, failure to meet these behaviorally determined diagnostic criteria does not preclude the possibility that faulty attention significantly contributes to a child's poor functioning. It is important for the clinician to recognize that ADHD and an attentional disorder not meeting specific criteria for ADHD according to DSM-IV criteria can exist separately and be of equal concern.

Research on DSM-IV subtypes of ADHD demonstrates that these differ in demographic characteristics, types of functional impairment, and profiles of comorbidity with other childhood disorders (Chabildas, Pennington et al., 2001), including a high proportion of children with comorbid learning disorders. Interpretation of ADHD, or attentional disorder, also depends on awareness of the child's developmental level with respect to patterns of objective test performance. For example, what might appear to be attentional disorder at age 6 might be interpreted as normal exploratory activity at age 3. Situational factors are also especially important. Thus, teacher concerns about a child's inattentive behaviors might not be replicated in a one-to-one testing situation that is highly structured, presents novel material in fairly rapid succession, and allows for a degree of motoric expression that exceeds what might be allowed in the classroom.

While the DSM-IV offers guidelines for diagnosis, it is a limited resource when its definitions are compared to those emerging as a result of recent empirical research and in context with controversy about whether ADHD has a unitary nature. In one study, the results on tests of processing speed, vigilance, and inhibition were examined to determine whether the subtypes differed in underlying neuropsychological deficits. The results were contrary to prediction since symptoms of inattention best predicted performance on all dependent measures and not just on processing speed and vigilance, and ADHD-Inattentive and ADHD-Combined children had similar profiles of impairment. In contrast, children with ADHD-Hyperactive/Impulsive were not significantly impaired on any dependent measures, once subclinical symptoms of inattention were controlled. These results did not support distinct neuropsychological deficits in ADHD-inattentive and ADHD-Combined children and suggested that symptoms of inattention, rather than symptoms of hyperactivity/impulsivity, were associated with neuropsychological impairment (Chabildas, Pennington et al., 2001).

However, support for the DSM-IV ADHD subtype classifications was found in another study. These results for four age-matched groups of 80 children, grouped by gender and ADHD subtype, found the ADHD-Combined group earning lower scores on tests requiring simple selection, automatic shifting, and executive control than a group without hyperactivity. Both the ADHD-Combined and ADHD-Inattentive groups had difficulty with effortful focusing, learning, and recall compared to age-standardized normative data. Five neuropsychological measures discriminated between the groups with 80% accuracy (Lockwood, Marcotte et al., 2001). Such research has added to a rich database supporting more extensive elaboration of attention subcomponents, neurobiological bases, and distributed neural circuit involvement. Some of these attention subdomains might overlap across models or be combined or considered jointly in different empiric studies. Altogether, current data lead to the conclusion that attention is not a unitary concept, and broad terminology only lessens the practical usefulness of a test, evaluation, or diagnosis, based on such global summary characteristics, and limits understanding of an individual case.

There is also a rapidly growing literature concerning the neuroanatomical networks and pathophysiological and neurobiological substrates related to the manifestation of attention deficits (Posner, Walker, et al., 1984; Posner and Peterson, 1990; Mirsky, Anthony et al., 1991; Heilman, Voeller et al., 1991; Mesulam, 2000), although the brain structures or mechanisms responsible for the cognitive/behavioral deficits remain at issue (Stefanatos and Wasserstein, 2001). The ideas posited in this literature are of interest, given the application of structural and functional neuroimaging techniques to child and adult populations. Brain-imaging studies of attention reveal intricate distributed neural networks, suggesting complex behavior depends on complex brain organization. The inferior parietal lobe's role in spatial selective attention is well documented (Mesulam, 1981; Posner, Walker et al., 1987; Heilman, Watson et al., 1988). There are also reports of the importance of the orbital frontal region (Fuster, 1989), limbic system (Cohen, 1993), subcortical systems (Petersen, Robinson et al., 1987), and midbrain systems (Pribram and McGuinness, 1975). Child study, using techniques of positron emission tomography (PET) and single photon emission computed tomography, found characteristic hypoperfusion of frontal and striatal regions and hyperperfusion of occipital regions, (SPECT; Lou, Henricksen et al., 1984). A corpus callosum contribution was suggested with volumetric study (Giedd, Castellanos et al., 1994). While, together, these data disprove the notion that there are merely discrete unitary brain areas responsible, a preponderance of data about ADHD implicate, more specifically, the prefrontal, striatal, and possibly the limbic regions (Zametkin, Nordahl et al., 1990; Benson, 1991; Heilman, Voeller et al., 1991; Zametkin, Liebenauer, et al., 1993).

Data also support the idea that, in adults, the right hemisphere is more involved than the left hemisphere in general attention processing (Cohen, Semple et al., 1988). The contribution of the right cerebral hemisphere to attention

was recognized early, but recent advances place even greater emphasis on the importance of the frontostriatal system of the right cerebral hemisphere. For example, activation studies found predominantly right frontal activation in healthy adults in sustained attention studies (Pardo, Pardo et al., 1991; Lewin, Friedman et al., 1996) supporting earlier hypotheses (Wilkins, Shallice et al., 1987) about this region's importance. Right frontal lobe abnormalities were suggested with both an event-related-potential study of children with ADHD (Harter, Anello-Vento et al., 1988) and with a magnetic resonance imaging (MRI) volumetric study (Filipek, Semrud-Clikeman et al., 1997).

Weintraub and Mesulam posited a right hemisphere (parietal) specialization for spatial attention to both sides of space, with right hemisphere lesions therefore resulting in a severe and persistent neglect (Weintraub and Mesulam, 1987). Yet it was suggested that this model may not account for left-neglecting patients who also demonstrate right-sided neglect or for the possibility that right hemisphere activation in right and left-field tasks is due to a nonlateralized sustained attention factor (Robertson, Tegner et al., 1995).

The relative contributions of each hemisphere continue to be the subject of investigation and speculation. For example, error-type analyses revealed a frontal lobe hemispheric distinction between bias (left hemisphere) and sensitivity (right hemisphere), the first such dissociation published (Stuss, Binns et al., 2002). For further discussion of the literature pertaining to ADHD as a right hemisphere syndrome, the reader is referred to a detailed review (Stefanatos and Wasserstein, 2001).

MODELS OF ATTENTION

A number of attention models are proposed to provide a context for understanding this most basic of functions. Four of these models are briefly noted here for the reader to consider in building his or her own conceptual framework for evaluating and interpeting this domain.

Mesulam divides attentional modulations into those that are domain-specific and domain-independent and refers to an overall attentional matrix that is the collective manifestation of both (Mesulam, 1981; Mesulam, 1985). Domain-specific attentional responses are mediated by modality-specific neurons, such as, face neurons for faces, posterior parietal neurons for spatial targets, visual neurons for visual stimuli. Domain-independent modulations are exerted through bottom-up influence by the ascending reticular activating system (ARAS) and top-down influence by the cerebral cortex, that is, from prefrontal parietal and limbic cortices. Thus, a clinical syndrome of impaired attention, such as an acute confusional state, refers to attentional matrix impairment, whereas a syndrome of contralesional neglect refers more discretely to domain-specific impairment of any cortical or subcortical component of the spatial system that distributes attention within extrapersonal space.

Mirsky and colleagues theorized about a brain-attention system and made tentative attribution of functional specialization to specific brain regions (Mirsky, Anthony et al., 1991). They initially proposed four major attention elements: focus/execute (scan and respond, selective attention, and psychomotor response), sustain (be vigilant, attend for a time interval), encode (sequential registration, recall, and mental manipulation of information), and shift (be flexible, change focus of attention). The tests factor analyses assigned to each element were then used to assess aspects of attentional capacity. These included the Wechsler Intelligence Scale for Children-III arithmetic and digit span subtests (encode), WISC-III coding subtest (focus/execute), visual search/cancellation tests (focus/execute), computer-assisted measures that provide sensitive data about reaction time and errors of omission and commission (sustain), the Trail Making Test (focus/execute), the Stroop test (focus/execute), and the Wisconsin Card Sorting Test (WCST) (shift). Stabilize, a fifth element, was subsequently added to the model (Mirsky, 1996). Stabilize was intended to capture the reliability or consistency of attentional effort, and was reflected in continuous performance test reaction time variability. As with the sustain element, the brain stem and midline thalamic structures were purported to correlate with this element. The model was incorporated in a study of children with myelomeningocele, who showed deficits across all four elements compared to sibling controls (Loss, Yeates et al., 1998).

Posner and Peterson posited the existence of three semiautonomous mechanisms or systems, that underlie human attention (Posner and Peterson, 1990). The first, *orienting,* is referred to as the posterior attention system, in part because of its basis in posterior brain regions, including the posterior parietal lobe, superior colliculus, and lateral pulvinar nucleus of the posteriolateral thalamus. This system has the capacity to direct spatial attention and is strongly implicated in neglect. It is also this system that can be influenced by its own mechanisms and the modulatory effects of a right hemisphere dominant, norepinephrine based alerting/sustained attention system (Robertson, Tegner et al., 1995). The second, *selection,* is linked to anterior cingulate and supplementary motor areas. It is the conscious attention system that is related to target selection and recognition, irrespective of spatial location.

The third, *alerting or sustained attention,* allows for continued response over time, when salient or novel external stimuli that engage attention are absent. Its neuroanatomical region is hypothesized to be right cerebral, especially anterior, prefrontal regions. Posner also posited a "spotlight," where attention is engaged, disengaged, and reengaged (Posner and Peterson, 1990). Preliminary support for this model was reported with a linkage of symptom domains, cognitive processes, and neural networks (Swanson, Posner et al., 1998).

Cohen conceptualizes attention as involving the interaction of four component processes influenced by multiple brain systems (Cohen, Semple et al., 1988; Cohen, 1993). These are sensory selective attention, response selection and control, capacity and focus, and sustained attention. According to this model, *sensory selective attention* is contingent on filtering sensory features, enhancement, and disengagement, or an attentional shift toward a new stimulus. *Response selection and control,* or intention, are generated by functional states of readiness, expectancy, and anticipatory response. In this model, the executive functions of intention, initiation, generative capacity, persistence, inhibition, and switching are linked to response selection and control. Attentional capacity and focus will determine the intensity of directed attention and, thus, the scope and quality of performance. *Sustained attention* refers to maintenance of performance over time and is dependent on the target : distractor ratio and influenced by reinforcement, such as an incentive and internal motivational state. This model has been applied in recent child neuropsychology studies (Lockwood, Bell et al., 1999; Lockwood, Marcotte et al., 2001), investigating differentiation of ADHD subtypes, with preliminary support found for identifying the inattentive and combined ADHD subtypes based on this model's attentional components. They found all four attentional components were represented in a discriminant analysis, which they interpreted to mean that heterogeneous attentional measures are needed to assess neuropsychological differences between ADHD subtypes. Interestingly, they found little influence of gender on neuropsychological performance in these children when comorbidity of learning and psychiatric conditions was well controlled.

Stuss and colleagues hypothesize a model of the "cognitive architecture of attention" and provide reaction time (RT) data supporting the existence of three separable attentional components in anterior cerebral regions (Stuss, Shallice et al., 1995; Stuss, Binns et al., 2002). One attentional system maintains a general state of readiness to respond. This activation state was associated with the superior medial frontal region, and in their study, lesions in this region affected simple RT speed. A second system sets a criterion level of response, or threshold, to a target or external stimulus and establishes a bias for responsiveness. This system was associated with the left dorsolateral frontal region, and lesions in this region altered response bias. A third system maintains the selection of the defined schema to allow for consistent target selection. This system of sustained attention was associated with right dorsolateral frontal regions, and lesions in this region decreased sensitivity in differentiating targets from nontargets. The authors suggested that this region is also important for inhibition of an incorrect response or irrelevant information.

NEUROPSYCHOLOGY'S CONTRIBUTION TO EVALUATION OF ATTENTION

There is a place for neuropsychological evaluation in the diagnosis and management of the child with ADHD, despite views that strongly emphasize the neurobehavioral features of this neuropsychiatric diagnosis (American Academy of Pediatrics, 2000). Importantly, neuropsychologists are very likely to see children referred for suspected or diagnosed ADHD. They can contribute to understanding a child who does not meet limited DSM-IV diagnostic criteria, but who does experience clinically significant attentional variability. As with any referral, it is necessary to understand the child's full range of behavioral and cognitive strengths and weaknesses and to consider the history, including any contributory but alternative primary disorder that might be explanatory for the presenting problem or comorbid problems that exacerbate the behavioral expression of attentional disorder.

It is the consideration of comorbid disorder that is of special purview for child neuropsychologists. Primary sensory impairment (e.g., hearing or vision), the family, medical, psychiatric and neurological histories, undiagnosed neurological disease (e.g., seizure disorder), late effects of prior neurological insult (e.g., trauma, infection, metabolic disorder), sleep disorder (Hansen and Vandenberg, 1997; Marcotte, Thacher et al., 1998; Chervin, Archbold, et al. 2002) allergies or asthma, and the full range of possible psychiatric disorders must be considered. The ability to exclude comorbid disorder or document alternative explanations through history taking, formal assessment, and careful integration of diverse personal, medical, and academic records is central to the day-to-day functioning of many clinical child neuropsychologists. It is they, along with other allied professionals interested in neurodevelopment, who are increasingly better able to contribute to defining and understanding separable attention subcomponents and how they influence a child's daily functioning.

It is also incumbent on child neuropsychologists to be familiar with related research directed toward linking discrete neurobehavioral manifestations of this global construct to specific brain regions or neural networks that will affect treatment recommendations and management decisions. A theoretical model is central to developing appropriate treatment or management procedures. Data were reported early concerning teaching children to self-alert and self-regulate their attention and behavior through self-instructional training intended to generalize to the everyday world (Meichenbaum and Goodman, 1971). A neuropsychological model of attention would appear to have the greatest salience for the clinician attempting to sort out the complexities of evaluating attention and attention disorder (Cooley and Morris, 1990).

In an effort to address the multifactorial etiological possibilities, psychology has produced numerous test instruments, including behavior rating scales, self-report inventories, checklists, parent and teacher questionnaires, structured interviews, and continuous performance tests of vigilance. Research paradigms have employed sophisticated procedural and statistical methods to determine which of the many standardized psychological and neuropsychological instruments will be most useful. Yet, despite all this attention, no definitive evaluation protocol has emerged as most effective, and the validity of currently used objective instruments has been questioned, particularly if used singly for ADHD diagnosis (Gordon and Barkley, 1990). The conclusions reached at the 1998 National Institutes of Health (NIH) Consensus Conference did not ultimately endorse one specific objective technique as confirmatory of an ADHD diagnosis, finding an independent diagnostic test does not exist (National Institutes of Health, 1998).

While the DSM-IV is relied on for diagnosis guidelines, it, too, fails to specify an objective instrument or procedure for diagnosis. More recently, the American Academy of Pediatrics released "Clinical Practice Guideline: Diagnosis and evaluation of the child with attention-deficit/hyperactivity disorder" (American Academy of Pediatrics, 2000). These guidelines for primary care clinicians are for the diagnosis, evaluation, and management of 6- to 12-year-old children with ADHD. The academy recommends that diagnosis meet DSM-IV criteria, and that assessment includes evidence obtained directly from parents or caregivers about the core ADHD symptoms in various settings, along with onset age, symptom duration, and degree of functional impairment. It also recommends that evidence be obtained directly from the teacher or school personnel about associated conditions, symptom duration, and functional impairment.

A related publication, "Clinical Practice Guideline: Treatment of the school-aged child with attention-deficit/hyperactivity disorder" (American Academy of Pediatrics, 2001), lists treatment guidelines for the pediatrician. These guidelines highlight the neurobehavioral nature of ADHD and the importance of history taking and direct information gathering from adults in different settings in which the child participates, and the use of questionnaires designed to identify inattention, hyperactivity, and impulsivity outside the range of normal functioning. The guidelines do not specify other diagnostic tests to establish the diagnosis of ADHD, but allude to their potential use in assessing coexisting conditions, such as learning disabilities and mental retardation. In limiting the scope of evaluation resources, these guidelines omit any specific reference to potential contributions by neuropsychology in both differential diagnosis and behavioral management.

There are many examples of the useful contributions of neuropsychological tests for children with ADHD (Denckla, 1985a; Yeates and Bornstein, 1992; Cahn, Marcotte et al., 1996; Ewing-Cobbs, 1998; Butler and Copeland, 2002). There is also a contrasting perspective that test administration has a limited role (Gordon and Barkley, 1990; Barkley, 1991) due to poor sensitivity of individual measures. Despite various viewpoints, it is quite clear that to answer the central questions, researchers need to specify an underlying model of attention, select tasks based on the model, and utilize multiple tasks with a well-defined clinical population (Fletcher, 1998).

SUBDOMAINS OF ATTENTION

Limited appreciation for the intricate and variable nature of attentional functioning in the individual is necessarily limiting. It is therefore useful to familiarize oneself with currently proposed clinical attention subdomains and appreciate how different manifestations of attention problems ultimately will lead to specific and more effective behavioral management techniques and treatment recommendations, a major goal of clinical evaluation.

A number of attention types, or subdomains, are described in the literature. Commonly, one sees reference to terms such as *focused attention, selective attention, sustained attention, switching or mental set shifting,* and *divided attention,* although other terminology is also encountered. Support for such differentiation is evident from a variety of studies, including those utilizing sophisticated statistical methodology. For example, a 3-factor model of sustained attention, selective attention, and central capacity was found to be a parsimonious fit, whereas the unitary model was a poor fit in a study of computerized, attention-test-performance patterns and general ability in second graders using structural equation modeling (SEM; Shapiro, Morris et al., 1998). Structural equation modeling also defined three factors in a study of 293 healthy children administered

the Test of Everyday Attention for Children (TEA-Ch), those of selective attention, sustained attention, and higher level executive control (Manly, Anderson et al., 2001).

Studies finding differential impairment of these subcomponents dependent on etiology also highlight the discriminability of attention subdomains. For example, dual task conditions proved especially sensitive to a variety of neurological conditions (Stuss, Stethem et al., 1989). Also, using logistic regression analyses, which do not assume population normality, children with ADHD-Inattentive or ADHD-Combined diagnoses had significantly higher ratings from parents and teachers than control children on the Behavior Rating Inventory of Executive Function Working Memory (WM) scale. The WM scale, however, did not distinguish between ADHD-Inattentive and ADHD-Combined subtypes. The Inhibit scale did prove useful in distinguishing between ADHD—Combined and ADHD—Inattentive and controls on the parent and teacher forms in 65%–68% of cases (Gioia, Isquith et al., 2000). Thus, continued study of separable attentional constructs is an avenue of particular

Table 7–1. Tests by Subtypes of Attention Assessed

Test	TYPE OF ATTENTION			
	Selective	Divided	Sustained	Shifting
Span	X			
Stroop Color-Word Test	X			
Symbol Digit Modalities Test	X			
d2 Test of Attention	X			
Trail Making Test	X	(Part B)		
Letter/Symbol Cancellation	X			
TEA-Ch Sky Search	X			
TEA-Ch Map Mission	X			
WISC Coding	X			
Consonant Trigrams Test		X		
CHIPASAT		X		
TEA-Ch Sky Search DT		X	X	
TEA-Ch Score DT		X	X	
Dichotic Listening	X	X	X	
WAIS-III Letter Number Sequencing		X		
Continuous Performance Tests			X	
TEA-Ch Score!			X	
TEA-Ch Walk-Don't Walk			X	
TEA-Ch Code Transmission			X	
TEA-Ch Opposite Worlds				X
TEA-Ch Creature Counting				X

interest. The subdomains of selective or fo-cused, divided, sustained, and alternating/shifting attention are described briefly below. Table 7–1 presents a listing of several tests dis-cussed later in this chapter along with their common subdomain assignment.

Selective or Focused Attention

Focused attention refers to vigilance in moni-toring information. When we attend, we orient physically toward a focus of attention. Focused attention is referred to as a discrete perceptual ability and response to a stimulus. It is some-times used interchangeably with the term *se-lective attention,* which refers to the ability to maintain a cognitive set in the presence of background "noise" or distraction. It also refers to a shifting of the focus of awareness from one extrapersonal event to another (Mesulam, 2000). Attention can shift overtly or covertly and in response to exogenous as well as en-dogenous events. Selective attention is mani-fest, for example, when one selects a target stimulus for enhanced processing from a larger array of stimuli. The terms *focus* and *execute* are combined in some theoretical models (Mirsky, Anthony et al., 1991). These authors defined *focus* as the visual perceptual ability to scan stimulus material, and *execute* as the ability to make a response. The parent–child interaction is considered crucial to the devel-opment of directed attention and to the regu-lation of behavior through outer speech inter-nalized to inner speech (Vygotsky, 1962) or metacognition (Borkowski and Burke, 1996).

This preference for some stimuli over oth-ers can be formally evaluated. Perceptual mo-tor speed can be a factor in such tests, irre-spective of modality. Examples of clinical tests (and the response modality required) that as-sess this capacity include the Stroop Color-Word Test (SCWT) (verbal), visual search and letter-cancellation tests (visuomotor), Symbol Digit Modalities Test (verbal and written), WISC-III Picture Completion (verbal) and Coding (visuomotor) subtests, and Trail Mak-ing Test (visuomotor). The TEA-Ch Sky Search and Map Mission subtests (both visuomotor) fit a selective attention factor using structural equation modeling (Manly, Anderson et al.,

2001). These two subtests were adapted for children and included in the TEA-Ch since two visual search tasks of the Test for Everyday Attention, adult version, had common factor loadings with the SCWT (Robertson, Ward et al., 1995).

Divided Attention

Divided attention refers to the ability to re-spond to more than one task or event simulta-neously. When attention is divided, it appears to influence performance significantly, and temporal factors appear influential. Research has demonstrated that divided attention has a negative effect on memory encoding in normal subjects and results in poor memory perfor-mance. Yet, divided attention at retrieval has minimal or no impact on memory perfor-mance. Also, free recall is affected more than cued recall by divided attention (Craik, Gov-oni et al., 1996).

Consistent with long-held suppositions about the importance of more anterior cerebral re-gions for intact attention and conceptual shift-ing, including prefrontal cortex and the stria-tum, neuroimaging studies reveal increased prefrontal cortex activation in the presence of switching demands, such as required in divided attention tasks (D'Esposito, Detre et al., 1995). This type of attention appears to resonate most with the practical realities that constitute our daily experiences, for which multitasking is prevalent.

The TEA-Ch Sky Search DT and Score DT subtests are examples of dual-task tests, as are the Auditory Consonant Trigrams Test, the Paced Auditory Serial Attention Test (Gron-wall, 1977), or Children's Paced Auditory Serial Addition Task (CHIPASAT), (Johnson, Roethig-Johnston et al., 1988), and reaction time tests. Also, the effects of concurrent tests are of interest with respect to the division of attention, for example, performing two tasks si-multaneously, such as tapping while respond-ing to a verbal fluency test (Kinsbourne and Cook, 1971; Kinsbourne and Hicks, 1978). Empirical data for the latter verbal–nonverbal pairings provided evidence supporting the no-tion of inhibitory interference, or, evidence of competition for functional space.

Interestingly, the effect is not always an inhibitory interference since facilitory interference can also occur, as resulted in a study of adult finger tapping concurrent with verbal and nonverbal motor and sensory tasks (Dalen and Hugdahl, 1986). In this study, a right-hand decrement occurred during a motor verbal task (reading aloud), as predicted, due to left-hemisphere dominance for language processing. However, left-hand tapping frequency above baseline was found during two sensory tasks (verbal watching, a list of nonsense syllables, and nonverbal viewing of complex figure patterns), evidence of facilitation. A significant increase above baseline was also found for the right hand during the motor nonverbal task (humming a melody with no lyric), although no difference was observed between hands.

Sustained Attention

Sustained attention refers to the ability to maintain vigilance and respond consistently during continuous or repetitive activity. A decrement in performance over time characterizes the sustained attention deficit. Sustained attention refers to maintaining performance over time, but not to the overall allocation of attention (van der Meere and Sergent, 1988). It is particularly dependent on mental control and working memory over a time interval. Children with ADHD appear to have particular difficulty with sustained attention (Seidel and Joschko, 1990; Shue and Douglas, 1992; Hooks, Milich et al., 1994; Barkley, 1997b). Sustained attention is commonly assessed with CPTs, but also with other tasks, such as dichotic listening. Vigilance tests can be presented by computer, but also by audiotape or orally. They are unlikely to be influenced by intelligence level. The TEA-Ch is an example of a noncomputerized test that includes sustained attention (vigilance) measures in the form of the TEA-Ch Score!, Score DT, Walk-Don't Walk, Code Transmission, and Sky Search DT subtests. These tests are of shorter duration and present quite different tasks than those of computerized CPTs, but sustained attention is still the identified factor of interest.

The minimal length required for a test to elicit failure to sustain attention is still debated. Sustained attention can be examined qualitatively as well, such observations serving as an additional marker for consideration within the overall profile. As an example, I describe below a scoring modification I routinely use for the Auditory Consonan Trigrams Test (ACTT) that adds another measure of sustained attention to the full profile.

Alternating Attention/Mental Shifting

Alternating attention refers to the ability to maintain mental flexibility in order to shift from one task requirement to another when these have different cognitive requirements. Tests that assess alternating attention or shifting capacity include the TEA-Ch Creature Counting and Opposite Worlds subtests. Verbal response inhibition is necessary for both these tests, and verbal response inhibition deficit has been noted in the presence of developmental disorders (Georgiou, Bradshaw et al. 1996). The WCST is a complex measure, dependent on many functional capacities. Of particular interest in this regard is the percent of conceptual responses and percent of perseverative errors scores. Tests of alternating and shifting attention cross sensory modalities. For example, tests of Reciprocal Motor Programs provide an index of motor shifting, while verbal and design fluency tests assess verbal and nonverbal generative function respectively. Both detect inability to shift in the form of perseverative errors. Children diagnosed as having autism tend to have particular difficulty shifting attention.

TESTS OF ATTENTION

Theoreticians, investigators, and clinicians may differ in the assignments of a particular test to the attention domain. This is largely due to the ambiguous nature of the construct of attention and that many tests considered useful in assessing attentional capacity were not developed in context with a strong theoretical basis. Validation studies of attention are not extensive, but in one study the construct validity of eight attention tests was examined. Loadings on three factors were identified that were similar for both normal and closed head injury (CHI) samples: visuomotor scanning (digit symbol, letter cancellation, Symbol Digit Modalities Test, Trail Making Test), sustained selective processing (Serial 7s and 13s, Stroop Interference) and visual/auditory spanning (digit forward, digit backward, Knox Cube) (Shum, McFarland et al., 1990). Such study is helpful in the discussion of test-domain assignment. In the section below, tests assigned to this domain are noted, although in some instances, a strong case could be presented for an equally appropriate assignment to another domain. I recognize the fluidity with which a test might move between domains, but my decisions were based on the predominant literature references and are not entirely arbitrary.

Span Tests

Span refers to the ability to hold an adequate amount of information in working memory (Baddeley, 1976). It refers to how much information can be held after a single presentation in correct serial order. The stimuli might be digits, words, or letters, for example. Traditionally, average span is considered 7 ± 2 (Miller, 1956). However, span is influenced by context, content, and culture. For example, the average span for recall of unrelated words is only five stimuli while sentence span (meaningful contextual information) can commonly reach 16 words (Baddeley, Vallar et al., 1987). Number span is also affected by linguistic factors (phonological length of the numbers or articulation length), and therefore, average span length will vary between cultures (Dehaene, 1997; Ardila, Rosselli et al., 2000). Average visuospatial span is four items, is affected by age and educational level, and males tend to excel, compared to females (Grossi, Orsini et al., 1979; Orsini, Schiappa et al., 1981; Orsini, Grossi et al., 1987). Active organization is necessary to exceed immediate memory span, including such executive function (EF) processes as chunking, clustering, and categorizing (Heubrock, 1999). These subjective organization processes, frequently taught as part of treatment interventions for brain impairment, are measurable (Tulving, 1962; Sternberg and Tulving 1977), are available in normal childhood, and are refined as the child matures

(Boyd, 1988). It is also noted that span and recency develop at different rates in normal children (Hitch and Halliday, 1983).

One of the most ubiquitous clinical screening measures is the digit span test with immediate repetition. Sequentially longer strings of numbers are presented orally, and the examinee must immediately repeat the sequence without interference, either in the identical order for the forward condition or in reverse order for the backward condition. Performance depends on a short-term, phonologically based storage system (Vallar and Baddeley, 1984) that tends to be spared with subcortical damage, but interrupted with left perisylvian region impairment. The literature suggests digit span is not affected by gender (Grossi, Matarese et al., 1980), but there is evidence in child studies of an influence of educational level (Orsini, Schiappa et al., 1981). Letter Number Span is a more complex, working memory task included in the Wechsler Adult Intelligence Scale-III (WAIS-III) and Wechsler Memory Scale-III. Another span task in use in adult research is the Alpha Span (Craik, 1990).

Two nonverbal test analogues of the digit span procedure are the Knox Cube Test (Knox, 1914; Arthur, 1947) and Corsi Blocks span test (Milner, 1971). These tests require the individual to tap a sequence of blocks in a given serial order after observing the examiner tapping the specific sequence. There was early evidence of impaired visuospatial span with posterior right cerebral hemisphere cortical lesions (De Renzi and Nichelli, 1975).

Supraspan is a term that refers to the retention of a greater number of items than meets the span capacity, and its impact was recognized early (Zangwill, 1943). It relies on the ability to form new memories and aids in the assessment of recent memory as contrasted with immediate memory (Loring, 1999). Supraspan is a technique that has application to material-specific and generalized amnesic disorders (Levin, 1986). Supraspan performance may be unimpaired in patients with anterograde amnesia, but impaired in the presence of a storage deficit (Drachman and Leavitt, 1974). A Serial Digit Learning Test measure of supraspan capacity for 8 or 9 digit sequences over a maximum of 12 learning trials was developed and adult normative data reported (Hamsher, Benton et al., 1980; Benton, Hamsher et al., 1983c). Word list learning tests such as the California Verbal Learning Test for Children, Rey Auditory Verbal Learning Test for children, and Verbal Selective Reminding Test are examples of supraspan learning tests that enable discrimination of efficiency of encoding, consolidation, storage, and retrieval.

Digit Span

Span tests are routinely included in many general intelligence tests, memory batteries, attention screening measures, and in adult dementia screening tests. The Wechsler series Digit Span subtest is considered a test of auditory attention and working memory. However, different functions may be attributed to both digit span forward and digit span backward (reverse digit span). A difference of three or more digits between forward and backward span is generally considered clinically significant. Digit span forward is considered a measure of efficiency of attention or "freedom from distractibility," while digit span backward is considered especially sensitive to working memory, as it requires the ability to hold in mind a sequence of numbers in order to respond effectively. Digit span backward also requires the additional processing components of mental manipulation of numbers, internal visual scanning, and/or visuospatial processing (Weinberg, Diller et al., 1972; Rudel and Denckla, 1974).

It is typical for digit span forward to exceed digit span backward. A forward span of 5 and backward span of 3 is expected of a 7- to 8-year-old, but not until 9 years old is forward span still expected to be 5, and backward span increased to 4 (Rudel and Denckla, 1974). A span of 5 forward and 4 backward is expected for an "average" adult. While some early studies refer to digit span as a short term memory task, the digit span test as a "memory test" is not empirically supported by factor analytic studies (Larrabee and Curtiss, 1995). Importantly, with respect to "memory," abnormal digit span scores are not characteristic of adult memory disordered patients (Iverson and Franzen, 1994; Leng and Parkin, 1995). Early study of digit span in learning-disabled children found those with right-sided signs and

presumable left cerebral hemisphere damage functioning more poorly on digit span forward, while those with left-sided signs and presumable right hemisphere damage functioning more poorly on digit span backward (Rudel and Denckla, 1974).

The literature includes a report of verbal and spatial immediate span normative data for 1112 four to ten-year-old Italian children (551 male, 561 female) (Orsini, Grossi et al., 1987). All children over 6 years old were in elementary school. The children were administered the verbal digit span procedure, following the Wechsler procedure of one digit/second presentation rate and using the WAIS sequences of 2 to 9 numbers (see Table 7–2). Trials continued until the failure of two equal-length sequences. The length of the longest sequence correctly recalled was recorded as the digit span score. The researchers identified the most effective linear model by reducing residual variance, using covariance analysis. They also corrected original scores for each subject by adding or subtracting the contribution of the concomitant variables and identified the corrected scores, ranking them in order of increasing magnitude with tolerance limits set at the 5th centile for the population. They found a mean verbal repetition scores of 4.4 ($SD = 1.0$) and 4.5 ($SD = 0.9$) for males and females, respectively. The nonparametric one-tailed lower 5% tolerance limits with 95% confidence was 3.0 for digit span.

To calculate a child's digit span performance, one must first correct the score for age according to the following: $+1$ for 4 years, $+0.75$ for 5 years, $+0.25$ for 6 years, $+0$ for 7 years, -0.25 for 8 years, -0.50 for 9 years and -1 for 10 years. For example, a 9-year-old repeats a maximum of 5 numbers. His score of 5 minus the correction (-0.50) results in a score of 4.5. Referring to normative data, presented as corrected scores in Table 7–3, this score corresponds to a cumulative percentage of 57.0 and falls higher than the one-tailed lower 5% tolerance limits score of 3.00.

Digit span means, standard deviations, and ranges for a cohort of 376 Australian school aged children are presented in Table 7–4, along with their results on the Corsi Block Span Test (see below).

Table 7–2. Digit and Block Sequences: Orsini et al. Study

Digit Span Sequences		Spatial Span Sequences
2–4	3–6	5–6
		4–7
		9–5
		5–7
		4–6
5–8–2	6–9–4	4–7–2
		8–1–5
		3–6–1
		4–1–5
		9–5–8
6–4–3–9	7–2–8–6	9–3–1–5
		6–5–4–8
		4–9–8–7
		1–6–5–3
		6–2–3–7
4–2–7–3–1	7–5–8–3–6	8–5–4–1–9
		2–3–5–4–1
		3–4–1–7–2
		7–9–3–4–1
		8–1–9–2–6
6–1–9–4–7–3	3–9–2–4–8–6	5–3–2–4–6–7
		9–8–1–4–6–5
		2–3–1–5–9–4
		2–4–6–3–5–1
		2–3–6–4–9–5
5–9–1–7–4–2–8	4–1–7–9–3–8–6	5–9–1–7–4–2–8
		4–1–7–9–3–8–6
		5–8–1–9–2–6–4
		3–8–2–9–5–1–7
		6–1–9–4–7–3–8
5–8–1–9–2–6–4–7	3–8–2–9–5–1–7–4	1–7–6–4–8–3–2–5
		5–8–3–2–6–7–1–9
		7–1–2–3–4–6–8–5
		9–4–7–3–1–8–2–5
		7–6–9–1–2–3–8–4
2–7–5–8–6–2–5–8–4	7–1–3–9–4–2–5–6–8	2–6–5–7–9–3–4–8–1
		8–2–3–4–1–7–9–6–5
		3–4–6–7–5–8–9–2–1
		8–6–7–3–4–9–5–2–1
		4–3–1–8–7–5–6–2–9

Source: Orsini, Grossi, Capitani, Laiacona, Papagno, & Vallar (1987); with permission of Masson Italia Periodici.

Adolescent normative data were reported for a high school cohort of 100 athletes with a mean age of 15.9 years ($SD = 0.98$), tested twice approximately 60 days apart (see Table 7–14 for demographic data and Tables 11–18, 11–19, and 11–20 for complete data) (Barr, 2003). While test–retest reliabilities were generally low ($r = 0.389$ to $r = 0.784$), no significant practice effects increases were found for the digit span subtest, although these were found for the WAIS-III Processing Speed Index, Trail Making Test, and Controlled Oral Word Association Test.

Table 7–3. Digit Span and Corsi Block Span Corrected Score Cumulative Frequency Data

DIGIT SPAN		CORSI BLOCKS	
Score[°]	Frequency	Score[°]	Frequency
1.25		1.25	0.2
1.50		1.50	0.4
1.75	0.1	1.75	1.0
2.00	0.4	2.00	1.3
2.25	0.4	2.25	2.3
2.50	0.8	2.50	4.3
2.75	1.7	2.75	7.7
3.00	5.9	3.00	12.7
3.25	8.9	3.25	22.7
3.50	12.5	3.50	36.4
3.75	22.3	3.75	47.8
4.00	40.6	4.00	59.6
4.25	50.5	4.25	76.6
4.50	57.0	4.50	88.7
4.75	69.2	4.75	93.3
5.00	81.7	5.00	95.6
5.25	84.5	5.25	97.9
5.50	88.5	5.50	99.6
5.75	93.8	5.75	99.8
6.00	97.5	6.00	100
6.25	98.3	6.25	
6.50	98.8	6.50	
6.75	99.6	6.75	
7.00	99.8	7.00	
7.25	99.8	7.25	
7.50	99.8	7.50	
7.75	99.9	7.75	
8.00	99.9	8.00	
8.25	99.9	8.25	
8.50	99.9	8.50	
8.75	100	8.75	

Source: Adapted from Orsini et al. (1987), with permission of Masson Italia Periodici.

[°]Corrected score

Corsi Block Span Test

A number of block or spatial span paradigms exist to test immediate repetition of visuospatial stimuli. The Corsi Block Span Test was developed as a nonverbal analog of the verbal supraspan technique in which a digit sequence recurred every third trial (Hebb, 1961). The subject observes the examiner tapping a sequence of fixed randomly arrayed blocks in a specific serial order and then must imitate the tapping sequence. In this block span version, nine 1 1/4 inch cubes are arrayed in a fixed random order on a 8 × 10 inch blackboard (Milner, 1971). The child must tap block sequences of increasing length, beginning with a three-block sequence. The Corsi Block Span Test has been adapted as a measure of visuospatial span in a number of test batteries, e.g., the Wechsler Memory Scale-III, and is analogous to the Wechsler auditory/verbal digit span test. The test was found sensitive to spatial short-term memory deficit in a study of Williams syndrome patients (Bellugi, Wang et al., 1994), and in a study of Down and Williams syndromes (Jarrold, Baddeley et al. 1999).

A variation of this test is part of a school-aged assessment battery for children in Australia (Anderson, Lajoie et al., 1995). This block span version was selected to collect current normative data on 376 Australian children between the ages of 7.0 and 13.11 years (Anderson, Lajoie et al., 1995). Two trials were administered at each difficulty level (7 taps maximum), and the final score reflected the maximum number of blocks tapped correctly.

Table 7–4. Mean, *SD* and Range for Block Span and Digit Span

Age	N	BLOCK SPAN			DIGIT SPAN		
		M	SD	Range	M	SD	Range
7	51	4.7	0.8	3–6	4.9	0.9	3–7
8	51	5.2	0.9	3–7	5.1	1.1	3–9
9	59	5.2	0.7	4–7	5.3	1.0	3–8
10	59	5.4	0.8	3–7	5.6	0.9	4–7
11	51	5.6	0.8	4–7	5.9	0.9	4–8
12	54	5.7	1.0	3–9	6.1	1.2	4–8
13	51	5.8	1.0	3–8	6.4	1.2	4–9

Source: Courtesy of Anderson, Lajoie and Bell (1995).

These normative data are presented in Table 7–4, along with the digit span means, standard deviations, and ranges.

The Corsi Blocks span test was also administered to 1112 four- to ten-year-old Italian children (551 males; 561 females) in a study that also included digit span performance (Orsini, Grossi et al., 1987). The blocks were tapped with the index finger at a rate of one block per 2 seconds. Sequences increased in length to a maximum of 9 taps per trial. There was a maximum of five sequences tapped out for each sequence length of two to nine numbers. The next sequence length was administered if at least three of five trials were correct within a sequence length block. The spatial span score was the length of the longest sequence correctly recalled for at least three of five trials.

They identified the most effective linear model by reducing residual variance, using covariance analysis. They also corrected original scores for each subject by adding or subtracting the contribution of the concomitant variables (age, sex, and education) and identified the corrected scores, ranking these in order of increasing magnitude with tolerance limits set at the 5th centile for the population. They found a sex difference favoring males, with mean spatial span scores of 4.0 (1.0) and 3.8 (0.8) for males and females, respectively. The nonparametric, one-tailed, lower 5% tolerance limits, with 95% confidence, was 2.75 for spatial span. These results were consistent with the child literature suggesting a male superiority for block span tests (Grossi, Orsini et al., 1979).

Thus, to obtain a spatial span score one must first correct for age and gender according to the following: Males: +0.75 for 4 years, +0.50 for 5 years, +0.25 for 6 years, +0 for 7 years, −0.50 for 8 years, −0.75 for 9 years and −1 for 10 years; Females: +1 for 4 years, +0.75 for 5 years, +0.50 for 6 years, +0.25 for 7 years, −0.25 for 8 years, −0.50 for 9 years and −0.75 for 10 years. The resulting corrected scores can then be compared to the table of density percentages and cumulative frequency percentages in Table 7–3. For example, a 9-year-old boy's maximum block span of 4 is corrected for age by gender (−0.75), for a score of 3.25. Re-

ferring to the corrected normative data in Table 7–3, one finds this score corresponding to a cumulative percentage of 22.7 and falling higher than the one-tailed, lower 5% tolerance limits score of 2.75.

Knox Cube Test

The Knox Cube Test (Knox, 1914; Arthur, 1947) is also a nonverbal analogue of the digit span test, and as for digit span, it is not empirically validated as a memory test (Iverson and Franzen, 1994). Knox developed this test of immediate memory to assess immigrants arriving in the United States. The Knox Cube Test was included as one of 15 subtests of the Pintner-Paterson Scale of Performance Tests (Pintner and Paterson, 1917). It was subsequently included as one of nine subtests in the 1930 Form I of the Arthur Point Scale of Performance Tests (Anastasi, 1968), and then with four other subtests in a revised Form II (Arthur, 1947). The latter was normed on 968 students from the same middle-class American district. It consists of four 1-inch wooden blocks, spaced two inches apart in a row, and attached to a piece of wood approximately 9 inches long. It is thus easily constructed and requires no purchase.

The cubes are placed in front of the child within easy reach and the examiner says, "I am going to touch these cubes in a certain order. Watch me carefully and when I stop, you touch them exactly the same way." The cubes are touched with the finger at the rate of 1 per second in the specified order (see Table 7–5). The first block is to the examiner's left. If the child is unsuccessful on the first item, he or she is told of the error and instructed to watch carefully for the exact order as the item is repeated. The first item may be presented up to three times, and if still not successful, the task is discontinued. If the child is successful on the second or third trial, the first trial is not scored, but the following sequences are then presented a single time only until three successive items are failed or until the test ends. The child is encouraged to watch as carefully as necessary. A second trial is administered 1 hour later. The test is scored by adding the number of correct items for each of the two trials and calculating

Table 7–5. Knox Cube Order of Administration

Trial	Pattern
1	14
2	23
3	124
4	134
5	214
6	341
7	1432
8	1423
9	1324
10	2431
11	13124
12	13243
13	14324
14	142341
15	132413
16	142314
17	143124
18	4132214

their mean. This raw score is converted to a mental age, see Table 7–6.

For individual administration, the materials include a board with nine blocks arranged in fixed position. The blocks are numbered when viewed from the examiner's position, enabling increasingly more difficult sequences to be tapped out in specified order and recorded accurately. The usual tapping rate is one block every 2 seconds.

Table 7–6. Point Value of Knox Cube Test Raw Scores

Raw Score	Mental Age
0 to 3.5	<4.5 years
4.0 to 5.0	4.5 years
5.5 to 7.0	5.5 years
7.5 to 8.0	6.5 years
8.5 to 9.0	7.5 years
9.5	8.5 years
10.0	9. 5 years
10.5	10.5 to 11.5 years
11.0	12.5 years
11.5	13.5 years
12.0	14.5 to 15.5 years
12.5 to 18.0	>15.5 years

Alpha Span

Another span test worth noting is one that has received attention in the adult literature, the Alpha Span Test (Craik, 1990). This short-term memory and mental tracking test requires an individual to listen to increasingly more difficult word lists and immediately recall the words in alphabetical order. Following the Wechsler digit span procedure, two trials of each list length are administered, the test is terminated when both items within a trial are failed, and a point is scored for completion of each trial of each list length.

Pattern Span

An experimental task of pattern span was developed to test a visual component in adults (Della Sala, Gray et al., 1999). The individual is shown a matrix in which half the cells are filled and is then required to immediately recall or recognize the pattern. The matrix size can be increased to reach the individual's visual span. Application to children is not reported.

Word Span

The Das-Naglieri Cognitive Assessment System includes a word series 27-item subtest. The test incorporates nine single-syllable, high-frequency words. The child must listen to a series of 2 to 9 words read at a rate of 1 word per second and then repeat the words in the exact serial order. Normative data are available for those 5 to 17 years old (Naglieri and Das, 1997).

Digit Ordering Test

The reader may also be interested in the Digit Ordering Test that was administered as a verbal working memory measure in an adult study (Hoppe, Müller et al. 2000). It requires memorization of 7 digits, presented in 5 seconds, and their immediate recall in ascending order. Test forms and instructions are presented in an appendix to this published report.

Test of Everyday Attention For Children

The Test of Everyday Attention for Children (TEA-Ch; Manly, Robertson et al., 1999) is a children's version of the adult 8-subtest Test of Everyday Attention (TEA; Robertson, Ward et al., 1995). It was developed to determine if the TEA could be successfully adapted downward for school-aged children and if the model of attention proposed for adults would be a valid construct for children. A pilot study version, or the current published version, was included in studies of males with Fragile X syndrome (Munir, Cornish et al., 2000), girls with Turner's syndrome (Skuse, James et al., 1997), children with head injury (Anderson and Pentland, 1998), and ADHD and learning disabilities (Manly, Anderson et al., 2001; Villella, Anderson et al., in press; Heaton and Fennell, 2001).

There is a screener version and a full nine-subtest administration, although individual subtests are studied as well. For example, the Same World-Opposite World task was administered as an indicator of the ability to inhibit a prepotent response (Bishop, Aamodt-Leeper et al., 2001). As noted earlier, structural equation modeling defined three factors in a study of 293 healthy children; selective attention, sustained attention, and higher level executive control (Manly, Anderson et al., 2001). Dual task performance is assessed for both auditory and visual modalities. See Table 7–7 for a listing of the TEA-Ch subtests for the abbreviated and full battery, and their respective attention factors.

The test materials are quite appealing to children, and administration procedures are both child- and examiner-friendly. For example, there are practice items that ensure compre-

hension of instructions, and the standardized instructions require the child to paraphrase directions to ensure comprehension. There are nine subtests, and a full administration takes approximately 1 hour. It is possible to use a four-subtest screener that on average takes 20–25 minutes or to select those individual tests that might best assist in a tailored evaluation.

The TEA-Ch measures different components of attention than do behavioral questionnaires or computerized CPTs and thus can be a supplement or can replace such tests (Baron, 2001). There are two parallel forms, allowing for retesting. Test–retest reliabilities were reported to range from .57 to .87 and percentage agreement from 71.0% to 76.2%. Of particular interest, IQ accounts for little of the variance in most TEA-Ch subtests for children with normal IQ scores, and thus, IQ scores do not predict well how a child will perform on the TEA-Ch (Manly, Robertson et al., 1999). The demand for memory or general knowledge that characterizes some other tests is also minimized.

Demographic data for the TEA-Ch are presented in Table 7–8 for 293 Australian children aged 6 to 16. The Daniel's Scale of Occupational Prestige (Daniel, 1983) ranks socioeconomic status (SES), with scores from 1 for high SES down to 7 for low SES. The mean SES ranking for the group was 4.04 (Manly, Anderson, et al., 2001). Normative data are presented by age band and gender, with raw scores con-

Table 7–7. TEA-Ch Subtests and Their Attention Factors

Subtest	Selective/Focused Attention	Sustained Attention	Sustained-Divided Attention	Attentional Control/ Switching
	ATTENTION FACTOR			
Sky Search	X			
Score!		X		
Creature Counting				X
Sky Search DT			X	
Map Mission	X			
Score DT		X		
Walk, Don't Walk		X		
Opposite Worlds				X
Code Transmission		X		

Bold subtests: Screening subtests of each attention factor and dual task performance.

Source: Adapted from Manly et al. (1999).

Table 7–8. Demographic data: Test of Everyday Attention for Children Normative Study

Subjects: 293 children in Australia
Age: 6 to 16 years; stratified in 6 age bands: 6–7, 7–9, 9–11, 11–13, 13–15, 15–16
Gender: 146 males; 147 females
Race: Not reported
SES: 4.04 on the Daniel's Scale of Occupational Prestige
Inclusion criteria: No history of head injury, neurological illness, developmental delay, sensory loss, referral for attention or learning problems, special educational needs

verted into age-scaled scores with a mean of 10 and a standard deviation or 3, and percentile bands.

The nine TEA-Ch subtests are:

Sky Search: A measure of selective/focused visual attention that requires that the child filters information to detect relevant information and rejects or inhibits distracting information. Specifically, the child must seek pairs of "spaceship" stimuli and rapidly circle all occurrences amid competing non-paired stimuli. A trial of rapid circling of only paired stimuli allows for interpretation of pure motor efficiency.

Score!: A measure of auditory sustained attention in which the child must count tones played on a tape recording, responding with the correct count at the end of each "game."

Creature Counting: A measure of attentional control and switching that requires executive functions such as working memory and mental flexibility in order to count stimuli according to visual cues to either count up or count down.

Sky Search DT: A sustained and divided attention task that requires circling paired spaceship stimuli, while also keeping a count of auditory tones, until all target stimuli are circled.

Map Mission: A measure of selective/focused attention requiring the child to seek a specific symbol on a detailed map and to circle each symbol found within one minute.

Score! DT: A measure of sustained auditory attention requiring the child to listen to and count tape-recorded tones while also listening for an animal named by the announcer in a news broadcast.

Walk, Don't Walk: A measure of sustained attention and response inhibition that requires the child to learn tones that allow progression (go) or require inhibition (no-go) and then make a mark accordingly. The speed of tone presentation increases as the task progresses, and the child must avoid making a mark in the no-go condition.

Opposite Worlds: A timed measure of attentional control and switching requiring the child to read sequenced chains of numbers as they appear (same world condition) or to inhibit the prepotent response and respond with an alternate number (i.e., 1 for 2 or 2 for 1 different world condition). This subtest makes the stimulus (a digit) and the response (the word "one" or "two") association explicit. In this respect, it is similar to the conflicting-response requirement for Stroop tests.

Code Transmission: An inherently uninteresting measure of sustained attention requiring the child to listen to a taped 12-minute recording of single-digit numbers presented at 2-s intervals and respond with the number that precedes the occurrence of all specific double-digit stimulus presentations. There are 40 target presentations. The subtest is a variation of an n-back task.

Trail Making Test

The Trail Making Test (TMT) was part of the Army Individual Test Battery (Army Individual Test Battery, 1944; Armitage, 1946) and was known as Partington's Pathways Test from the Leiter-Partington Adult Performance Scale (Partington and Leiter, 1949). It was subsequently incorporated into the Halstead-Reitan Neuropsychological Test Battery (Halstead, 1947; Reitan, 1958; Reitan and Davison, 1974) and later adapted for children (Reitan, 1971). The TMT has became one of the most widely used neuropsychological tests because of its sensitivity to general brain dysfunction and to impairment in a variety of cognitive domains (Reitan, 1971; Lezak, 1995). Sensitivity to general frontal lobe dysfunction (Pontius and Yudowitz, 1980; Amieva, Lafont et al., 1998) and to diverse etiologies (Stuss, Stethem et al., 1987) was reported in adults, but neither Part A nor Part B have proven to be dependable for localization of cerebral dysfunction (Lezak, 1995) in adults or children. Reliability as measured by the coefficient of concordance was reported as 0.98 for Part A and 0.67 for Part B (Cohen, Paul et al., 2001). The TMT is sensitive to the EF subdomains of shift and sustain, and inhibitory control reflected by improved Trails B scores was reported for 7- to 13-year-old children (Kelly, 2000).

The TMT is a timed paper-and-pencil test. There are two parts. Part A requires the child to draw a line in sequence between numbered circles scattered across the page. Part B is more complex and requires the child to draw a line while alternating between numbers and letters in sequence. Children aged 9 to 14 use a version with 15 numbers on Part A and 15 numbers and letters on Part B, the Reitan Intermediate version. Those aged 15 or older receive the adult version with 25 numbers on Part A and a total of 25 numbers and letters on Part B. The examinee's errors are immediately pointed out and a correction requested. This procedure adds to the time-to-completion score, and the speed with which the examiner catches and requests this correction can affect the final score. The test should not be administered to those whose alphabet is not European, but a variation such as the Color Trails Test might substitute (see below).

Significant associations were found between TMT and age and education (Spreen and Strauss, 1998). Gender difference was investigated (Lezak, 1995) and found not significant for either adults or children (Reitan, 1971; Kennedy, 1981; Heaton, Grant et al., 1986), although at least one study found girls completing the Trail Making Test-Part B and Color Trails Test-2 (CTT) faster than boys (Williams, Rickert et al., 1995). The effects of different language backgrounds on both the TMT and CTT were studied using Chinese- and English-speaking adults (Lee, Cheung et al., 2000). These data found the TMT and CTT generally culturally fair, but suggested that a temporally loaded language like English might confer an advantage.

The most common scoring procedure documents time to completion, including time taken to correct the subject's errors (Boll and Reitan, 1973; Reitan and Wolfson, 1993). Number of errors is a qualitative score in this administration. Relative slowing of Part B compared to Part A may provide another index of cognitive efficiency (Wheeler and Reitan, 1963). While some question the usefulness of a B–A difference score (Schreiber, Goldman et al., 1976), others suggest that a derived B/A ratio is useful, controls for age and education, and may be another index of EF (Arbuthnott and Frank, 2000).

Data from three early studies that provide normative data for Part A and Part B times-to-completion in seconds are presented in Table 7–9. The data are for ages 8 to 13 (Spreen and

Table 7–9. Trail Making Test Means and *SD*s in Seconds By Age

Age	TMT, PART A[1] Mean	SD	TMT, PART B[1] Mean	SD	TMT, PART A[2]		TMT, PART B[2] Mean	SD	TMT, PART A[3] Mean	SD	TMT, PART B[3]	
8					34.5	15.9	74.7	37.0				
9	21.5	8.9	49.5	19.7	25.1	8.8	54.6	19.0				
10	18.6	4.6	42.5	12.2	19.8	5.7	47.5	15.4				
11	15.5	4.5	35.7	16.8	17.4	6.3	41.7	15.8				
12	15.9	6.5	27.6	9.0	16.3	5.7	35.7	12.5				
13	14.7	4.6	29.4	11.2	14.9	7.6	35.4	19.5				
14	14.8	6.2	26.9	12.8								
15–17									23.4	5.9	47.7	10.4
18–23									26.7	9.4	51.3	14.6

Source: Adapted from [1]Knights (1966); [2]Spreen & Gaddes (1969); and [3]Fromm-Auch & Yeudall (1983) © Swets & Zeitlinger.

Gaddes, 1969), ages 9 to 14 (Knights, 1966), and also for age blocks of 15 to 17 years and 18 to 23 years as part of an adolescent and adult study (Fromm-Auch and Yeudall, 1983). Normative data by age and gender, for a total normal sample of 272 children, for time-to-completion of Part A and Part B in seconds for children 8- to 15-years-old, using the standard administration of the Halstead-Reitan Intermediate version, are presented in Table 7–10 (Spreen and Gaddes, 1969).

More recent normative data are available. Metanormative data means, based on the performance of 417 children, 9- to 13-years-old, are presented in Table 7–11 (Findeis and Weight, 1994). An explanation of this study along with a table of demographic data for these meta-norms are provided in Chapter 6.

Mean time-to-completion, standard deviation, and number of errors by age level for Parts A and B for 392 Australian children, 7- to 13-years-old, administered the standard version TMT, are presented in Table 7–12 (Anderson, Lajoie et al., 1995).

Adolescent TMT normative data are reported for a small sample as part of a study of 16- to 69-year-olds with no history of neurological or psychiatric disorders (Stuss, Stethem et al., 1988). Data were reported for thirty 16- to 29-year-olds, with a mean age of 22.43 years ($SD = 2.67$). The subjects were tested twice, at a 1-week interval. The time in seconds to complete the task is reported in Table 7–13. These data are for the adult 25-circle version. Another small adolescent group was reported as part of an adult study (Fromm-Auch and Yeudall, 1983), and these data for thirty-two 15- to 17-year-olds and seventy-six 18- to 23-year olds are presented in Table 7–9. Data from 100 high school athletes from two suburban New York City schools were also reported prior to the start of the competitive season as part of a brief screening battery for sports-related concussion (Barr, 2003). The demographic data for the latter study of high school athletes (mean age = 15.9 years ($SD = 0.98$) are presented in Table 7–14. A subset of 48 subjects (32 male, 16 female) were retested at approximately 60 days. The means and standard deviations for both test sessions, for both studies, are presented in Table 7–13 and closely parallel one another. Table 7–13 also includes the means and standard deviations for the entire 100 subjects in the Barr (2002) study by gender as female exceeded male TMT Part B performance, as it did for digit-symbol and COWAT measures (see also Tables 11–18; 11–19; and 11–20 for the full data set).

Delis-Kaplan Executive Function System Trail Making Test

As anyone who has routinely administered the standard TMT knows, the reason for a poor time-to-completion score can be puzzling. An examiner must consider a number of possibilities, including whether poor performance is due to slowed information processing, slow psychomotor speed, fine motor impairment, poor visual scanning, or impaired ability to sequence numbers and/or letters. The availability of the Delis-Kaplan Executive Function System Trail Making Test (D-KEFS TMT) is therefore a welcome modification that appears to address some of these issues, although empiric data are still needed to confirm its sensitivity and specificity across diagnostic groups and with normal subjects.

The D-KEFS TMT is normed for persons 8- to 89-years old, and whether its norms are weak for the younger ages remains to be determined. Instead of only the two standard conditions of number sequencing in Part A and letter-number sequencing in Part B, the D-KEFS TMT requires completion of 5 separate conditions: 1—visual scanning, 2—number sequencing, 3—letter sequencing, 4—number-letter switching, and 5—motor speed (in that order). As a result, there is the ability to discriminate whether more basic visual or motor components, or deficit in automatic language sequences, influence results on a more complex cognitive shifting task that is procedurally similar to the original TMT, Part B.

Each condition has a maximum time limit: 150 seconds for Conditions 1, 2, 3, and 5, and 240 seconds for Condition 4. The stimuli are printed over two pages rather than the single $8\frac{1}{2} \times 11$ page for each part of the standard version, also aiding in recognition of hemispace inattention or neglect. While empirical data comparing the usefulness of this version and

Table 7–10. Trail Making Test Normative Data by Age and Gender

TIME IN SECONDS FOR PART A

Age	MALE					FEMALE					ALL NORMALS				
	N	Mean	SD	Median	Range	N	Mean	SD	Median	Range	N	Mean	SD	Median	Range
8	11	32.4	11.7	30.5	16–55	12	36.4	18.7	33.5	16–86	23	34.5	15.9	30.5	16–86
9	22	26.8	8.9	25.5	13–45	19	23.1	8.1	21.0	13–48	41	25.1	8.8	23.0	13–48
10	26	21.3	6.1	20.5	13–42	25	18.2	4.6	17.8	10–28	51	19.8	5.7	19.4	10–42
11	21	16.4	5.6	14.8	9–30	30	18.0	6.6	17.2	9–37	51	17.4	6.3	16.3	9–37
12	48	16.6	5.9	15.1	10–43	44	16.0	5.4	14.7	7–32	92	16.3	5.7	14.9	7–43
13	7	16.0	10.1	15.3	9–39	7	13.7	1.9	13.3	12–18	14	14.9	7.6	13.3	9–39
14–15		16.0			8–30		13.0			12–17		14.0			8–30

TIME IN SECONDS FOR PART B

Age	MALE					FEMALE					ALL NORMALS				
	N	Mean	SD	Median	Range	N	Mean	SD	Median	Range	N	Mean	SD	Median	Range
8	11	77.8	34.5	76.5	32–159	12	71.8	39.0	77.5	26–176	23	74.7	37.0	76.5	26–176
9	22	58.0	21.6	57.5	22–120	19	50.7	14.5	50.8	24–76	41	54.6	19.0	51.3	22–120
10	26	51.6	14.7	52.5	18–82	25	43.2	15.0	42.0	25–84	51	47.5	15.4	45.8	18–84
11	21	43.3	20.0	38.8	25–122	30	40.6	11.8	38.5	15–62	51	41.7	15.8	38.8	15–122
12	48	39.6	13.3	37.8	14–90	44	33.5	11.1	31.3	20–74	92	35.7	12.5	34.0	14–90
13	7	40.1	25.5	39.0	17–99	7	30.7	6.9	29.3	22–43	14	35.4	19.5	29.5	17–99
14–15		29.0			13–45		31.0			13–50		31.0			13–50

Source: O. Spreen and W. H. Gaddes (1969) Developmental norms for 15 neuropsychological tests age 6 to 15, *Cortex*, *V*: 171–191, Tables XLIV and XLV. Reprinted with Permission.

Table 7–11. Trail Making Test Meta-Norm Means and *SD*s

Age	N	TMT, PART A		TMT, PART B		TMT, TOTAL TIME	
		Mean	SD	Mean	SD	Mean	SD
9	76	25.09	9.4	54.77	20.0	79.85	28.9
10	93	21.04	5.9	49.80	20.0	70.84	30.4
11	89	18.87	6.2	41.20	15.6	60.07	20.3
12	124	17.19	5.8	37.14	14.1	54.33	22.6
13	35	16.00	5.7	32.73	10.9	48.73	10.3

Source: Unpublished data, courtesy of Findeis & Weight (1994).

the standard administration are as yet limited, the D-KEFS TMT has immediate appeal in the child clinical setting, and especially for children whose conditions result in visuomotor or fine motor difficulties that might otherwise be inaccurately attributed to cognitive flexibility impairment. These features make the test worth serious consideration as a new standard for children.

Trail Making Test Error Analysis

As noted above, there are different ways to do poorly on the TMT. Yet, until the D-KEFS was published, normative data rarely accounted for these diverse error types. According to standard TMT instructions, timing proceeds even as the examiner instructs the child that an error has been made, and correction is encouraged. Thus, the influence of number of errors on timing presents a qualitatively different profile than when a slowed time to completion is error free. The different types of errors that

might be made are also of clinical interest. For example, children might lose mental set due to poor attention, lose their place on the paper and become spatially confused, cover a circle with the hand holding the paper and therefore incur inordinate delay finding the hidden circle, or omit circles on the periphery due to ineffective visual search.

Quantifying TMT error types is now becoming routine as recognition of the clinical importance of accounting for stylistic difference increases. For example the, D-KEFS TMT includes procedural and scoring adaptations that include optional error scores for which cumulative percentile ranks can be derived (Delis, Kaplan et al., 2001). Errors of omission (an unmarked target) and commission (marked incorrect foil) are scored for the Visual Scanning condition, which requires a search for a target number 3. Sequencing errors, set-loss errors, and time-discontinue errors are scored for each of the conditions of

Table 7–12. Mean Time, *SD* and Range for Trail Making Test

Age	N	TRAIL MAKING TEST: PART A			TRAIL MAKING TEST: PART B		
		M	SD	Errors	M	SD	Errors
7	56	30.9	15.9	0.2	97.9	113.4	0.9
8	56	26.6	11.5	0.3	69.0	32.2	0.0
9	62	22.8	11.8	0.2	58.1	29.5	0.4
10	62	18.1	0.5	0.1	44.5	19.9	0.7
11	51	15.8	4.9	0.1	43.6	29.1	0.4
12	54	20.1	17.0	0.1	33.6	19.3	0.4
13	51	15.7	9.1	0.1	30.6	11.6	0.4

Source: Courtesy of Anderson, Lajoie and Bell (1995).

Table 7–13. Trail Making Test Data for Adolescents

	FIRST TESTING		SECOND TESTING	
	M	*SD*	*M*	*SD*
Part A[1]	21.48	6.44	19.68	7.32
Part B[1]	48.77	18.66	42.18	15.54
Part A[2]	21.4	5.4	19.3	5.4
Part B[2]	50.1	17.3	44.9	15.6

MEAN (*SD*) TOTAL HIGH SCHOOL SAMPLE

	Total	Males	Females
Part A[2]	22.5 (6.7)	23.2 (7.6)	21.4 (4.9)
Part B[2]	52.5 (17.1)	56.1 (18.9)	47.2 (12.4)

Source: Adapted from [1]Stuss et al. (1988), © Swets and Zeitlinger; and, [2]Barr (2003), with permission from Elsevier Science.

number sequencing, letter sequencing, and number-letter switching. The latter is possible since a time limit is imposed on the D-KEFS, and targets might be uncompleted. Number of time-discontinue errors are scored for the motor speed condition. For number-letter switching (Condition 4) the total number of all sequencing, set-loss, and time-discontinue errors are converted to a scaled score ($M = 10$; $SD = 3$) corrected for each of the 16 age groups.

Another approach to quantifying TMT error types was defined and examined in adults with dementia of the Alzheimer type (DAT) along with a modification of the administration procedure (Amieva, Lafont et al., 1998), and the results were interpreted to reveal an inhibitory processing deficit in those with DAT. This study has heuristic interest as a potential means of further studying children's inhibitory capacity through similar test modification and error analysis. The TMT procedure was altered so that only errors made during the first four connections were corrected by the examiner, and the subject continued the test without further examiner help. An error was coded as a *sequential error* (SE) or a *perseverative error* (PE). An error was a SE if there were a failure to continue the sequence due to an omission, or skipping, of a number or letter.

Subtypes of SE were also elaborated. A *proximity* SE involves spatial proximity of the circles on the page: the connected target is one of the five nearest to where the pencil is and can be reached without crossing another. The authors note that proximity errors are most likely due to an inhibitory deficit. An SE to rectify was coded if the subject recognized an error had been made and attempted correction. A *displacement* SE referred to a Part B error consecutive to a previous SE, which then involved continued displacement error. *Unexplained* SE did not obey the above rules. *Perseverative Error* was failure to alternate between the number and letter series on Part B. By making these distinctions, the authors identified error profiles that suggested an inhibitory deficiency, even on Part A. That is, compared to normal subjects, the DAT subjects found it more difficult to suppress a tendency to connect with the nearest circles and had more difficulty su-

Table 7–14. Demographic Data for High School Athlete Study: Barr (2003)

Subjects: 100 adolescent high school athletes in New York City surburban schools
Age: Mean of 15.9 years ($SD = 0.98$)
Gender: 60 males; 40 females
Race/Ethnicity: 88% Caucasian, 10 African-Americans, 2 Hispanic, 2 Asian-American
SES: Not reported
Handedness: 90% right handed
Inclusion criteria: English speaking, good academic standing. 13 with previous history of concussion, 3 reported ADHD, 3 others reported dyslexia or LD

pressing the overlearned and irrelevant number or letter sequence in order to make the required shifts.

Part A vs. Part B

The differences between TMT Part A and Part B have received investigators' attention (Reitan and Tarshes, 1959; Fitzhugh, Fitzhugh et al., 1963). Both parts depend on visual acuity. Part A is considered a test of attention and visuomotor speed and tracking and depends on visual field integrity and intact visual directional scanning. In contrast, while also requiring attentional control (Arbuthnott and Frank, 2000) and directional scanning, factor analysis found Part B had a stronger association with spatial intelligence or nonverbal ability than with attention or information processing (Larrabee and Curtiss, 1995; Larrabee, 2000). Part B is also considered more complex because it requires divided attention and additional executive function capabilities (Lamberty, Putnam et al., 1994; Arbuthnott and Frank, 2000). These include planning (Golden, 1981), cognitive flexibility (Bechtold, Horner et al., 2001), and/or the ability to maintain a complex response set for the two automatic language or symbolic sequences (Lezak, 1995; Reitan, 1971).

For children, it is often appropriate to consider both Trails A and B as attention measures, but then also to consider the differential results between the two parts as well as the profile that emerges when it is compared to other EF tests. Besides these additional cognitive requirements, there is also an increased demand for motor speed and visual search on Part B. Therefore, the assumption of equal trail length and equal complexity of visual search between the two parts might be inaccurate (Gaudino, Geisler et al., 1995) and could lead to faulty conclusions about reason for impairment (Crowe, 1998).

Color Trails Test

The Color Trails Test (CTT), also has its origin in the Partington Pathways nonlanguage measure of ability in the Leiter-Partington Adult Performance Scale (Partington and Leiter, 1949; Maj, D'Elia et al., 1993; Williams, Rick-

ert et al., 1995). Designed with the intention that it be culture free, the CTT minimizes dependence on knowledge of the English alphabet by using colored circles (13 yellow, 12 pink) for letters and requires alternation between colors and 25 numbers. The equivalence of the TMT and CTT is not firmly established. The TMT and CTT have been found to be an equivalent construct only when specific age and education parameters are considered, with stronger correlation between TMT and CTT scores found for older and higher intelligence level Chinese subjects (Lee and Chan, 2000). Instructions can be presented nonverbally through gestures or sign language.

Progressive Figures Test and Color Form Test

The Progressive Figures Test is printed on an $8\frac{1}{2}'' \times 11''$ paper and has eight stimulus figures, each with a large outside geometric form and a smaller internal form. The child is instructed to use the small inside figure as the cue about which large figure will come next in a progressive sequence. That is, the child traces a path with a finger from one shape to the next, with the smaller internal shape cueing which larger external shape is next in the sequence. The Color Form Test stimuli employ color and shape. The child is instructed to follow a progressive sequence from one figure to the next, shifting between shape and color. That is, from the initial stimulus, the child moves to one with the same shape but different color, and then to one with the same color but of a different shape, alternating for the duration of the trial. Both of these tests were included in a meta-analysis (see Chapter 6 for details), and normative data are provided in Table 7–15, with means, standard deviations for Progressive Figures Test time, and Color Form Test time and errors.

Auditory Consonant Trigrams Test

The Auditory Consonant Trigrams Test (ACTT), also known as the Brown-Peterson Auditory Short-Term Memory Test (Brown, 1958; Peterson and Peterson, 1959), is a test of divided attention and rapid information processing (Stuss,

Table 7–15. Reitan-Indiana NTB Meta-Norm Means, (*SD*), [*N*] for 5 to 8 years old

SUBTEST:	AGE (YEARS)			
	5	6	7	8
Progressive Figures (seconds)	96.12 (57.4) [208]	73.43 (50.4) [208]	51.74 (31.0) [190]	41.50 (21.4) [184]
Color Form (seconds)	44.61 (.3) [206]	32.00 (19.1) [190]	28.34 (12.0) [218]	19.58 (8.9) [184]
Color Form (errors)	2.31 (2.6) [206]	0.86 (1.4) [160]	0.43 (.9) [188]	.33 (.9) [154]

Source: Unpublished data courtesy of Michael K. Findeis & David G. Weight, Brigham Young University (1994).

Stethem et al., 1987; Stuss, Stethem et al., 1988). Paniak and colleagues (1997) made two modifications in the adult administration procedure to accommodate a younger age, that is, interval length was shortened to 0, 3, 9, and 18 seconds from the adult version's 0, 9, 18, and 36 seconds, and children counted backward by 1's instead of by 3's.

The ACTT procedure specifically requires the child to listen to an oral recitation of three consonants followed by a specified number. The child must immediately count aloud backward by 1s from the number without repeating the letters until the specified time interval has elapsed. The child is then asked to recall the three consonant letters in any order. It is especially important that the child restate the number and count backward immediately to avoid subvocal rehearsal. To ensure the instructions are followed, I immediately re-state the number when the child delays responding, compelling the child to respond quickly. At the conclusion of that trial, I re-state the instructions and insist that the number be stated immediately. There are 15 trials, including the initial 5 trials with no interval delay. The directions, consonants, and time intervals are presented in Table 7–16. Demographic data for an ACTT normative data study of 9- to 15-year-old children are presented in Table 7–17 (Paniak, Miller et al., 1997), and the normative data are presented in Table 7–18 (Paniak, Miller et al., 1997). Data for total score are presented in Table 7–19.

Adolescent normative data for 16 years and older were obtained with a limited sample and using the adult Consonant Trigrams Test form and procedure of counting backward by 3s. ACTT normative data were reported for 30 subjects aged 16 to 29, with a mean age of 22.43 (*SD* = 2.67) (Stuss, Stethem et al., 1988; see Table 7–20 for demographic data). There were 16 males, 14 females, 22 right-handers, 8 left-handers, with a mean education of 14 years (*SD* = 1.34). The subjects were tested twice, at a 1-week interval. Data about the time-in-seconds to complete the task's three conditions are reported in Table 7–21.

Index of Sustained Effort and Attention for the ACTT

Sustained effort on the ACTT can be examined qualitatively. I routinely use a scoring modification for the ACTT that provides another index about performance over time, as in the following example:

N. V. was a 16-year-old male. His ACTT scores were recorded as indicated below. The headings 9, 18, 36, are the interference seconds duration per trial, and each line includes the score for each set of three interval durations, in the order of their presentation. Thus, the first line includes the first three test items, and N. V. was correct twice at the 9-second interval, 3 times at the 18-second interval, and 3 times at the 36-second interval. Line two includes items 4 to 6. The total correct for items 1 to 6 equalled 15. Skipping the middle trials of items 7 to 9 (between the lines), I then added the number correct for the final six trials (items 10 to 15), and his score equalled 8. Therefore, in the first part of the test N. V. ob-

Table 7–16. Directions and Stimuli for the Auditory Consonant Trigrams Test

"I am going to say three letters and when I am through I am going to knock like this. When I do I want you to say the letters back."

Stimulus	Start #	Delay (Seconds)
XTN		0
TQJ		0
LNP		0
SJH		0
KPW		0

"This time, I am going to say three letters followed immediately by a number. As soon as you get the number, I want you to start counting backward by ones out loud, like this: 29–28–27. Continue counting out loud until I knock as before. (Demonstrate knocking on the desk). When I knock, I want you to recall the three letters. Do you have any questions?"

Stimulus	Start #	Delay (Seconds)	Response	# Correct
NKR	94	18		
FBM	69	9		
KXQ	53	3		
GQS	46	9		
DLX	47	18		
BFM	48	3		
ZGK	55	18		
WGP	62	9		
ZDL	38	3		
RLB	22	9		
QDH	35	3		
GWB	47	18		
CSJ	39	9		
FMH	77	18		
HFZ	49	3		

correct
   0 second delay   ____
   3 second delay   ____
   9 second delay   ____
   18 second delay   ____
   Total Correct   ____

Source: Paniak, Miller & Murphy, (1997), © Swets & Zeitlinger.

tained 15 of 18 points, but at the end he obtained only 8 of 18 points. It is apparent that there was a decline in efficiency of performance over the time course of this test with the reason yet to be determined. Clinically, a decline of 3 or 4 points does not appear worrisome. This child's decline of 7 points represents a real decline over time. Since either a decline or improvement is possible, his particular pattern highlights his inability to exert structure or strategy in order to perform consistently well.

Inspection of performance within time intervals is also possible. In the above example, there was no decline over time for responses following a 9-second interval: 4/6 correct responses in the first part and 4/6 correct responses in the latter part. However, 6/6 correct responses in the first part was reduced to only 1/6 correct responses on the final trials for 18-second interval items. The 36-second interval found him responding correctly 5/6 times early, but 3/6 times towards the end. Such data are suggestive with respect to when, in the length-

Table 7–17. Demographic Data for the Auditory Consonant Trigrams Test: Paniak et al. (1997)

Subjects: 714 children in Edmonton, Canada, public schools
Age: 9 to 15 years
Gender: 326 males; 388 females
Handedness: Not reported
Race: Not reported
SES: Not reported
Inclusion criteria: Reported group's estimated verbal intelligence to be near the WISC-III normative sample's mean

Table 7–19. Normative Data for Total Score[*]

Age	n	M	SD
9	82	37.1	6.2
10	140	38.2	6.0
11	132	40.3	6.0
12	122	42.8	6.2
13	96	45.8	6.5
14	115	46.4	5.6
15	28	47.4	5.5

Source: Paniak, Miller & Murphy, 1997, © Swets & Zeitlinger.

[*]Total score = Total no. correct consonants after 0-, 3-, 9-, and 18-second time intervals.

ening time interval, a child may experience critical performance failure. In this instance, the problem did not emerge for the generally easier 9-second interval items, but did for later and longer interval items.

	9	18	36	
	2	3	3	
	2	3	2	} 15
	3	2	3	
	2	0	2	
	2	1	1	} 8
Total	11	9	11	

Importantly, when scored in the traditional way on the answer sheet (see Table 7–16), N.V. earned a score of 11 for the 9-second interval, 9 for the 18-second interval, and 11 for the 36-second interval. Referring to the age-appropriate normative data (see Table 7–21), his scores fell within normal limits for each time interval. The traditional summary scores did not reveal the qualitative features with respect to sustained attention as did this scoring

alternative. There are no empiric data using this scoring modification to assess sustained attention on the ACTT.

Children's Paced Auditory Serial Addition Test

The Children's Paced Auditory Serial Addition Test (CHIPASAT; (Johnson, Roethig-Johnston et al., 1988) is a downward extension of the original Paced Auditory Serial Addition Test (PASAT) developed for adults (Sampson, 1954; Gronwall and Sampson, 1974; Gronwall, 1977; Gronwall and Wrightson, 1981). These tests are considered measures of information-processing speed, sustained auditory attention, and divided attention (Kinsella, 1998) and are especially sensitive to traumatic brain damage and other brain dysfunction etiologies. They also require intact math calculation skill (Sherman, Strauss et al., 1997) and working memory. While age (Johnson, Roethig-Johnston et

Table 7–18. Means and SD for Auditory Consonant Trigrams Test

Age	N	DELAY INTERVAL IN SECONDS			
		0″	3″	9″	18″
9	81	15.0 (0.2)	9.9 (2.7)	6.6 (2.6)	5.7 (2.5)
10	140	14.9 (0.3)	10.5 (2.6)	6.9 (2.7)	6.0 (2.1)
11	131	14.9 (0.4)	10.9 (2.3)	7.8 (2.4)	6.7 (2.4)
12	123	14.9 (0.4)	11.5 (2.5)	8.6 (2.6)	7.8 (2.6)
13	96	14.9 (0.4)	12.2 (2.0)	9.9 (2.8)	8.7 (2.9)
14	115	15.0 (0.1)	12.1 (2.0)	10.1 (2.6)	9.3 (2.6)
15	28	14.9 (0.3)	12.1 (1.9)	10.9 (2.2)	9.5 (2.8)

Source: Paniak, Miller & Murphy (1997), © Swets & Zeitlinger.

Table 7–20. Brown-Peterson Auditory Memory Demographic Data: Stuss et al. Study (1988)

Subjects: 30 Ss with mean education of 14.1 years
  (SD = 1.34); range 11–18
Age: 16 to 29 years; mean = 22.43 (2.67)
Gender: 16 males; 14 females
Handedness: 22 right-handed; 8 left-handed
Race: Not reported
SES: Not reported
Inclusion criteria: No history of neurological and/or
  psychiatric disorders

al., 1988) and intelligence (Brittain, LaMarche et al., 1991; Wiens, Fuller et al., 1997) affect PASAT performance, these effects were not found for the CHIPASAT (Johnson, Roethig-Johnston et al., 1988). Age and, to a lesser extent, the child's arithmetical ability ($r = 0.29$) had a significant influence on information processing capacity, while general intellectual ability ($r = 0.10$) and gender were unrelated to CHIPASAT performance. The CHIPASAT has good split-half reliability ($r = 0.9165$), indicating good internal reliability and assurance that it assesses the same function in all trials.

The CHIPASAT procedure requires the child to listen to a random series of tape-recorded, single-digit numbers presented at different speeds for five trials. There are 61 digits in each trial. Presentation is one digit every 2.8, 2.4, 2.0, 1.6, or 1.2 seconds. The child must add successive pairs of numbers and respond aloud, so that each number is added to the one immediately preceding it, that is, dropping the answer to add the next number to the previous number. The 2.8-second data were eliminated since score distribution did not fall

Table 7–21. Brown-Peterson Auditory Memory Test Data for 16- to 29-years-old

	FIRST TESTING		SECOND TESTING	
Interval	M	SD	M	SD
9″	12.03	2.24	12.57	2.03
18″	11.37	2.82	12.27	2.41
36″	9.43	2.71	10.93	2.88

Source: Stuss, Stethem & Pelchat (1988), © Swets & Zeitlinger.

within the expected normal curve on this trial, but it is recommended that it be included as a practice trial (Johnson, Roethig-Johnston et al., 1988). An examiner should be cautious in interpreting CHIPASAT performances for those below 9. 5 years of age since information processing speed increased exponentially with age, and the greatest changes occurred in those below 10 years old. A sample ($N = 315$) of normal school children was assessed with the CHIPASAT to establish normative data, and these data along with demographic data are presented in Table 7–22.

PASAT administration is appropriate for adolescents 16 and older, and normative data were reported for an adult sample that included breakdown into a 16–29 year age sample (Stuss, Stethem et al., 1988; see Table 7–20 for demographic data and Table 7–23 for normative data). A number of adult normative studies were also reported (Stuss, Stethem et al., 1987; Stuss, Stethem et al., 1988; Roman, Edwall et al., 1991.

Symbol Digit Modalities Test

The Symbol Digit Modalities Test (SDMT; Smith, 1973; Smith, 1982) is a measure of visual scanning, visual tracking, and sustained visual attention. It requires rapid and accurate information processing. Like many other tests that have a long history in assessment, it is still selectively useful. The test page has a key at the top with divided blocks pairing numbers and symbols. The test items are divided blocks with symbols, but no numbers. On the first trial the child refers to the key in order to write in rapidly the number that is correctly paired with each symbol. The second trial requires oral production of the numbers. The child is instructed to say the number aloud for each block while the examiner writes the responses. Each trial is 90 seconds. Thus, a comparison of written and oral productions is possible. Demographic data for 3680 children are presented in Table 7–24 and normative data in Table 7–25.

The SDMT oral trial was administered as part of a battery to children with Duchenne Muscular Dystrophy (DMD) as an index of complex attention not requiring motor control (Cotton, Crowe et al., 1998). The DMD chil-

Table 7–22. Demographic and Normative Data: CHIPASAT

Subjects: 315 children from primary, middle and secondary schools
Age: 8 to 14 years, 6 months
Gender: 148 males; 167 females
Race or SES: Not reported

Age (years)	N	2.4 INTERVAL CORRECT RESPONSES			TIME	2.0 INTERVAL CORRECT RESPONSES			TIME	1.6 INTERVAL CORRECT RESPONSES			TIME	1.2 INTERVAL CORRECT RESPONSES			TIME	CHIPASAT OVERALL RESPONSE SPEED		CORRECT RESPONSES		
		M	SD	%	X Sec	M	SD	%	X Sec	M	SD	%	X Sec	M	SD	%	X Sec	X Sec	SD	M	SD	%
8–9	51	22.5	5.5	37.5	6.8	19.4	6.5	32.4	7.0	16.4	6.4	27.4	7.0	9.9	5.2	16.5	11.6	8.1	5.0	17.1	5.5	28.5
9–10	58	27.1	7.1	45.2	5.7	23.0	6.6	38.3	5.9	19.8	6.5	33.0	5.7	13.1	5.9	21.8	7.9	6.3	3.1	20.7	5.8	34.6
10–11	60	30.5	8.3	50.9	5.1	26.2	7.1	43.7	5.0	20.8	6.3	34.6	5.3	14.9	5.9	24.8	5.9	5.3	1.9	23.1	6.2	38.5
11–12	51	33.8	8.5	56.3	4.6	28.3	7.2	47.2	4.5	23.1	6.2	38.4	4.5	16.6	5.4	27.7	5.0	4.6	1.4	25.5	6.2	42.4
12–13	36	32.3	9.1	53.8	5.1	29.6	7.9	49.4	4.9	24.4	7.4	40.6	5.3	16.1	6.8	26.8	4.7	4.4	1.2	25.6	7.0	42.7
13–14	51	37.4	9.4	62.4	4.2	33.4	10.1	55.7	4.1	27.7	9.1	46.1	3.9	19.3	7.4	32.2	4.7	4.2	1.8	29.4	8.4	49.1
14–15	8	41.1	9.9	68.5	3.7	38.3	8.0	63.8	3.3	31.5	6.8	52.5	3.2	20.6	5.7	34.4	3.8	3.5	0.9	32.9	6.9	54.8

Johnson, D. A., Roethig-Johnston, K. & Middleton, J. (1988). Development and evaluation of an attentional test for head injured children—1. Information processing capacity in a normal sample. *Journal of Child Psychology and Psychiatry, 29,* 199–208. Adapted with permission of Pergamon Press.

Table 7–23. PASAT Data for 16 to 29-years-old

	FIRST TESTING		SECOND TESTING	
Interval	M	SD	M	SD
2.4	47.40	10.12	53.73	7.30
2.0	42.00	12.50	50.23	9.17
1.6	35.97	12.97	43.37	11.02
1.2	27.40	9.86	31.20	10.24

Source: Stuss, Stethem & Pelchat (1988), © Swets & Zeitlinger.

dren functioned more poorly than controls on this measure and on tests of verbal fluency and nonverbal memory that also did not require motor control.

Spanish normative data for the SDMT are now available (Arribas, 2002), under the title *Test de Símbolos y Dígitos* (Digit and Symbol Test). The written portion was recently administered to 1,249 boys and girls (see Table 7–26 for age and gender data) and the oral version to 1079 children from several cities, in Spain, including Madrid, Bilbao, Barcelona, and Sevilla, in order to obtain a representative sample. Ages of the normative group were 8 to 17 years old (M = 12.24; SD = 2.84).

Correlation coefficients for the SDMT and WISC-R Spanish version coding subtest (Arribas, D., 1992) are reported in the validity chapter of the Spanish Manual. They found a correlation coefficient of 0.53 for the written SDMT and 0.45 for the oral SDMT. Differ-

Table 7–24. Symbol Digit Modalities Test Demographic Data

Subjects: 3680 children from Omaha, Nebraska, public schools
Age: 8 to 17 years; mean = 22.43 (2.67)
Gender: 1874 males, 1806 females (Written SDMT: 1090 males, 1011 females, Oral SDMT: 784 males, 795 females
Education: Normal classes, grades 3 to 12
Race: Not reported
SES: Proportional representation of low, middle and upper income neighborhoods
Exclusion criteria: History of mental retardation, brain damage, emotional disturbance, severe visual impairment

Source: Smith (1982).

ences between boys' written SDMT performance (Mean = 45.26, SD = 13.40) and girls' written SDMT performance (Mean = 44.71, SD = 13.44) or boys' oral SDMT performance (Mean = 54.80, SD = 16.17) and girls' oral SDMT performance (Mean = 53.86, SD = 13.97) were not statistically significant. Differences between right-handed (Mean = 46.51, SD = 11.86) and left-handed (Mean = 45.34, SD = 12.95) children for written SDMT performance were not statistically significant. Differences between right-handed (Mean = 57.31, SD = 14.60) and left-handed (Mean = 55.00, SD = 13.42) children for oral SDMT performance were not statistically significant. The Spanish normative data are presented in Table 7–27.

Dichotic Listening

The dichotic listening paradigm has wide applicability to the assessment of attention. It has principally been utilized in studies of selective attention, but it also applies to investigations of divided and sustained attention. The dichotic listening technique involves the presentation of two different auditory messages simultaneously, one to the right ear, and one to the left. Normal right-handed individuals typically demonstrate a right ear advantage (REA) when listening to linguistic stimuli since the left hemisphere has principal dominance for language processing. One possibility is that left ear input is suppressed by competition or attenuated because it reaches the left hemisphere via callosal transfer from right auditory cortex. Another is that basic attention and activation mechanisms are responsible for the ear-advantage effect, and not structural constraints.

Presurgical evaluation of epilepsy patients who are candidates for resection of epileptogenic foci has provided strong support for the empirical validity of dichotic listening procedures as an index of hemispheric dominance. The procedure is especially useful in predicting language lateralization and noting change or adaptation in superior temporal lobe function, or possibly recognizing change in hearing integrity in the ear contralateral to the lesion. Although it is not always considered anything more than an experimental technique, the

Table 7–25. Written and Oral Symbol Digit Modalities Test Means and SDs

| | WRITTEN SDMT | | | | | | ORAL SDMT | | | | | |
| | BOYS | | | GIRLS | | | BOYS | | | GIRLS | | |
Age	N	Mean	SD	N	Mean	SD	N	Mean	SD	N	Mean	SD
8	72	23.31	6.99	97	23.65	5.67	69	28.63	8.49	76	30.57	7.86
9	122	26.46	8.07	123	26.88	8.13	79	29.63	8.77	79	30.50	7.83
8–9	194	25.29	6.72	220	25.45	7.32	148	29.17	7.32	155	30.54	7.86
10	114	28.08	7.26	110	29.90	8.55	73	34.30	8.91	78	37.33	9.27
11	94	30.96	8.10	93	33.27	9.09	89	41.06	8.46	67	42.15	9.75
10–11	208	29.39	7.86	203	31.45	8.97	162	38.01	9.33	145	39.56	9.08
12	104	37.58	9.87	83	38.02	10.87	79	41.69	8.97	86	45.70	10.38
13	97	41.69	9.18	83	43.04	10.05	71	46.43	10.35	63	47.58	9.90
12–13	201	39.56	9.75	166	40.53	10.79	150	43.94	9.96	149	46.50	10.20
14	106	45.49	8.49	88	50.93	9.97	87	48.98	9.57	105	50.90	7.89
15	134	48.73	9.69	114	53.20	11.01	115	49.30	10.32	105	53.32	11.16
14–15	240	47.30	9.33	202	52.21	10.63	202	49.16	9.81	210	52.11	9.62
16	130	49.27	11.08	130	54.13	7.74	70	49.33	8.10	78	51.72	10.76
17	117	53.01	12.27	90	56.61	11.56	52	50.35	7.56	58	58.00	8.28
16–17	247	51.04	11.53	220	55.15	11.06	122	49.76	7.86	136	54.40	10.26

technique has proved sensitive to changes in cerebral organization occurring with recovery from an aphasia, with a typical shift from left ear advantage to REA as recovery proceeds.

Visual Search Cancellation Tests

Paper-and-pencil visual search cancellation tests aid in the determination of hemispatial inattention, often by calculation of the number of omission and commission errors in each hemispace. A simple marking response is required, minimizing the need for more integrated visuomotor integrative performance and praxis. These tests have a number of different target stimuli (e.g., lines, letters, shapes, recognizable symbols, nonsense forms, words), present single or double stimuli, may measure time-to-completion, and vary in format (e. g., solely lines or target stimuli embedded in a competing visual array). Some require a search in a random or scattered array, while others require a search of an organized array in which the stimuli are printed in defined rows and columns. The former procedure is documented as more challenging. Qualitatively, the direction of the visual search, typically left to right, is of

interest, as is whether there is a systematic or disorganized search. Three cancellation tests are described below along with their child normative data.

Verbal Cancellation Test for Children

A procedure for evaluating children in Grades 1 to 5, based on the methods developed for organized and random array cancellation tests, has been developed and is referred to as Ver-

Table 7–26. Test de Símbolos y Dígitos: Normative Sample Age and Gender Distribution

| | GENDER | | |
Age	Boys	Girls	Total
8	51	55	106
9	68	93	161
10	63	104	167
11	63	74	137
12	51	69	120
13	53	71	124
14	42	45	87
15	57	44	101
16	83	66	149
17	64	33	97
TOTAL	595	654	1.249

Table 7–27. Normative Data for the Test de Símbolos y Dígitos

	Age	SCORE LEVEL[*]				Mean	SD	N
		Very Low	Low	Normal	High			
Written SDMT	8	0–18	19–21	22–36	37–110	29,04	7,07	106
	9	0–21	22–25	26–40	41–110	33,07	7,66	161
	10	0–24	25–29	30–47	48–110	38,61	9,29	167
	11	0–30	31–34	35–52	53–110	43,37	8,62	137
	12	0–25	26–32	33–60	61–110	46,36	13,86	120
	13	0–34	35–39	40–60	61–110	50,19	10,31	124
	14	0–35	36–40	41–60	61–110	50,36	9,76	87
	15	0–36	37–41	42–63	64–110	52,69	10,89	100
	16	0–39	40–45	46–66	67–110	55,90	10,71	149
	17	0–41	42–46	47–68	69–110	57,40	10,66	97
Oral SDMT	8	0–22	22–26	22–44	45–110	35,50	8,75	106
	9	0–27	28–32	33–49	50–110	40,97	8,69	152
	10	0–33	34–38	39–59	60–110	49,23	10,40	145
	11	0–37	38–42	43–63	64–110	53,02	10,12	126
	12	0–38	39–44	45–67	68–110	55,87	11,69	101
	13	0–45	46–50	51–70	71–110	60,32	10,12	114
	14	0–45	46–50	51–70	71–110	60,21	9,79	81
	15	0–46	47–52	53–76	77–110	64,57	11,85	68
	16	0–52	53–58	59–80	81–110	69,15	11,07	107
	17	0–51	52–57	58–83	84–110	70,75	12,85	79

Source: Reproduced with permission and authorization of TEA Ediciones, S.A. Madrid, Spain. 2002.
[*]Score level intervals: Very Low: [0, Mean − 1.5 (SD)]; Low: [Very Low, Mean − 1 (SD)]; Normal: [Low, High]; High: [Mean + 1.5 (SD), Max].

bal and Nonverbal Cancellation Tests for Children. The stimuli pages were from the Tests of Directed Attention and Memory (Weintraub and Mesulam, 1985). Included was a letter cancellation test that required the child to search for a target letter A within a randomized array on one trial and for a target within a random array on another. Each trial includes 60 target letters, half on the right and half on the left half of the page. For older children and adults, there are also more difficult random and orderly shape-target trials, in which one searches for a circle with 8 external radii and an oblique diameter (Weintraub and Mesulam, 1985). Just as for the Rey-Osterrieth Complex Figure procedure, colored pens can be used later to reconstruct the subject's path, for example, by changing colors every time the child has cancelled 10 targets.

Preliminary child normative data were obtained on 123 children from Texas with average to above average ability. There were 65 females and 58 males equally distributed by grade from a private parochial school, with no exclusionary criteria. The study used two par-

allel letter targets (A and E) and two geometric figure targets, each presented in an organized or random array. A ninth task required the child to underline boxes. The authors found effects of age, stimulus, format, and practice in the childrens' performance. The normative data for the trials using the letter A in both organized and random arrays, each administered for 45-seconds, are presented in Table 7–28 (K. Thorstad, J. M. Fletcher, J. Andrews, & R. Morris, 2002, personal communication). It is also noted that the random array format was

Table 7–28. Means (SDs) for Number Correct on Letter A Cancellation Task

Grade	Organized Array	Random Array
1	16.76 (4.75)	20.40 (5.31)
2	23.12 (4.75)	23.36 (8.69)
3	26.10 (4.11)	29.67 (6.15)
4	26.54 (3.49)	27.13 (4.39)
5	30.21 (3.78)	32.57 (7.06)

Source: K. G. Thorstad, J. M. Fletcher, J. Andrews, & R. Morris, personal communication.

Table 7–29. Latency and Error Scores for Cancellation of Targets Test

Age		LIF Controls	Non-Dyslexic	Dyslexic	592 Controls	Non-Dyslexic	Dyslexic	DIAMOND SHAPE Controls	Non-Dyslexic	Dyslexic
4–5	*M* errors				13			12		
	(*SD*)				(3.4)			(4.0)		
6–7	*M* Time	153.9	122.1	186.0	200.8	158.4	207.3	103.4	128.0	98.4
	(*SD*)	(57.8)	(41.4)	(62.3)	(81.5)	(87.3)	(81.4)	(46.3)	(76.1)	(20.2)
	M errors				6			5		
	(*SD*)				(2.6)			(2.8)		
8–9	*M* Time	93.2	108.5	119.4	116.0	127.8	144.2	66.3	67.0	74.5
	(*SD*)	(26.4)	(40.7)	(48.8)	(33.7)	(46.8)	(58.8)	(21.6)	(21.1)	(26.4)
	M errors				2			4		
	(*SD*)				(1.8)			(2.4)		
10–11	*M* Time	73.9	81.5	99.8	90.7	103.5	118.8	70.1	68.2	66.9
	(*SD*)	(25.4)	(29.4)	(20.9)	(24.7)	(37.1)	(35.6)	(24.6)	(30.5)	(21.9)
	M errors				2			3		
	(*SD*)				(1.9)			(2.5)		
12–13	*M* Time	53.7	94.0	95.4	67.1	106.8	124.1	40.9	67.0	73.7
	(*SD*)	(12.8)	(27.9)	(17.2)	(15.8)	(28.1)	(36.9)	(8.9)	(21.4)	(34.7)
	M errors				2			2		
	(*SD*)				(1.8)			(2.3)		

Source: Adapted from Rudel, Denckla, and Broman (1978).

adapted for Chinese adults using 374 Chinese characters (words), in the Random Chinese Word Cancellation Test (Chen Sea, Cermak et al., 1993).

Cancellation of Targets

The Cancellation of Targets Test is a visual search and cancellation test (Rudel, Denckla et al., 1978) that has limited normative data for 4 to 13 years old, but is easily administered. It has the potential to detect dissociation between the ability to search for linguistic symbols (i.e., a number or letter trigram) and a geometric shape amid a competing visual array. Intact shape search, but poor letter and/or number search is potentially indicative of a language-learning disability or of dysfunction in the language-dominant hemisphere and a marker that further evaluation of language functions is required. Or, a child might perform within intact limits for each trial of a letter and number trigram search, but demonstrate many omission errors on shape search. This pattern might suggest a nonverbal disorder or dysfunction in the non–language-dominant hemisphere that

then requires further investigation. Besides the time to completion and error scores, the test is also useful when ability to sustain performance is observed to deteriorate from trial to trial.

A pattern of neglect might also be evident in either right or left hemispace, or for upper or lower quadrants. Commission errors might indicate impulsivity, and omission errors suggest inattention to visual detail; both errors reflect behavior that may complicate academic functioning. Poor performance across all three trials should be evaluated differently than performance that worsens over each subsequent trial. While originally consisting of three parts, search for three letters, the "LIF" trigram, three numbers, the "592" trigram, and the geometric shape of a diamond, some now administer only "592" and the geometric shape trials (Martha B. Denckla, 2002, personal communication). The normative data are presented in Table 7–29. Modifications are possible. For example, in one study, each subjects' completion time was divided by total number of correct hits for an additional index score (Lockwood, Marcotte et al., 2001).

d2 Test of Attention

The d2 Test of Attention (Brickenkamp and Zillmer, 1998) is a measure of an individual's ability to differentiate visual stimuli rapidly and accurately. It is a timed, visual search, attention, and concentration test that is considered a measure of both selective and sustained attention, visual perception, and visuomotor speed. The d2 test loads with other tests of selective attention such as the Stroop Color Word Test and the Symbol Digit Modalities Test in a factor analytic study supporting construct validity (Davis and Zillmer, 1998). The test takes between 4 and 8 minutes to administer and can be administered individually or to groups of individuals without visual acuity impairment.

The test stimuli are printed lines of lower case p's and d's with one to four apostrophes either below or above the letters (see Figure 7–1). There are 14 lines of 47 letters/line on a test page (total $N = 658$ items). The subject has 20 seconds per line to cross out all d2 stimuli, that is, a "d" with two apostrophes above or below the letter. After each 20-second trial, the subject moves on to the next line of stimuli. Template scoring allows for easy calculation of a number of critical variables. Included is CP, concentration performance (the number of correct responses minus commission errors). Also scored are TN = total number of items marked; E1 = omission errors; E2 = commission errors; E% = error percentage; FR = fluctuation rate; S-syndrome = skipping syndrome, and TN-E/C = overall performance.

The d2 Test of Attention has been translated into six languages, and in the original German version it is in its eighth revision. The U. S. version is normed on individuals 9 to 59 years old. Normative data in the United States is limited to a small number, but since the first German edition in 1962, normative data have been collected on a German sample of over 6,000 individuals (Eric Zillmer, 2002, personal communication). Preliminary adult U.S. normative data were also collected on 506 college-educated individuals aged 18 to 32.

Child normative data are presented for a German standardization sample of 3132 school children (see Table 7–30), and preliminary norms are also reported for Concentration Performance (CP) on a sample of 900 children and for a small subset of American children (see Table 7–31). The American norms include TN-E and CP scores for 56 middle-class, primarily Caucasian (96%) children (28 male, 26 female), rated as average or better academically, and without a history of behavioral problems, psychotropic medication, psychotherapy, special education, or remedial academic assistance. The standard scores and percentile ranks for male and female combined are reported for ages 7 to 9 years ($N = 28$) and 10 to 12 years ($N = 28$), with a SD of 10. TN-E data are also reported for 40 primarily Caucasian children with ADHD using DSM-IV criteria, 32 males and 8 females aged 7 to 9 years ($N = 18$) and 10 to 12 years ($N = 22$). WISC-III IQ scores based on selected subtests were equal to or greater than 80. Children were ex-

Figure 7—1. Practice line of d2 Test. The test items consist of the letters d and p with one to four dashes, arranged either individually or in pairs above and below the letter. The subject must scan across each line to identify and cross out each d with two dashes. In the manual, these items (correct hits) are called "relevant items." All other combinations of letters and lines are considered "irrelevant," because they should not be crossed out. The one-page d2 Test form provides sections for recording indentifying data and test scores, and provides a practice sample. On the reverse side is the standardized test, consisting of 14 lines, each with 47 characters, for a total of 658 items. The subject is allowed 20 seconds per line (From R. Brickenkamp and E. A. Zillmer, *d2 Test of Attention*, Göttingen, Germany: Hogrefe & Huber, p. 7; reprinted by permission)

Table 7–30. German Sample Child and Adolescent Norms for d2 Test of Attention

PR	SS	AGE IN YEARS					
		9–10	11–12	13–14	15–16	17–18	19–29
	70	40	57	65	72	88	81
	80	60	78	89	99	115	109
10		75	94	106	120	136	130
	90	80	99	113	126	142	137
25		87	106	122	135	151	147
50	100	100	120	137	153	169	165
75		113	134	152	171	187	183
	110	120	141	161	180	196	193
90		125	147	168	188	204	199
	120	140	162	185	207	223	221
	130	160	183	209	234	250	249

Note: PR = percentile rank; SS = standard score.

Adapted from Brickenkamp and Zillmer (1998). The *d2 Test of Attention. Manual*, 36 (Table 7–15). © Hogrefe & Huber Publishers.

cluded if there was documented brain injury, seizures, or psychiatric disability.

Norms for 3132 German children and adolescents are presented in tables by two-year age blocks from 9 to 18 years and in a single 10-year block for ages 19 to 29. Gender distribution was 1601 males and 1531 females who were placed in elementary to middle school ($N = 1054$), vocational school ($N = 438$), and junior high to high school ($N = 1640$). Internal consistency results are reported to reflect high reliability, $r = .70$ to $>.90$. Test–retest reliability for German children ranged from .37 to .88, the lower score obtained on child

Table 7–31. Preliminary U. S. Population Child Norms for the d2 Test of Attention

PR	SS	AGE IN YEARS					
		7–9 N = 28 TN-E Normal	10–12 N = 28 TN-E Normal	7–9 N = 28 CP Normal	10–12 N = 28 CP Normal	7–9 N = 18 TN-E ADHD	10–12 N = 22 TN-E ADHD
	70	<186	<233	<71	<99	<94	<199
	80	186	233	71	99	94	199
10		202	296	83	116	175	215
	90	218	301	91	124	192	230
25		237	315	97	131	165	335
50	100	248	350	103	137	251	301
75		266	390	108	154	287	359
	110	290	414	119	165	308	374
90		307	433	125	175	332	404
	120	331	450	135	180	>332	>404
	130	>331	>450	>135	>180		

Note: PR = percentile rank; SS = standard score; ADHD = Attention Deficit Hyperactivity Disorder; TN = total number; E = errors; CP = concentration performance.

Source: Reprinted from Brickenkamp and Zillmer (1998). *The d2 Test of Attention. Manual*, 38 (Table 7–18). © Hogrefe & Huber Publishers.

samples of behaviorally disturbed German children over an 11-month interval and therefore possibly underestimating true test–retest reliability.

The d2 test procedure can be adapted for specific uses. For example, in an adult study, the subject was asked to mark quickly and precisely, within 5 minutes, as many "d"'s that carried the two apostrophes (either above or below) (Gendolla, Abele et al., 2001).

The Underlining Test

The reader may also be interested in the Underlining Test, adapted from work by D. G. Doehring (Rourke and Orr, 1977), a timed test of visuomotor speed and self-paced attention that provides data about speed and accuracy of visual search for target stimuli printed in rows amid distractors. There are 14 subtests. Targets include number, letter, irregular design, geometric form, combinations of letters, groups of shapes, and a control subtest intended to provide an indication of underlining speed. Scores are: net correct (correct targets − errors); errors not self-corrected; and time (seconds for a subtest/net correct for that subtest). Subtests 2 (Greek cross), 4 (geometric figure), and 9 (letters "fsbm") were included in a study of *Haemophilus influenzae* Type b meningitis (Taylor, Barry et al., 1993).

Continuous Performance Tests

The Continuous Performance Test (CPT) was originally developed as a test of vigilance that required attention to a visual or auditory presentation of randomly occurring letters and a response to a target stimulus (Rosvold, Mirsky et al., 1956). Sensitivity to attentional deficit is based on the rapid presentation of stimuli over an extended time period (Halperin, Sharma et al., 1991). Speed of stimulus presentation and target and complexity of stimuli are methodological variables chosen by experimenters that have made this type of test difficult to standardize across settings. As a result, it is difficult to confidently define a neuroanatomical substrate for CPT performance (Beebe, Ris et al., 2000). Yet, data to date suggest CPTs are sensitive to anterior cortical lesions and to disruption of EF subdomains such as the ability

to inhibit, sustain attention, and be vigilant (Mirsky, 1996; Pennington, 1997).

The CPT paradigm has particular salience in the evaluation of children with ADHD (Seidel and Joschko, 1991) and is in wide use, although it has not been shown to be diagnostic as a single instrument (National Institutes of Health, 1998). It was not endorsed as sufficiently sensitive to attentional problems in the NIH consensus meeting (National Institutes of Health, 1998) but it does give indices of sustained attention. Limitations include a child's unwillingness to persevere for the duration of the CPT. These tests tend to have poor specificity for ADHD, including relatively common false negatives.

While CPTs receive increasing application because of face validity, they appear to assess more pure aspects of attention independent of other cognitive processes. Their strength may lie more in the discrimination between psychiatric groups and controls than in the ability to discriminate between clinical patient groups (Halperin, Sharma et al., 1991). CPT as a diagnostic instrument, has been investigated and comparisons have been made with other procedures, but such data are limited. CPT tests are valued for their ability to provide information about an attention subdomain that is not easily obtained from other cognitive tests. For example, CPT test scores were found to represent a unique factor that was independent of indices from the WCST (Mirsky, 1996).

There are many CPT versions, and these vary by length, stimulus modality, and stimulus complexity. A review and comparison of CPTs was published (Riccio, Reynolds et al., 2001). There are many CPT versions; only a few are noted below for those readers wishing to further investigate their merits. However, the concepts underlying these tests are worth reviewing, and a definition of some related terms follows to familiarize the reader with the vocabulary of CPTs.

Included as dependent CPT measures are the percentage of correct responses to target, the percentage of erroneous responses to nontargets (commission errors or false alarms), and reaction time. Commission errors are more frequent in children than omission errors (Halperin, Sharma et al., 1991). These errors are typically viewed as a measure of impulsivity, but in at least one study, distinct measures of inattention and impulsivity were generated within an "A–X" CPT paradigm, making it more difficult to explain commission errors as inattention (Halperin, Wolf et al., 1988).

The Conners' Continuous Performance Test (CPT) evaluates concentration, sustained vigilance, and attention for a simple task over a time interval (Conners, 1992). The database includes individuals aged 4 years to adulthood. The child must press a key when a letter appears on the computer screen, except when it is the letter X. The test lasts approximately 14 minutes. The 324 non-X stimuli are interspersed with 36 X stimuli, presented in blocks of trials with interstimulus intervals of 1, 2, and 4 seconds, which vary between blocks.

Common measures reported for the Conners' version include number of hits and number of omissions reported in percentiles, and T scores and percentiles for number of commissions, hit reaction time (RT), and standard error (SE), variability of standard errors, attentiveness (d') and risk taking (B). Other measuers include: hit RT block change, hit SE block change, hit RT interstimulus interval (ISI change), and hit SE ISI change. A combination of variables is entered to obtain an overall index score (OIS), which ranges from 0.00 to 20.74, with any value above 4.00 indicating significant attentional disturbance.

Overall hit reaction time or overall processing speed represents the average speed of correct responses for the entire test. An averaged slow response time and neglect of responding would suggest the person was not paying close attention to the task.

Overall standard error is indicative of overall attentional variability. High levels of variability indicate inconsistency in speed of responding, a sign of fluctuating attention from trial to trial.

Speed decrement over time or the pattern of hit reaction time is an indication of the ability to maintain speed of responding over time, suggesting loss of effort or energy.

Variability over time or the pattern of standard error is also of interest. Greater variability over time in the speed of response indicates a graduated loss of sustained attention.

Omissions indicative of inattentiveness may be caused by temporary blocks in responding, or actual looking away from the test when signals are presented. A high number of omission errors indicates this loss of attentiveness. Omission error refers to the frequency of non-X stimuli which do not elicit response.

Commissions errors may represent an inability to withhold motor responses as a result of an impulsive response tendency. Commission error refers to the frequency of an X stimulus eliciting response. Omission and Commission errors load on a single factor, and this is distinct from other EF measures (Mirsky, 1996).

Perceptual Sensitivity (d') is another index. Errors in responding may represent difficulties in discriminating the perceptual features of signals (all letters except X) and non-signals (Xs). A value of d' is obtained that suggests average or atypical perceptual sensitivity.

Response bias (B) or Beta (β) represents an individual's response tendency. Some individuals are cautious and choose not to respond very often. These will obtain high Beta T scores. Others are more risk-taking or impulsive and respond more frequently than they should, obtaining low Beta T scores. This score, for example, might show the person having a response style that emphasizes the minimization of commission errors more than omission errors relative to the general population.

Activation/arousal provides inter-stimulus statistics. Individuals will adjust their reaction speed according to how fast the stimuli occur. When stimuli are presented quickly, brain activation/arousal is high and responses tend to be fast. When stimuli are presented slowly, brain activation/arousal is low and responses tend to be slower and less consistent.

All component CPT measures need not be abnormal. If none or only one is atypical, this is rarely an indication of an attention problem. If two or more are atypical, a possibility of an attention problem should be considered. A greater number of atypical responses provides more evidence for an attention problem. Percentile values must be much higher than T-scores to be considered atypical. For B, high and low scores are noteworthy. Low scores indicate too frequent responding, which is usually related to impulsivity; high scores indicate an atypically low number of responses, usually related to inattention.

The Gordon Diagnostic System (GDS; Gordon, 1983; Gordon, McClure et al., 1996) is a portable electronic device with microprocessor whose indices of delay provide an efficiency ratio, vigilance, and distractibility. For its delay condition, impulsivity is measured with a differential reinforcement of low rates of responding paradigm, that is, as the child tries to earn points by pressing a button a light goes on, and a point is recorded by a visible counter. If the child presses the button the next time too early, no point is earned, and the interval resets. Variables include total correct and an efficiency ratio for the proportion of correct responses compared to the total number of responses. For the vigilance condition, a series of digits is flashed in the center column of the computer screen at a rate of 1/second. A stimulus is presented for 800 msec, with 200 msec intervals between stimuli. The child presses a button every time the alerting stimulus, 1, is followed by the target, 9. The child must inhibit responding to the alerting stimulus, to non-target digits, and to the target digit if it does not follow the alerting stimulus. Total correct indicates sustained attention; commission errors is the index of impulsivity.

For the distractibility condition, similar to the vigilance task, a distraction of random digits flashed at random intervals on the left and right sides of the central stimuli, is added. The child must ignore the numbers in these outer portions of the screen. As for the vigilance condition, the total correct is considered a measure of sustained attention, and commission errors are indices of impulsivity. Support for use of the GDS with ADHD children resulted from analysis of the performance of 165 referred children with ADHD-Combined type and 46 non-ADHD children, aged 6 to 16 (Mayes, Calhoun et al., 2001).

The Test of Variables of Attention (TOVA; Greenberg, 1996) is a go-no-go CPT with both auditory and visual versions. The stimuli for the former are nonlinguistic. For the latter, the child must respond or withhold responding to a target and non-target geometric design. It uses a 2 per second interstimulus interval and presents stimuli over a 3.5:1 ratio. Target-infrequent and target-frequent paradigms are employed, resulting in measures of omission, commission, response time, and response time variability. Age and gender normative data were collected on 775 children aged 6 to 16

(Greenberg and Waldman, 1993). The test's utility in child studies was examined, including for those with ADHD and/or Tourette syndrome, when examining omission errors, commission errors, reaction time to correct responses, and variability of reaction time (Harris, Singer et al., 1995; Shucard, Benedict et al., 1997; Forbes, 1998; Mahone, Cirino et al., 2002), and for children with complex partial seizures with and without ADHD (Semrud-Clikeman and Wical, 1999). It receives criticism for limited reported reliability (Riccio, Reynolds et al., 2001).

For the Auditory Continuous Performance Test (ACPT; Keith, 1994), the child indicates the presence of a target word during six consecutive tape-recorded readings of a 96-item word list containing 76 distractor words and the target word repeated 20 times. The child raises a thumb every time the target word is perceived, and the examiner records the number of false negative and false positive responses. The test is approximately 10 minutes long. Norms are based on 510 6 to 11 years, 11-month-old children. Two measures of attention are obtained: selective attention (missed target words plus mistaken words) and, sustained attention (first and final trial error score difference). High scores indicate impaired attention.

The Adaptive Rate Continuous Performance Test (ARCPT) is a CPT modification. It is a computer-generated test that requires the person to identify target combinations (letter A followed by the letter X). The person presses a key on a keyboard each time the combination is identified. The test provides an estimate of deviations of attention that extend beyond a normal range. The three primary measures are detection accuracy (ARCPT-d'), response bias (ARCPT-β), and an inconsistency index (ARCPT-II; Cohen, Kaplan et al., 1999).

Another CPT modification is the Immediate Memory Task/Delayed Memory Task (IMT/DMT; Dougherty, 1999). It has primarily been used to investigate impulsive behavior in adult psychiatric groups, such as conduct-disordered adults, bipolar disorder and borderline personality disorder. The Microcomputer Test of Attention (MTA) is a vigilance test that requires the child to press a space bar when a target form appears in a box in the center of the computer screen, but to refrain from pressing when another form appears inside the box or when the target appears outside the box (Murphy-Berman and Wright, 1987). The Continuous Attention Test (CAT) presents 12 capital letters singly and centrally on the screen at a rate of 1.5 seconds and for a duration of 0.2 seconds. Each of two subtests presents 600 randomized letters, including 90 targets. There are three 5-minute blocks for each subtest in which the child must press a key each time the target appears, i.e., an X in the first subtest and an X if immediately preceded by an A on the second subtest (Seidel and Joschko, 1990; 1991).

The development of CPTs for preschoolers resulted in a visual CPT (Corkum, Byrne et al., 1995) and an auditory CPT, named "Zoo Runner" (Prather, Sarmento et al., 1995), both of which were administered in a study of 25 preschool children with ADHD and 25 controls (De Wolfe, Byrne et al., 1999). In the latter study, the ADHD group had significantly more omission and commission errors on the visual attention task. They did not make significantly more omission or commission errors on the auditory attention test. A visual search task was also administered, and ADHD children made significantly more commission errors and took a longer time to complete the test compared to the control subjects. Thus, these young children did produce a pattern of performance consistent with that typically observed in older children with ADHD and distinctly different than their normal controls.

Behavior Questionnaires

A wide variety of questionnaires that provide information related to attentional capacity are also published. A few of these are noted below although there is a wide range of such measures. The Behavior Rating Inventory of Executive Function (Gioia, Isquith et al., 2000) has subscales of interest in the assessment of the child with an attentional problem, and is discussed in Chapter 6.

The Attention Deficit Hyperactivity Disorder Rating Scale-IV—Home Version (DuPaul 1991; DuPaul, Anastopoulos et al. 1992; DuPaul, Power et al., 1998) is an 18-item scale based on DSM-IV diagnostic criteria for ADHD. There are 9 inattention items and 9

hyperactivity/impulsivity items. Parent report on a 4-step Likert scale, ranging from 0 to 3, is related to the child's behavior over the past 6 months. Normative data are based on 2000 children based on the 1990 U. S. census data. Test–retest reliability is 0.85 for the total score, 0.78 for Inattention and 0.86 for Hyperactivity-Impulsivity. Strong correlation with the Conners Parent Rating Scales was found.

The Behavior Assessment System for Children (BASC; Reynolds and Kamphaus, 1992) is useful to assess DSM-IV-listed and broad behavioral disorders. It includes questions about internalizing and externalizing behaviors, inattention, hyperactivity, social behavior, and adaptive skills in a true-or-false format. There are parent and teacher rating forms. There is a parent rating scale (BASC-PRS) normed on 3483 U. S. children, (Reynolds and Kamphaus, 1998a) and a self-report version, normed on 9861 U. S. children, that the child completes (Reynolds and Kamphaus, 1998b).

The Diagnostic Rating Scale (DRS; Weiler, Bellinger et al., 1999) has published reliability and validity data (Weiler, Bellinger et al., 2000). There are parent and teacher versions of this DSM-IV-based ADHD questionnaire. The items include questions for the 18 DSM-IV criteria for predominantly inattentive and predominately hyperactive-impulsive ADHD subtypes, eight oppositional defiant disorder criteria, seven conduct disorder criteria and seven questions from the Depression-Anxiety scale of the Pediatric Behavior Scale (Lindgren and Koeppl, 1987; Weiler, Bernstein et al., 2000). "The DRS Attention scale correlates .65 and .59 with the Attention Problems and Hyperactivity scales of the BASC, respectively; .75 and .59 with the Hyperactivity and Impulsive-Hyperactive scales of the CPRS-48, respectively; and .61 with the Attention Problems scale of the CBCL. The Hyperactivity scale of the DRS correlates .73 and .48 with the Hyperactivity and Attention Problems scales of the BASC, respectively; .65 and 59 with the Impulsive-Hyperactive and Hyperactivity scales of the CPRS-48, respectively; and .54 with with the Attention Problems scale of the CBCL." (Weiler, Bernstein et al., 2000, 221).

The Conner's Rating Scales-Revised (Conners, 1996) has long and short parent, teacher, and adolescent (12–17 years old) self-report forms for children aged 3 to 17. In addition to assessing a range of psychopathology and problem behaviors, an ADHD index for at-risk children can be calculated. The ADHD/DSM-IV scales are linked to the DSM-IV diagnostic criteria. The Conners' Global Index has parts for Restless/Impulsive and Emotional Lability.

The Brown Attention-Deficit Disorder Scales (Brown, 2001) has forms for the primary/preschool, school-age, adolescent and adult ages, enabling assessment of those 3-years old and older. Six cluster scores can be obtained: *(1)* Organizing, Prioritizing and Activating to Work, *(2)* Focusing, Sustaining and Shifting Attention to Tasks, *(3)* Regulating Alertness, Sustaining Effort and Processing Speed, *(4)* Managing Frustration and Modulating Emotions, *(5)* Utilizing Working Memory and Accessing Recall, and *(6)* Monitoring and Self-Regulating Action. A Total Score indicates overall impairment from a range of symptoms.

CONCLUSION

The assessment of attention is but one component within a neuropsychological evaluation that contributes to understanding the child's overall neurocognitive competence. We are now more able to appreciate the subtypes of attention and how they are reflected in a wider variety of test instruments than was true in the earlier days of child assessment. Within this chapter are normative data enhanced by computations that express the reliable change or statistical regression indices that allow for detection of meaningful change over time. This trend toward including such calculations along with normative data stratified by age and other appropriate demographic characteristics is a very positive development. It is demonstrated, for example, by the normative data for adolescents presented by William Barr (Barr, 2003). Normative data have a usefulness that extends beyond comparisons of a child's performance to a peer group. Such data provide a more cogent means for evaluating development, decline, or progress over time.

REFERENCES

American Academy of Pediatrics. (2000). Clinical Practice Guideline: Diagnosis and evaluation of the child with attention-deficit/hyperactivity disorder. *Pediatrics, 105,* 1158–1170.

American Psychiatric Association. (1994). *Diagnostic and statistical manual of mental disorders,* Fourth edition. Washington, D. C.: American Psychiatric Association.

Amieva, H., Lafont, S., Auriacombe, S., Rainville, C., Orgogozo, J., Dartigues, J., et al. (1998). Analysis of error types in the Trail Making Test evidences an inhibitory deficit in dementia of the Alzheimer type. *Journal of Clinical and Experimental Neuropsychology, 20,* 280–285.

Anastasi, A. (1968). *Psychological Testing* (3rd Ed.). London: The Macmillan Company.

Anderson, V., Lajoie, G., & Bell, R. (1995). *Neuropsychological Assessment of the School-Aged Child.* Melbourne: University of Melbourne.

Anderson, V., & Pentland, L. (1998). Residual attention deficits following childhood head injury: Implications for ongoing development. *Neuropsychological Rehabilitation, 8,* 283–300.

Arbuthnott, K., & Frank, J. (2000). Trail Making Test, Part B as a measure of executive control: Validation using a set-switching paradigm. *Journal of Clinical and Experimental Neuropsychology, 22,* 518–528.

Ardila, A., Rosselli, M., Ostrosky-Solis, F., Marcos, J., Granda, G., & Soto, M. (2000). Syntactic comprehension, verbal memory, and calculation abilities in Spanish-English bilinguals. *Applied Neuropsychology, 7,* 3–16.

Armitage, S. G. (1946). An analysis of certain psychological tests used for the evaluation of brain injury. *Psychological Monographs, 60,* 30–34.

Army Individual Test Battery. (1944). Army Individual Test Battery: Manual of directions and scoring. Washington, D.C.: War Department, Adjutant General's Office.

Arribas, D. (2002). *SDMT, Digit and Symbol Test (Test de Símbolos y Dígitos).* Madrid: TEA Ediciones.

Arthur, G. (1947). *A point scale of performance tests* (Rev. Form II). New York: The Psychological Corporation.

Baddeley, A. D. (1976). *The psychology of memory.* New York: Basic Books.

Baddeley, A. D. (2001). Is working memory still working. *American Psychologist, 56,* 851–864.

Baddeley, A. D., Vallar, G., & Wilson, B. A. (1987). Sentence comprehension and phonological memory: Some neuropsychological evidence. In M. Coltheart (Ed.), *Attention and performance XII:*

The psychology of reading (pp. 509–529). Hove, England: Erlbaum.

Barkley, R. A. (1990). *Attention Deficit Hyperactivity Disorder: A Handbook for Diagnosis and Treatment.* New York: Guilford Press.

Barkley, R. A. (1991). The ecological validity of laboratory and analogue assessment methods of ADHD symptoms. *Journal of Abnormal Child Psychology, 19,* 149–178.

Barkley, R. A. (1997). Behavioral inhibition, sustained attention, and executive functions: Constructing a unifying theory of ADHD. *Psychological Bulletin, 121,* 65–94.

Baron, I. S. (2001). Test Review: Test of Everyday Attention for Children. *Child Neuropsychology, 7,* 190–195.

Barr, W. B. (2003). Neuropsychological testing of high school athletes: Preliminary norms and test-retest indices. *Archives of Clinical Neuropsychology, 18,* 91–101.

Bechtold, K. T., Horner, M. D., & Windham, W. K. (2001). *The Trail Making Test, Part B: Cognitive flexibility or ability to maintain set.* Paper presented at the 29th Annual Meeting of the International Neuropsychological Society, Chicago, IL.

Beebe, D. W., Ris, M. D., & Dietrich, K. N. (2000). The relationship between CVLT-C process scores and measures of executive functioning: Lack of support among community-dwelling adolescents. *Journal of Clinical and Experimental Neuropsychology, 22,* 779–792.

Bellugi, U., Wang, P. P., & Jernigan, T. L. (1994). Williams syndrome: An unusual neuropsychological profile. In S. H. Brodman & J. Grafman (Eds.), *Atypical cognitive deficits in developmental disorders: Implications for brain function* (pp. 23–56). Hillsdale, NJ: Erlbaum.

Benson, D. F. (1991). The role of fontal dysfunction in attention deficit hyperactivity disorder. *Child Neurology, 6,* 9–12.

Benton, A. L., Hamsher, K., Varney, N. R., & Spreen, O. (1983c). *Contributions to neuropsychological assessment: A clinical manual.* New York: Oxford University Press.

Bishop, D. V. M., Aamodt-Leeper, G., Creswell, C., McGurk, R., & Skuse, D. H. (2001). Individual differences in cognitive planning on the Tower of Hanoi task: Neuropsychological maturity or measurement error? *Journal of Child Psychology and Psychiatry, 42,* 551–556.

Boll, T., & Reitan, R. (1973). Effect of age on performance of the Trail Making Test. *Perceptual and Motor Skills, 36,* 691–694.

Borkowski, J. G., & Burke, J. (1996). Trends in the development of theories, models, and measurement of executive functioning: Views from an in-formation processing perspective. In G. R. Lyon & N. A. Krasnegor (Eds.), *Attention, memory and executive functioning.* Baltimore: Paul H. Brooke.

Boyd, T. (1988). Clinical assessment of memory in children. A developmental framework for practice. In M. G. Tramontana & S. R. Hooper (Eds.), *Assessment issues in child neuropsychology* (pp. 177–204). New York: Plenum Press.

Brickenkamp, R., & Zillmer, E. (1998). *d2 Test of Attention* (1st U.S. ed.) Seattle: Hogrefe and Huber Publishers.

Brittain, J. L., LaMarche, J. A., Reeder, K. P., Roth, D. L., & Boll, T. (1991). Effects of age and IQ on Paced Auditory Serial-Addition Task (PASAT) performance. *The Clinical Neuropsychologist, 5,* 163–175.

Brown, J. (1958). Some tests of the decay of immediate memory. *Quarterly Journal of Experimental Psychology, 10,* 12–21.

Brown, T. E. (2001). *Brown Attention-Deficit Scales.* San Antonio, TX: The Psychological Corporation.

Butler, R. W., & Copeland, D. R. (2002). Attentional processes and their remediation in children treated for cancer: A literature review and the development of a therapeutic approach. *Journal of the International Neuropsychological Society, 8,* 115–124.

Cahn, D. A., Marcotte, A. C., Stern, R. A., Arruda, J. A., Akshoomoff, N. A., & Leshko, I. C. (1996). The Boston qualitative scoring system for the Rey-Osterrieth Complex Figure: A study of children with attention deficit hyperactivity disorder. *The Clinical Neuropsychologist, 10,* 397–406.

Chabildas, N., Pennington, B. F., & Willcutt, E. G. (2001). A Comparison of the Neuropsychological Profiles of the DSM-IV Subtypes of ADHD. *Journal of Abnormal Child Psychology, 29,* 529–540.

Chen Sea, M.-J., Cermak, S. A., & Henderson, A. (1993). Performance of normal Chinese adults and right CVA patients on the Random Chinese Word Cancellation Test. *The Clinical Neuropsychologist, 7,* 239–249.

Chervin, R. D., Archbold, K. H., Dillon, J. E., Panahi, P., Pituch, K. J., Dahl, R. E., et al. (2002). Inattention, hyperactivity, and symptoms of sleep-disordered breathing. *Pediatrics, 109,* 449–456.

Cohen, R., Kaplan, R. F., Moser, D. J., Jenkins, M. A., & Wilkinson, H. (1999). Impairments of attention after cingulotomy. *Neurology, 53,* 819–824.

Cohen, R. A. (1993). *Neuropsychology of attention.* New York: Plenum.

Cohen, R. A., Paul, R., Zawacki, T., Moser, D., Sweet, L., & Wilkinson, H. (2001). Emotional and personality changes following cingulotomy. *Emotion, 1,* 38–50.

Cohen, R. M., Semple, W. E., Gross, W., Holcomb, H. J., Dowling, S. M., & Nordahl, T. E. (1988).

Functional localization of sustained attention. *Neuropsychology and Behavioral Neurology, 1,* 3–20.

Conners, C. K. (1992). *Manual for the Conners' continuous performance test.* Toronto: Multi-Health Systems, Inc.

Conners, C. K. (1996). *Conners' Rating Scales-Revised.* San Antonio, TX: The Psychological Corporation.

Cooley, E. L., & Morris, R. D. (1990). Attention in children: A neuropsychologically based model for assessment. *Developmental Neuropsychology, 6,* 239–274.

Corkum, P., Byrne, J. M., & Ellsworth, C. (1995). Clinical assessment of sustained attention in preschoolers. *Child Neuropsychology, 1,* 3–18.

Cotton, S., Crowe, S., & Voudouris, N. (1998). Neuropsychological profile of Duchenne Muscular Dystrophy. *Child Neuropsychology, 4,* 110–117.

Craik, F. I. M. (1990). Changes in memory with normal aging: A functional view. In R. J. Wurtman, S. Corkin, H. H. Growdon & E. Ritter-Walker (Eds.), *Advances in neurology:* Vol. 51. Alzheimer's disease (pp. 201–205). New York: Raven Press.

Craik, F. I. M., Govoni, R., Naveh-Benjamin, M., & Anderson, N. D. (1996). The effects of divided attention on encoding and retrieval processes in human memory. *Journal of Experimental Psychology: General, 125,* 159–180.

Crowe, S. (1998). The differential contribution of mental tracking, cognitive flexibility, visual search, and motor speed to performance on Parts A and Part B of the Trail Making Test. *Journal of Clinical Psychology, 54,* 585–591.

Dalen, K., & Hugdahl, K. (1986). Inhibitory versus facilitory interference for finger-tapping to verbal and nonverbal, motor and sensory tasks. *Journal of Clinical and Experimental Neuropsychology, 8,* 627–636.

Daniel, A. (1983). *Power, privilege and prestige: Occupations in Australia.* Melbourne: Longman-Cheshire.

Davis, K. L., & Zillmer, E. (1998). Contrasts between the d2 Test of Attention and intelligence measures from a normative sample. *[?abstract] Archives of Clinical Neuropsychology, 1,* 72.

Dehaene, S. (1997). *The number sense.* New York: Oxford University Press.

Delis, D., Kaplan, E., & Kramer, J. (2001). *The Delis-Kaplan Executive Function System: Examiner's Manual.* San Antonio, TX: The Psychological Corporation.

Della Sala, S., Gray, C., Baddeley, A. D., Allamano, N., & Wilson, L. (1999). Pattern span: A means of unwelding visuo-spatial memory. *Neuropsychologia, 37,* 1189–1199.

Denckla, M. B. (1985). Motor proficiency in dyslexic children with and without attentional disorders. *Archives of Neurology, 42,* 228–231.

Denckla, M. B. (1989). Executive function, the overlap zone between attention deficit hyperactivity disorder and learning disabilities. *International Pediatrics, 4,* 155–160.

De Renzi, E., & Nichelli, P. (1975). Verbal and nonverbal short-term memory impairment following hemispheric damage. *Cortex, 11,* 341–354.

D'Esposito, M., Detre, J., Alsop, D., Shin, R., Atlas, S., & Grossman, M. (1995). The neural basis of the central executive system of working memory. *Nature, 378,* 279–281.

De Wolfe, N. A., Byrne, J. M., & Bawden, H. N. (1999). Early clinical assessment of attention. *The Clinical Neuropsychologist, 13,* 458–473.

Dougherty, D. M. (1999). *IMT/DMT, Immediate Memory Task and Delayed Memory Task: A research tool for studying attention and memory processes.* Houston, TX: The University of Texas Health Science Center at Houston.

Drachman, D. A., & Leavitt, J. (1974). Human memory and the cholinergic system. *Archives of Neurology, 30,* 113–121.

DuPaul, G. J. (1991). Parent and teacher ratings of ADHD symptoms: Psychometric properties in a community based sample. *Journal of Clinical and Child Psychology, 20,* 243–253.

DuPaul, G. J., Anastopoulos, A. D., Shelton, T. L., Guevremont, D. C., & Metevia, L. (1992). Multimethod assessment of attention deficit hyperactivity disorder: The diagnostic utility of clinic-based tests. *Journal of Clinical Child Psychology, 21,* 394–402.

DuPaul, G. J., Power, T. J., Anastopoulos, A. D., & Reid, R. (1998). *ADHD Rating Scale-IV.* New York: Guilford Press.

Ewing-Cobbs, L. (1998). Attention after pediatric traumatic brain injury: A multidimensional assessment. *Child Neuropsychology, 4,* 35–48.

Fernandez-Duque, D., & Posner, M. I. (2001). Brain imaging of attentional networks in normal and pathological states. *Journal of Clinical and Experimental Neuropsychology, 23,* 74–93.

Filipek, P., Semrud-Clikeman, M., Steingard, R. J., Benshaw, P. F., Kennedy, D. N., & Biederman, J. (1997). Volumetric MRI analysis comparing attention-deficit hyperactivity disorder and normal controls. *Neurology, 48,* 589–601.

Findeis, M. K., & Weight, D. G. (1993). *Meta-norms for Indiana-Reitan Neuropsychological Test Battery and Halstead-Reitan Neuropsychologial Test Battery for Children, ages 5–14.* Unpublished manuscript.

Fitzhugh, K. B., Fitzhugh, L. C., & Reitan, R. (1963). Effects of "chronic" and "current" lateralized and non-lateralized cerebral lesions upon Trail Making Test performance. *Journal of Nervous and Mental Disease, 137*, 82–87.

Fletcher, J. (1998). Attention in children: Conceptual and methodological issues. *Child Neuropsychology, 4*, 81–86.

Forbes, G. (1998). Clinical utility of the Test of Variables of Attention in the diagnosis of attention-deficit/hyperactivity disorder. *Journal of Clinical Psychology, 54*, 461–476.

Fromm-Auch, D., & Yeudall, L. T. (1983). Normative data for the Halstead-Reitan Neuropsychological Tests. *Journal of Clinical Neuropsychology, 5*, 221–238.

Fuster, J. M. (1989). *The prefrontal cortex: Anatomy, physiology and neuropsychology of the frontal lobe* (2nd ed.). New York: Raven Press.

Gaudino, E. A., Geisler, M. W., & Squires, N. K. (1995). Construct validity in the Trail Making Test: What makes Part B harder? *Journal of Clinical and Experimental Neuropsychology, 17*, 529–535.

Gendolla, G. H. E., Abele, A., & Krüsken, J. (2001). The informational impact of mood on effort mobilization: A study of cardiovascular and electrodermal responses. *Emotion, 1*, 12–24.

Georgiou, N., Bradshaw, J. L., Phillips, J. G., & Chiu, E. (1996). The effect of Huntington's disease and Gilles de la Tourette's syndrome on the ability to hold and shift attention. *Neuropsychologia, 34*, 843–851.

Giedd, J. N., Castellanos, F. X., Casey, B. J., Eckburg, P., & Marsh, W. I. (1994). Qualitative morphology of the corpus callosum in attention deficit hyperactivity disorder. *American Journal of Psychiatry, 151*, 665–669.

Gioia, G. A., Isquith, P. K., Guy, S. C., & Kenworthy, L. (2000). *Behavior Rating Inventory of Executive Function*. Odessa, FL: Psychological Assessment Resources, Inc.

Golden, C. J. (1981b). A standardized version of Luria's neuropsychological tests. In S. Filskov & T. Boll (Eds.), *Handbook of Clinical Neuropsychology*. New York: Wiley-Interscience.

Gordon, M. (1983). *The Gordon Diagnostic System*. DeWitt, NY: Gordon Systems.

Gordon, M., & Barkley, R. A. (1990). Tests and Observational Measures. In R. Barkley (Ed.), *Attention Deficit Hyperactivity Disorder: A Handbook for Diagnosis and Treatment* (pp. Chapter 9). New York: Guilford Press.

Gordon, M., McClure, F. D., & Aylward, G. P. (1996). *Gordon Diagnostic System interpretive guide* (3rd ed.). DeWitt, NY: GSI Publications.

Greenberg, L. M. (1996). *Tests of Variables of Attention*. St. Paul, MN: Attention Technology, Inc.

Greenberg, L. M., & Waldman, I. D. (1993). Developmental normative data on the Test of Variables of Attention (T.O.V.A.). *Journal of Child Pschology and Psychiatry, 34*, 1019–1030.

Gronwall, D. (1977). Paced Auditory Serial-Addition Task: A measure of recovery from concussion. *Perceptual and Motor Skills, 44*, 367–373.

Gronwall, D., & Sampson, H. (1974). *The Psychological Effects of Concussion*. Auckland, NZ: Auckland University Press/Oxford University Press.

Gronwall, D., & Wrightson, P. (1981). Memory and information processing capacity after closed head injury. *Journal of Neurology, Neurosurgery and Psychiatry, 44*, 889–895.

Grossi, D., Matarese, V., & Orsini, A. (1980). Sex differences in adults' spatial and verbal memory span. *Cortex, 15*, 339–340.

Grossi, D., Orsini, A., Monetti, C., & De Michele, G. (1979). Sex differences in children's spatial and verbal memory span. *COrtex, 15*, 667–670.

Halperin, J. M., Sharma, V., Greenblatt, E., & Schwartz, S. T. (1991). Assessment of the Continuous Performance Test: Reliability and validity in a nonreferred sample. *Psychological Assessment, 3*, 603–608.

Halperin, J. M., Wolf, L. E., Pascualvaca, D. M., Newcorn, J. H., Healey, J. M., O'Brien, J. D., et al. (1988). Differential assessment of attention and impulsivity in children. *Journal of the American Academy of Child and Adolescent Psychiatry, 27*, 326–329.

Halstead, W. C. (1947). *Brain and Intelligence*. Chicago, IL: University of Chicago Press.

Hamsher, K. d., Benton, A., & Digre, K. (1980). Serial digit learning: Normative and clinical aspects. *Journal of Clinical Neuropsychology, 2*, 39–50.

Hansen, D. E., & Vandenberg, B. (1997). Neuropsychological features and differential diagnosis of sleep apnea syndrome in children. *Journal of Clinical and Child Psychology, 26*, 304–310.

Harris, E. L., Singer, H. S., Reader, M. J., Brown, J., Cox, C., Mohr, J., et al. (1995). Executive function in children with Tourette syndrome and/or attention deficit hyperactivity disorder. *Journal of the International Neuropsychological Society, 1*, 511–516.

Harter, M. R., Anello-Vento, L., Wood, F. B., & Schroeder, M. M. (1988). Separate brain potential characteristics in children with reading disability and attention deficit disorder. *Brain and Cognition, 7*, 115–140.

Heaton, R. K., Grant, I., & Matthews, C. G. (1986). Differences in neuropsycholgical test performance asociated with age, education, and sex. In I. Grant & K. M. Adams (Eds.), *Neuropsychologial assessment of neuropsychiatric disorders (pp. 100–120). New York: Oxford University Press.

Heaton, S., Reader, S. K., Preston, A. S., Fennell, E. B., Puyana, O. E., Gill, N., et al. (2001). The Test of Everyday Attention for Children (TEA-Ch): Patterns of performance in children with ADHD and clinical controls. Child Neuropsychology, 7, 251–264.

Hebb, D. O. (1961). Distinctive features of learning in the higher animals. In J. F. Delafresnaye (Ed.), Brain Mechanisms and Learning. London: Oxford University Press.

Heilman, K. M., Voeller, K. K. S., & Nadeau, S. E. (1991). A possible pathophysiological substrate of attention deficit hyperactivity disorder. Journal of Child Neurology, 6, 76–81.

Heilman, K. M., Watson, R. T., Valenstein, E., & Goldberg, M. (1988). Attention: Behavior and neural mechanisms. Attention, II (461–481).

Helland, T., & Asbjørnsen, A. (2000). Executive functions in dyslexia. Child Neuropsychology, 6, 37–48.

Heubrock, D. (1999). Subjective organization of verbal memory and learning in adolescents with brain damage. Child Neuropsychology, 5, 24–33.

Hitch, G. J., & Halliday, M. S. (1983). Working memory in children. Philosophical Transactions of the Royal Society of London, 302, 325–340.

Hooks, K., Milich, R., & Lorch, E. (1994). Sustained and selective attention in boys with attention deficit hyperactivity disorder. Journal of Clinical and Child Psychology, 23, 69–77.

Hoppe, C., Müller, U., Werheid, K., Thöne, A., & von Cramon, D. Y. (2000). Digit Ordering Test: Clinical, psychometric, and experimental evaluation of a verbal working memory test. The Clinical Neuropsychologist, 14, 38–55.

Iverson, G. L., & Franzen, M. D. (1994). The Recognition Memory Test, Digit Span, and Knox Cube Test as markers of malingered memory impairment. Assessment, 1, 323–334.

Jarrold, C., Baddeley, A., & Hewes, A. K. (1999). Genetically dissociated components of working memory: Evidence from Downs and Williams syndrome. Neuropsychologia, 37, 637–651.

Johnson, D. A., Roethig-Johnston, K., & Middleton, J. (1988). Development and evaluation of an attentional test for head injured children. I. Information processing capacity in a normal sample. Journal of Child Psychology and Psychiatry, 29, 199–208.

Keith, R. W. (1994). Auditory Continuous Performance Test Examiner's Manual. New York: Harcourt Brace & Company.

Kelly, T. (2000). The development of executive function in school-aged children. Clinical Neuropsychological Asessment, 1, 38–55.

Kennedy, K. J. (1981). Age effects on Trail Making Test performance. Perceptual and Motor Skills, 52, 671–675.

Kinsbourne, M., & Cook, L. (1971). Generalized effects of concurrent verbalization on a unimanual skill. Quarterly Journal of Experimental Psychology, 23, 341–345.

Kinsbourne, M., & Hicks, R. E. (1978). Functional cerebral space: A model for overflow, transfer and interference effects in human performance. In J. Requin (Ed.), Attention and Performance VII (pp. 345–362). New York: Academic Press.

Kinsella, G. (1998). Assessment of attention following traumatic brain injury: A review. Neuropsychological Rehabilitation, 8, 351–375.

Knights, R. M. (1966). Normative data on tests evaluating brain damage in children 5–14 years of age. Research Bulletin No. 20. London, Ontario: Department of Psychology, University of Western Ontario.

Knox, H. A. (1914). Mental defectives. New York Medical Journal, 99, 215–222.

Lamberty, G. J., Putnam, S. H., Chatel, D. M., Bieliauskas, L. A., & Adams, K. M. (1994). Derived Trail Making Test indices: A preliminary report. Neuropsychiatry, Neuropsychology, and Behavioral Neurology, 7, 230–234.

Larrabee, G. J. (2000). Association between IQ and neuropsychological test performance: commentary on Tremont, Hoffman, Scott and Adams (1998). The Clinical Neuropsychologist, 14, 139–145.

Larrabee, G. J., & Curtiss, G. (1995). Construct validity of various verbal and visual memory tests. Journal of Clinical & Experimental Neuropsychology, 17, 536–547.

Lee, T. M. C., & Chan, C. C. H. (2000). Are Trail Making and Color Trails tests of equivalent constructs? Journal of Clinical and Experimental Neuropsychology, 22, 529–534.

Lee, T. M. C., Cheung, C. C. Y., Chan, J. K. P., & Chan, C. C. H. (2000). Trail making across languages. Journal of Clinical and Experimental Neuropsychology, 22, 772–778.

Leng, N. R. C., & Parkin, A. (1995). The detection of exaggerated or simulated memory disorder by neuropsychological methods. Journal of Psychosomatic Medicine, 39, 767–776.

Levin, H. S. (1986). Learning and Memory. In H. J. Hannay (Ed.), Experimental techniques in human neuropsychology (pp. 309–362). New York: Oxford University Press.

Lewin, J. S., Friedman, L., Wu, D., Miller, D. A., Thompson, L. A., Klein, S. K., et al. (1996). Cortical localization of human sustained attention:

Detection with functional MR using a visual vigilance paradigm. *Journal of Computer Assisted Tomography, 20,* 695–701.

Lezak, M. (1995). *Neuropsychological Assessment,* (3rd Edition). New York: Oxford University Press.

Lindgren, S. D., & Koeppl, G. K. (1987). Assessing child behavior problems in a medical setting: Development of the pediatric behavior scale. *Advances in Behavioral Assessment of Children and Families, 3,* 57–90.

Lockwood, K. A., Bell, T. S., & Colegrove, R. W. (1999). Long-term effects of cranial radiation therapy on attention functioning in survivors of childhood leukemia. *Journal of Pediatric Psychology, 24,* 55–66.

Lockwood, K. A., Marcotte, A. C., & Stern, C. (2001). Differentiation of Attention-Deficit/Hyperacitivy Disorder Subtypes: Application of a neuropsychological model of attention. *Journal of Clinical and Experimental Neuropsychology, 23,* 317–330.

Loring, D. (Ed.). (1999). *INS dictionary of neuropsychology.* New York: Oxford University Press.

Loss, N., Yeates, K. O., & Enrile, B. G. (1998). Attention in children with myelomeningocele. *Child Neuropsychology, 4,* 7–20.

Lou, H. C., Henricksen, L., & Bruhn, P. (1984). Focal cerebral hypoperfusion in children with hysphasia and/or attention deficit disorder. *Archives of Neurology, 46,* 48–52.

Mahone, E. M., Cirino, P. T., Cutting, L. E., Cerrone, P. M., Hagelthorn, K. M., Hiemenz, J. R., et al. (2002). Validity of the Behavior Rating Inventory of Executive Function in children with ADHD and/or Tourette syndrome. *Archives of Clinical Neuropsychology, 17,* 643–662.

Maj, M., D'Elia, L., Satz, P., Janssen, R., Zaudig, M., Uchiyama, C., et al. (1993). Evaluation of two new neuropsychological tests designed to minimize cultural bias in the assessment of HIV-1 seropositive persons: A WHO study. *Archives of Clinical Neuropsychology, 8,* 123–135.

Manly, T., Anderson, V., Nimmo-Smith, I., Turner, A., Watson, P., & Robertson, I. H. (2001). The differential assessment of children's attention: The Test of Everyday Attention for Children (TEA-Ch), normative sample and ADHD performance. *Journal of Child Psychology and Psychiatry, 42,* 1065–1081.

Manly, T., Robertson, I. H., Anderson, V., & Nimmo-Smith, I. (1999). *The Test of Everyday Attention for Children: Manual.* Bury St. Edmunds, UK: Thames Valley Test Company, Ltd.

Marcotte, A. C., Thacher, P. V., Butters, M., Bortz, J., Acebo, C., & Carskadon, M. A. (1998). Parental report of sleep problems in children with attentional and learning disorders. *Journal of Developmental and Behavioral Pediatrics, 19,* 178–186.

Mayes, S. D., Calhoun, S. L., & Crowell, E. W. (2001). Clinical validity and interpretation of the Gordon Diagnostic System in ADHD assessments. *Child Neuropsychology, 7,* 32–41.

Meichenbaum, D., & Goodman, J. (1971). Training impulsive children to talk to themselves: A means of developing self control. *Journal of Abnormal Psychology, 77,* 115–126.

Mesulam, M.-M. (1981). A cortical network for directed attention and unilateral neglect. *Annals of Neurology, 10,* 309–325.

Mesulam, M.-M. (1985). *Principles of behavioral neurology.* Philadelphia: F. A. Davis Co.

Mesulam, M.-M. (2000). *Principles of behavioral and cognitive neurology.* New York: Oxford University Press.

Miller, G. A. (1956). The magical number seven, plus or minus two: Some limits on our capacity for processing information. *Psychological Review, 63,* 81–97.

Milner, B. (1971). Interhemispheric differences in localization of psychological processes in man. *British Medical Bulletin, 27,* 272–277.

Mirsky, A. (1996). Disorders of attention: A neuropsychological perspective. In G. R. Lyon & N. A. Krasnegor (Eds.), *Attention, memory, and executive function.* Baltimore, MD: Paul H. Brookes.

Mirsky, A. F., Anthony, B. J., Duncan, C. C., Ahearn, M. B., & Kellam, S. G. (1991). Analysis of the elements of attention: A neuropsychological approach. *Neuropsychology Review, 2,* 109–145.

Munir, F., Cornish, K., & Wilding, J. (2000). A neuropsychological profile of attention deficits in young males with fragile X syndrome. *Neuropsychologia, 38,* 1261–1270.

Murphy-Berman, V. A., & Wright, G. (1987). Measures of attention. *Perceptual and Motor Skills, 64,* 1139–1143.

Naglieri, J., & Das, J. P. (1997). *Das-Naglieri: Cognitive assessment system.* Itasca, IL: Riverside.

National Institutes of Health Consensus Development Conference. (1998). *Diagnosis and treatment of attention deficit hyperactivity disorder* (Vol. 16, pp. 1–37). Bethesda, MD: National Institutes of Health/Foundation for Advanced Education in the Sciences.

Orsini, A., Grossi, D., Capitani, E., Laiacona, M., Papagno, C., & Vallar, G. (1987). Verbal and spatial immediate memory span: Normative data from 1355 adults and 1112 children. *Italian Journal of Neurological Sciences, 8,* 539–548.

Orsini, A., Schiappa, O., & Grossi, D. (1981). Sex and cultural differences in children's spatial and

verbal memory span. *Perceptual and Motor Skills,
53,* 39–42.

Paniak, C. E., Miller, H. B., Murphy, D., Andrews,
A., & Flynn, J. (1997). Consonants Trigrams Test
for children: Development and norms. *The Clinical Neuropsychologist, 11,* 198–200.

Pardo, J. V., Pardo, P., Janer, K., & Raichle, M. E.
(1991). Localization of a human system for sustained attention by positron emission tomography.
Nature, 349, 61–64.

Partington, J., & Leiter, R. (1949). Partington's Pathways Test. *Psychological Service Center Bulletin,
1,* 11–20.

Pediatrics, A. A. o. (2001). Clinical Practice Guideline: Treatment of the school-aged child with at-
tention-deficit/hyperactivity disorder. *Pediatrics,
108,* 1033–1044.

Pennington, B. F. (1997). Dimensions of executive
functions in normal and abnormal development.
In N. A. Krasnegor, G. R. Lyon & P. S. Goldman-
Rakic (Eds.), *Development of the prefrontal cortex: Evolution, neurobiology and behavior* (pp.
265–281). Baltimore, MD: Paul H. Brookes.

Petersen, S. E., Robinson, D. L., & Morris, J. D.
(1987). Contributions of the pulvinar to visual spatial attention. *Neuropsychologia, 25,* 97–105.

Peterson, L. R., & Peterson, M. J. (1959). Short-
term retention of individual verbal items. *Journal
of Experimental Psychology, 58,* 193–198.

Pintner, R., & Paterson, D. G. (1917). *A scale of performance tests.* New York: Appleton.

Pontius, A., & Yudowitz, B. (1980). Frontal lobe system dysfunction in some criminal actions shown
in the Narratives Test. *The Journal of Nervous and
Mental Disease, 168,* 111–117.

Posner, M. I., Walker, J. A., Friedrich, F. J., & Rafal,
R. D. (1984). Effects of parietal injury on covert
orienting of attention. *Journal of Neuroscience, 4,*
1863–1874.

Posner, M. I., & Peterson, S. E. (1990). The attention system of the human brain. *Annual Review
of Neuroscience, 13,* 25–42.

Posner, M. I., Walker, J. A., Friedrich, F. J., & Rafal,
R. D. (1987). How do the parietal lobes direct
covert attention? *Neuropsychologia, 25,* 135–145.

Prather, P. A., Sarmento, N., & Alexander, A. (1995).
Development of vigilance in preschoolers. *Journal of the International Neuropsychological Society, 1,* 153.

Pribram, K. H., & McGuinness, D. (1975). Arousal,
activation, and effort in the control of attention.
Psychological Review, 82, 116–149.

Reitan, R. (1958). The validity of the Trail Making
Test as an indication of organic brain damage. *Perceptual and Motor Skills, 8,* 271–276.

Reitan, R. (1971). Trail Making Test results for normal and brain-damaged children. *Perceptual and
Motor Skills, 33,* 575–581.

Reitan, R., & Davison, L. (1974). *Clinical neuropsychology: Current status and applications.* New
York: Hemisphere.

Reitan, R., & Tarshes, E. L. (1959). Differential effects of lateralized brain lesions on the Trail Making Test. *Journal of Nervous and Mental Disease,
129,* 257–262.

Reitan, R., & Wolfson, D. (1993). *The Halstead-
Reitan Neuropsychological Test Battery: Theory
and clinical interpretation.* Tucson, AZ: Neuropsychology Press.

Reynolds, C. R., & Kamphaus, R. W. (1992). *Behavior Assessment System for Children.* Circle
Pines, MN: American Guidance Service.

Reynolds, C. R., & Kamphaus, R. W. (1998a).
*Behavior Assessment System for Children. Parent
Rating Scale.* Circle Pines, MN: American Guid-
ance Services, Inc.

Reynolds, C. R., & Kamphaus, R. W. (1998b). *Behavior Assessment System for Children. Self-
report Version.* Circle Pines, MN: American
Guidance Services, Inc.

Riccio, C. A., Reynolds, C. R., & Lowe, P. A. (2001).
*Clinical Applications of Continuous Performance
Tests: Measuring attention and impulsive re-
sponding in children and adolescents.* New York:
John Wiley & Sons, Inc.

Robertson, I. H., Tegner, R., Tham, K., Lo, A., &
Nimmo-Smith, I. (1995). Sustained attention
training for unilateral neglect: Theoretical and rehabilitation implications. *Journal of Clinical and
Experimental Neuropsychology, 17,* 416–430.

Robertson, I. H., Ward, A., Ridgeway, V., & Nimmo-
Smith, I. (1995). *Test of Everyday Attention.* Bury
St. Edmunds, UK: Thames Valley Test Company,
Ltd.

Roman, D. D., Edwall, G. E., Buchanan, R. J., &
Patton, J. H. (1991). Extended norms for the
Paced Serial Addition Task. *The Clinical Neu-
ropsychologist, 5,* 33–40.

Rosvold, H., Mirsky, A., Sarason, I., Bransome, E.,
& Beck, L. (1956). A continuous performance test
for brain damage. *Journal of Clinical and Consulting Psychology, 20,* 343–350.

Rourke, B. P., & Orr, R. R. (1977). Prediction of the
reading and spelling performances of normal and
retarded readers: A four-year follow-up. *Journal
of Abnormal Child Psychology, 5,* 9–20.

Rudel, R., & Denckla, M. B. (1974). Relationship of
forward and backward digit repetition to neurological impairment in children with learning disabilities. *Neuropsychologia, 12,* 109–118.

Rudel, R. G., Denckla, M. B., & Broman, M. (1978). Rapid silent response to repeated target symbols by dyslexic and nondyslexic children. *Brain and Language, 6,* 52–62.

Sampson, H. (1954). Correlations between performance on serial addition tests of general and arithmetical ability. *Cited in D. Gronwall and H. Sampson (1974).* The Psychological Effects of Concussion. Auckland, NZ: Auckland University Press/Oxford University Press.

Schreiber, D. J., Goldman, H., Kleinman, K. M., Goldfader, P. R., & Snow, M. Y. (1976). The relationship between independant neuropsychological and neurological detection of cerebral impairment. *Journal of Nervous and Mental Disease, 162,* 360–365.

Seidel, W. T., & Joschko, M. (1990). Evidence of difficulties in sustained attention in children with ADDH. *Journal of Abnormal Child Psychology, 18,* 217–229.

Seidel, W. T., & Joschko, M. (1991). Assessment of attention in children. *The Clinical Neuropsychologist, 5,* 53–66.

Semrud-Clikeman, M., & Wical, B. (1999). Components of attention in children with complex partial seizures with and without ADHD. *Epilepsia, 40,* 211–215.

Shapiro, M., Morris, R., Morris, M., Flowers, C., & Jones, R. (1998). A neuropsychologically based assessment model of the structure of attention in children. *Developmental Neuropsychology, 14,* 657–677.

Sherman, E. M. S., Strauss, E., & Spellacy, F. (1997). Validity of the Paced Auditory Serial Addition Test (PASAT) in adults referred for neuropsychological assessment after head injury. *The Clinical Neuropsychologist, 11,* 34–45.

Shucard, D. W., Benedict, R. H. B., Tekok-Kilic, A., & Lichter, D. G. (1997). Slowed reaction time during a continuous performance test in children with Tourette's syndrome. *Neuropsychology, 11,* 147–155.

Shue, K. L., & Douglas, V. I. (1992). Attention deficit hyperactivity disorder and the frontal lobe syndrome. *Brain and Cognition, 20,* 104–124.

Shum, D., McFarland, K., & Bain, J. (1990). Construct validity of eight tests of attention: Comparison of normal and closed head injured samples. *The Clinical Neuropsychologist, 4,* 151–162.

Skuse, D. H., James, R. S., Bishop, D. V. M., Coppin, B., Dalton, P., Aamodt-Leeper, G., et al. (1997). Evidence from Turner's syndrome of an imprinted X-linked locus affecting cognitive function. *Nature, 387,* 705–708.

Smith, A. (1973). *Symbol Digit Modalities Test.* Los Angeles, CA: Western Psychological Services.

Smith, A. (1982). *Symbol Digit Modalities Test (SDMT) Manual—Revised.* Los Angeles: Western Psychological Services.

Spreen, O., & Gaddes, W. H. (1969). Developmental Norms for 15 neuropsychological tests age 6 to 15. *Cortex, 5,* 171–191.

Spreen, O., & Strauss, E. (1998). *A compendium of neuropsychological tests: Adminstration, norms, and commentary* (2nd ed.). New York: Oxford University Press.

Stefanatos, G. A., & Wasserstein, J. (2001). Attention deficit/hyperactivity disorder as a right hemisphere syndrome: Selective literature review and detailed neuropsychological case studies. *Annals of the New York Academy of Sciences, 931,* 172–195.

Sternberg, R. J., & Tulving, E. (1977). The measurement of subjective organization in free recall. *Psychological Bulletin, 84,* 539–556.

Stuss, D. T., Stethem, L. L., Hugenholtz, H., Picton, T. W., Pivik, J., & Richard, M. T. (1989). Reaction time after head injury: Fatigue, divided and focused attention and consistency of performance. *Journal of Neurology, Neurosurgery and Psychiatry, 79,* 81–90.

Stuss, D. T., Stethem, L. L., & Pelchat, G. (1988). Three tests of attention and rapid information processing: An extension. *The Clinical Neuropsychologist, 2,* 246–250.

Stuss, D. T., Stethem, L. L., & Poirier, C. A. (1987). Comparison of three tests of attention and rapid information processing across six age groups. *The Clinical Neuropsychologist, 1,* 139–152.

Swanson, J., Posner, M. I., Cantwell, D., Wigal, S., Crinella, F., Filipek, P., et al. (1998). Attention-deficit/hyperactivity disorder: Symptom domains, cognitive processes and neural networks. In R. Parasuraman (Ed.), *The attentive brain* (pp. 445–460). Cambridge, MA: The MIT Press.

Taylor, H. G., Barry, C. T., & Schatschneider, C. (1993). School-age consequences of Haemophilus influenzae Type b meningitis. *Journal of Clinical Child Psychology, 22,* 196–206.

Thorstad, K. G., Fletcher, J. M., Andrews, J., & Morris, R. Verbal and Nonverbal Cancellation Tests for Children. Unpublished manuscript.

Tulving, E. (1962). Subjective organization in free recall of "unrelated words". *Psychological Review, 69,* 344–354.

Vallar, G., & Baddeley, A. (1984). Fractionation of working memory: Neuropsychological evidence for a phonological short-term store. *Journal of Verbal Learning and Verbal Behavior, 23,* 151–161.

van der Meere, J., & Sergent, J. (1988). Controlled processing and vigilance in hyperactivity: Time will tell. *Journal of Abnormal Child Psychology, 16,* 641–656.

Villella, S., Anderson, J., Anderson, V., Robertson, I. H., & Manly, T. (in press). Sustained and selective attention in children with Attention Deficit/Hyperactivity Disorder and Specific Learning Disabilites. *Clinical Neuropsychological Asessment.*

Weiler, M. D., Bellinger, D., Marmor, J., Rancier, S. A., & Waber, D. P. (1999). Mother and teacher reports of ADHD symptoms: DSM-IV questionnaire data. *Journal of the American Academy of Child and Adolescent Psychiatry, 38,* 1139–1147.

Weiler, M. D., Bellinger, D., SImmons, E., Rappaport, L., Urion, D., Mitchell, W., et al. (2000). Reliability and validity of a DSM-IV based ADHD screener. *Child Neuropsychology, 6,* 3–23.

Weiler, M. D., Bernstein, J. H., Bellinger, D., & Waber, D. P. (2000). Processing speed in children with Attention Deficit/Hyperactivity Disorder, Inattentive Type. *Child Neuropsychology, 6,* 218–234.

Weinberg, J., Diller, L., Gerstman, L., & Schulman, P. (1972). Digit span in right and left hemiplegics. *Journal of Clinical Psychology, 28,* 361.

Weintraub, S., & Mesulam, M.-M. (1985). Mental state assessment of young and elderly adults in behavioral neurology. In M.-M. Mesulam (Ed.), *Principles of behavioral neurology* (pp. 71–123). Philadelphia: F. A. Davis.

Weintraub, S., & Mesulam, M.-M. (1987). Right cerebral dominance in spatial attention: Further evidence based on ipsilateral neglect. *Archives of Neurology, 44,* 621–625.

Wheeler, L., & Reitan, R. (1963). Discriminant functions applied to the problem of predicting cerebral damage from behavioral tests: A cross validation study. *Perceptual and Motor Skills, 16,* 681–701.

Wiens, A. N., Fuller, K. H., & Crossen, J. R. (1997). Paced Auditory Serial Addition Test: Adult norms and moderator variables. *Journal of Clinical & Experimental Neuropsychology, 19,* 473–483.

Wilkins, A. J., Shallice, T., & McCarthy, R. (1987). Frontal lesions and sustained attention. *Neuropsychologia, 25,* 359–365.

Williams, J., Rickert, V., Hogan, J., Zolten, A., Satz, P., D'Elia, L., et al. (1995). Children's Color Trails. *Archives of Clinical Neuropsychology, 10,* 211–223.

Yeates, K. O., & Bornstein, R. A. (1992). Attention deficit disorder and neuropsychological performance in children with Tourette's syndrome. *Journal of Clinical and Experimental Neuropsychology, 14,* 109.

Zametkin, A., Liebenauer, L. L., Fitzgerald, G. A., King, A. C., Minkunas, D. V., Herscovitch, P., et al. (1993). Brain metabolism in teenagers with attention-deficit hyperactivity disorder. *Archives of General Psychiatry, 50,* 333–340.

Zametkin, A., Nordahl, T., Gross, M., King, A. C., Semple, W. E., Rumsey, J., et al. (1990). Cerebral glucose metabolism in adults with hyperactivity of childhood onset. *New England Journal of Medicine, 323,* 1361–1366.

Zangwill, O. L. (1943). Clinical tests on memory impairments. *Proceedings of the Royal Society of Medicine, 36,* 576.

8

Language

A suspicion that a child has a language impairment is one of the most frequent reasons a neuropsychological evaluation is requested in the outpatient setting. It may emerge as a concern when a young child fails to master the usual language developmental milestones consistent with expectation for chronological age or when a language-learning disability is suspected for a school-age child. Manifestation of language impairment may be an immediate concomitant of a traumatic brain injury; the aphasia may be prominent in the acute stages, but often is a transient phenomenon that may evolve into a subtle deficit or become part of a complex neurobehavioral profile. Thus, an inpatient referral is often made in the presence of such overt impairment. Further, language impairment in a child may often resolve faster and more completely after acute injury than would be observed in an adult. For example, an anomia or expressive aphasia following injury may disappear within days, while other residual language deficits may persist far longer. Thus, there needs to be conscientious investigation of the possibility that a subtle linguistic deficit may persist, one that may complicate the child's readjustment to the academic setting's demands.

Even observant adults, looking for reasons why a child experiences delayed academic achievement or failure in a highly verbal academic setting, might miss the clues that signal a persisting, acquired language deficit, mild developmental language deficit, or language learning disability. Formal evaluation can be conducted to consider the range of etiological possibilities and highlight the most likely explanatory factor(s). It is also possible that an earlier precipitating incident is no longer consciously recalled by the parent. When the behavior emerges incompletely or is deficient at a later developmental stage, the etiology may be obscure, underscoring the need for careful history taking as one means of linking disparate incidents and exposures in the course of the child's developmental history.

There is a distinction between speech and language. Speech is the mechanical aspect of oral communication. Language refers to the communication of meaningful symbols (Benson and Ardila, 1996). The speech and language portion of a neuropsychological evaluation generally includes screening of the following components: conversational fluency, phonological processing, generative fluency, comprehension, repetition, naming, reading, writing, spelling, calculation, and praxis. Initially, engaging the child or adolescent in discussion about non-test matters is useful in evaluating his or her spontaneous speech characteristics, such as fluency or fluidity of word usage in meaningful speech, articulation and clarity, rate and rhythm, prosody or intonation, grammar or syntax, level of vocabulary sophistication, length of utterances, and comprehension.

Qualitative features of the child's linguistic skill are important to observe and to inquire about. Some abnormal features have a higher likelihood of being present than others. For example, paraphasias are commonly observed in adults with acquired language deficit, but these are rarely observed in childhood. Impaired word finding, dyscalculia, or impaired written formulation are far more likely to be evident and to be signs of acquired abnormality. It is therefore important to confirm with parents whether the observed and worrisome errors noted during testing are indeed characteristic behaviors for their child. It is important to establish that what was observed was not a function of shyness, fearfulness, stranger anxiety, or deliberate manipulative and elective action taken to control the immediate testing situation.

Any need for the examiner to change voice volume while engaged in conversation with the child or to repeat directions should be noted. The former may suggest a hearing impairment, and the latter may be a marker of an auditory comprehension deficit. Special consideration is necessary for language testing and interpretation when there is a known or suspected hearing impairment, when expressive language is immature or inconsistent with the child's chronological age, when there is a documented receptive or production deficit, or when English is not the child's first or primary home language. Results from tests that do not require explicit verbal responses are usefully compared with results from those that do assess expressive language in order to obtain a better understanding of the child's relative efficiency with speech and language function. These competencies can then be further compared with the test results from other cognitive domains that may confound results. Initial screening measures that detect potential problematic function require formal follow-up evaluation with more detailed instruments, including nonlanguage testing for dyspraxia and agnosia, perceptual dysfunction, and personality and mood.

Documentation of a language deficit should not automatically lead one to suppose the abnormality is due to dysfunction in the language-dominant hemisphere since other explanations are entirely possible. An analysis of test structure-function relationship is required at an individual level to determine the likely correct etiology. The underlying deficit may be due to impairment in brain regions not usually directly intimated as mediating language, such as

in the presence of associated prominent visuospatial dysfunction. For example, a specific deficit in verbal-spatial function can be documented in individuals who otherwise have generally intact language. Williams syndrome is a genetic syndrome of neurological maldevelopment characterized by excellent language ability (Bellugi, Bihrle et al., 1990). Despite this proficiency, children with Williams syndrome have difficulty processing sentences involving spatial syntactic forms such as "inside" and "outside" or "above" and "below" (Baddeley, 2001), highlighting a need to consider the extended range of contributory deficits that may be reflected in overt language dysfunction in the individual child.

Ambidexterity or ambiguous handedness may affect suppositions of the usual left hemisphere language mediation for right handers (see Chapter 9). Family history is also highly relevant. The implications of poor handwriting and language delay for a young boy whose family has a strong history of left-handedness in immediate family members may be different than for a child without such a history. Scrutiny of each test's factor structure for all possible contributory reasons for a poorer than expected performance is necessary since tests often rely on multiple factors for successful performance. Which of these has the most salience for the particular child under evaluation may be misleading or cryptic in individual cases. Profile analysis of language behavior is also useful in considering the differential diagnostic possibilities. For example, comprehension deficits and language formulation deficit, without impaired single-word production, may characterize the language profile of the autistic child. Yet, prosody (vocal intonation that may change a word's literal meaning) and pragmatic language may be impaired for both children with autism and those with Asperger's syndrome.

A long history of study of brain-injured individuals, through case analysis or with clinical population groups, continues and elaborates on the intricate cortical and subcortical contributions to intact and dysfunctional language. The thalamus, basal ganglia, and afferent tracts to auditory speech regions are characteristically implicated in the presence of signs of subcortical aphasia, whereas specific cortical regions and underlying white matter tracts are long established as crucial for intact language function. Functional neuroimaging studies of language after focal brain injury contribute to our expanding knowledge of which cerebral regions are activated by different language tasks. (At least, these studies suggest that some of our long-held notions might need revision or re-evaluation.) Some of these notions relate to the differences between how the child and adult brains adapt to interference. For example, children, younger than 5 years old when they incurred focal left hemisphere injury, organized language in homotopic areas of the unaffected right cerebral hemisphere (Müller, Rothermel et al., 1998; 1999; Booth, Macwhinney et al., 1999). These data supported the notion of considerable opportunity for cerebral plasticity at very early ages, but this result would be unexpected with damage in adulthood.

Newer imaging techniques provide a means for us to appreciate the restructuring that occurs in a way that prior imaging techniques did not allow. A functional imaging study also revealed that there are multiple dispersed midbrain, cerebellar, cortical, and subcortical brain regions activated when reading (Shaywitz, Shaywitz et al., 1998), an intricate network visualized that highlights the functioning brain's interregional communication pattern. Yet, it is also apparent that the integrity of these underlying and interconnected pathways for reading must be concomitant with rapid processing rates, an "automaticity" (LaBerge and Samuels, 1974; Wolf and O'Brien, 2001; Wolf, in press).

The range of available psychological, educational, and neuropsychological tests within the language domain is more extensive than can be reasonably summarized in one chapter. Further, these test instruments often have detailed accompanying manuals with extensive stratified normative data that exceed what is reasonable to reproduce here. A few of these many existent tests are noted below, but the reader is encouraged to explore these resources about speech and language development, dysfunction, assessment, and treatment further as they relate to his or her own clinical population and research interests. The tests mentioned in this chapter do not cover all aspects of a formal

speech and language evaluation, but they do present a representative range for functions routinely evaluated by child neuropsychologists, and, when possible, their normative data are included. These tests are discussed under the general categories of aphasia screening, phonological processing, naming, receptive and expressive vocabulary, and written formulation. Generative verbal fluency is discussed in Chapter 6, along with design fluency. Praxis is discussed in Chapter 9. Repetition of meaningful auditory/verbal information as assessed with sentence memory tests is included in Chapter 11.

APHASIA SCREENING TESTS AND LANGUAGE BATTERIES

Aphasia refers to an acquired impairment in symbolic linguistic processing that is not due to a perceptual disorder. Specific dysfunctional brain regions are associated with the presence of aphasia. Aphasia encompasses disorders of word retrieval, motor speech implementation, syntax and morphology, auditory comprehension, repetition, reading, and writing. Commonly, aphasia is classified broadly into subtypes, although the shortcomings of the syndrome approach are acknowledged (Goodglass, 1993). The following subtypes are described with their central defining features and typical brain localization, if applicable:

Broca's Aphasia—characterized by nonfluent speech, intact comprehension, impaired repetition, associated with a right hemiparesis and the left inferior posterior frontal lobe

Wernicke's Aphasia—characterized by fluent speech, impaired comprehension, impaired repetition, no motor signs, associated with the left superior posterior temporal lobe

Conduction Aphasia—characterized by fluent speech with articulation difficulty, intact comprehension, impaired repetition, associated with left auditory cortex and insula, the left supramarginal gyrus

Transcortical Motor Aphasia—characterized by nonfluent speech, intact comprehension, intact repetition, associated with disruption anterior or superior to, or including, Broca's region

Transcortical Sensory Aphasia—characterized by fluent speech, impaired comprehension, intact repetition, associated with regions posterior or inferior to Wernicke's area

Global Aphasia—characterized by limited speech, impaired comprehension, impaired repetition, with or without right hemiplegia, associated with the left perisylvian region with hemiplegia or separate frontal and temporoparietal lesions without hemiplegia

Anomic Aphasia—characterized by fluent speech, but with word-finding problems, especially for nouns, circumlocutory speech, associated with diverse lesions

Pure-modality, specific aphasias such as pure word-deafness, subcortical motor aphasia, and pure word blindness are also described. *Dysarthria,* an articulation disorder, is not appropriately classified as an aphasia. Among the many screening tests and formal speech and language test batteries are many commonly selected by child neuropsychologists, in whole or in part, to obtain direct information about receptive and expressive language. These are "screening" instruments, and any abnormal responses need to be thoroughly evaluated in context with what else is known about the child to determine the significance of the results. More specific tests may need to be conducted to appreciate better why the screening test error was made and to place the error in appropriate context, given the overall neurobehavioral profile. A discussion of these tests follows.

Halstead-Wepman Aphasia Screening Test

The Halstead-Wepman Aphasia Screening Test (Reitan and Heineman, 1968) is a widely used instrument that samples a number of receptive and expressive language functions. It is perhaps the most widely used as it was incorporated as part of the Halstead Reitan Neuropsychological Test Battery (HRNTB) in two age-based forms. The form for older children (9 to 14 years old) includes the following items: five naming, three oral spelling, two writing (of a word and a sentence), three multisyllabic word repetition, one sentence repetition, six number, letter, word, and sentence reading, three simple geometric shape copy, one skeleton key copy, two calculation (oral and written), and four comprehension of verbal instructions. A downward extension for younger children (5 to 8 years old) (Reitan and Heineman, 1968) includes four naming, two writing, three reading, three drawing, four calculation, four body orientation, and two right-left discrimination items.

This screening test can detect both acquired impairment and responses suggestive of language developmental delay. There are certain items that have particular salience. Using the older child version, oral and written spelling items enable comparison by modality and may provide evidence of a tendency toward producing letter reversal, letter sequencing, or rotational errors. Phonetic spelling errors are contrasted with dysphonetic errors, and one must determine whether the error is common or a marker of a more profound dysfunction for a child of that chronological age. With frequent administration of this task to many children, common misspellings are easily recognized and evaluated in relation to the child's chronological age or grade placement. More unusual errors will stand out as signs of a potentially fundamental problem requiring further investigation. The letter identification and reading items may highlight developmental delays in letter recognition or single-word and sentence reading, but this screening test does not assess reading for comprehension. It is necessary to administer one of the numerous academic achievement tests that more specifically assess such functioning.

When calculation problems are encountered with either the oral or written problem, it is useful to examine performance with a similar but simpler calculation. For example, if an older child incorrectly multiplies 17×3, I ask for the easier 6×3, or if $85 - 27$ is calculated incorrectly, I request a simpler double digit problem that does not involve carrying. Limited or constrained written production is often indicative of a general reluctance that accompanies a writing deficit. Erasures often underscore the child's intent to do well and to improve on a performance incompatible with the child's own expectations. Thus, one will interpret differently the motivation of a child who produces a poorly written sentence that remains uncorrected compared to a child who produces an equivalently incorrect sentence, but who then erases and deliberately attempts to improve the output. Whether the child succeeds or fails to make the needed correction will be useful adjunct information with respect to the difference between the visuomotor and linguistic components.

Aspects of the screening extend beyond linguistic features. For example, the geometric figure-copying items may reveal a tremulous line quality for the non-linguistic written production. Planning and organizational difficulties may be reflected in poor spacing, overlapping designs, or designs colliding with other written responses. There may be a failure to follow the three-part instructions—use a single line, keep the pencil on the page, make it about the same size—to maintain symmetry, or to close the drawing, or there may be evidence of rotational or reversal errors.

In instances where language dysfunction is suspected, it is useful to add additional items to refine the identified problem. With the young-child version, it is useful to ask for color naming (e.g., "What color is your shirt?" "What color is my book?"), oral and written alphabet production, and number recitation and writing as additional screening items. If a young child refuses to state the alphabet, I ask her to sing it and often find that this results in successful performance. Items from other tests may be included. The Comprehension of Oral Spelling and Phrase Repetition (for sentences with high and low word probability) subtests from the Boston Diagnostic Aphasia Examination (BDAE) are useful for older children. Also, selected subtests from the Multilingual Aphasia Examination (MAE), the Boston Naming Test (BNT), or one of the many available reading, writing, spelling, and arithmetic academic achievement subtests may be administered.

The Aphasia Screening Test requires experience for valid interpretation, especially since there is no useful "score" in routine use. Some scoring paradigms were proposed, principally for research purposes as the test (or parts selected) is most sensitive when there is flexibility in interpretation and recognition of the critical features that signal receptive or expressive language disturbance. It is possible to limit its administration to items that have the highest payoff, although the full test itself is relatively brief in its entirety. For a partial administration, the older-child form contains items that, in general, have the highest likelihood of detecting problems include the shape copying, naming, oral and written spelling, sentence reading ("He is a friendly animal, a famous winner of dog shows"), calculations, key drawing, and right–left orientation. The younger-child form is so brief that administration of all items is worthwhile.

Boston Diagnostic Aphasia Examination

The Boston Diagnostic Aphasia Examination (3rd ed.) (BDAE) (Goodglass and Kaplan, 1983; Goodglass, Kaplan et al., 2000) was developed for adults and is not especially useful in its entirety with children. However, it includes a number of subsections that do have practical clinical utility with children and adolescents. As noted above, Comprehension of Oral Spelling and Phrase Repetition are useful as gross screening items. The Paragraph Formulation task requires a child to respond to the "cookie theft picture," which is an appealing way to obtain an estimate of a child's ability to formulate thoughts and expressively communicate through written and oral channels. Whether the child restricts written language and prefers oral expression is often a helpful dichotomy to observe.

In contrast, the child who writes a considerable amount, but limits verbalization, provides useful clinical information about inherent motivation to do well and suggests the need for a more thorough investigation. This is accomplished in part through evaluation of the form, grammar, spelling, punctuation, capitalization, and emotional content of the written production, but it will also require formal testing of aspects of receptive and expressive language. The BDAE also recommends tests of constructional drawing, finger identification, clock drawing, directional orientation, and arithmetic screening as part of the Parietal Lobe Battery. All of these areas may be screened with more specific tests or in accord with other normative data sets, as detailed elsewhere in this book, and, of course, the influence of more anterior cerebral regions to successful selective performances on the "parietal" lobe tests is now well documented.

Spreen-Benton Aphasia Test, or Neurosensory Center Comprehensive Examination for Aphasia

The Spreen-Benton Aphasia Test for adults, also known as the Neurosensory Center Comprehensive Examination for Aphasia, (Spreen and Benton, 1977) includes 20 language subtests, along with four visual and tactile function tests (see Table 8–1). A linear developmental pattern was found in a study of 353 5- to 13-year-old children of "slightly above average intelligence" (Gaddes and Crockett, 1975). The authors concluded that the battery was generally discriminating for children between 6 and 8 or 9 years old, but less helpful for older children. Most subtests resulted in a premature "ceiling" at around age 9 or 10. This low-ceiling effect may obscure subtle linguistic-processing deficits. These authors found no gender differences for 11 of 20 subtests. When present, female superiority was generally transient or isolated. However, two subtests produced extended female superiority: word fluency at ages 9 to 13 and spelling written names at ages 7, 9, 10, and 11.

Multilingual Aphasia Examination

The Multilingual Aphasia Examination (MAE) includes nine subtests and two rating scales, the latter for articulation and writing praxis. The Visual Confrontation Naming subtest requires naming 30 pictures, ranging from easy to middle-level difficulty. The Sentence Repetition subtest requires repetition of 14 sentences from 3 to 16 words in length, terminated after four consecutive failures. There are two forms for this measure of immediate recall of linguistic information (see Chapter 11 for normative data). Two forms to measure Controlled Oral Word Association require word production for each of three letters (see Chapter 6 for normative data). The Oral, Written, and Block Spelling subtests each consist of 11 words in ascending order of difficulty. Each spelling test is terminated after three consecutive failures. These tests are administered to children in grade 4 or higher. The Token Test is an abbreviated 22-item version of the original (De Renzi and Vignolo, 1962), and there are two alternate forms (see below). The Aural Comprehension of Words and Phrases subtest requires a pointing response to all 18 items. The Reading Comprehension of Words and Phrases subtest requires a pointing response to a picture of printed words or phrases and is administered to children in grade 2 and above. It is terminated after four consecutive failures. Rating of Speech Articulation and Rating of Praxic Quality of Writing each have a 9-point scale (Benton and Hamsher, 1976; Benton and Hamsher, 1983a; Benton, Hamsher et al., 1994). Standardization was conducted with 265 children from rural areas or small towns in Iowa. Intelligence was assessed with the Peabody Picture Vocabulary Test-Revised, Form L, (PPVT-R) and children with standard scores between 80 and 120 were included. Children receiving special education services or diagnosed as learning disabled were excluded. The MAE Visual Confrontation Naming normative data are presented in Table 8–2.

Table 8–1. Spreen-Benton Aphasia Tests (Neurosensory Center Comprehensive Examination for Aphasia): Language Subtests

Visual Naming
Description of Use
Tactile Naming–Right Hand
Tactile Naming–Left Hand
Sentence Repetition
Repetition of Digits (Forward)
Reversal of Digits (Backward)
Word Fluency
Sentence Construction
Identification by Name
Indentification by Sentence (Token Test)
Oral Reading, Names
Oral Reading, Sentences
Reading Names for Meaning, Pointing
Reading Sentences for Meaning, Point
Visual-Graphic Naming
Writing Names
Writing to Dictation
Writing from Copy
Articulation

Table 8–2. Norms for MAE Visual Confrontation Naming

Age	N	Grade	Mean	SD
6.3	35	K	30.1	4.7
7.3	34	1	32.2	5.0
8.2	32	2	37.4	4.8
9.3	43	3	40.3	5.6
10.2	33	4	43.4	4.1
11.3	31	5	45.0	4.4
12.3	21	6	46.2	3.1

Source: Schum, Sivan and Benton (1989); © Swets & Zeitlinger.

Additional data were subsequently collected for 32 children in seventh grade (17 male, 15 female) and 33 in eighth grade (15 male, 18 female), and these previously unpublished data are presented in Table 8–3. Visual naming was highly correlated with IQ, and a high false positive rate was found in an inner city sample, making corrections necessary (Roberts and Hamsher, 1984).

Normative data for children in Kindergarten to Grade 6 for the MAE Token Test are presented in Table 8–41 and for grades 7 and 8 in Table 8–4. Reading comprehension normative data are presented in Table 8–5 for Grade 2 to Grade 6 and in Table 8–6 for Grades 7 and 8. Data for aural comprehension for children in Kindergarten to Grade 6 are presented in Table 8–7. Additional normative data for aural comprehension obtained for 65 seventh and eighth graders are presented in Table 8–8. Grade 4 to Grade 6 normative data for oral, written, and block spelling are presented in Table 8–9. Additional normative data for oral, written, and block spelling were obtained for 65 seventh and eighth graders, and these unpublished data are presented in Table 8–10. Other language screening tests may be appli-

Table 8–3. MAE Normative Data for Visual Naming: 7th and 8th Graders

Age	N	Grade	Mean	SD
13	32	7	44.19	5.26
14	33	8	46.97	5.81

Source: Unpublished data, courtesy of Steven Zorich and Kerry Hamsher.

Table 8–4. Normative Data for MAE Token Test: 7th and 8th Grade

Age	N	Grade	Mean	SD
13	32	7	43.41	0.84
14	33	8	43.64	0.55

Source: Unpublished data, courtesy of Steven Zorich and Kerry Hamsher.

cable for the reader's specific clinical populations. For example, the Western Aphasia Battery is intended for adolescents and adults and includes some items adapted from the BDAE as part of the assessment of spontaneous speech, naming, repetition and comprehension (Kertesz, 1982). An Aphasia Quotient may be computed.

PHONOLOGICAL PROCESSING

Phonological processing refers to "the use of phonological information (i.e., the sounds of one's language) in processing written and oral language" (Wagner and Torgeson, 1987, p. 197). *Phonological awareness,* one kind of phonological processing, refers to an individual's awareness of and access to the sound structure of oral language and an ability to recognize phonemes and segment the structure underlying spoken words. The linguistic units or phonemes provide the basis for constructing a vocabulary. Deficits in two other kinds of phonological processing, *phonological memory* and *rapid naming,* are commonly observed, along with poor phonological awareness, in children experiencing difficulty reading (Wag-

Table 8–5. Norms for MAE Reading Comprehension

Age	N	Grade	Mean	SD
8.2	32	2	12.3	2.4
9.3	43	3	13.9	1.8
10.2	33	4	15.2	1.4
11.3	31	5	16.5	1.3
12.3	21	6	16.6	1.0

Source: Schum, Sivan and Benton (1989); © Swets & Zeitlinger.

Table 8–6. Norms for MAE Reading Comprehension: 7th and 8th Grade

Age	N	Grade	Mean	SD
13	32	7	16.31	1.31
14	33	8	17.24	0.94

Source: Unpublished data, courtesy of Steven Zorich and Kerry Hamsher.

Table 8–8. Norms f⸍ 7th and 8th Grade

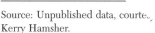

Age	N
13	32
14	33

Source: Unpublished data, courte⸍ Kerry Hamsher.

ner, Torgesen et al., 1999), and some of the tests assessing these capacities are described below or under the section, Naming.

The path from acoustic signal to phonetic level to phonological level is only briefly summarized here. Words are represented by waves of acoustic energy, and spectrographic analysis visually reveals the separation of words into distinct sounds, or phones. Our speech consists of strings of these basic language sounds, that is, phones that represent a combination of articulatory gestures. Related phones (*allophones*) are combined into groups of phonemes, or individual sound units. These phonemes represent differences in speech sounds that signal differences in meaning. Phonemes can be combined into onsets (initial consonant or consonant cluster of a syllable), rimes (remaining vowel and consonant or consonant cluster), syllables, or words. With maturation, children become more aware of smaller phonological units, from words, to syllables, to onsets and rimes (Wagner, Torgesen et al., 1999).

There are a number of commonly used tests of phonological processing. These appear especially useful in predicting who will eventually demonstrate a language learning disability, that is, a neuropsychological disorder charac-

terized by a specific processing problem (⸍ dman, Biederman et al., 2001). Such tests may assist in the identification of those who have developmental dyslexia since phonological processing is a precursor skill for how well a child will read and comprehend written language. Phonological processing is considered a core deficit for children unable to read successfully, that is, children with developmental dyslexia. In some models, speeded processing is considered but one core deficit; another is speeded naming. Proponents of the "double-deficit model" cite the importance of both of these core deficits in understanding reading acquisition failure (Wolf, Bowers et al., 2000). Reading fluency is integral to reading comprehension. Studies confirm that reading fluency, even pseudoword reading (reading pronounceable letter combinations), enables differentiating more capable from less capable readers (Siegel, 1992). Besides pseudoword reading, it is also useful to study lexical-decision, spelling, and peudoword-recognition tasks (Vandervelden and Siegel, 1996). Thus, dyslexia involves impairment in single-word reading, reading fluency, and reading comprehension, often the result of deficient phonological processing (Pennington, Grossier et al., 1993). Interestingly, bright, reading-disabled children achieved average reading levels in adulthood, but continued to exhibit weak phonological processing and rapid naming skills (Flowers, Wood et al., 1991). Current research suggests that dyslexia is not only a reading disability that is a result of phonological awareness weaknesses, but one that also includes time-and fluency-related deficits. Thus, children who are dyslexic are thought of as belonging to one of three categories: those with phonological deficits; those with naming speed and subsequent comprehension weaknesses without phonological is-

Table 8–7. Norms for MAE Aural Comprehension

Age	N	Grade	Mean	SD
6.3	35	K	12.3	1.8
7.3	34	1	12.3	1.6
8.2	32	2	13.7	1.7
9.3	43	3	13.7	1.6
10.2	33	4	14.7	1.8
11.3	31	5	15.6	1.6
12.3	21	6	15.6	1.6

Source: Schum, Sivan and Benton (1989); © Swets & Zeitlinger.

Table 8–9. Norms for MAE Oral, Written, Block Spelling

Age	N	Grade	OS Mean	OS *SD*	WS Mean	WS *SD*	BS Mean	WS *SD*
10.2	33	4	7.7	1.8	7.9	1.7	7.6	2.1
11.3	31	5	8.5	1.9	8.5	1.7	8.3	1.7
12.3	21	6	9.0	1.4	8.8	1.1	9.1	1.4

Source: Schum, Sivan and Benton (1989); © Swets & Zeitlinger.

sues; and those with both deficits, resulting in the most impaired reader. The latter category is the "double deficit."

There exists a group of children who do not have phonological awareness issues and, instead, have processing-rate and naming-speed weaknesses. The multiple components necessary for fluent reading are not fully integrated and automatic for these children. Consequently, they read text in a slow, dysfluent fashion that, in turn, negatively impacts their comprehension. It is likely that the reason traditional phonics reading intervention is not successful for these children is that fluency issues are not specifically addressed.

Studies of reading-disabled children with poor phonological memory who had a specific deficit in phonological coding of familiar verbal material, such as digits or words, found no impairment of short-term memory for nonverbal stimuli, long-term memory, or listening comprehension. Yet, these children had severe impairment in decoding visually presented nonsense syllables. Long-term follow-up found persisting memory impairment and no improvement in reading skill, and, as adults, the children with poor phonological memory had low Wechsler vocabulary scores but intact Wechsler block-design scores (Torgesen and

Houck, 1980; Torgesen, Rashotte et al., 1988; Torgesen, 1988; Torgesen, 1996).

Most phonological processing tests are normed on young children, and relatively few provide norms that extend into adolescence. Among measures assessing phonological processing are the Test of Phonological Awareness (Torgesen and Bryant, 1994), the NEPSY Phonological Awareness subtest (Korkman, Kirk et al., 1997), the Wepman's Auditory Discrimination Test (Reynolds, 1987), the Auditory Analysis Test (Rosner and Simon, 1971), and the Comprehensive Test of Phonological Processing (Wagner, Torgesen et al., 1999). The latter two are described below.

Auditory Analysis Test *no need for speed.*

The Auditory Analysis Test (AAT; Rosner and Simon, 1971) assesses how well a child can repeat a word after being told to eliminate certain sounds within that word, that is, omit phonemes or syllables. In this initial study, the test proved related to reading performance after controlling for IQ in a group of 284 elementary school children. The AAT has withstood the test of time for many clinicians, *for* myself included, as an indicator of potential language or reading impairment.

Table 8–10. Norms for MAE Oral, Written, Block Spelling: 7th and 8th Grades

Age	N	Grade	OS Mean	OS *SD*	WS Mean	WS *SD*	BS Mean	WS *SD*
13	32	7	8.53	1.41	8.91	1.35	8.16	1.59
14	33	8	8.76	1.68	9.30	1.49	9.03	1.85

Source: Unpublished data, courtesy of Steven Zorich and Kerry Hamsher.

Two demonstration test cards are presented as practice items. The first card has pictures of a cow and a boy. The child is asked to repeat "cowboy." After the child responds correctly, the picture of the boy is covered and the examiner says, "Now say it again, but without the boy," the correct answer being "cow." Similarly, pictures of a tooth and brush are presented next; the child is asked to say "toothbrush"; the tooth picture is covered, and the instruction given, "Say it again, but without the tooth"; the correct answer being "brush." The test proceeds if the child responds correctly for both demonstrations.

The child repeats each test word and then responds without the word part or sound indicated by the examiner. The portion to be omitted is indicated within parentheses on the examiner's record form. For example, item 1 is "birth(day)". The child first repeats "birthday" and then must say it without the "day," the correct response being "birth." Importantly, the sound(s) to be omitted are pronounced by the examiner, not the letter name. An articulation problem is not penalized. A second trial is allowed if the child does not respond the first time. The test is discontinued after four consecutive errors. There are 40 items, and one point is given for each correct response, for a maximum of 40. The test stimuli words are pre-

Table 8–11. Auditory Analysis Test: Stimulus Words

1. birth(day)	21. (sh)rug
2. (car)pet	22. g(l)ow
3. bel(t)	23. cr(e)ate
4. (m)an	24. (st)rain
5. (b)lock	25. s(m)ell
6. to(ne)	26. Es(ki)mo
7. (s)our	27. de(s)k
8. (p)ray	28. Ger(ma)ny
9. stea(k)	29. st(r)eam
10. (l)end	30. auto(mo)bile
11. (s)mile	31. re(pro)duce
12. plea(se)	32. s(m)ack
13. (g)ate	33. phi(lo)sophy
14. (c)lip	34. s(k)in
15. ti(me)	35. lo(ca)tion
16. (sc)old	36. cont(in)ent
17. (b)reak	37. s(w)ing
18. ro(de)	38. car(pen)ter
19. (w)ill	39. c(l)utter
20. (t)rail	40. off(er)ing

Table 8–12. Auditory Analysis Test Demographic Data: Rosner & Simon Study (1971)

Subjects: 284 suburban elementary school children in western Pennsylvania

Grade: Kindergarten through Grade 6

Gender: Male/female Ns not specified

Race: White

SES: Middle class

sented in Table 8–11. The demographic data for the AAT normative study are presented in Table 8–12. Normative data for Kindergarten through sixth grade were collected on 284 children and are presented in Table 8–13. The mean score for Kindergarten children was 3.5 ($SD = 3.5$). The number correct for first graders jumped to 17.6 ($SD = 8.4$) and increased gradually with sixth graders obtaining a mean of 29.9 ($SD = 6.9$).

A lowered score on the AAT for a child referred for poor academic performance is often an excellent indication that further investigation of language function will prove useful in delineating the etiology for the academic problems. The AAT can be a valuable screening tool for underlying linguistic deficit, making alternative behavioral (emotional) explanations, for example, less likely, although still requiring exploration. (See Appendix A in Chapter 3 for an example of this in an evaluation of an 8-year-old child with highly developed manipulative and interpersonal skills. This child's difficulty was also reflected in his spontaneous conversation, by comprehension errors for oral directions, and on academic achievement testing.)

Table 8–13. Auditory Analysis Test Normative Data: Raw Score Correct by Grade

Grade	N	Mean	SD	Median	Range
K	50	3.5	3.5	3.1	0–14
1	53	17.6	8.4	17.6	2–35
2	41	19.9	9.3	17.6	1–36
3	37	25.1	8.5	25.5	6–37
4	29	25.7	7.9	28.7	9–35
5	35	28.1	7.6	30.8	11–38
6	39	29.9	6.9	32.3	15–38

Source: Rosner and Simon (1971), courtesy of Sage Publishing.

The AAT served as a model and was modified for inclusion in a battery of tests of phonological processing, phonological memory, and rapid naming, the Comprehensive Test of Phonological Processing (CTOPP) Elision subtest (Wagner, Torgesen et al., 1999). This subtest is described below, following a brief description of the CTOPP.

Comprehensive Test of Phonological Processing

The Comprehensive Test of Phonological Processing (CTOPP; Wagner, Torgesen et al., 1999) is intended for ages 5 to 24. The authors list four principal uses: to identify those who are significantly below their peers in phonological abilities, to determine strengths and weaknesses among developed phonological processes, to document progress in phonological processing following specific intervention programs, and to serve as the measurement instrument for research studies investigating phonological processes. The demographic data for the normative sample are presented in Table 8–14. Norms are presented in standard scores, with a mean of 10 and a standard deviation of 3, and composite scores are based on a distribution having a mean of 100 and a standard deviation of 15. Percentiles are included for subtests and composite scores. Age and grade equivalents are provided, with appropriate cautions about their use.

Content sampling reliability study results found averaged coefficient alpha (a measure of

Table 8–14. CTOPP Demographic Data for School Age Population

Subjects: 1656 individuals from 30 states representing four major U.S. geographic regions; Northeast = 293, Midwest = 363, South = 566, West = 322

Age: 7 to 24 years. 1544 of these are school age, 5 to 17 years old.

Gender: 770 male; 774 female

Race: 1265 White, 212 Black, 67 Other

Ethnicity: 215 African American; 135 Hispanic; 48 Asian; 4 Native American; 1142 Other

Residence: 1203 Urban; 341 Rural

Income: 214 under $15,000; 237 $15,000–24,999; 264 $25,000–34,999; 356 $35,000–49,999; 307 $50,000–74,999; 166 $75,000 and over

Parent Education: 1056 less than Bachelor's degree; 356 Bachelor's degree; 132 Graduate degree

internal consistency) for the unspeeded subtests ranged from .77 to .90, averaged coefficient alphas for the composite scores ranged from .83 to .95, and all 69 coefficients that relate to the composite scores exceeded .80. Standard errors of measurement were low, supporting a high degree of test reliability. Subgroup alphas were studied for selected gender, racial, ethnic, and disability categories. Alphas are presented that indicate the CTOPP is about equally reliable for all groups and contains little or no bias toward these groups. Test–retest reliability calculations (over a 2-week interval) ranged from .68 to .95. Error due to test scorer variability was measured and ranged from .95 to .99.

There are well-documented validity studies for CTOPP's use as a measure of phonological processes presented in the manual, including confirmatory factor analysis for two age ranges (5–6 years and 7–24 years) that both support construct validity, that is, the factor structure matched the model on which it was based. Criterion concurrent and prediction validity were examined using the Woodcock Reading Mastery Tests (rev.) (Woodcock, 1987), Gray Oral Reading Tests (3rd ed.) (Wiederholt and Bryant, 1992), Wide Range Achievement Test (3rd ed.) (Wilkinson, 1995), Test of Word Reading Efficiency (Torgesen, Wagner et al., 1999), and Lindamood Auditory Conceptualization Test (Lindamood and Lindamood, 1971).

The 13 subtests of the CTOPP are:

Elision. 20-item variation of the 40-item AAT, requires statement of a word, and then restatement with a designated sound omitted (see below)

Blending Words. 20-items requiring combination of sounds to form real words

Sound Matching. 20 items; child points to picture that matches 10 items of beginning sounds and 10 items of ending sounds

Memory For Digits. 21-item standard digit repetition subtest with audiocasette recorded numbers presented at a rate of 2/second

Rapid Digit Naming. 72-item subtest assessing speed of naming randomly arranged numbers

Nonword Repetition. 18-item subtest requiring repetition of 3 to 15 sounds for nonwords played on an audiocasette recording[1]

Rapid Letter Naming. 72-item subtest assessing speed of naming randomly arranged letters

Rapid Color Naming. 72-item subtest assessing speed of naming printed colored blocks

Phoneme Reversal. 18-item subtest measuring the ability to reorder speech sounds presented as audiotaped nonwords to form real words

Rapid Object Naming. 72-item subtest assessing speed of naming objects.

Blending Nonwords. 18-item subtest requiring the combination of speech sounds presented by audiocassette recorder to make nonwords

Segmenting Words. 20-item subtest requiring statement of individual phonemes that comprise a word

Segmenting Nonwords. 20-item subtest assessing the ability to say separate phonemes that make up a nonword presented by audiocassette recorder

Five composite scores can be computed: Phonological Awareness, Phonological Memory, Rapid Naming, Alternate Phonological Awareness and Alternate Rapid Naming. Phonological Awareness and Phonological Memory scores are obtained for all individuals. Rapid color naming and rapid object naming together make up the Rapid Naming Composite for 5- and 6-year-olds, while rapid digit naming and rapid letter naming are used for the Rapid Naming Composite for 7 through 24 years old. For 5 to 6 years old, Elision, Blending Words, and Sound Matching result in the Phonological Awareness composite and Memory for Digits and Nonword Repetition result

in the Phonological Memory Composite. For 7 to 24 years old, Elision and Blending Words scores result in the Phonological Awareness composite, and Memory for Digits and Nonword Repetition scores result in the Phonological Memory Composite. The Alternate Phonological Awareness and Alternate Rapid Naming Composites are only obtained for those 7 to 24 years old. The former is based on Blending Nonwords and Segmenting Nonwords. The latter is based on Rapid Color Naming and Rapid Object Naming.

Comprehensive Test of Phonological Processing—Elision Subtest

The CTOPP Elision subtest consists of 20 test items, instead of 40 items as in the AAT. CTOPP normative data are available for 1656 individuals between the ages 5 to 24 (1544 between 5 and 17), and thus these data are more extensive than for the original and longer AAT. Clinical experience suggests the longer AAT continues to be an exceptionally dependable measure. CTOPP demographic data are presented for geographic area, gender, race, residence, ethnicity, family income and parents' educational attainment, see Table 8–14 for a summary.

NAMING

Speeded naming is considered a core deficit in reading-impaired children, along with poor phonological processing. Speeded naming tests vary by task demand. Some require word generation in response to a phoneme or category, others to a drawing (visual confrontation), and still others to word definition. It should be emphasized that intelligence level affects naming performance (Rudel, Denckla et al., 1980), and determination of abnormality should therefore consider this confounding variable.

One description of the naming task cites the requirement for distinguishing between five stages. The first two stages are visual processing of the stimulus and recognition of the picture, with difficulty at either of these stages not generally considered indicative of an aphasic disorder. The remaining three stages are retrieval of the semantic representation, access

---

[1]It is of interest that the capacity to hear and repeat an unfamiliar pseudoword (nonword repetition) was found to predict level of vocabulary development in normal children (Gathercole, S. E., and Baddeley, A., 1989). These data were interpreted as providing evidence of the phonological loop (see Chapter 5) and long-term memory interaction, that is, language acquisition is facilitated by maintaining the representation of a new word to optimize learning (Baddeley, A. D., 2001).

of a corresponding phonological word form, and recognition of the sequence of articulated phonemes (Basso, Corno et al., 1996). Confrontation naming ability is an aspect of semantic memory that has been examined extensively in a temporal lobe epilepsy (TLE) population, and an association between intractable mesial TLE and impaired object naming or dysnomia is well documented in the adult literature (Bell, Hermann et al., 2001).

Naming Errors

While it is intended that the examiner transcribe the subject's verbatim responses on a confrontation naming test for free retrieval and when phonemic and semantic cues are offered, these tests do not specify error types for routine quantification as part of the scoring; these often remain qualitative indicators. It is therefore of interest to consider some naming errors that have been studied. For example, 10 error types were defined in a study of aphasic adults secondary to a vascular etiology: *(1)* no response (refused or could not produce speech); *(2)* word-finding difficulty (attempted to answer but could not); *(3)* semantic paraphasia (superordinates, in class coordinates, or contextual associates); *(4)* unrelated paraphasia; *(5)* phonemic/orthographic paraphasia; *(6)* neologism (nonwords); *(7)* paraphasic jargon (using real but semantically inappropriate words); *(8)* phonemic/neologistic jargon (strings of phonemes); *(9)* stereotypy (repetition of the same syllable sequence or words), and; *(10)* other (Basso, Corno et al., 1996). Such error differentiation is not routinely considered for children or formalized as part of the procedures for naming-test scoring.

Color Naming

Color naming and color name recognition impairment are possible concomitants of developmental dyslexia (Denckla and Rudel, 1972). Color association performance in normal children and those with developmental dyslexia was examined, and young normal children quickly achieved performance comparable to normal adults for color-association skill and a

relatively high functioning group of dyslexic children had normal performance (Varney and Sivan, 1985). It should be noted that acquired, rather than developmental, reading problems in association with aphasia are associated with color association problems. Thus, color association appears to precede development of color naming or color name recognition skill.

Boston Naming Test

The Boston Naming Test (BNT) was originally designed for use with adults (Kaplan, Goodglass et al., 1983), and its utility as a test of visual confrontation naming and word retrieval for adults with aphasia is well established. The test was subsequently applied to children and is considered useful in the assessment of children with dysphasia or language learning disability when supplemented with additional language and reading measures. It is associated with reading comprehension and written comprehension (Berninger and Colwell, 1985). The BNT is a measure of word knowledge (vocabulary) (Halperin, Healey et al., 1989), verbal learning, word retrieval, and semantic language. It also has a perceptual element since the child must distinguish the drawn-line stimuli. Yet, naming difficulty has not been fully explained on the basis of vocabulary deficit (Wolf, 1984; Wolf and Goodglass, 1986). Since naming depends on word acquisition, age at acquisition is an important variable to consider in the interpretation of test scores. Unfortunately, child and adolescent normative data are not available for all the ages for which it is applicable.

In adult studies, an Object Definition Test (ODT) that required the subject to define words was used to assess the integrity of conceptual (semantic) knowledge about a subset of items from the BNT (Hodges, Salmon et al., 1992; Hodges, Patterson et al., 1996). Although not part of child studies to date, the test has interest and is described briefly here.

Word definitions were requested after completion of the BNT for the following stimuli: beaver, stethoscope, cactus, accordian, rhinoceros, and pyramid. Adapted instructions were, "I will read the name of something and ask you to describe it in as much detail as possible. Please define the object as if you were explaining it to someone from a different country who has never seen or hear of such a thing." The word "horse" is used as practice, and the subject is encouraged to be thorough and to include the object's physical appearance, uses, and habitat/location in addition to other facts. Six different types of information are scored: general physical feature, specific physical feature, general associative feature, specific associative feature, superordinate category label, and intrusion error (Hodges, Patterson et al., 1996). One point is scored for each instance of a type provided, and multiple types are each scored (see Bell, Hermann et al., 2001, for an additional scoring example).

The clinical usefulness of the BNT has been investigated with small groups of children diagnosed as having language disorder/dysphonetic dyslexia (N = 12), visuospatial/dyseidetic dyslexia (N = 3) and left temporal lobe brain tumor (N = 3) (Cohen, Town et al., 1988). The visuospatial/dyseidetic group exhibited average or above average confrontational naming ability contrasted with the language disorder/dysphonetic group. The tumor group demonstrated similar performance to the language disorder/dysphonetic group, but their profile was more severe. The authors concluded there was support for a left temporal lobe contribution to the etiology of the language disorder/dysphonetic reading disorder subtype.

The BNT procedure requires the child to name spontaneously a series of two-dimensional black-and-white line drawings. One can begin testing with item 30 for children at least 10 years old. Testing is discontinued after six consecutive errors. If unable to respond within 20 seconds, or if there is a misperception, a semantic cue is offered as specified on the record form. If the correct name is not produced, a phonemic cue (initial sound) is then presented as an additional cueing strategy. Several scores may be computed: spontaneous number of correct responses, number of semantic cues and number of correct responses to semantic cues, number of phonemic cues and number of correct responses to phonemic cues, total correct, total correct for spontaneous and semantic

cues, and termination point item number. Standard practice is to sum the scores for total spontaneous and total postsemantic cueing for the total score, omitting the number correct after phonemic cueing.

The original 85-item version was administered to eighty-two 6- and 7-year-old children. A normal distribution was found, with boys having better performance than girls for total correct, spontaneous responses, and upper-limit variables (Kindlon and Garrison, 1984). In the revised publication of a 60-item version (Kaplan, Goodglass et al., 1983), normative data were presented for only 30 children across six grade levels from Kindergarten to fifth grade, aged 5 to 10 (see Table 8–15).

The following BNT phonemic cueing scores were obtained for 241 children from suburban New York City elementary schools in regular classes following standard administration instructions. These children had not repeated a grade, were not believed to have a learning disability, and did not have non-English speaking parents (Halperin, Healey et al., 1989). These data were reported by gender and age, see Table 8–16. The highest age group had a very small number of subjects, only two and eight 12-year-old boys and girls, respectively. Adolescent BNT normative data remain a persisting gap in the literature. However, cross-cultural application of the BNT includes report of normative data on a Korean version of the BNT, including data on thirty-five 15- to 19-year-olds (Kim and Na, 1999).

Normative data were collected for varying sample sizes: 70 children aged 6 to 12 (Cohen, Town et al., 1988; see Table 8–17 for demo-

Table 8–15. Boston Naming Test Provisional Means (*SDs*) for the 60-item Test

Grade	Mean Age	N	Mean	SD	Range
K	5.5	5	29.6	5.78	20–37
1	6.5	5	29.0	5.55	20–34
2	7.5	5	37.0	4.15	34–45
3	8.5	5	38.4	2.94	33–41
4	9.5	5	41.6	3.56	37–47
5	10.5	5	43.2	4.07	37–48

Source: Adapted from Kaplan, Goodglass & Weintraub (1983).

Table 8–16. BNT Performance Following Phonemic Cueing

	BOYS			GIRLS			TOTAL GROUP		
Age	N	M	SD	N	M	SD	N	M	SD
6	16	38.50	5.6	18	34.78	4.7	34	36.53	5.4
7	18	41.67	4.3	22	39.95	6.3	40	40.73	5.5
8	23	42.96	4.0	15	41.33	3.9	38	42.32	4.0
9	20	45.95	4.0	25	45.68	4.8	45	45.80	4.4
10	16	46.69	5.8	22	48.45	3.3	38	47.71	4.6
11	16	50.44	3.9	20	49.55	4.6	36	49.94	4.3
12	2	55.50	0.7	8	51.75	2.9	10	52.50	3.0

Source: Halperin et al. (1989), © Swets & Zeitlinger.

graphic data, Table 8–18 for normative data); 357 children aged 5 to 12 (Guilford and Nawojczyk, 1988); 241 children aged 6 to 12 (Halperin, Healey et al., 1989) (see Table 8–16 for normative data); and 382 children 5 to 13 (Kirk, 1992). Along with the BNT manual data on 30 children, these normative studies were subjected to analyses of variance, and mean levels of performance at each age level from 5 to 13 years were compared (Yeates, 1994). The resulting differences were of a sufficiently small magnitude to allow the norms to be combined. The resulting demographic data are presented in Table 8–19, and the metanorm compilation is presented in Table 8–20.

Rapid Automatized Naming

One of the more useful screening tests to detect the processing problems that place a child at risk for academic problems is the Rapid Automatized Naming (RAN) test. The origin of the RAN is traced to Norman Geschwind's seminal description of the disconnection syn-

drome (Geschwind, 1965; Denckla and Cutting, 1999): the disconnection syndrome in Dejerine's case of "pure alexia without agraphia." The RAN was developed to assess the contribution of both language (a specific visual–verbal connection) and executive (a general processing speed) domains to reading. Whereas color naming might serve as a marker for visual–verbal disconnection in the adult, long latencies, hesitancy, or a lack of automaticity was observed to be the salient behavior in children (Denckla and Rudel, 1972).

Color naming, object naming, lower-case letter naming and number (digit) naming comprise the four parts of the 50-item RAN. Studies of normal and reading disabled children (Denckla and Rudel, 1974; 1976) established the RAN as a reliable predictor of reading skill and a diagnostic indicator of risk for reading disability (Waber, Wolff et al., 2000). Both reading-disabled children and learning-disabled children without reading disability performed poorly compared to controls

Table 8–17. Boston Naming Test Demographic Data: Cohen et al. Study (1988)

Subjects: 70 children in the South
Age: 6 to 12 years
Gender: 35 Male; 35 Female
Handedness: Not reported
Race: 83% White, 17% Black
SES:
IQ: Mean of 105.1 (SD = 10.7)
Inclusion: Regular education, normal intelligence, reading at grade level, no grade repetition, no behavior abnormalities

Table 8–18. Boston Naming Test Means and Standard Deviations

Age	N (Male/Female)	Mean	SD
6.0–6.11	10 (5/5)	31.5	6.12
7.0–7.11	10 (5/5)	33.8	6.39
8.0–8.11	10 (5/5)	35.9	5.76
9.0–9.11	10 (5/5)	38.5	6.52
10.0–10.11	10 (5/5)	44.0	5.56
11.0–11.11	10 (5/5)	43.2	4.10
12.0–12.11	10 (5/5)	47.8	4.19

Source: Cohen, Town and Buff (1988); Courtesy of Lawrence Erlbaum Associates.

Table 8–19. Compiled Demographic Data for
5 Boston Naming Test Studies: Yeates
Meta-Analysis (1994)

Subjects: 1080 children compiled from 5 developmental
   normative studies; geographically represented across
   the U.S. Northeast and South
Age: 5 to 13 years
Gender: Fairly equal but not reported for 1 study
Handedness: Not reported
Race: Principally Caucasian for 3 studies; not reported
   for 2 studies
SES: Middle class for 3 studies; not reported for
   2 studies
Inclusion criteria: Urban or suburban children without
   learning or language disability

(Denckla and Rudel, 1976). Recent data confirm the use of the RAN for discriminating children with dyslexia from those with learning disabilities, but also highlight this instrument's reliability in discriminating between children with general learning problems and controls (Waber, Wolff et al., 2000) and between ADHD-Inattentive type and controls (Weiler, Bernstein et al., 2000). Additional study supports the RAN's ability to discriminate between children with the hyperactive form of ADHD, but without learning disabilities and controls (Semrud-Clikeman, Steingard et al., 2000). Other child studies found slower response rates in the presence of left hemisphere lesions, raising question about the efficiency of lexical retrieval in these children (Aram, Ekelman et al., 1987; Aram, Meyers et al., 1990).

The RAN has a clear linguistic component and requires visual-verbal connections, but an executive mental control aspect has also been proposed through a processing speed contribution (Denckla and Cutting, 1999). The test should be appreciated for its multiple subcomponent processes that can be differentially affected by various processing problems (Denckla and Cutting, 1999). Research has demonstrated slow naming speed to be an effective indicator of vulnerability to neurocognitive problems in learning and processing in general but not specifically of reading or attention disorders as currently defined by DSM-IV (Waber, Wolff et al., 2000). In the latter Waber et al. (2000) study the RAN detected risk for learning problems in general, but was less effective distinguishing learning-impaired children with and without reading disability from each other. The RAN was also part of a study of late effects of perinatal complications (Korhonen, Vaehae-Eskeli et al., 1993). Rapid automatized naming and gesture tasks were administered to language-impaired children, and their age and IQ matched control subjects, at ages 4, 6, and 8 years. The language-impaired group's impairment on both tasks suggested a generalized disability in processing rapid, sequential information, and a relationship between language and praxis in childhood (Katz, Curtiss et al., 1992).

The RAN consists of four cards with 50 stimuli per card. Each card presents five stimuli in random sequence within one semantic domain, either letters, numbers, colors, or objects. The child must rapidly name the stimuli. A continuous format results in total time scores for consecutively naming all items on each card. A mean score on any of the subtests greater than one standard deviation above the mean for age is considered indicative of the slowness associating with a naming-speed deficit and, consequently, suggestive of learning impairment (Waber, Wolff et al., 2000).

The RAN, first developed by Martha Denckla and Rita Rudel, has subsequently been modified, and subtests have been created within a number of standardized child tests that stem from this early work, but no studies have compared the variations to the original. For example, there is a criterion-referenced RAN subtest in the Clinical Evaluation of Language Fundamentals (3rd ed.) with norms for 6 to 21

Table 8–20. Boston Naming Test Compiled
Norms for 5 Studies

Age	Weighted M	Estimated SD	Total N
5	27.76	5.95	62
6	33.56	4.90	150
7	36.87	5.22	153
8	38.99	4.59	147
9	41.74	4.59	152
10	45.10	4.53	167
11	46.84	4.80	146
12	48.55	3.95	80
13	49.55	4.68	22

Source: Yeates (1994), © Swets & Zeitlinger.

years old (Semel, Wiig et al., 1995). The tasks are shape naming, color naming, and color-shape naming, under timed conditions. There is a NEPSY Speeded Naming subtest requiring rapid naming of size-color-shape combinations normed for ages 5–12 years (Korkman, Kirk et al., 1997). Normative data are published in the respective manuals of these batteries.

Unpublished RAN normative data from Wolf and Biddle for 115 children (1995) are in the process of being updated along with data for the Rapid Alternating Stimulus (RAS) (Maryanne Wolf, 2002, personal communication; Wolf and Biddle, 1985). For example, while a child is timed on how fast he or she reads a page of 50 individual letters, numbers, and pictures for the RAN, he or she reads a page of 50 stimuli that change categories for the RAS (color swatches, numbers, two or three different stimuli). The score is the time it takes to name all of the items. Essentially, the RAS is a subset of the RAN, not a separate test. These previously unpublished RAN and RAS normative data by age are presented in Tables 8–21 to 8–38.

The MAE Visual Confrontation Naming data for children from Kindergarten to fifth grade are presented in Table 8–2, and for seventh and eighth graders in Table 8–3.

RECEPTIVE AND EXPRESSIVE LANGUAGE

In addition to items screening for aspects of receptive and expressive language as noted above there are individual tests that specifically address such competencies. Among these are the Peabody Picture Vocabulary Test-III, Receptive One-Word Picture Vocabulary Test, Expressive Vocabulary Test, and the Gardner Expressive One-Word Vocabulary Test. The Test of Word Knowledge is also noted, along with component subtests from Wechsler IQ tests that add to our knowledge of the child's verbal linguistic efficiency. The Wechsler vocabulary subtest is perhaps the most frequently administered screening measure of the child's semantic knowledge and expressive language. Versions of the Token Test, a test of auditory comprehension requiring a motoric response, are also described.

Peabody Picture Vocabulary Test-III and Expressive Vocabulary Test

The Peabody Picture Vocabulary Test-III (PPVT-III; Dunn and Dunn, 1997) is an individually administered measure of receptive or hearing vocabulary, or the child's internal dictionary of words. It can be interpreted as an achievement test of the child's vocabulary acquisition that does not require a verbal response and as a screening measure of verbal ability. There is supportive data for the validity of the PPVT as a screening measure of intelligence and achievement, although lower scores for low socioeconomic minority children have led to questions about its use with these populations (Washington and Craig, 1992). Additionally, it has been studied along with the K-ABC in 416 African American children of low socioeconomic status and correlated .58

Table 8–21. RAN Age Norms: Objects—Errors

Age	ALL			FEMALE			MALE		
	N	Mean	SD	N	Mean	SD	N	Mean	SD
8	13	0.23	0.44	6	0.17	0.41	7	0.29	0.49
9	11	0.36	0.67	5	0.60	0.89	6	0.17	0.41
10	22	?	0.29	9	0.00	0.00	13	0.15	0.38
11	19	0.32	0.67	11	0.36	0.67	8	0.25	0.71
12	17	?	0.24	8	0.00	0.00	9	0.11	0.33
13	9	0.44	0.88	6	0.33	0.82	3	0.67	1.15
14	19	0.21	0.54	11	0.27	0.65	8	0.13	0.35
15	5	0.20	0.45				5	0.20	0.45
Total	115	0.22	0.53	56	0.23	0.57	59	0.20	0.48

Table 8–22. RAN Age Norms: Color—Errors

Age	ALL			FEMALE			MALE		
	N	Mean	SD	N	Mean	SD	N	Mean	SD
8	13	0.54	0.97	6	0.67	1.21	7	0.43	0.79
9	11	0.18	0.40	5	0.20	0.45	6	0.17	0.41
10	22	?	0.21	9	0.00	0.00	13	?	0.28
11	19	0.16	0.50	11	0.18	0.60	8	0.13	0.35
12	17	0.12	0.49	8	0.00	0.00	9	0.22	0.67
13	9	0.22	0.67	6	0.00	0.00	3	0.67	1.15
14	19	0.16	0.37	11	?	0.30	8	0.25	0.46
15	5	0.00	0.00				5	0.00	0.00
Total	115	0.17	0.52	56	0.14	0.52	59	0.20	0.52

Table 8–23. RAN Age Norms: Numbers—Errors

Age	ALL			FEMALE			MALE		
	N	Mean	SD	N	Mean	SD	N	Mean	SD
8	13	0.00	0.00	6	0.00	0.00	7	0.00	0.00
9	11	0.00	0.00	5	0.00	0.00	6	0.00	0.00
10	22	0.23	0.69	9	0.44	1.01	13	?	0.28
11	19	?	0.23	11	?	0.30	8	0.00	0.00
12	17	0.00	0.00	8	0.00	0.00	9	0.00	0.00
13	9	0.00	0.00	6	0.00	0.00	3	0.00	0.00
14	19	0.00	0.00	11	0.00	0.00	8	0.00	0.00
15	5	0.20	0.45				5	0.20	0.45
Total	115	?	0.33	56	?	0.44	59	?	0.18

Table 8–24. RAN Age Norms: Letters—Errors

Age	ALL			FEMALE			MALE		
	N	Mean	SD	N	Mean	SD	N	Mean	SD
8	13	0.23	0.83	6	0.00	0.00	7	0.43	1.13
9	11	0.00	0.00	5	0.00	0.00	6	0.00	0.00
10	22	0.00	0.00	9	0.00	0.00	13	0.00	0.00
11	19	0.11	0.46	11	0.18	0.60	8	0.00	0.00
12	17	0.00	0.00	8	0.00	0.00	9	0.00	0.00
13	9	0.00	0.00	6	0.00	0.00	3	0.00	0.00
14	19	?	0.23	11	0.0	0.00	8	0.13	0.35
15	5	0.00	0.00				5	0.00	0.00
Total	115	?	0.35	56	?	0.27	59	?	0.41

Table 8–25. RAS Two Age Norms: Errors

Age	ALL N	ALL Mean	ALL SD	FEMALE N	FEMALE Mean	FEMALE SD	MALE N	MALE Mean	MALE SD
8	13	0.46	0.78	6	0.67	0.82	7	0.29	0.76
9	11	0.64	0.81	5	0.80	1.10	6	0.50	0.55
10	22	0.14	0.47	9	0.00	0.00	13	0.23	0.60
11	19	0.11	0.32	11	0.18	0.40	8	0.00	0.00
12	17	0.12	0.33	8	0.13	0.35	9	0.11	0.33
13	9	0.33	0.71	6	0.50	0.84	3	0.00	0.00
14	19	?	0.23	11	?	0.30	8	0.00	0.00
15	5	0.00	0.00				5	0.00	0.00
Total	115	0.21	0.52	56	0.27	0.59	59	0.15	0.45

Table 8–26. RAS Three Set Age Norms: Errors

Age	ALL N	ALL Mean	ALL SD	FEMALE N	FEMALE Mean	FEMALE SD	MALE N	MALE Mean	MALE SD
8	13	?	0.28	6	0.00	0.00	7	0.14	0.38
9	11	?	0.30	5	0.20	0.45	6	0.00	0.00
10	22	0.27	0.46	9	0.11	0.33	13	0.38	0.51
11	19	0.21	0.54	11	0.36	0.67	8	0.00	0.00
12	17	0.12	0.33	8	0.00	0.00	9	0.22	0.44
13	9	0.00	0.00	6	0.00	0.00	3	0.00	0.00
14	19	0.16	0.37	11	0.00	0.00	8	0.38	0.52
15	5	0.20	0.45				5	0.20	0.45
Total	115	0.16	0.39	56	0.11	0.37	59	0.20	0.41

Table 8–27. RAN Age Norms: Objects—Latency

Age	ALL N	ALL Mean	ALL SD	FEMALE N	FEMALE Mean	FEMALE SD	MALE N	MALE Mean	MALE SD
8	13	42.62	8.51	6	43.83	7.88	7	41.57	9.50
9	11	43.00	4.36	5	41.20	4.87	6	44.50	3.62
10	22	41.09	7.47	9	39.00	5.24	13	42.54	8.59
11	19	36.42	6.57	11	36.18	6.11	8	36.75	7.57
12	17	35.47	4.40	8	33.38	3.54	9	37.33	4.42
13	9	33.67	6.02	6	32.00	6.36	3	37.00	4.36
14	19	32.53	3.66	11	32.18	4.19	8	33.00	2.98
15	5	29.60	6.58				5	29.60	6.58
Total	115	37.35	7.24	56	36.27	6.55	59	38.37	7.77

Table 8–28. RAN Age Norms: Color—Latency

Age	ALL			FEMALE			MALE		
	N	Mean	SD	N	Mean	SD	N	Mean	SD
8	13	42.46	11.89	6	44.17	11.13	7	41.00	13.19
9	11	43.09	6.88	5	40.20	3.27	6	45.50	8.41
10	22	38.27	7.08	9	39.56	6.52	13	37.38	7.57
11	19	34.05	6.96	11	34.18	7.36	8	33.88	6.88
12	17	32.00	5.10	8	29.75	4.65	9	34.00	4.85
13	9	31.11	7.70	6	29.50	7.58	3	34.33	8.39
14	19	30.05	4.38	11	29.82	4.87	8	30.38	3.89
15	5	26.80	5.02				5	26.80	5.02
Total	115	35.17	8.49	56	34.66	8.25	59	35.64	8.75

Table 8–29. RAN Age Norms: Numbers—Latency

Age	ALL			FEMALE			MALE		
	N	Mean	SD	N	Mean	SD	N	Mean	SD
8	13	28.00	7.84	6	31.00	9.59	7	25.43	5.44
9	11	26.18	3.95	5	26.20	5.54	6	26.17	2.56
10	22	25.18	5.20	9	28.11	5.44	13	23.15	4.08
11	19	21.32	3.90	11	21.27	3.82	8	21.38	4.27
12	17	21.06	3.42	8	20.50	4.21	9	21.56	2.70
13	9	18.56	3.09	6	18.83	3.71	3	18.00	1.73
14	19	18.95	2.82	11	18.45	3.05	8	19.63	2.50
15	5	16.20	3.96				5	16.20	3.96
Total	115	22.41	5.58	56	22.93	6.52	59	21.92	4.51

Talbe 8–30. RAN Age Norms: Letter—Latency

Age	ALL			FEMALE			MALE		
	N	Mean	SD	N	Mean	SD	N	Mean	SD
8	13	25.92	5.74	6	27.00	6.10	7	25.00	5.72
9	11	25.45	3.14	5	24.80	3.11	6	26.00	3.35
10	22	25.00	5.30	9	27.22	6.34	13	23.46	4.01
11	19	21.84	4.02	11	22.18	4.07	8	21.38	4.17
12	17	21.94	3.13	8	20.50	3.96	9	23.22	1.39
13	9	18.89	2.52	6	18.17	2.86	3	20.33	0.58
14	19	18.42	3.63	11	17.64	3.59	8	19.50	3.63
15	5	15.80	3.03				5	15.80	3.03
Total	115	22.21	5.05	56	22.18	5.62	59	22.24	4.48

Table 8–31. RAS Two Age Norms: Latency

Age	ALL			FEMALE			MALE		
	N	Mean	SD	N	Mean	SD	N	Mean	SD
8	13	34.54	8.50	6	38.50	9.35	7	31.14	6.52
9	11	30.73	6.42	5	30.40	5.50	6	31.00	7.62
10	22	30.14	5.63	9	32.33	6.34	13	28.62	4.75
11	19	25.68	4.87	11	26.45	5.39	8	24.63	4.14
12	17	25.06	4.29	8	23.75	5.50	9	26.22	2.68
13	9	21.22	2.28	6	20.33	2.25	3	23.00	1.00
14	19	20.37	2.91	11	19.64	2.66	8	21.38	3.11
15	5	17.00	4.42				5	17.00	4.42
Total	115	26.32	7.09	56	26.66	8.01	59	26.00	6.14

Table 8–32. RAS Three Set Age Norms—Latency

Age	ALL			FEMALE			MALE		
	N	Mean	SD	N	Mean	SD	N	Mean	SD
8	13	39.08	11.09	6	44.33	12.39	7	34.57	8.18
9	11	35.00	4.88	5	36.20	5.02	6	34.00	4.98
10	22	33.91	6.08	9	36.89	4.99	13	31.85	6.07
11	19	30.16	6.16	11	31.27	6.81	8	28.62	5.15
12	17	28.94	5.24	8	26.13	4.67	9	31.44	4.56
13	9	25.11	4.94	6	24.50	5.21	3	26.33	5.13
14	19	25.11	3.73	11	23.64	3.53	8	27.13	3.14
15	5	19.40	2.19				5	19.40	2.19
Total	115	30.47	7.83	56	31.05	9.04	59	29.92	6.50

Table 8–33. RAN Age Norms: Objects—Self Corrections

Age	ALL			FEMALE			MALE		
	N	Mean	SD	N	Mean	SD	N	Mean	SD
8	13	0.85	0.99	6	0.83	0.98	7	0.86	1.07
9	11	1.00	0.77	5	0.40	0.55	6	1.50	0.55
10	22	0.59	0.80	9	0.44	0.73	13	0.69	0.85
11	19	0.47	0.70	11	?	0.30	8	1.00	0.76
12	17	0.71	1.10	8	1.00	1.41	9	0.44	0.73
13	9	0.78	0.97	6	0.83	1.17	3	0.67	0.58
14	19	0.79	0.92	11	0.82	0.98	8	0.75	0.89
15	5	0.40	0.89				5	0.40	0.89
Total	115	0.70	0.88	56	0.61	0.93	59	0.78	0.83

Table 8–34. RAN Age Norms: Color—Self Corrections

Age	ALL			FEMALE			MALE		
	N	Mean	SD	N	Mean	SD	N	Mean	SD
8	13	0.31	0.63	6	0.33	0.52	7	0.29	0.76
9	11	0.36	0.50	5	0.00	0.00	6	0.67	0.52
10	22	0.45	0.60	9	0.56	0.53	13	0.38	0.65
11	19	0.42	0.84	11	0.36	0.67	8	0.50	1.07
12	17	0.35	0.49	8	0.38	0.52	9	0.33	0.50
13	9	0.56	0.73	6	0.50	0.55	3	0.67	1.15
14	19	0.32	0.48	11	0.27	0.47	8	0.38	0.52
15	5	0.20	0.45				5	0.20	0.45
Total	115	0.38	0.60	56	0.36	0.52	59	0.41	0.67

Table 8–35. RAN Age Norms: Numbers—Self Corrections

Age	ALL			FEMALE			MALE		
	N	Mean	SD	N	Mean	SD	N	Mean	SD
8	13	0.38	0.87	6	0.67	1.21	7	0.14	0.38
9	11	0.27	0.47	5	0.40	0.55	6	0.17	0.41
10	22	0.41	0.50	9	0.44	0.53	13	0.38	0.51
11	19	0.16	0.37	11	0.18	0.40	8	0.13	0.35
12	17	0.18	0.39	8	0.25	0.46	9	0.11	0.33
13	9	0.22	0.67	6	0.33	0.82	3	0.00	0.00
14	19	0.16	0.37	11	?	0.30	8	0.25	0.46
15	5	0.20	0.45				5	0.20	0.45
Total	115	0.25	0.51	56	0.30	0.60	59	0.20	0.41

Table 8–36. RAN Age Norms: Letters—Self Corrections

Age	ALL			FEMALE			MALE		
	N	Mean	SD	N	Mean	SD	N	Mean	SD
8	13	?	0.28	6	0.00	0.00	7	0.14	0.38
9	11	0.36	0.67	5	0.00	0.00	6	0.67	0.82
10	22	0.23	0.43	9	0.22	0.44	13	0.23	0.44
11	19	?	0.23	11	0.00	0.00	8	0.13	0.35
12	17	0.41	0.51	8	0.50	0.53	9	0.33	0.50
13	9	0.22	0.44	6	0.33	0.52	3	0.00	0.00
14	19	0.11	0.32	11	?	0.30	8	0.13	0.35
15	5	0.20	0.45				5	0.20	0.45
Total	115	0.20	0.42	56	0.16	0.37	59	0.24	0.47

Table 8–37. RAS Two Age Norms: Self Corrections

Age	ALL			FEMALE			MALE		
	N	Mean	SD	N	Mean	SD	N	Mean	SD
8	13	0.31	0.48	6	0.33	0.52	7	0.29	0.49
9	11	0.36	0.92	5	0.00	0.00	6	0.67	1.21
10	22	0.45	0.60	9	0.67	0.50	13	0.31	0.63
11	19	0.21	0.54	11	0.36	0.67	8	0.00	0.00
12	17	0.53	0.62	8	0.38	0.52	9	0.67	0.71
13	9	0.22	0.44	6	0.17	0.41	3	0.33	0.58
14	19	0.16	0.37	11	0.18	0.40	8	0.13	0.35
15	5	0.00	0.00				5	0.00	0.00
Total	115	0.31	0.57	56	0.32	0.51	59	0.31	0.62

with the K-ABC Mental Processing Composite (MPC) score. The children scored significantly lower on the PPVT-III than on the MPC. While receiver operating characteristic analyses supported its use as a screening of intelligence and achievement, the authors expressed caution about use of a single cutoff score (Campbell, Bell et al., 2001). Nonetheless, it has long appeared to be one of the more useful screening measures for verbal IQ as measured with a Wechsler intelligence test, and statistically significant discrepancies between PPVT-III and VIQ are taken seriously as markers of language discordance requiring explanation.

The test can be administered beginning at age 2½ years. Two alternative forms, with 204 items each, are available: III–A and III–B. The child listens to the examiner's stimulus word and must choose the picture that best describes the word from a 4-picture multiple choice array. A pointing response is all that is required. A standard score with a mean of 100 ($SD = 15$)

is computed. Internal consistency reliability and temporal stability are high ($r = .95$ and $r = .92$, respectively; Campbell, 1998). The most recent normative database demographics are presented in Table 8–39.

The PPVT-III is co-normed with the Expressive Vocabulary Test (Williams, 1997), a measure of expressive language similarly normed on 2725 individuals aged 2 to 90 years, stratified to match the 1994 U.S. Census data. The test is similar to the BNT in its initial items. The Expressive Vocabulary Test includes 38 labeling items and 152 synonym items, and the child must respond with a one-word answer. Split-half reliabilities are reported to range from .83 to .97, with a median of .91. Alphas range from 90 to .98, with a median of .95. Test–retest reliability coefficients assessing test stability ranged from. 77 to .90.

There is support for interpreting a discrepancy between PPVT and BNT results as clini-

Table 8–38. RAS Three Set Age Norms—Self Corrections

Age	ALL			FEMALE			MALE		
	N	Mean	SD	N	Mean	SD	N	Mean	SD
8	13	0.23	0.44	6	0.33	0.52	7	0.14	0.38
9	11	0.36	0.81	5	0.40	0.89	6	0.33	0.82
10	22	0.36	0.49	9	0.22	0.44	13	0.46	0.52
11	19	0.32	0.58	11	0.45	0.69	8	0.13	0.35
12	17	0.35	0.70	8	0.25	0.71	9	0.44	0.73
13	9	0.22	0.44	6	0.33	0.52	3	0.00	0.00
14	19	0.16	0.50	11	0.00	0.00	8	0.38	0.74
15	5	0.20	0.45				5	0.20	0.45
Total	115	0.29	0.56	56	0.27	0.56	59	0.31	0.56

Table 8–39. Peabody Picture Vocabulary Test-III Normative Data Sample

Subjects: 2725 individuals
Age: 2.6 to 90+ years
Gender: 1284 male; 1441 female
Handedness: Not reported
Race: 18.1% African American, 12.9% Hispanic,
    64.3% White, 4.6%Other
SES: Not reported
Geographic Area: 19.4% Northeast, 27.8% North Central,
    33.1% South, 19.7% West

cally useful for identifying a learning disability subtype, that of reading disability (Halperin, Healey et al., 1989). Independent of research data, it is abundantly clear from clinical practice that a receptive language test is valuable as a screening index of a child's internal lexicon. It provides an expectation for what the overall VIQ might be if the WISC-III intelligence test were administered. Should the VIQ differ from the receptive language IQ, the discrepancy requires satisfactory resolution through further investigation.

Expressive One-Word Picture Vocabulary Test (2000 ed.) and Receptive One-Word Picture Vocabulary Test (2000 ed.)

In contrast to the pointing response accepted for the PPVT-III, the Expressive One-Word Picture Vocabulary Test (2000 ed.) (EOWPVT; Gardner, 2000) requires the child to verbalize, that is, to express a single-word response to colored illustrations. The stimuli are progressively more difficult depictions of an object, action, or concept. The EOWPVT is a useful measure to use in association with the PPVT-III or the Receptive One-Word Picture Vocabulary Test (ROWPVT), with which it is co-normed, to compare receptive and expressive language. The co-normed tests included a standardization sample of more than 2000 individuals aged 2 years to 18 years, 11 months. The PPVT-III presents stimuli in a 2 × 2 matrix, while the ROWPVT (2000) presents items in a 1 × 4 array.

Test of Word Knowledge

The Test of Word Knowledge (Wiig and Secord, 1992) is normed for children 5 to 17 years old. It examines semantic skill (attachment of meaning to words and sentences) and knowledge of figurative language, multiple meanings, conjunctions, and transition words. There are two levels, one for 5- to 8-year-olds and one for 8- to 17-year-olds. Receptive and expressive composite scores can be calculated along with age equivalents, percentile ranks, stanines and subtest means.

Token Test for Children

The Token Test for Children is a measure of the consistency of listening skill. It requires the child to listen to increasingly lengthy and complex verbal directions in order to carry out a requested action. The test was originally developed to measure decoding, along with awareness of abstract relationships, in adults (De Renzi and Vignolo, 1962), but was subsequently extended downward into child and adolescent ages. There are numerous versions, and these vary by shape of tokens, color of tokens, verbal commands, and number of items. It is useful as both a screening assessment of auditory/verbal comprehension and as a sensitive measure of impairment in the presence of increasing grammatical complexity and verbal abstraction, such as in the final section's syntactically complex commands. A statistically significant correlation ($r = .71$, $p < .001$) was found for the Token Test and the PPVT, establishing its validity as a receptive language measure (Lass and Golden, 1975). The test is also an index of the child's facility with immediate memory for sequenced, contextual words. It has the additional advantage of potential usefulness with children suspected as having contributory attentional deficits since, as part of the procedure, the child must sustain effort and attention in response to increasingly more lengthy oral instructions.

The Token Test was reduced in length from the original 5-part, 62-item test to 36-items (De Renzi and Faglioni, 1978). For this short form the following colored token arrangement (circle, square, circle, square, in order from top to bottom) for red (R), blue (B), yellow (Y), white (W) and green (G) tokens is used:

R	B	Y	W	G
B	R	W	G	Y
W	B	Y	R	G
Y	G	R	B	W

There are 20 Tokens. All 20 tokens are presented for Parts I, III, and V. The small tokens are removed for Parts II, IV, and VI. The items for the short version Token Test (De Renzi and Faglioni, 1978) are as follows:

Part 1. All 20 tokens as shown above.
1. Touch a circle
2. Touch a square
3. Touch a yellow token
4. Touch a red one
5. Touch a blue one
6. Touch a green one
7. Touch a white one

Part 2. Small tokens removed.
8. Touch the yellow square
9. Touch the blue circle
10. Touch the green circle
11. Touch the white square

Part 3. Replace small tokens.
12. Touch the small white circle
13. Touch the large yellow circle
14. Touch the large green square
15. Touch the small blue circle

Part 4. Remove small tokens.
16. Touch the red circle and the green square
17. Touch the yellow square and the blue square
18. Touch the white square and the green circle
19. Touch the white circle and the red circle

Part 5. Replace the small tokens.
20. Touch the large white circle and the small green square
21. Touch the small blue circle and the large yellow square
22. Touch the large green square and the large red square
23. Touch the large white square and the small green circle

Part 6. Remove small tokens.
24. Put the red circle on the green square
25. Touch the blue circle with the red square
26. Touch the blue circle and the red square

27. Touch the blue circle or the red square
28. Put the green square away from the yellow square
29. If there is a black circle, touch the red square
30. Put the green square next to the red circle
31. Touch the square slowly and the circles quickly
32. Put the red circle between the yellow square and the green square
33. Touch all the circles except the green one
34. Touch the red circle—no—the white square
35. Instead of the white square, touch the yellow circle
36. In addition to touching the yellow circle, touch the blue circle

The raw score is the maximum 36 points, minus the number of errors. The impairment ratings based on raw scores for the aphasic patient sample are presented in Table 8–40.

The task is considered sufficiently important as a measure of receptive language so that it is modified and included in a number of batteries, including the Clinical Evaluation of Language Fundamentals (3rd ed.) (ELF-3) (Semel, Wiig et al., 1995) in which black-and-white geometric figures are used. The CELF-3 is nationally normed on 2400 individuals aged 6 to 21. It is available in Spanish as a parallel version and not as a translation. A total language score can be computed based on six subtests, with additional supplemental subtests available. A CELF-Screening Test is also available along with observational rating scales. A

Table 8–40. Levels of Comprehension Deficit in Aphasics for Token Test Scores

Score	Impairment	# Patients In Each Group
29–36	Nil	14 (7%)
25–28	Mild	20 (10%)
17–24	Moderate	76 (38%)
9–16	Severe	58 (29%)
0–8	Very Severe	32 (16%)

Source: Adapted from De Renzi & Faglioni (1978).

separate five part Token Test for Children is also available (DiSimoni, 1978).

A 39-item token test version is included in the Neurosensory Center Comprehensive Examination for Aphasia (NCCEA; Spreen, 1977). A 22-item version is included in the MAE. Of 56 children and adolescents examined following closed head injury during the subacute stage of recovery, 25% of those with moderate/severe injuries and 9% of those with mild injuries had impaired performance on the NCCEA Identification by Sentence (token) subtest (two adolescents took the MAE version). But receptive language was less impaired than naming, expression, and written language (Ewing-Cobbs, Levin et al., 1987).

Multilingual Aphasia Examination: Token Test

The Multilingual Aphasia Examination (MAE) includes a 22-item version of the Token Test (Benton, Hamsher et al., 1994). The test items were selected from the De Renzi and Faglioni (1978) Token Test described above and are listed below.

1. Point to a circle
2. Point to a square
3. Point to a black circle
4. Point to a yellow square
5. Point to the small white circle
6. Point to the large yellow square
7. Pick up the large green square and the large red square
8. Pick up the small red circle and the small white circle
9. Pick up the large white square and small green circle
10. Pick up the small yellow circle and the large black square

Remove small tokens

11. Pick up the white square and the green circle
12. Touch the green square with the black circle
13. Touch the white circle with the green square
14. Touch all squares except the green one
15. Touch the green square of the yellow circle

16. Touch all circles except the yellow one
17. Pick up the white circle and the red circle
18. Pick up the green square or the white square
19. Put the yellow square on the white circle
20. Touch the black circle with the red square
21. Pick up the black circle or the red square
22. Put the white circle on the red square

The items are scored 0, 1, or 2 points. There are 22 items, for a maximum of 44 points.

There are associated child normative data from Kindergarten to Grade 6 (Schum, Sivan et al., 1989). These normative data are presented in Table 8–41. The normative data were subsequently expanded to include seventh and eighth graders (Steven Zorich and Kerry Hamsher, 2002, personal communication) and these data are presented in Table 8–4.

WRITTEN LANGUAGE AND HANDWRITING

Written language and handwriting are interesting, but sometimes overlooked, aspects of a cognitive evaluation that may be evaluated informally as well as formally. Writing is a complex linguistic function that is expected to develop rapidly around age 5 to 7, paralleling those years when formal elementary schooling begins. Informal observations made about the way a child writes may include how well the child grasps the writing instrument, hand choice and position, letter size, including how well uniform size is maintained, letter forma-

Table 8–41. Normative data for MAE Token Test

Mean Age	N	Grade	Mean	SD
6.3	35	K	37.5	3.3
7.3	34	1	38.6	3.3
8.2	32	2	40.2	3.4
9.3	43	3	40.3	3.4
10.2	33	4	41.1	2.7
11.3	31	5	41.3	2.5
12.3	21	6	40.5	3.0

Source: Schum, Sivan and Benton (1989); © Swets & Zeitlinger.

tion, spatial characteristics or writing placement, and the extent of overwriting and erasures. These are observed, along with form, content, grammar, punctuation, capitalization, spelling, and production length, when there is a production of written language.

Routine administration of a particular stimulus picture to assess written paragraph formulation allows for a standard administration protocol that provides the examiner with an internal database enabling determination about whether a production is normal, indicative of developmental delay, or reflecting specific dysfunction. A clinician needs to dissociate the visuomotor component from the linguistic component. Chronological age and task specifics will affect such determination. For example, writing "squaer" instead of "square," when copying the printed word, is a significant error for an adolescent. A young child writing a phonetically correct error such as "showted" for "shouted" may not be as worrisome as when an older child writes "shoated" or "showlted." An impoverished written production in response to such a picture may contrast markedly with the child's facility for oral production. Thus, it is useful to follow up the poor written response, or outright refusal to write, by asking the child, "Now tell me about this picture." The BDAE "cookie theft" picture is especially useful in this regard.

Of course, other writing subtests from diverse tests and language batteries also lend themselves to such routine use. One standardized written production test is the Test of Written Language-3, an 8-subtest battery for young people 7 years, 6 months to 17 years that incorporates both spontaneous and contrived formats for two alternative equivalent forms. It was standardized on 2000 public and private school students from 26 states in Grades 2 through 12. The eight subtests are Vocabulary (write a sentence with a specific word), Spelling (from dictation), Style, Logical Sentences (edit and improve an illogical sentence), Sentence Combining, Contextual Convention (write a story for a picture), Contextual Language (vocabulary, sentence construction, and grammar are evaluated), and Story Construction (Hammill and Larsen, 1996).

Another measure is the Woodcock-Johnson Psychoeducational Battery (rev.) Tests of Achievement Supplemental Battery: Writing Fluency task that tests the child's ability to formulate and write sentences within a time limit. The sentences are based on stimulus pictures, and three words are specified for inclusion. The Wechsler Individual Achievement Test (WIAT) includes a Written Expression subtest for Grades 3 to 12 with a fixed time limit of 15 minutes (Wechsler Individual Achievement Test, 1992). The child writes in response to a prompt presented orally and in print. The production is scored for analytical elements, including (1) Ideas and Development, (2) Organization, Unity and Coherence, (3) Vocabulary, (4) Sentence Structure and Variety, (5) Grammar and Usage, and (6) Capitalization and Punctuation. It may also be scored with a rapid holistic method.

The clinical implications of differential capacity to communicate through oral or written channels are directly relevant to academic performance. Indications of impoverished written production often parallel a child's reluctance to write and may contrast dramatically with the child's capacity for oral production. The teacher needs to be acutely aware of this disparity. Also, a child with a speech impairment may find it much easier to communicate knowledge and comprehension through writing, but become blocked if requested to communicate the same information orally. Again, this discrepancy is critically useful information for the teacher. Too often, personality or temperament may be implicated by teachers before they recognize the true nature of the child's incapacitating cognitive problems.

In serial evaluation it is also possible to make note of any change in handwriting efficiency to supplement objective test data. For example, I have long considered increased writing problems to be an early marker of physiological decompensation in a child who has hydrocephalus. Rough comparisons over time can be made by merely looking at the child's handwriting and evaluating whether there is improvement with increased chronological age, stability, or loss of efficiency. It also has become evident that handwriting is sometimes the earliest indicator of successful neurosurgical intervention. Shunt placement to reduce the deleterious influences of increased intracranial pressure could result in dramatically different handwriting samples between preoperative and postoperative evaluations.

AUDITORY PERCEPTION

Speech Sounds Perception Test

The Speech Sounds Perception Test is part of the Halstead-Reitan NTB (Reitan, 1969). It is considered a test of the ability to discriminate phonemes, but it also depends on attentional capacity and requires single-word reading. The child is required to listen to 30 tape-recorded nonsense syllables and to read and select the correct response from three choices printed on the answer sheet. The score is the number correct. Normative data from a meta-analysis of existing research (Findeis and Weight, 1994; see Chapter 6 for detail) are presented in Table 8–42. Along with these data are normative data for 15- to 17-year olds and 18- to 23-year olds, published as part of a larger adolescent and adult normative data study (Fromm-Auch and Yeudall, 1983).

Seashore Rhythm Test

The Seashore Rhythm Test (Seashore, Lewis et al. 1960) is a component of the Halstead-Reitan Neuropsychological Test Battery (HRNTB) (Reitan, 1969; Reitan and Wolfson, 1989). Its usefulness has been called into ques-

Table 8–42. Speech Sounds Perception Test Error Means and *SD*s

	SPEECH SOUNDS PERCEPTION TEST			
Age	N	Mean	SD	Range
9	72	7.23	4.7	
10	97	6.58	3.3	
11	90	5.36	2.6	
12	122	5.50	2.9	
13	36	5.04	1.3	
14	N/A			
15–17	32	4.6	2.4	1–13
18–23	76	4.2	2.0	1–10

Source: 9- to 14-year-old data, courtesy of Findeis & Weight (1994); 15- to 23-year-old data adapted from Fromm-Auch and Yeudall (1983), © Swets and Zeitlinger.

tion. It was intended as a measure of the ability to sustain responding under speeded conditions to paired auditory tones, discriminating whether the patterns of the tones are similar or dissimilar. There are three subsections, each with 10 sets of paired tones. The tones vary by length (5, 6, and 7 tones for Parts A, B, and C, respectively) and by rate of delivery (2/4, 3/4, and 4/4 time). Early studies of reliability were criticized for omitting normal subjects or for not computing the reliabilities of the diagnostic groups separately (Charter and Webster, 1997). In their own study, these authors provided data from item analysis, considered subject fatigue and inability to sustain attention, and computed internal consistency reliabilities for total score and for each of the three subparts. The total test score reliability of .78 was similar to that of earlier studies (Bornstein, 1983; Moses, 1985).

The test was criticized for its low reliability for each subpart and because too many subjects had scores no different than chance responding. This has led to a recommendation that these serious deficiencies be considered before one chooses to use the test (Charter and Webster, 1997). Presumption that the test is sensitive to right cerebral hemisphere dysfunction has not always held up in adult studies (Boone and Rausch, 1989). Also, caution is advised in administering the test to individuals with a musical background since these individuals may function normally on the test despite other evidence of cognitive impairment (Karzmark, 2001).

The Rhythm Test has weaknesses that make it less desirable in a flexible battery approach. These limitations were addressed in an adult study that also examined the Speech Sounds Perception Test, an interesting refutation of nonempirically based statements supporting their use (Sherer, Parsons et al., 1991). Both measures failed to discriminate right- and left-hemisphere damage, and discriminant analyses failed to support their use in a battery context. However, those who maintain a strict HRNTB battery approach or want to compute a HRNTB Impairment Index or a general neuropsychological deficit scale (Reitan and Wolfson, 1993) will continue to include this test in their battery, perhaps as one more general in-

Table 8–43. Rhythm Test Means and *SD*s

Age	N	Mean	SD	Range
RHYTHM TEST—NO. CORRECT				
9	43	14.23	5.5	
10	42	18.85	6.3	
11	46	19.10	6.3	
12	47	19.66	5.3	
13	38	20.85	4.9	
14	51	19.54	5.4	
RHYTHM TEST—NO. ERRORS				
15–17	32	2.1	1.4	0–5
18–23	75	2.5	2.1	0–9

Source: 9- to 14-year-old data, courtesy of Findeis & Weight (1994); 15- to 23-year-old data, adapted from Fromm-Auch and Yeudall (1983), © Swets & Zeitlinger.

dicator of cortical function. Rhythm Test normative data were part of a meta-analysis of 20 data sets (Findeis and Weight, 1993; see Chapter 6 for description of the meta-analysis and Table 8–43 for data).

The reader may also be interested in the Preschool Language Scale–3, a test that is appropriate from birth to 6 years, with recommended modifications for hearing or physical impairments. It includes Auditory Comprehension and Expressive Communication subscales. There is an optional Articulation Screener, Language Sample Checklist and Parent Questionnaire. Also, the Test of Word Reading Efficiency (Torgesen, Wagner et al., 1999) proved useful in a study comparing reading accuracy with word-list reading and reading rate (Waber, Wolff et al., 2000). The sight word subtest requires the child to read real words of increasing difficulty in 45 seconds. The phonologic decoding subtest requires the child to decode nonsense words of increasing difficulty in 45 seconds.

CONCLUSION

The existence of many well-standardized language measures, along with many measures that depend on clinical judgment of specific performance errors, makes the language domain a very interesting and essential portion of the neuropsychological evaluation. There

are many available language batteries that the reader may wish to consider further. Most of the tests included in this chapter were selected because they included specific normative data that were either unpublished or individually distributed across diverse references. Other tests that tend to appear with greater frequency in child neuropsychology research publications were also mentioned. It is important, however, to emphasize that there are many easily obtainable tests of the diverse aspects of language function, including academic achievement tests, to assess integrated function appropriate for grade level. Clinicians need to choose the measures that will best match the characteristics associated with their own clinical practice population.

REFERENCES

Aram, D., Ekelman, B., & Whitaker, H. (1987). Lexical retrieval in left and right brain lesioned children. *Brain and Language, 31,* 61–87.

Aram, D., Meyers, S. C., & Ekelman, B. (1990). Fluency of conversational speech in children with unilateral brain lesions. *Brain and Language, 38,* 105–121.

Baddeley, A. D. (2001). Is working memory still working? *American Psychologist, 56,* 851–864.

Basso, A., Corno, M., & Marangolo, P. (1996). Evolution of oral and written confrontation naming errors in aphasia: A retrospective study on vascular patients. *Journal of Clinical and Experimental Neuropsychology, 18,* 77–87.

Bell, B. D., Hermann, B. P., Woodward, A. R., Jones, J. E., Rutecki, P. A., Sheth, R., et al. (2001). Object namng and semantic knowledge in temporal lobe epilepsy. *Neuropsychology, 15,* 434–443.

Bellugi, U., Bihrle, A., Jernigan, T. L., Trauner, D., & Doherty, S. (1990). Neuropsychological, neurological, and neuroanatomical profile of Williams syndrome. *American Journal of Medical Genetics Supplement, 6,* 115–125.

Benson, D. F., & Ardila, A. (1996). *Aphasia: A clinical perspective.* New York: Oxford University Press.

Benton, A., & Hamsher, K. (1976). *Multilingual Aphasia Examination.* Iowa City: University of Iowa.

Benton, A., & Hamsher, K. (1983a). *Multilingual Aphasia Examination.* Iowa City, IA: Department of Neurology, University of Iowa Hospitals and Clinics.

Benton, A., Hamsher, K., & Sivan, A. B. (1994). *Mul-*

tilingual Aphasia Examination: Manual of instructions (3rd ed.). Iowa City: AJA Associates, Inc.

Berninger, V. W., & Colwell, S. O. (1985). Relationships between neurodevelopmental and educational findings in children aged 6 to 12 years. *Pediatrics, 75*, 697–702.

Boone, K. B., & Rausch, A. (1989). Seashore rhythm test performance in patients with unilateral temporal lobe damage. *Journal of Clinical Psychology, 45*, 614–618.

Booth, J. R., Macwhinney, B., Thulborn, K. R., Sacco, K., Voyvodic, J., & Feldman, H. M. (1999). Functional organization of activation patterns in children: Whole brain fMRI imaging during three different cognitive tasks. *Progress in Neuro-Psychopharmacology and Biological Psychiatry, 23*, 669–682.

Bornstein, R. L. (1983). Reliability and item analysis of the Seashore Rhythm Test. *Perceptual and Motor Skills, 57*, 571–574.

Campbell, J. M. (1998). Review of the Peabody Picture Vocabulary Test, Third Edition. *Journal of Psychoeducational Assessment, 16*, 334–338.

Campbell, J. M., Bell, S. K., & Keith, L. K. (2001). Concurrent validity of the Peabody Picture Vocabulary Test-Third Edition as an intelligence and achievement screener for low SES African American Children. *Assessment, 8*, 85–94.

Charter, R. A., & Webster, J. S. (1997). Psychometric structure of the Seashore Rhythm Test. *The Clinical Neuropsychologist, 11*, 167–173.

Cohen, M. J., Town, P., & Buff, A. (1988). Neurodevelopmental differences in confrontational naming in children. *Developmental Neuropsychology, 4*, 75–81.

Denckla, M. B., & Cutting, L. E. (1999). History and significance of rapid automatized naming. *Annals of Dyslexia, 49*, 29–42.

Denckla, M. B., & Rudel, R. (1972). Color naming in dyslexic boys. *Cortex, 8*, 164–176.

Denckla, M. B., & Rudel, R. (1974). Rapid "automatized" naming of pictured objects, colors, letters and numbers by normal children. *Cortex, 10*, 186–202.

Denckla, M. B., & Rudel, R. (1976). Rapid "Automatized" Naming (R.A.N.): Dyslexia differentiated from other learning disabilities. *Neuropsychologia, 14*, 471–479.

De Renzi, E., & Faglioni, P. (1978). Normative data and screening power of a shortened version of the Token Test. *Cortex, 14*, 41–49.

De Renzi, E., & Vignolo, L. A. (1962). The Token Test: A sensitive test to detect receptive disturbances in aphasics. *Brain, 85*, 665–678.

DiSimoni, F. (1978). *The Token Test for Children*. Hingham, MA: Teaching Resources Corporation.

Dunn, L. M., & Dunn, L. M. (1997). *Examiner's manual for the Peabody Picture Vocabulary Test* (3rd ed.). Circle Pines, MN: American Guidance Service.

Ewing-Cobbs, L., Levin, H. S., Eisenberg, H. M., & Fletcher, J. M. (1987). Language functions following closed-head injury in children and adolescents. *Journal of Clinical and Experimental Neuropsychology, 9*, 593–621.

Findeis, M. K., & Weight, D. G. (1994). *Meta-norms for Indiana-Reitan Neuropsychological Test Battery and Halstead-Reitan Neuropsychologial Test Battery for Children, ages 5–14*. Unpublished manuscript.

Flowers, D. L., Wood, F. B., & Naylor, C. E. (1991). Regional cerebral blood flow correlates of language processes in reading disability. *Archives of Neurology, 48*, 637–643.

Fromm-Auch, D., & Yeudall, L. T. (1983). Normative data for the Halstead-Reitan Neuropsychological Tests. *Journal of Clinical Neuropsychology, 5*, 221–238.

Gaddes, W. H., and Crockett, D. J. (1975). The Spreen-Benton aphasia tests: Normative data as a measure of normal language development. *Brain and Language, 2*, 257–280.

Gardner, M. F. (2000). *Expressive One-Word Picture Vocabulary Test-2000 Edition*. Novato, CA: Academic Therapy Publications.

Gathercole, S. E., & Baddeley, A. (1989). Development of vocabulary in children and short-term phonological memory. *Journal of Memory and Language, 28*, 200–213.

Geschwind, N. (1965). Disconnection syndromes in animals and man. I. [Review]. *Brain, 88*, 237–294.

Goodglass, H. (1993). *Understanding aphasia*. San Diego, CA: Academic Press.

Goodglass, H., & Kaplan, E. (1983). *Assessment of aphasia and related disorders* (2nd ed.). Philadelphia: Lea and Febiger.

Goodglass, H., Kaplan, E., & Barresi, B. (2000). *Boston Diagnostic Aphasia Examination* (3rd ed.). San Antonio, TX: The Psychological Corporation.

Guilford, A. M., & Nawojczyk, D. C. (1988). Standardization of the Boston Naming Test at the kindergarten and elementary school levels. *Language, Speech and Hearing Services in Schools, 19*, 395–400.

Halperin, J. M., Healey, J. M., Zeitchik, E., Ludman, W. L., & Weinstein, L. (1989). Developmental aspects of linguistic and mnestic abilities in normal children. *Journal of Clinical and Experimental Neuropsychology, 11*, 518–528.

Hammill, D. D., & Larsen, S. C. (1996). *Test of Written Language* (3rd ed.). Los Angeles, CA: Western Psychological Services.

Hodges, J., Patterson, K., Graham, N., & Dawson, K. (1996). Naming and knowing in dementia of Alzheimer's type. *Brain and Language, 54,* 302–325.

Hodges, J., Salmon, D. P., & Butters, N. (1992). Semantic memory impairment in Alzheimer's disease: Failure of access or degraded knowledge? *Neuropsychologia, 30,* 301–314.

Kaplan, E., Goodglass, H., & Weintraub, S. (1983). *Boston Naming Test (Revised 60-item version).* Philadelphia: Lea & Febiger.

Karzmark, P. (2001). Impact of musical experience on the Seashore Rhythm Test. *The Clinical Neuropsychologist, 15,* 305–308.

Katz, W. F., Curtiss, S., & Tallal, P. (1992). Rapid automatized naming and gesture by normal and language-impaired children. *Brain and Language, 43,* 623–641.

Kertesz, A. (1982). *Western Aphasia Battery.* San Antonio, TX: The Psychological Corporation.

Kim, H., & Na, D. L. (1999). Normative data on the Korean version of the Boston Naming Test. *Journal of Clinical and Experimental Neuropsychology, 21,* 127–133.

Kindlon, D. J., & Garrison, W. (1984). The Boston Naming Test: Norm data and cue utilization in a sample of normal 6- and 7-year old children. *Brain and Language, 21,* 255–259.

Kirk, U. (1992). Confrontation naming in normally developing children: Word-retrieval or word knowledge? *The Clinical Neuropsychologist, 6,* 156–170.

Korhonen, T. T., Vaehae-Eskeli, E., Sillanpaeae, M., & Kero, P. (1993). Neuropsychological sequelae of perinatal complications: A 6-year follow-up. *Journal of Clinical Child Psychology, 22,* 226–235.

Korkman, M., Kirk, U., & Kemp, S. (1997). *NEPSY: A developmental neuropsychological assessment.* San Antonio: The Pyschological Corporation.

LaBerge, D., & Samuels, S. J. (1974). Toward a theory of automatic information processing in reading. *Cognitive Psychology, 6,* 293–323.

Lass, N., & Golden, S. (1975). A correlational study of children's performance on three tests for receptive language abilities. *Journal of Auditory Research, 15,* 177–182.

Lindamood, C., & Lindamood, P. (1971). *Lindamood Auditory Conceptualization Test.* Austin, TX: PRO-ED.

Moses, J. A. (1985). Internal consistency of standard and short forms of the Halstead-Reitan Neuropsychological Test Battery. *The International Journal of Clinical Neuropsychology, VII,* 164–166.

Müller, R. A., Rothermel, R. D., Behen, M. E., Muzik, O., Chakraborty, P. K., & Chugani, H. T. (1999). Language organization in patients with early and late left-hemisphere lesion: A PET study. *Neuropsychologia, 37,* 545–557.

Müller, R. A., Rothermel, R. D., Behen, M. E., Muzik, O., Mangner, T. J., & Chugani, H. T. (1998). Differential patterns of language and motor reorganization following early left hemisphere lesion: A PET study. *Archives of Neurology, 55,* 1113–1119.

Pennington, B. F., Grossier, D., & Welsh, M. C. (1993). Contrasting cognitive deficits in attention deficit hyperactivity disorder versus reading disability. *Developmental Psychology, 29,* 511–523.

Reitan, R. (1969). *Manual for Administration of Neuropsychological Test Batteries for Adults and Children.* Unpublished manuscript.

Reitan, R., & Heineman, C. (1968). Interactions of neurological deficits and emotional disturbance in children with learning disorders: Methods for their differential assessment. In J. Hellmuth (Ed.), *Learning Disorders* (Vol. 3, pp. 93–135). Seattle, WA: Special Child Publications.

Reitan, R., & Wolfson, D. (1989). The Seashore Rhythm Test and brain functions. *The Clinical Neuropsychologist, 3,* 70–77.

Reitan, R., & Wolfson, D. (1993). *The Halstead-Reitan Neuropsychological Test Battery: Theory and clinical interpretation.* Tucson, AZ: Neuropsychology Press.

Reynolds, W. (1987). *Wepman's Auditory Discrimination Test Manual* (2nd ed.): Los Angeles, CA: Western Psychological Services.

Roberts, R. J., & Hamsher, K. d. (1984). Effects of minority status on facial recognition and naming performance. *Journal of Clinical Psychology, 40,* 539–545.

Rosner, J., & Simon, D. P. (1971). The auditory analysis test: An initial report. *Journal of Learning Disability, 4,* 384–392.

Rudel, R., Denckla, M. B., Broman, M., & Hirsch, S. (1980). Word-finding as a function of stimulus context: Children compared with aphasic adults. *Brain and Language, 10,* 111–119.

Schum, R. L., Sivan, A. B., & Benton, A. (1989). Multilingual Aphasia Examination: Norms for Children. *The Clinical Neuropsychologist, 3,* 375–383.

Seashore, C. E., Lewis, D., & Saetveit, D. L. (1960). *Seashore measures of musical talent.* New York: The Psychological Corporation.

Seidman, L. J., Biederman, J., Monuteaux, M. C., Doyle, A. E., & Faraone, S. V. (2001). Learning disabilities and executive dysfunction in boys with Attention-Deficit/Hyperactivity Disorder. *Neuropsychology, 15,* 544–556.

Semel, E., Wiig, E. H., & Secord, W. (1995). *Clinical Evaluation of Language Fundamentals* (3rd ed.). San Antonio, TX: The Psychological Corporation.

Semrud-Clikeman, M., Steingard, R. J., Filipek, P., Biederman, J., Bekken, K., & Renshaw, P. F. (2000). Using MRI to examine brain-behavior relationships in males with attention deficit disorder with hyperactivity. *Journal of the American Academy of Child and Adolescent Psychiatry, 39,* 477–484.

Shaywitz, S. E., Shaywitz, B. A., Pugh, K., Fulbright, R., Constable, R. T., Mencl, W. W., et al. (1998). Functional disruption in the organization of the brain for reading in dyslexia. *Neurobiology, 95,* 2636–2641.

Sherer, M., Parsons, O. A., Nixon, S. J., & Adams, R. L. (1991). Clinical validity of the Speech Sounds Perception Test and the Seashore Rhythm Test. *Journal of Clinical & Experimental Neuropsychology, 13,* 741–751.

Siegel, L. S. (1992). Phonological processing deficits as the basis of a reading disability. *Developmental Review, 13,* 246–257.

Spreen, O., & Benton, A. (1977). *Neurosensory centre comprehensive examination for aphasia. Manual of instructions.* Victoria, B.C.: University of Victoria.

Torgesen, J. K. (1988). Studies of children with learning disabilities who perform poorly on memory span tasks. *Journal of Learning Disability, 21,* 605–612.

Torgesen, J. K. (1996). A model of memory from an information processing perspective: The special case of phonological memory. In G. R. Lyon & N. A. Krasnegor (Eds.), *Attention, memory and executive function* (pp. 157–184). Baltimore: Paul H. Brookes.

Torgesen, J. K., & Bryant, B. R. (1994). *Test of Phonological Awareness.* Austin, TX: PRO-ED.

Torgesen, J. K., & Houck, G. (1980). Processing deficiencies in learning disabled children who perform poorly on the digit span task. *Journal of Educational Psychology, 72,* 141–160.

Torgesen, J. K., Rashotte, C. A., & Greenstein, J. (1988). Language comprehension in learning disabled children who perform poorly on memory span tests. *Journal of Educational Psychology, 80,* 480–487.

Torgesen, J. K., Wagner, R. K., & Rashotte, C. A. (1999). *Test of Word Reading Efficiency.* Austin, TX: PRO-ED, Inc.

Vandervelden, M. C., & Siegel, L. S. (1996). Phonological recoding deficits and dyslexia: A developmental perspective. In J. H. Beitchman, N. J. Cohen, M. M. Konstantareas & R. Tannock (Eds.), *Language, learning, and behavior disorders* (pp. 224–246). Cambridge, U.K.: Cambridge University Press.

Varney, N. R., & Sivan, A. B. (1985). Color association performances of dyslexic and normal children. *Journal of Clinical and Experimental Neuropsychology, 7,* 314–316.

Waber, D. P., Wolff, P. H., Forbes, P. W., & Weiler, M. D. (2000). Rapid automatized naming in children referred for evaluation of heterogeneous learning problems: How specific are naming speed deficits to reading disability? *Child Neuropsychology, 6,* 251–261.

Wagner, R. K., & Torgesen, J. K. (1987). The nature of phonological processes and its causal role in the acquisition of reading skills. *Psychological Bulletin, 101,* 192–212.

Wagner, R. K., Torgesen, J. K., & Rashotte, C. A. (1999). *Examiner's Manual: The Comprehensive Test of Phonological Processing.* Austin, TX: PRO-ED, Inc.

Washington, J. A., & Craig, H. A. (1992). Performances of low-income, African-American preschool and kindergarten children on the Peabody Picture Vocabulary Test-Revised. *Language, Speech and Hearing Services in the Schools, 23,* 329–333.

Wechsler Individual Achievement Test: Manual. (1992). San Antonio, TX: The Psychological Corporation.

Weiler, M., Bernstein, J. H., Bellinger, D., & Waber, D. P. (2000). Processing speed in children with Attention Deficit/Hyperactivity Disorder, Inattentive Type. *Child Neuropsychology, 6,* 218–234.

Wiederholt, J. L., & Bryant, B. K. (1992). *Gray Oral Reading Tests* (3rd ed.). Austin, TX: PRO-ED.

Wiig, E. H., & Secord, W. (1992). *Test of Word Knowledge.* San Antonio, TX: The Psychological Corporation.

Wilkinson, G. S. (1995). *Wide Range Achievement Test administration manual* (3rd ed.). Wilmington, DE: Wide Range, Inc.

Williams, K. T. (1997). *Expressive Vocabulary Test. Manual.* Circle Pines, MN: American Guidance Service.

Wolf, M. (1984). Naming, reading, and the dyslexias: A longitudinal overview. *Annals of Dyslexia, 34,* 87–115.

Wolf, M. (in press). *Time, Fluency, and Dyslexia.* New York: York Press.

Wolf, M., & Biddle, K. R. (1985). *Normative data for RAN and RAS tasks.* Unpublished manuscript. Tufts University, Boston.

Wolf, M., Bowers, P., & Biddle, K. R. (2000). Naming-speed processes, timing, and reading: A conceptual review. *Journal of Learning Disabilities, 33,* 322–324.

Wolf, M., & Goodglass, H. (1986). Dyslexia, dysnomia, and lexical retrieval: A longitudinal investigation. *Brain and Language, 28,* 154–168.

Wolf, M., & O'Brien, B. (2001). On issues of time, fluency, and intervention. In A. Fawcett & R. Nicolson (Eds.), *Dyslexia: Theory and Best Practice* (pp. 124–140.). London: Whur Publishers.

Woodcock, R. W. (1987). *Woodcock Reading Mastery Tests-Revised.* Circle Pines, MN: American Guidance Service.

Yeates, K. O. (1994). Comparison of developmental norms for the Boston Naming Test. *The Clinical Neuropsychologist, 8,* 91–98.

9

Motor and Sensory-Perceptual Examinations

Motor and sensory-perceptual data are distinctly useful to the neuropsychologist. Yet, these data and their contribution in child evaluation are sometimes minimized, omitted entirely, or examined cursorily. Motor and sensory-perceptual data aid in the determination of severity of an acute or chronic neurological insult and extension of impairment across brain regions and in documenting developmental versus acquired impairment. Laterality data that highlight major inconsistencies between the two sides of the body aid in the assessment of differential cerebral hemisphere function when interpreted in context with other data.

Caution, however, must be advised for individual cases. Assumptions based on level of performance about a child's motor and sensory laterality data and their correlation to lateralized cerebral function in the absence of outright brain damage may be open to question since this approach leads to a high rate of false positive errors due to absent discriminant validity. Other modes of clinical interpretation cannot be ruled invalid, including a widely discrepant score that might be pathognomonic of brain dysfunction and a differential score approach in which inferences are made from overall patterns of function rather than solely right–left disparities (Francis, Fletcher et al., 1988). Also, it should be noted that, in the presence of lateralized impairment, a clinician must confirm that the dysfunction is not the result of recent or chronic peripheral limb injury or some other noncentral nervous system etiology.

As for the adult, a poor performance in some aspect of a child's motor and/or sensory examination can highlight a persisting impairment that may be functionally intrusive but subtle enough to remain undetected to the casual observer. For example, general clumsiness or awkwardness on the sports field may indicate residual fine or gross motor deficit long after a precipitating neurological insult such as acquired brain injury or an early and successfully treated posterior fossa brain tumor. While sensory-perceptual deficit can also be subtle and undetected in daily living activities, the assessment and identification of such disturbance is useful in documenting both static and progressive neuropsychological conditions. For example, the presence of a moderate number of sensory-perceptual errors on fingertip number-writing perception and finger recognition testing may be one indication of decompensating hydrocephalus in a young child, whereas a relatively unchanged number of errors across a time interval suggests stability of function and of physiological status over that time span.

MOTOR SOFT SIGNS AND SEQUENCING TESTS

Soft signs are those features that may occur in normal individuals but with greater frequency in those who are neurologically compromised. They are considered possible indicators of a compromised central nervous system, but may be of unclear etiology. Recognizing them on a clinical neurological examination, an examiner makes a formal attempt to quantify their presence in order to determine their significance. Among the signs that have usually been considered soft signs are skull or limb asymmetry, paresis, incoordination, anosmia, dysarthria, and synkinesia (motor overflow movements), generally in a mild form. Mirror movements, directly observable involuntary movements in homologous muscles of the resting limb that mirror voluntary movement of the other limb, are observed in children without neurological impairment, especially when very young. By themselves, motor overflow or mirror movements are not always a worrisome finding; in other instances they may be highlighted as a soft sign (Waber, Mann et al., 1985). The child's chronological age is a factor in interpretation of the significance of such movements. Their presence is expected to diminish around 8 or 9, and they should no longer be observed by age 11, while type and frequency of motor overflow varies greatly among same-aged children (Wolff, Gunne et al., 1983).

Neuroimaging techniques are helping us learn more about motor sequencing and more general motor function. For example, functional imaging study found motor function localizing to secondary areas of the contralesional hemisphere, rather than to primary or homotopic areas, as was found for language function after early focal brain injury (Müller, Rothermel et al., 1998). In other studies it was concluded that the left parietal cortex represents higher order aspects of movements seen by activation during performance of learned movements and during mental rotation of the hands (Bonda, Petrides et al., 1995; Shadmehr and Holcomb, 1997). A distinction is made between anterior and posterior left cerebral function. Deficits in hand posture sequencing are more common after left parietal than frontal damage (Kolb and Milner, 1981), and the parietal lobe has a special role in encoding relationships among abstract properties of sequential movements (Harrington, Rao et al., 2000).

Repetitive and alternating movement tests assess the ability to coordinate the performance of fast movements (Denckla, 1973;

Denckla, 1974). Typically, the preferred hand or foot is tested before the nonpreferred side. Some quantitative procedures or tests of motor planning, sequencing, or incidental motor movements exist to supplement clinical observation and informal evaluation. Child normative data are reported for some of these, while other tests might be clinically useful but have limited or no normative data. The Timed Motor Examination provides normative data for a series of actions (Denckla, 1985), while other data are available for individual tasks.

Timed Motor Examination

The Timed Motor Examination (Denckla, 1985) assesses the time to complete 20 instances of each of a number of actions. Included are foot tapping, finger tapping, alternate heel and toe tapping, hand pronation-supination, hand patting, and successive finger opposition (touching each finger to the thumb in order). Normative data for right handed males and females respectively, aged 5 to 17, are presented in Table 9–1 and Table 9–2. Normative data for left handed males and females aged 5- to 10-years are presented in Table 9–3 and Table 9–4.

Finger Sequencing

A unimanual finger sequencing task was adapted from the Luria Nebraska Neuropsychological Battery for Adults (Golden, 1981), and normative data were published for children 3 to 12 years old (Welsh, Pennington et al., 1991). The task requires the child to touch each of four fingers to the thumb in order (ring finger to pinky) without missing a finger or striking any finger twice, as does the successive finger opposition task noted above on the Timed Motor Examination. However, the score reflects the number of correct sequences completed within 10 seconds rather than 20 seconds required for the Timed Motor Examination. It has been noted that this task continues to develop into adolescence as the eldest children in this study (12 years old) did not achieve adult levels of responding (Welsh, Pennington et al., 1991). These normative data are presented in Table 9–5.

Table 9–1. Timed Motor Examination Means (*SDs*) for Right-handed Males: Denckla Data

Age(Hand)	Foot Tapping	Foot/Heel°	Hand Patting	Pron/Sup°	Finger Tap	Finger App°
5 (Right)	8.57 (2.16)	15.03 (3.75)	6.25 (2.67)	9.32 (1.67)	7.30 (1.08)	16.70 (4.08)
5 (Left)	8.66 (1.86)	14.50 (3.40)	5.93 (1.19)	9.35 (1.64)	7.95 (1.00)	16.88 (5.32)
6 (Right)	6.83 (0.82)	12.16 (1.49)	5.57 (1.27)	8.76 (1.17)	6.69 (0.82)	14.48 (3.23)
6 (Left)	7.13 (1.31)	12.93 (3.45)	5.79 (1.41)	8.59 (1.90)	7.44 (0.91)	14.26 (2.66)
7 (Right)	6.31 (1.63)	10.23 (2.27)	4.82 (1.06)	8.87 (1.93)	5.94 (0.81)	12.22 (2.92)
7 (Left)	6.82 (1.40)	11.70 (2.90)	5.26 (1.42)	6.83 (1.43)	6.60 (0.83)	12.60 (3.05)
8 (Right)	4.71 (0.58)	9.44 (2.36)	4.17 (0.96)	6.83 (1.43)	5.99 (0.98)	10.41 (2.03)
8 (Left)	5.15 (0.71)	10.14 (2.74)	4.74 (0.82)	7.27 (1.08)	6.31 (0.64)	10.84 (2.70)
9 (Right)	5.75 (0.88)	9.21 (1.84)	4.57 (1.13)	7.59 (1.91)	5.97 (0.72)	10.45 (2.95)
9 (Left)	6.08 (0.90)	9.84 (2.25)	4.60 (0.62)	7.66 (1.76)	6.35 (1.23)	10.94 (3.82)
10 (Right)	5.84 (1.39)	8.07 (1.56)	4.31 (1.17)	7.09 (1.54)	5.55 (1.22)	10.22 (2.74)
10 (Left)	6.31 (1.10)	8.61 (1.57)	4.48 (1.26)	7.41 (1.73)	6.09 (1.11)	10.19 (2.65)
11 (Right)	5.1 (0.8)	7.1 (1.4)	3.8 (0.5)	5.8 (1.7)	5.1 (1.3)	9.7 (2.6)
11 (Left)	5.9 (1.1)	7.5 (1.8)	4.1 (0.5)	6.3 (1.9)	6.0 (1.1)	9.8 (2.6)
12 (Right)	4.7 (0.8)	6.6 (1.8	3.7 (0.5	5.6 (1.8)	4.9 (1.2)	8.8 (2.0)
12 (Left)	5.4 (1.3)	7.0 (2.1)	4.0 (0.5)	6.0 (1.8)	5.3 (1.3)	9.2 (2.1)
13 (Right)	4.5 (0.7)	6.2 (1.6)	3.7 (0.5)	5.3 (1.6)	4.7 (0.9)	7.3 (2.3)
13 (Left)	5.2 (1.2)	6.5 (2.3)	4.0 (0.5)	5.7 (1.6)	5.2 (1.0)	7.7 (2.3)
14 (Right)	4.3 (0.7)	5.9 (1.6)	3.6 (0.5)	5.1 (1.3)	4.1 (0.7)	6.2 (1.5)
14 (Left)	4.8 (0.9)	6.1 (1.3)	3.9 (0.5)	5.3 (1.6)	4.6 (0.7)	6.8 (1.5)
15–17 (Right)	4.0 (0.7)	5.6 (1.4)	3.5 (0.4)	4.9 (0.9)	3.5 (0.5)	5.6 (0.9)
15–17 (Left)	4.3 (0.7)	5.6 (1.7)	3.8 (0.6)	5.1 (1.1)	4.1 (0.7)	6.0 (1.4)

Source: Courtesy of Martha Bridge Denckla, M.D., Kennedy Krieger Institute, Johns Hopkins University School of Medicine.

°Foot/Heel = foot heel tapping; Pron/Sup = pronate supinate alternation; Finger App = finger apposition.

Hand Pronation–Supination Test

Bimanual movement is required on the Hand Pronation–Supination Test. The child must make alternating movements, with one hand in a pronation position and the other in a supination position. Instances of reverting to symmetrical movements or any failure to alternate successfully are actions that indicate developmental delay or impairment. This task is useful, along with fist-palm alternation (see Oseretskii Test below) and alternate tapping, as a screening test for cerebellar integrity and as part of the assessment of motor maturity. Normative data are provided as part of the Timed Motor Examination. Qualitative impressions are generally based on attempts to produce a series of correct alternations at least five times consecutively.

Fist-Edge-Palm Test

The Fist-Edge-Palm test is a three-part unimanual motor sequencing task. The task is part of the Luria investigation of dynamic motor functions (Christensen, 1975) and requires successive placement of the hand in three positions. The child must touch the table with a fist, switch to the ulnar edge of the outstreched hand with extended fingers, and then place of the outstretched hand palm down on the table. Repetition of the sequence as an example is acceptable. The movements should be produced as quickly as possible. The sequenced actions are demonstrated for the child and the preferred upper extremity is examined first.

I aim for five correct three-part sequences and keep track of errors, allowing the child to restart after an error. Start-up errors are common, and it might be misleading to consider these early errors as definitive evidence of premotor cerebral impairment or immaturity. Once the preferred side is examined, the child is asked to perform the actions with the other upper extremity, and without examiner demonstration. This enables clinical notation of in-

Table 9–2. Timed Motor Examination Means (*SD*s) for Right-handed Females: Denckla Data

Age(Hand)	Foot Tapping	Foot/Heel°	Hand Patting	Pron/Sup°	Finger Tap	Finger App°
5 (Right)	8.49 (1.35)	12.71 (4.07)	5.91 (1.26)	9.57 (1.56)	7.85 (1.78)	14.40 (2.94)
5 (Left)	9.74 (3.38)	13.16 (3.94)	6.45 (1.25)	10.28 (1.61)	8.56 (1.86)	14.33 (2.20)
6 (Right)	6.79 (1.45)	11.75 (3.44)	5.48 (0.72)	9.38 (1.51)	6.51 (1.01)	13.13 (2.61)
6 (Left)	8.01 (2.53)	12.36 (4.11)	6.00 (1.02)	9.02 (1.26)	7.15 (0.97)	13.18 (3.21)
7 (Right)	6.26 (3.01)	9.22 (3.00)	5.22 (1.44)	7.69 (0.88)	5.99 (0.70)	11.29 (3.18)
7 (Left)	5.95 (1.61)	9.71 (3.14)	5.16 (1.18)	7.54 (1.01)	6.83 (0.82)	11.68 (3.30)
8 (Right)	6.14 (0.96)	8.71 (2.06)	4.55 (0.48)	7.29 (1.33)	5.50 (0.80)	9.25 (2.69)
8 (Left)	6.04 (1.09)	8.43 (1.72)	4.63 (0.64)	7.69 (1.15)	6.14 (0.88)	9.89 (2.76)
9 (Right)	5.62 (0.84)	7.44 (1.02)	4.26 (0.72)	6.76 (1.30)	5.84 (1.25)	9.59 (2.10)
9 (Left)	5.91 (1.21)	8.11 (2.33)	4.50 (0.67)	7.05 (1.19)	6.43 (0.90)	9.84 (2.20)
10 (Right)	6.32 (2.03)	6.90 (1.57)	5.43 (1.81)	7.05 (1.36)	5.77 (1.38)	8.41 (2.37)
10 (Left)	6.34 (1.88)	7.00 (1.49)	5.37 (1.72)	7.04 (1.55)	6.27 (1.79)	7.99 (2.11)
11 (Right)	4.8 (0.6)	6.3 (2.9)	3.8 (0.8)	5.7 (1.6)	5.4 (1.4)	7.7 (2.2)
11 (Left)	5.3 (1.1)	7.7 (2.1)	4.3 (0.7)	6.1 (1.6)	5.9 (1.5)	7.8 (2.3)
12 (Right)	4.7 (0.4)	6.0 (2.8)	3.6 (0.8)	5.5 (1.3)	4.8 (1.2)	7.3 (1.0)
12 (Left)	5.2 (1.1)	6.9 (2.4)	4.2 (0.7)	5.8 (1.4)	5.2 (1.0)	7.4 (1.0)
13 (Right)	4.5 (0.2)	5.6 (1.2)	3.5 (0.8)	5.3 (1.2)	4.7 (1.1)	6.8 (0.5)
13 (Left)	4.9 (0.9)	5.9 (2.0)	4.2 (0.6)	5.6 (1.3)	5.1 (0.7)	6.9 (0.5)
14 (Right)	4.3 (0.2)	4.9 (0.7)	3.5 (0.7)	4.8 (0.7)	4.4 (0.8)	6.4 (0.2)
14 (Left)	4.6 (0.9)	5.3 (1.4)	4.1 (0.6)	5.4 (0.5)	4.7 (0.5)	6.5 (0.2)
15–17 (Right)	4.0 (0.1)	3.9 (0.5)	3.4 (0.6)	4.3 (0.4)	3.8 (0.5)	5.1 (0.1)
15–17 (Left)	4.4 (0.4)	4.7 (0.4)	4.0 (0.6)	4.6 (0.5)	4.1 (0.2)	4.8 (0.4)

Source: Courtesy of Martha Bridge Denckla, M.D., Kennedy Krieger Institute, Johns Hopkins University School of Medicine.

°Foot/Heel = foot heel tapping; Pron/Sup = pronate supinate alternation; Finger App = finger apposition.

terhemispheric transfer of this information along with useful clinical observation of the methods the child uses to accomplish the task, such as, vocal cueing, trial and error, and reference back to movement of the other side.

Oseretskii Test of Reciprocal Coordination

The Oseretskii Test of Reciprocal Coordination (Buchanan and Heinrichs, 1989), or fist-palm alternation, requires alternating movements

Table 9–3. Timed Motor Examination Means (*SD*s) for Left-handed Males: Denckla Data

Age(Hand)	Foot Tapping	Foot/Heel°	Hand Patting	Pron/Sup°	Finger Tap	Finger App°
5 (Right)	10.25 (2.26)	11.42 (2.02)	5.56 (1.49)	11.28 (6.57)	6.89 (1.06)	19.99 (6.29)
5 (Left)	9.54 (2.00)	10.71 (2.72)	5.91 (1.75)	8.92 (2.77)	7.19 (1.06)	19.12 (4.50)
6 (Right)	8.30 (1.60)	13.30 (3.23)	5.81 (1.05)	9.75 (1.59)	7.75 (1.40)	16.49 (5.30)
6 (Left)	9.39 (2.51)	12.48 (1.82)	5.28 (0.76)	9.38 (1.27)	7.00 (0.97)	16.20 (4.80)
7 (Right)	8.05 (1.94)	11.04 (3.09)	5.28 (0.80)	9.39 (2.64)	6.74 (0.86)	14.40 (3.06)
7 (Left)	9.00 (2.49)	10.41 (2.44)	4.58 (0.59)	7.70 (0.80)	6.58 (0.89)	13.90 (3.10)
8 (Right)	6.29 (1.07)	8.55 (2.22)	4.92 (0.43)	7.81 (1.14)	6.52 (0.84)	12.69 (2.58)
8 (Left)	6.96 (1.25)	10.05 (4.39)	4.54 (0.57)	7.18 (1.60)	6.19 (0.78)	12.00 (2.51)
9 (Right)	6.48 (1.79)	8.35 (3.36)	4.85 (1.11)	7.39 (2.49)	5.31 (0.79)	9.61 (2.46)
9 (Left)	4.94 (1.10)	8.70 (4.30)	4.51 (0.66)	6.88 (2.58)	4.64 (0.89)	10.06 (2.51)
10 (Right)	5.34 (1.48)	6.31 (2.36)	3.95 (0.67)	7.02 (1.29)	5.46 (0.96)	11.10 (2.12)
10 (Left)	5.22 (1.16)	6.18 (2.57)	3.74 (0.77)	6.39 (0.96)	4.74 (1.39)	9.41 (2.21)

Source: Courtesy of Martha Bridge Denckla, M.D., Kennedy Krieger Institute, Johns Hopkins University School of Medicine.

°Foot/Heel = foot heel tapping; Pron/Sup = pronate/supinate alternation; Finger App = finger apposition.

Table 9–4. Timed Motor Examination Means (*SDs*) for Left-handed Females: Denckla Data

Age(Hand)	Foot Tapping	Foot/Heel°	Hand Patting	Pron/Sup°	Finger Tap	Finger App°
5 (Right)	12.55 (3.52)	15.55 (2.64)	6.22 (1.09)	10.36 (1.46)	7.61 (0.93)	17.84 (4.44)
5 (Left)	13.39 (4.41)	16.31 (5.30)	5.90 (0.90)	9.22 (0.53)	7.18 (0.43)	17.34 (5.76)
6 (Right)	6.95 (1.46)	8.98 (3.05)	5.64 (1.38)	8.58 (1.00)	7.42 (1.08)	16.49 (5.30)
6 (Left)	7.64 (2.06)	10.51 (3.63)	5.52 (1.05)	8.54 (1.78)	6.79 (1.01)	15.15 (3.59)
7 (Right)	8.72 (2.54)	9.16 (2.36)	5.18 (1.03)	8.70 (1.27)	6.71 (0.57)	13.69 (3.16)
7 (Left)	7.88 (1.77)	9.62 (2.95)	4.95 (0.83)	8.25 (1.28)	6.65 (0.89)	13.14 (2.27)
8 (Right)	6.36 (1.15)	7.56 (3.13)	4.75 (0.78)	7.19 (0.98)	6.35 (0.68)	11.70 (2.38)
8 (Left)	6.46 (0.86)	6.46 (1.89)	4.04 (0.83)	6.88 (1.06)	5.46 (0.61)	10.72 (2.29)
9 (Right)	6.71 (1.35)	6.80 (2.40)	4.84 (1.05)	6.61 (1.09)	5.59 (0.90)	9.54 (2.76)
9 (Left)	6.31 (0.95)	6.66 (2.09)	4.36 (0.92)	6.30 (1.36)	5.04 (0.72)	9.06 (1.88)
10 (Right)	6.65 (1.86)	7.29 (2.67)	4.61 (1.46)	7.14 (1.51)	4.80 (1.19)	9.66 (1.90)
10 (Left)	6.11 (1.82)	7.06 (1.98)	4.32 (1.19)	6.94 (1.41)	4.28 (0.96)	8.94 (1.42)

Source: Courtesy of Martha Bridge Denckla, M.D., Kennedy Krieger Institute, Johns Hopkins University School of Medicine.

°Foot/Heel = foot heel tapping; Pron/Sup = pronate/supinate alternation; Finger App = finger apposition.

when one hand is in an outstretched position and the other is fisted. The Oseretskii Test of Reciprocal Coordination was administered as part of a cross-sectional study examining the performances of 219 3- to 8-year old children on several bimanual and unimanual coordination tasks (Tupper, 1983a; 1983b) (see Table 9–6 for demographic data). The test is one of the tasks in the Luria investigation of motor functions (Christensen, 1975). There were an approximately equal number of males and females, and the age groups were equivalent demographically. About 80% were right-side dominant. Children with hearing, visual, or learning difficulties were excluded. The Porac-Coren Lateral Preference Inventory (Coren, Porac et al., 1979; Coren, Porac et al., 1981; Porac and Coren, 1981) was used. Tasks administered to dominant, nondominant, and both hands in this specific order included the Purdue Pegboard Test and bilateral alternating finger tapping and associated movements testing (see below).

The child was first asked to open and close the dominant hand as fast as possible for a 10-second trial while seated at a table with the elbow on the table and the hand up in the air. The instructor said, "I want you to hold your hand up like this. Let me see you open and close your hand as fast as you can. Good. Now, when I say Go, do that as fast as you can until I tell you to Stop. Okay. Go." The second trial

Table 9–5. Means and *SDs* of Motor Sequencing Raw Scores by Age: 10-second trials

Age	Mean	SD	N
3	1.50	.85	10
4	2.60	1.35	10
5	3.10	2.23	10
6	2.70	.675	10
7	4.00	.943	10
8	4.00	1.05	10
9	5.40	1.43	10
10	5.70	1.49	10
11	5.90	1.52	10
12	6.60	1.35	10

Source: Adapted from Welsh et al. (1991), with permission of Lawrence Erlbaum Associates.

Table 9–6. Bimanual and Unimanual Performance: Tupper Study

Subjects: 219 children in Western Canada
Age: 3 to 8 years
Gender: 114 male (52%), 105 female (48%)
Handedness: 80% right handed
Race: Mostly Caucasian
SES: Middle- to upper-middle class
Exclusion criteria: hearing, visual, or learning difficulties

Source: Unpublished data courtesy of David E. Tupper (1983), personal communication.

required nondominant hand performance. The number of alternations (complete opening and closing) was recorded.

The third trial was of bilateral performance. The child was instructed to alternate opening and closing hands so that while one hand was open, the other was closed: "Now I want you to put both hands up and to start with one hand open and one hand closed, like this. I want you to close this hand, and open this one, then open this one and close that one, and keep going, like this. Now you try. That's good. When I say Go, do that as fast as you can until I tell you to stop. Okay. Go." The number of alternations for both hands was scored. Alternations were defined as a complete sequence of one hand opening and closing and then the other hand opening and closing. The hands had to be in the same position as the starting position to count as an alternation.

Scoring for children who could not alternate was the number of simultaneous movements divided by 2. Also, a 1 was scored if the child was able to complete the both-hands trial correctly, and a 0 was scored if the child could not alternate hands. The means and standard deviations by age and gender on the Oseretskii Test of Reciprocal Coordination performance are presented in Table 9–7.

It was concluded that lateral preference patterns did not change significantly from ages 3 to 8, while unilateral motor skills of both the preferred and nonpreferred hands did increase linearly. Nondominant hand functioning was at about 90% of dominant hand performance at all ages. This is of interest, given clinical lore that a 10% to 20% differential is within normal limits. The preferred hand was superior for motor skills across ages most of the time (60%–70%) for both right- and left-preferring children. These data were interpreted to mean that it is most appropriate to conceptualize unilateral motor abilities in young children with a strict dissociation of lateral preference versus lateral proficiencies or skill. They also supported the conclusions of an earlier study of young children, but with combined age groups, that compared the relationship between lateral preference pattern and manual skill distribution (Annett, 1971).

Associated Movements

Associated-movements testing in the Tupper study (Tupper, 1983a; 1983b) involved the untimed administration of ipsilateral and contralateral finger trials for the right or left side, for a total of 20 trials. Unintended movements were scored. The task consisted of having the child place both hands palms downwards on a piece of paper. The examiner then drew a line around each hand, explaining to the child that

Table 9–7. Oseretskii Test of Reciprocal Coordination Means (*SDs*) by Age and Gender: Tupper Data

Age	Sex	N	Dominant Hand	Nondominant Hand	Both Hands
			NUMBER OF ALTERNATIONS		
3	Male	15	20.33 (3.04)	19.73 (2.76)	9.40 (1.59)
	Female	15	20.60 (2.87)	18.80 (3.34)	9.87 (3.78)
4	Male	15	23.67 (3.06)	22.80 (2.86)	12.73 (2.96)
	Female	15	22.47 (3.62)	21.27 (3.49)	10.27 (2.68)
5	Male	16	26.44 (3.65)	25.06 (2.35)	13.38 (4.86)
	Female	15	24.47 (3.76)	22.40 (2.90)	11.00 (3.05)
6	Male	23	27.17 (2.72)	25.61 (3.12)	14.00 (4.35)
	Female	19	26.68 (3.27)	25.00 (2.16)	15.95 (3.72)
7	Male	22	29.59 (2.99)	28.55 (3.00)	18.09 (3.02)
	Female	21	27.90 (4.02)	26.43 (3.42)	17.95 (3.01)
8	Male	23	30.91 (3.49)	29.09 (3.03)	17.74 (3.33)
	Female	20	28.05 (4.35)	26.35 (3.42)	17.50 (2.84)

Source: Unpublished data courtesy of David. E. Tupper (1983), personal communication.

her hands were being traced and that the hands must remain on the paper. The examiner then pointed to a finger with a pencil and the child was asked to lift that finger. The examiner demonstrated lifting the designated finger with his own hands, while keeping the other fingers unmoving. The child was instructed to lift the finger pointed to, but was not specifically told to refrain from moving the other fingers. Examination consisted of pointing to each finger of the dominant hand in order (thumb, middle finger, index finger, ring, little finger) and then to the fingers of the nondominant hand in the same order. The finger lifted was always replaced before the next trial.

The directions are: "I want you to put both of your hands on this paper, and I will trace them. When I finish tracing them, I want you to leave your hands where they are. Now, I am going to point to your fingers like this (demonstrate on self), and whenever I point to one, I want you to lift that finger for me, like this. We'll start on this hand." Instructions before starting the second part: "Now we will go through this one more time so leave your hands there. Lift the finger I point to."

To score, the examiner first marks with a slash the number of other fingers that were lifted at the same time as the designated finger, for each finger of both hands. Second, the both-hand sequence was repeated, and the number of contralateral hand movements were recorded with a cross mark. Different marks made it possible to later examine the pattern, that is, total slash marks indicated the number of homolateral (same side) movements, and total crosses indicated number of contralateral (opposite side) movements for both hands. The means and standard deviations for associated movements by age and gender are presented in Table 9–8.

LATERAL DOMINANCE: HANDEDNESS

Handedness is an important component of cerebral lateralization in humans. Two common approaches used to define and measure handedness are examination of manual skill and observation of manual preference for a specific task. In clinical practice, handedness is most often defined by hand preference on a specific task such as writing.

Handedness is generally firmly established by age 9, and often is clearly evident earlier. Right-handedness is preponderant, with an incidence of approximately 90%, or slightly higher, in the general population. Age differences are associated with handedness incidence, that is, about 10% to 13% of the normal young adult population is left-handed for writing (Spiegler and Yeni-Komishian, 1983)

Table 9–8. Associated Motor Movements Means (*SDs*) by Age and Gender: Tupper Data

			NUMBER OF MOVEMENTS	
Age	Sex	N	Contralateral	Homolateral
3	Male	15	4.27 (1.87)	9.53 (3.72)
	Female	15	4.00 (2.33)	9.67 (3.39)
4	Male	15	2.00 (1.65)	8.67 (3.31)
	Female	15	2.40 (1.96)	6.87 (2.56)
5	Male	16	2.50 (2.00)	6.38 (2.66)
	Female	15	1.67 (1.11)	5.40 (1.30)
6	Male	23	1.17 (0.94)	5.39 (1.92)
	Female	19	1.05 (1.47)	4.89 (2.26)
7	Male	22	0.95 (1.09)	3.68 (1.94)
	Female	21	0.33 (0.58)	3.24 (2.55)
8	Male	23	0.17 (0.39)	3.22 (2.73)
	Female	20	0.40 (0.94)	2.95 (1.76)

Source: Unpublished data, courtesy of David. E. Tupper (1983), personal communication.

while very young children may demonstrate a greater proportion of left handedness. This is often clinically apparent in evaluating infants or preschoolers, when reaching with the left arm is more commonly observed than for school age children. Such a tendency is recognized as normal and not proof of eventual left-handedness, but perhaps of more import if there is a close family history of left-handedness, in a grandparent, parent, or sibling.

A higher incidence of left-handedness is also associated with certain population subgroups. Some neurological populations are associated with high percentages of left-handedness, including persons with hydrocephalus (Baron and Goldberger, 1993). There are data supporting a higher incidence of left-handedness in the creative arts community (Peterson, 1979). There is also continued interest in the concept of pathological left-handedness (Satz, 1972), in which left-handedness results from a trauma or early development circumstance that makes the left cerebral hemisphere brain regions or networks less capable of sustaining right-side preference.

The literature contains a number of approaches to handedness documentation and proposed functional and genetic models (Chapman and Chapman, 1987; see review by Fennell, 1986). Commonly, one of a number of standardized hand-preference questionnaires is routinely used. Simply asking for self-report of hand preference is not ideal because the intensity of preference is not documented, and self-report may not correlate well with actual manual performance. This is particularly true in cases of ambidexterity, when handedness was changed secondary to injury, or in now rare instances when an adult's or culture's preference is for the child to switch to right-handedness. Thus, in some cultures, a low incidence of left-handedness is reported that might be due to an environmental rather than biological basis.

In infants and young children hand "preference" must also be defined within the context of a specific task. It is likely that neural networks subserving attention, vision and head position, praxis, corticospinal motor control, and language are somehow integrated into handedness. Interestingly, there is evidence of right thumb-sucking in most fetuses starting around the 15th gestational week. After birth, reaching movements are noted earlier than prehension. The hand preferred for unimanual use at 7 months corresponds to the dominant hand used in bimanual activities at 13 months (Ramsay, 1980). By around 9 months, the majority of babies have settled on the right hand (Harris, 1982). However, a unilateral hand preference may be interspersed with ambidexterity until the baby is close to 24 months, and these fluctuations may be related to specific events in language development [see review by (Butterworth and Hopkins, 1993)].

Anomalous early or late hand preference suggests neuromotor dysfunction. A striking preference for one hand before age 1 may be a marker of lateralized cerebral damage. An early sign of a hemiparesis is a consistent lateralized hand preference at around 6 months for all tasks (without the fluctuations seen in normal children). Prolonged ambidexterity, that is, no sign of hand preference by age 3, is another marker of a possible neurodevelopmental problem. Since determining hand preference by relying on either parental observation or self-report may be misleading, it is valuable to ask the child to perform a series of actions and to observe directly and quantify hand use and praxis.

Handedness will directly influence interpretive conclusions about neuropsychological data. For example, right hemisphere dysfunction in the presence of lowered performance IQ, together with impaired function on visuoperceptual and visuomotor and visuospatial tests, cannot be reliably ascribed when the child is left-handed or if right-handedness is not strongly established. About 96% of right-handed, but only 70% of left-handed epilepsy patients had left hemisphere control of language, using the Wada sodium amytal technique and results of a handedness questionnaire. Of the remaining 30% left-handers, about 15% had right hemisphere language representation and 15% had bilateral language representation (Rasmussen and Milner, 1977).

Thus, although the probability is high that even left-handers have language mediated principally by the left cerebral hemisphere, a proportion of individuals will have either contralateral mediation or crossed control, or bilateral influences without clear strong lateralization. A distinction is made between *ambidextrous* hand preference in which the person uses one hand consistently for certain tasks, but varies hand use for other tasks and *ambiguous* hand preference in which there is inconsistent hand use within a type of task and across different tasks (Elliott and Watkins, 1998). Ambiguous hand preference is common among the mentally retarded, possibly due to bilateral cortical damage that makes neither hemisphere dominant for motor function (Sopher, Satz et al., 1987).

A variety of lateral dominance tests or procedures are available, and only a few are noted here. These take the form of questionnaires, action tasks, observations, and self-report. One of the more widely used is the Reitan-Klove Lateral Dominance Examination that is routinely administered as part of the Halstead-Reitan Neuropsychological Test Battery (HRNTB; Reitan and Davison, 1974) or individually included by some endorsing a flexible battery approach. Right–left discrimination for four personal and four extrapersonal body parts and a request for demonstration of seven transitive movements for apraxia screening and strength of laterality are included. A request for transitive movements requires the demonstration of pretend action for an object and therefore serves as a screening for dyspraxia as well.

Intransitive or nonrepresentational movements are not sampled on this test. A small number of eye and foot dominance screening items are included. For example, using the Miles ABC Test of Ocular Dominance, the child views a picture through a conical form that allows the examiner to see the eye preferred. The child also demonstrates how to kick a ball or step on a bug. Frequently, however, children will demonstrate inconsistent laterality for hand, eye, and foot preference, and failure to demonstrate one-sided preference should not be automatically interpreted as indicative of pathology.

The Handedness Inventory (Briggs and Nebes, 1975) is a hand-preference questionnaire that measures strength of laterality. Scoring is published for 12 actions: write a letter legibly, throw a ball to hit a target, play a game requiring the use of a racquet, place at the top of a broom to sweep dust from the floor and

at the top of a shovel to move sand, hold a match when striking it, hold scissors to cut paper, hold thread to guide it through the eye of the needle, deal playing cards, hammer a nail into wood, hold a toothbrush while cleaning teeth, and unscrew the lid of a jar. The actions are scored for always left (-2), usually left (-1), no preference (0), usually right (1), always right (2). Scores of $+9$ or above $=$ right-handed, -9 to $+8 =$ mixed-handed, -9 to $-24 =$ left-handed.

The Hand Preference Demonstration Test (Llorente, Satz et al., 1998) assesses hand preference by asking the child to demonstrate the use of nine objects, presented three times each in a counterbalanced order for a total of 27 presentations. Completion by a parent for an indirect quantitative measure of premorbid hand preference is possible. Another such measure is the Harris Test For Lateral Dominance (Harris, 1947), which screens for left–right discrimination with three items, hand preference with ten unilateral actions (and thus dyspraxia as well), simultaneous writing, timed handwriting, one trial tapping, coordination while dealing cards, and grip strength. There are also screening items for foot dominance, eye dominance with monocular and binocular tests, and optional stereoscopic testing. Using this measure's 10 unilateral actions in a longitudinal study of over 200 males, handedness at age 5 was found predictive of handedness at age 11, unless there was evidence of ambidexterity (Fennell, Satz et al., 1983).

The Edinburgh Handedness Inventory (Oldfield, 1971) questionnaire inquires about ten unimanual items, with the respondent checking off degree of hand preference strength, or indicating no preference. It allows for a computation of a laterality quotient. The Porac Coren Lateral Preference Inventory (Porac and Coren, 1981), which assesses eye, hand, ear, and foot preference with behavioral items appropriate for young children is also available.

Another short-hand preference screening procedure requires the child to demonstrate writing, ball throwing, cutting with scissors, hammering, drinking from a cup, picking up a piece of candy, eating with a spoon, and tooth brushing. Requests for picking up a dime and pointing to the examiner's nose are included (Green, Satz et al., 1989). The requests are made over two to three trials. If there is 100% accuracy for the right or left side, then handedness is assigned as right or left, respectively. Inconsistent responses between trials for three or more tasks can be considered indicative of ambiguous-handedness, while within-item inconsistent responses on two or fewer tasks lead to a decision of ambidextrous (Elliott and Watkins, 1998).

The PIN Test (Satz and D'Elia 1989) provides a ratio of the dominant-hand fine motor skill to the nondominant-hand fine motor skill—the Pin Advantage Index or Pin AI. This index provides a continuum of relative motor advantage for each upper extremity. The individual must insert a pin through a small holes arranged in a serpentine line on a metal plate, producing holes in an underlying paper template. Each hand performs the task twice, alternating each trial. The number of punched holes for each trial is recorded and averaged for the two trials by hand.

There is also a history of examination of writing posture in investigation of cerebral hemisphere specialization and functional integration. Inverted versus noninverted posture and their relative contribution to language lateralization was a focus of study (Levy and Reid, 1976). It is noted that most right-handers have a noninverted posture, that is, the right hand is positioned beneath the line of writing, and the pencil points toward the top of the page. About two-thirds of left-handers used an inverted writing posture, that is, the hand is positioned above the line of writing, and the pencil points downward. The implications of these differences is not firmly established (Levy, 1982), yet of particular clinical interest when the child neuropsychologist is faced with a left-handed, and far more rarely, a right-handed child who inverts hand posture.

RIGHT–LEFT ORIENTATION

Directional orientation learning develops over years, and is a hierarchical complex of abilities that also is associated with intelligence level (Benton, 1962). The average 7 year old can cor-

rectly discriminate right and left on his own body, but may still fail to make extrapersonal discriminations for several years. Further, once able to make these 180-degree judgments about lateral body parts, a 10-year-old child may still make errors when required to make a more complex response requiring simultaneous self and extrapersonal orientation "Place your right hand to my left shoulder." (Benton, 1962). Tests such as the Money Road Map Test depend on right–left orientation (see Chapter 10). A 20-item right–left orientation subtest is included in the Benton Laboratory of Neuropsychology Tests (Benton, Sivan et al., 1994). Right–left orientation questions are also included on aphasia screening tests. Further, one may simply ask the child to point to his or her own right- and left-sided body parts and then to the examiner's body directly across from the child, a screening for orientation in extrapersonal space.

PRAXIS

Praxis refers to the ability to perform skilled movements. Movement representations (praxicons or visuokinesthetic movement engrams) are stored in the inferior parietal lobe, and usually, but not always, in the dominant hemisphere. Thus, praxis involves association cortex and is firmly linked to the dorsal occipitoparietal pathway, the "where" system that requires an appreciation for the spatial locations of objects and that is differentiated from the ventral occipitotemporal pathway, "what" system, important for object identification. Both of these pathways interact with prefrontal cortex. Apraxia refers to an inability to perform learned skilled movements that is not explained by weakness, incoordination, sensory loss, or inability to understand instructions (Liepmann, 1920; Geschwind, 1975). Apraxia is a loss of, or inability to access or evoke movement representations of skilled forelimb actions that involve three-dimensional motor sequences in time.

Praxis assessment involves asking the child for a pantomime of these skilled acts. Pantomime request provides minimal cues and therefore depends on stored learned movement representations. A child is considered *apraxic* if, despite an otherwise normal neurological examination, a simple learned movement cannot be performed. One should request both transitive movements and intransitive movements. Examples of transitive movements, which require tool or instrument use, are: using a scissors, combing hair, hammering a nail, brushing teeth, hitting with a hammer, throwing a ball, cutting with a knife, eating with a spoon, writing with a pencil, using an eraser. Examples of intransitive movements, those that demonstrate a familiar gesture, include: making a hitchhike sign, saluting, demonstrating the "OK" or victory symbols, waving goodbye, snapping fingers, making a fist, crossing fingers, praying, and applauding.

Normal adults typically make more errors when producing transitive than intransitive pantomimes and also have greater difficulty selecting correct postures for transitive than intransitive movements, suggesting intransitive gesture representations are stored or activated differently than those for transitive pantomimes (Mozaz, Gonzalez-Rothi et al., 2002). These authors developed a recognition test of praxis knowledge that does not rely on verbal command comprehension or require pantomime or gesture production, the Postural Knowledge Test.

Both limbs should be tested in the clinical evaluation. When pantomime errors are made, the examiner should model the gesture and request that the child then imitate the action. If needed, the actual tool may be provided for use. A thorough apraxic examination might also include testing of the ability to comprehend pantomimes and associate tools with specific tasks and functions. Apraxia and aphasia can coexist, but are also dissociable. Also, dyspraxia was also dissociable from intellectual ability in a study of 9- to 12-year-old children (Deuel and Doar, 1992).

Apraxic deficits can occur at a production as well as at a conceptual level. Several types of apraxia are described. *Ideomotor apraxia* refers to impaired pantomime and imitation. *Dissociation apraxia* is also referred to as callosal apraxia. *Ideational apraxia* refers to the impaired use of common objects, with preserved pantomime and imitation. *Conceptual apraxia*

refers to difficulty with tool–object knowledge (Ochipa, Rothi et al., 1989; 1992). When a body part is used to represent the imagined object, the response is a "body-part-as-object" (BPO) error (Goodglass and Kaplan, 1963) or "body-part-as-tool" (BPT) error (Raymer, Maher et al., 1997). The latter authors suggested that BPT errors (when pantomiming transitive gestures to verbal command) made by normal subjects are usually corrected on a second trial, while limb apraxic subjects do not correct on a second attempt. In one study, normal adults of any age were able to correct BPO errors on subsequent trials, attesting to the integrity of these gestural representations in both young and older adult groups (Peigneux and van der Linden, 1999). Such data support good clinical practice of asking the child to repeat an action that was performed incorrectly. For example, the request, "Show me how you would use a scissors" often initially results in a two-fingered scissors motion, but when the command is repeated, the child recognizes the error and converts the action to the appropriate tool-use position. Accepting the first response would lead to inappropriate characterization of the motor action.

A child is considered apraxic if unable to perform a simple learned movement such as brushing teeth, combing hair, or waving goodbye, despite an otherwise normal neurological examination. The dyspraxic child is often described as clumsy or incoordinated, but it is often unlikely that impaired skilled motor movements will be observed incidentally and recognized as the deficit they represent. Therefore, direct examination is required. Reports of dyspraxic children often do not separate motor system deficit from apraxic deficit.

It is suggested that a functioning motor system is required to learn appropriate movement sequences. An integration of a brain-behavior model of apraxia and dyspraxic children identified six impairment patterns in dyspraxic children: (*1*) difficulty learning general rules or schemata about classes of motor actions; (*2*) using perceptual cues such as spatial location or object speed/trajectory; (*3*) organizing somatosensory/vestibular information; (*4*) problem solving or adaption to new situation; (*5*) analyzing task requirements and components, using knowledge in an effective fashion; and (6) preparing for upcoming actions. These deficits involve both praxis and meta knowledge about properties and execution of motor movements, that is, prefrontal cognition (Goodgold-Edwards and Cermak, 1990).

The neurological substrate of limb apraxia is well researched, and it is recognized that frontoparietal circuits control these complex skilled actions. Parietal cortex damage disrupts kinematic and spatiotemporal aspects of movement. More specifically, damage to left middle frontal gyrus (Brodmann areas 46, 9, 8, and 6) and the inferior and superior parietal cortex (areas 7, 39, 40) surrounding the intraparietal sulcus commonly produces ideomotor limb apraxia (Haaland, Harrington et al., 2000). The classic view of a left hemisphere contribution is supported by functional imaging data. That is, the left cerebral hemisphere of right-handers controlled cognitive motor tasks of both arms (Haaland and Harrington, 1996). Left motor cortex and association areas of either hemisphere were activated by ipsilateral and contraleteral movements while right hemisphere motor regions were not activated. Left premotor cortex was involved in the selection of movements of either hand, but in the left hand only after right premotor cortex stimulation, and the disruption was specific to response selection rather than motor activation (Haaland, Harrington et al., 2000). Also, the left hemisphere plays a more central role in the storage and retrieval of motor representations (Bonda, Petrides et al., 1995). Haaland and her colleagues' data support the view that frontal and parietal cortex are equally implicated as formerly proposed (Heilman, Rothi et al., 1982), but contradicts another view (Geschwind, 1965) that subcortical parietal lobe damage to fibers connnecting frontal and occipital cortex is primarily responsible for ideomotor limb apraxia.

Frontal lobe regions and their relationship to apraxia were investigated. The supplementary motor area (SMA) and limb apraxia are associated in some studies, but not in others. Questions about their relationship is not easily answered since focal SMA damage is rare. However, limb apraxia in stroke patients with SMA damage is reported (Haaland, Harring-

ton et al., 2000). While the middle frontal gyrus role in limb apraxia is as yet unknown, its association with aspects of working memory are recognized. Area 6 was associated with short-term storage and areas 9 and 46 related to active manipulation of the stored information (Smith and Jonides, 1999). It was also found that areas 9 and 46 were activated when preparing to imitate simple movements (Krams, Rushworth et al., 1998).

Pantomime Recognition Test

Pantomime recognition deficits are associated with left hemisphere lesions. A Pantomime Recognition Test was developed (Benton, Hamsher et al., 1983a) and administered to 80 children aged 3 to 8 years old from schools around Iowa City, Iowa (Sivan and Varney, 1985). The test requires the child to identify the object whose use was pantomimed on a color videotape. There are 30 pantomimes of the use of common objects, such as a pen. The child chooses each object pantomimed from among four presented black-and-white line drawings. The adult mean score was 28.7, and a score of 26 fell at the fifth percentile. The results for children were as follows: Age 3 years ($N = 10$), mean of 20.8, range of 17–24. Age 4 years ($N = 10$), mean of 24.6, range of 18–28. Age 5 years ($N = 20$), mean of 25.3, range of 20–30. Age 6 years, ($N = 15$), mean of 28.0, range 26–30. Age 7 years ($N = 15$), mean of 29.1, ranged of 27–30. Age 8 years ($N = 10$), mean of 29.8, range 29–30. Thus, children as young as 6 already demonstrated performance comparable to that of adults.

MOTOR SPEED, DEXTERITY, AND STRENGTH

Motor performance tests provide continuous measure data that supersedes the usefulness and reliability of pathognomonic sign data in child evaluation (Kaspar and Sokolec, 1980). Motor function evaluation typically includes tests of speed, dexterity, and/or strength. These do not always include all factors one may be interested in. The experimental literature provides data about force and timing of motor action, variables not routinely assessed with current clinical instrumentation. For example, sequential tapping was studied in 15 children with motor incoordination and 15 control subjects matched for age, gender, and verbal IQ. The "clumsy" children had longer reaction time and left their finger on the tapping plate longer for each tap than did the controls—a mechanical movement feature of interest. The groups did not differ for time taken between taps or on mean average force. The authors concluded that clumsy children do have a timing deficit, but that implementation is critical, and it is peripheral rather than central nervous system processes that may the most important contributors to these timing deficits (Piek and Skinner, 1999).

Some motor function studies controlled for lowered IQ and therefore provided data for normal children of lowered intelligence. For example, motor speed effects subsequent to brain damage and in the presence of borderline IQ was studied in 39 brain-injured children and 38 matched for age, IQ, and gender control children 5 to 8 years old. Both the brain-damaged and borderline-IQ children related independently to diminished motor efficiency. The neurologically impaired children were slower than control children with each hand, especially with the nonpreferred hand (Kaspar and Sokolec, 1980). More commonly, data were presented without reference to IQ. Perhaps the most widely used motor measure is the Finger Tapping Test, but it is also a test that is associated with many methodological variations. These affect interpretation of various normative data sets and research data comparability across studies when uniformity is not maintained.

Finger Tapping Test

The Finger Tapping Test (FTT) measure of fine motor speed (Halstead, 1947; Reitan, 1969) is also referred to as the Finger Oscillation Test, or Index Finger Tapping Test. The child is encouraged to tap rapidly, using only the index finger on a tapping apparatus for a specified number of trials. Trials are conducted independently for the right and left side. A comparison of preferred and nonpreferred upper extremity efficiency results from calculation of the mean tapping rate for each side.

An electric finger tapper is recommended for the "Kiddie" version for 5 to 8 year olds. A manual finger tapper is used for children age 9 and older. Exceptions are noted: the Spreen and Gaddes (1968) 8- to 12-year-old data for the manual finger tapper and the more commonly referenced Spreen and Gaddes (1969) 6- to 13-year-old electric tapper data, reported along with 9- to 15-year-old data for the manual tapper. However, the latter data are presented as total number of taps across six trials, and are not prorated for five trials or presented as averaged scores consistent with procedures for the Reitan-Indiana Neuropsychological Test Battery for young children and Halstead Intermediate Neuropsychological Test Battery for older children.

Administration rules vary widely with respect to number of trials, inclusion of rest breaks, acceptable standards for averaging, and hand-alternation patterns. Hand position is rarely specified, that is, whether fisted or fingers spread out, although position can affect speed. The considerable confounds to standardized test administration and scoring criteria are well described (Snow, 1987). For example, Knights and Norwood (1980) reported on the average of the best three of four 10-second trials within 5 points, with the child allowed to attempt 10 trials. Knights and Moule used a Meylan finger counter, mounted on a board, instead of the Reitan-type tapper (Knights and Moule, 1967). As noted above, Spreen and Gaddes (1969) included a 50-tap, warm-up period and six 10-second trials, not the more common five trials per hand. Fromm-Auch & Yeudall (1983) used a manual tapper, and Reitan's procedure of five consecutive 10-second trials per hand for 193 adolescents and adult subjects, including adolescent age-range blocks of 15 to 17 years and 18 to 23 years.

Further, administration instructions for the FTT are not uniform, and instructions might vary across settings. For example, in an early manual (Reitan 1969) the instructions stated:

Measurements are made first with the subject using the index finger of the preferred hand, and a comparable set of measurements are obtained with the

Table 9–9. Sample Tapping Data Interpretation by Source

Source	Standard Score: Preferred	Standard Score: Non-Preferred
Klonoff & Low, 1974	100	100
Finlayson & Reitan, 1976	116	116
Knights & Norwood, 1980	86	98
Spreen & Gaddes, 1969	101	108

Source: Courtesy of Lynn Bennett Blackburn and Tara V. Spevack.

non-preferred hand. The subject is given 5 consecutive 10-second trials with the hand held in a constant position in order to require movements of only the finger rather than the whole hand and arm. Every effort is made to encourage the subject to tap as fast as he possibly can (p. 5).

In later directions, the objective was to obtain five trials within five taps of one another. Later still, a maximum of 10 trials was recommended. More recently, a standardized record form directs a practice trial, then two trials, a rest break, and then three additional tapping trials for each side. Should these five consecutive trials not yield scores within a five-tap range, the directions are to continue to 10 trials (three additional trials, a rest, and the final two trials) and compute the mean for all 10 trials (Psychological Assessment Resources, 1992). What is important, irrespective of any set of instructions is that timing begin when the child makes the first tap, and not when the examiner says "go" or "start." The delay between the start command and the actual tapping can skew mean rate downward.

As a result of these many procedural and methodological variations, uniformity of administration has not been obtained across settings, interpretation of normative data cannot be expected to be uniform as a result, and one's data may require prorating, depending on which normative reference data set is chosen. Further complicating the picture is the availability of primarily old normative data, with different interpretations resulting, dependent on which older data set one chooses to use. It is incumbent on the current examiner to realize there is considerable disparity in procedures and normative data bases that profoundly complicate FTT interpretation. For example, it has been pointed out (Blackburn and Spevack,

2000; Lynn Blackburn and Tara Spevack, 2000, personal communication) that one neuropsychologist might use one set of norms and describe a child as intact on finger tapping, while another neuropsychologist might refer to a different set of norms and characterize the child as impaired. To illustrate their point, they point out the disparity between normative data and standard scores for preferred and nonpreferred upper extremity tapping speed by comparing an 8 year old's average performance according to various norms (see Table 9–9 for these calculations).

Older FTT normative data were relied on, and some of these data sets are presented here for comparative purposes. For example, early FTT normative data were obtained on 120 children: 20 at each age level for 6, 7, 8, 12, 13, and 14 years (Finlayson and Reitan, 1976) (see Table 9–10 for demographic data). These normative data are presented by age, gender and handedness in Table 9–11, and leave a gap for children below 6, from 9 to 11, and 15 and older. An older data set for 5- to 14-year-old children (Knights, 1966) are presented in Table 9–11 along with data for 8- to 12-year olds (Spreen and Gaddes, 1968). A small adolescent group was included as part of an adult study, and the tapping data using the manual tapper for these 15 to 17 year olds (Fromm-Auch and Yeudall, 1983) are also presented in Table 9–11. Normative data on 231 children aged

Table 9–10. Demographic Data for Finger Tapping Test: Finlayson and Reitan Study (1976)

Subjects: 120 children, 20 at each of 6 age levels
Age: 6–8 and 12–14 years old
Gender: 60 male; 60 female (20 children/age level; 10 per cell)
Handedness: All right-handed

Table 9–11. Finger Tapping Test Normative and Reference Group Means and SDs

Age	MALE RIGHT HAND[1]		MALE LEFT HAND[1]		FEMALE RIGHT HAND[1]		FEMALE LEFT HAND[1]		DOMINANT HAND[2]		NON-DOMINANT HAND[2]		DOMINANT HAND[3]		NON-DOMINANT HAND[3]		DOMINANT HAND[4]		NON-DOMINANT HAND[4]		DOMINANT HAND[5]		NON-DOMINANT HAND[5]	
	M	SD	M	SD	M	SD	M	SD	M	SD	M	SD	M	SD	M	SD	M	SD	M	SD	M	SD	M	SD
5									22.6	3.0	21.5	4.9					28.56	2.88	26.00	3.04	26.98	5.14	23.99	4.18
6	35.60	4.06	32.00	4.32	33.10	4.07	30.10	3.45	25.8	3.4	21.6	2.8					32.66	4.44	29.85	3.98	28.15	3.48	25.36	3.01
7	37.00	3.83	33.40	3.34	36.90	5.57	32.50	5.06	26.6	3.8	24.4	2.8					36.09	4.28	33.01	3.96	29.78	4.72	26.82	4.17
8	39.90	5.15	35.20	5.09	38.80	4.95	33.30	4.55	29.3	3.6	27.3	3.1	41.6	5.2	36.0	6.1	37.98	4.49	34.02	5.55	33.75	5.09	29.86	4.71
9									31.8	4.2	29.2	3.7	34.3	4.3	30.7	3.7					33.90	4.12	30.20	3.27
10									34.8	5.3	32.6	5.2	37.6	4.9	33.1	4.7					37.37	5.43	33.20	4.86
11									38.5	4.9	35.5	5.4	37.9	5.5	34.1	4.7					40.90	4.79	36.48	4.75
12	41.00	6.34	36.40	4.95	41.40	5.83	35.50	3.92	39.7	5.3	36.6	5.4	41.3	5.4	36.7	3.8					41.61	4.89	36.89	3.88
13	45.80	3.99	38.90	5.36	40.70	5.17	35.40	4.33	43.2	4.5	38.9	5.8									45.97	5.80	42.01	4.58
14	47.30	7.13	40.70	6.72	44.70	4.83	39.30	4.95	45.3	4.5	40.8	4.5									46.32	6.04	42.18	5.45
15–17[6]	47.6	5.8	43.6	4.9	42.7	7.9	41.1	6.2																
18–23[6]	49.5	6.9	45.4	6.9	43.6	7.5	41.2	6.5																

Adapted from: [1] = Finlayson, M. A. J. & Reitan, R. M. Handedness in relation to measures of motor and tactile-perceptual functions in normal children. *Perceptual and Motor Skills*, 1976, 43, 475–481. © Perceptual and Motor Skills 1976; [2] = Spreen & Gaddes (1966); [3] = Knights (1966); [4] = Fromm-Auch & Yeudall, (1983); © Swets & Zeitlinger. [5] = Klonoff and Low (1994); [6] = Gray et al. Reference Group (2000).

2 years, 8 months, to 15 years, 10 months were obtained, without report of gender, socioeconomic status, or handedness. These children had a mean IQ of 11.71 to 113.79 across the ages (SD = 8 to 10) (Klonoff and Low, 1974). A subset of these data are also included in Table 9–11.

Normative data were also published for 462 children aged 6 to 13 years old, consecutively, by age and gender (Spreen and Gaddes, 1969) using the electric tapper. Normative data using the manual tapper for ages 9 to 15 were also published in this report. It should be noted that these data were obtained under a procedural variation of the Halstead-Reitan Neuropsychological Test Battery (HRNTB): a 50-tap warm-up, followed by six 10-second trials. The trials are administered in this order: three dominant hand trials, three nondominant hand trials, three dominant hand trials and three nondominant hand trials. The data were total number of taps for six trials, and therefore the totals need to be prorated to be equivalent to the five trials per hand HRNTB procedure.

Findeis and Weight meta-normative data
Unpublished meta-normative data on 3225 children that included the FTT for children aged 5 to 14 (Findeis and Weight, 1994) are less well known. However, they are in use clinically by a number of child neuropsychologists with access to these data and judged useful by those familiar with these norms. Informally, it would appear that merging data across studies has clinical merit, but this requires empiric validation. (See Chapter 6 for a listing of the 20 studies used to calculate these meta-norms and

for the demographic data.) The FTT results of the meta-analysis are presented in Table 9–12.

A reference group sample of 219 children, aged 5 to 8, with academic or behavioral problems, from rural or suburban Texas was administered the FTT (Gray, Livingston et al., 2000) as part of the administration of a larger number of Reitan-Indiana Neuropsychological Test Battery measures. The tapping scores were reported as the mean of five tapping trials. These reference data are included along with normative data sets in Table 9–11.

Bilateral Alternating Finger Tapping Test

As noted above, an unpublished study provided normative data for bilateral alternating finger tapping for children 3 to 8 years old (see Table 9–6 for demographic data) (Tupper, 1983a; 1983b). The apparatus for this test was a painted plywood board with two standard telegraph keys (3 cm in diameter) mounted 12 cms apart, graduated for a travel of 2 mm and a 50 gram force, and connected to electric counters. Three trials were obtained in this order: dominant hand, nondominant hand, both hands. For the unilateral trials, the child was asked to tap as fast as possible with his or her index finger on the key, and the other fingers spread out on the board. Approximately 30 practice taps were given. Each actual trial was 10 seconds in duration. For the both-hands-alternating trial, the child placed the index fingers of both hands on the keys and first tapped with one finger, then the other. The instructor said, "This time I want you to place both hands

Table 9–12. Findeis & Weight Meta-Norms: Finger Tapping Test

Age	DOMINANT HAND			NONDOMINANT HAND		
	N	Mean	SD	N	Mean	SD
5	339	29.39	4.2	311	26.32	4.6
6	226	29.87	3.3	221	27.22	3.3
7	288	33.67	4.6	288	30.01	3.9
8	265	36.40	4.6	265	32.03	3.8
9	49	34.01	4.1	49	30.31	3.3
10	95	37.52	5.4	95	34.04	4.8
11	93	40.72	4.8	93	35.06	4.8
12	143	41.36	5.4	143	36.66	4.1
13	41	44.64	5.2	41	39.64	4.7
14	52	44.38	6.8	52	40.67	6.1

Source: Unpublished data, courtesy of the authors, Findeis & Weight (1994).

on the buttons. What I want you to do is to tap with one hand, then the other, like this [demonstrating]. You try. That's it. When I say 'Go,' do that as fast as you can until I tell you to stop. Okay. Go." The score was the combined left- and right-hands scores, provided they were within three taps of each other. If a young child could not alternate and only made simultaneous taps, his or her total score was divided by two and a notation made on the score sheet. The trial was included only if the difference between the two hands was three taps or less, to ensure adequate alternation. In addition to scoring the number of taps for each 3-trial portion, a 1 was scored if the child completed the bilateral alternating trial correctly, and a 0 if alternation was not correct. The results of bilateral alternating finger tapping test performance are presented in Table 9–13.

Grooved Pegboard Test

The Grooved Pegboard Test (Klove, 1963; Reitan, 1969) is a widely used dexterity test that assesses speed and accuracy of eye–hand coordination. It has a long history of usefulness in child neuropsychology. It produces data different than those obtained from other commonly administered motor function tests, such as the FTT. While this difference may relate to involvement of different neuroanatomical pathways, such a distinction is likely not based solely on such dissociation for the neurologically impaired child.

Determining the child's relative efficiency of speed and dexterity on both tests is useful. For example, a child with maximal subcortical dysfunction might evidence poor dexterity, impaired motor go-no-go inhibitory behavior, impaired motor sequencing, poor rapid alternating movements, and/or poor handwriting, along with other indicators of impairment from tests within different domains while maintaining intact gross motor tapping speed. Motor slowness might be secondary to a mood disorder and reflected in unilaterally or bilaterally poor performance on tests of speed, strength, and/or dexterity. For example, nineteen depressed school-aged right-handed boys between 9 and 11 failed to demonstrate the expected asymmetry for grip strength, while 19 nondepressed boys exhibited the preferred right upper extremity grip strength. A trend was noted for more rapid right upper extremity fatigue across the four dynamometer trials for nondepressed boys, but depressed boys maintained the left upper extremity grip longer across trials than nondepressed boys (Emerson, Harrison et al., 2001). Intact dexterity— but lateralized tapping speed impairment— might indicate residual cortical dysfunction such as that associated with a traumatic brain injury or cerebrovascular insult. Evaluation of these differential patterns (see convergence profile analysis in Chapter 1 for discussion) contributes to a more complete and accurate interpretive conclusion.

Table 9–13. Bilateral Alternating Finger Tapping Means (*SDs*) by Age and Gender: Tupper Data

| Age | Sex | N | NUMBER OF TAPS | | |
			Dominant Hand	Nondominant Hand	Both Hands
3	Male	15	24.07 (4.22)	22.73 (4.42)	32.87 (10.13)
	Female	15	23.87 (4.84)	23.00 (5.82)	32.67 (10.14)
4	Male	15	28.07 (4.70)	26.93 (3.41)	42.67 (10.91)
	Female	15	28.80 (4.68)	26.60 (4.26)	42.53 (11.58)
5	Male	16	32.39 (3.59)	28.81 (3.27)	38.38 (8.55)
	Female	15	28.80 (4.68)	26.67 (4.47)	36.27 (9.43)
6	Male	23	32.39 (3.59)	28.78 (3.77)	41.96 (6.49)
	Female	19	33.47 (4.29)	30.68 (3.87)	47.32 (12.63)
7	Male	22	35.55 (2.42)	32.14 (2.90)	48.77 (9.85)
	Female	21	35.33 (3.64)	32.38 (3.40)	47.10 (7.91)
8	Male	23	40.26 (4.09)	37.00 (3.67)	55.61 (11.13)
	Female	20	36.90 (5.46)	35.95 (4.50)	52.75 (10.52)

Source: Unpublished data, courtesy of David. E. Tupper (1983), personal communication.

The grooved pegboard is placed midline with the child so that the board is at the edge of the table and the peg tray immediately above the board. The older child (9 years old and up) places 25 keyhole shaped pegs into holes on a $4'' \times 4''$ board, beginning at the left side with the right hand and at the right side with the left hand. The child is encouraged to place the pegs quickly. Three scores are reported: (1) time to completion with each upper extremity, (2) the number of unintentional peg drops during each trial, and (3) the number of pegs correctly placed in each trial. Younger children, 5 years to 8 years, 11 months, need only place pegs into the two upper rows, that is, 10 pegs.

The instructions for children are:

This is a pegbaord and these are the pegs (Examiner points). All the pegs are the same. They have a groove. That is, a round side and a square side, and so do the holes in the board. What you must do is match the groove of the peg with the groove of the board and put these pegs into the holes like this (Examiner does top row). When I say "go," begin here and put the pegs into the boards as fast as you can, using only your (dominant) hand. Fill the top row completely from this side to this side. Do not skip any. Fill each row the same way you filled the top row. Any questions? Ready, as fast as you can, Go!

Note that the dominant hand trial precedes the nondominant hand trial, the examiner can tell the child to speed up if necessary, and the examiner can point out the first hole of a new row. Although the printed directions do not specify this, only one peg should be picked up at a time and only one hand used. If a peg is dropped on the floor, one of the first pegs placed is taken out and used again so as not to interfere with timing. Timing begins when the child starts the task, and a trial can be discontinued after 5 minutes.

The printed material that accompanies the purchase of the pegboard cites normative data as part of those obtained from a clinical neuropsychological test battery administered to over 2500 adults and children (Trites, 1977). Normative data for the Lafayette Instrument Company pegboard were published for 184 children 5 to 14 years old (Knights and Moule, 1968), see Table 9–14. The norms are for 61 children, 5 to 8 years old, and 123 older children and adolescents, 9 to 14 years old. The cell sizes were small, ranging from 10 to 22 children per cell for 5- to 8-year-olds and 18 to 24 children per cell for 9- to 14-year-olds. These data were subsequently updated as "smoothed" data (see Table 9–15). Because the raw data plotted over age levels resulted in sawtooth patterns, the means and SDs were smoothed statistically to provide consistent standard scores from age level to age level (Knights, 1970).

More current normative data are also available for 358 Canadian adolescents (152 male and 206 female), aged 12 to 15 (Christopher Paniak and colleagues, personal communication, unpublished norms) (see Table 9–16).

Purdue Pegboard Test

The Purdue Pegboard Test was developed to aid in selection of employees for industrial jobs

Table 9–14. Grooved Pegboard Test: Means (SDs) for Time in Seconds and Errors

Age	N	DOMINANT HAND Mean (SD)	ERRORS Mean (SD)	NONDOMINANT HAND Mean (SD)	ERRORS Mean (SD)
5	10	60.8 (26.0)	0.30 (0.48)	61.6 (22.5)	0.70 (1.30)
6	11	50.9 (17.8)	0.09 (0.30)	59.4 (21.7)	0.18 (0.40)
7	22	34.9 (7.2)	0.05 (0.21)	38.0 (8.0)	0.09 (0.29)
8	18	34.3 (12.5)	0.06 (0.24)	39.6 (21.0)	0.06 (0.24)
9	21	66.7 (11.5)	0.24 (0.24)	79.3 (13.7)	0.24 (0.54)
10	24	71.7 (8.0)	0.25 (0.53)	77.1 (10.0)	0.08 (0.28)
11	18	65.5 (9.5)	0.22 (0.43)	71.2 (8.7)	0.11 (0.32)
12	21	65.9 (8.7)	0.19 (0.40)	71.8 (10.0)	0.40 (0.36)
13	20	62.2 (7.0)	0.15 (0.37)	66.9 (9.1)	0.10 (0.31)
14	19	66.5 (13.3)	0.05 (0.23)	70.1 (7.5)	0.05 (0.23)

Reproduced with permission of authors and publisher. Knights, R. M. & Moule, A. D. Normative data on the Motor Steadiness Battery for children. *Perceptual and Motor Skills*, 1968, 26, 643–650. © Southern Universities Press, 1968.

Table 9–15. Grooved Pegboard Test Smoothed Normative Data

Age	N	DOMINANT HAND Mean (SD)	ERRORS Mean (SD)	NONDOMINANT HAND Mean (SD)	ERRORS Mean (SD)
5	10	60.8 (26.0)	0.30 (0.48)	61.6 (22.54)	0.70 (1.25)
6	11	50.9 (17.79)	0.20 (0.30)	52.0 (21.69)	0.18 (0.41)
7	22	43.0 (10.0)	0.20 (0.29)	45.0 (17.0)	0.00 (0.29)
8	18	36.0 (8.0)	0.20 (0.24)	39.0 (10.0)	0.00 (0.15)
9	21	74.0 (15.0)	0.22 (0.40)	80.0 (15.1)	0.23 (0.50)
10	24	72.0 (10.0)	0.17 (0.35)	78.0 (10.0)	0.18 (0.40)
11	18	70.0 (8.0)	0.15 (0.33)	76.0 (8.32)	0.11 (0.33)
12	21	68.0 (7.5)	0.13 (0.30)	74.0 (7.8)	0.05 (0.30)
13	20	66.0 (7.2)	0.11 (0.29)	72.0 (7.54)	0.00 (0.29)
14	19	64.0 (6.86)	0.09 (0.29)	70.0 (7.2)	0.00 (0.29)

Source: Adapted from Knights (1970).

(Tiffin and Asher, 1948). Peg placement on the Purdue Pegboard Test of Manual Dexterity (PTT) is a useful measure of finger dexterity. After a practice trial with the right hand, the child is instructed to pick up the pegs with the right hand, one at a time and place them rapidly in holes on the right side of the board until told to stop at 30 seconds elapsed time. A practice trial with the left hand precedes the 30 second left-hand trial for holes on the left side of the board. The third trial allows the child to use both hands simultaneously, picking up a peg with each hand and placing the pegs at the same time. Scores are obtained for number of pegs placed for each unilateral trial and for the number of pairs of pegs placed for the both hands trial.

Purdue Pegboard Test performance was studied with respect to its ability to discriminate children with learning disabilities, including 150 children with learning problems who did not receive any remedial intervention and 45 children enrolled in a program for children with minimal brain dysfunction who had received at least 6 months of remedial reading, perceptual training, controlled physical and motor coordination exercises and special class placement (Kane and Gill, 1972). The results of these analyses are provided in the test manual, Instructions and normative data for Model 32020 Purdue Pegboard, (undated). Early normative data for 5- to 15-year-old children were published (Gardner and Broman, 1979), for boys and girls from New Jersey aged 5 to 15 years, 11 months, in 6-month increments, approximately 30 subjects in each cell (663 boys and 671 girls). Normative data were also reported for a right-handed preschool population with a modified version of the PPT (Wilson, Iacovello, et al., 1982). The Gardner and Broman data are also published elsewhere, stratified by gender and age (Spreen and Strauss, 1998). Ex-

Table 9–16. Grooved Pegboard Test Mean (SD): Time in Seconds: Paniak et al. Data

		MALE			FEMALE	
Age	N	Right Hand Mean (SD)	Left Hand Mean (SD)	N	Right Hand Mean (SD)	Left Hand Mean (SD)
12	38	64.61 (10.08)	70.03 (10.85)	56	66 05 (8.64)	71.61 (9.37)
13	39	61.82 (6.74)	67.33 (10.85)	57	62.93 (6.27)	70.60 (9.57)
14	46	64.00 (10.54)	70.09 (10.88)	70	62.43 (9.12)	67.30 (10.06)
15	29	62.21 (7.04)	68.34 (8.95)	23	64.78 (9.52)	67.48 (10.72)

Source: Unpublished data, courtesy of Christopher Paniak, Harry Miller & Deirdre Murphy personal communication.

Table 9–17. Purdue Pegboard Demographic Data: Wilson et al. Study (1982)

Subjects: 206 children in Nassau County, New York
Age: 2 years 6 months to 5 years 11 months
Gender: 105 male, 101 female
Handedness: Right-handed, determined by three criteria
Race 186 Caucasian (90.4%); 30 non-Caucasian (9.6%)
SES: Heterogeneous sample with majority from two income families
Inclusion criteria: Normal learning skills, psychosocial development, absence of motor clumsiness

amination of performance for overlapping age levels between the Wilson et al. and Gardner and Broman studies found no significant differences for either males or females, supporting the use of the modified PPT as a finger dexterity measure, for right handers. The 1982 study by Wilson and colleagues involved an adaptation of the standard 25-pair PPT, reducing it to 15 pairs. Table 9–17 presents the demographic data for 206 children, aged 2 years, 6 months to 5 years, 11 months, and Table 9–18 presents the normative data means, standard deviations, and ranges for these children stratified by age.

An unpublished study of young children's bimanual and unimanual motor function also provided normative data for children 3 to 8 (see Table 9–6 for these demographic data) (Tupper 1983a; 1983b). An adapted version with 15 pairs of holes was also used for 3- to 5-year-old children, and the full size version with 24 pairs of holes was used for children 6 to 8 years old. The adaptation was accomplished by sawing off

the lower portion of the pegboard to obtain a 29.5 × 29.5 cm board, making it easier for the children to reach the pegs. For this study, three trials were given for each of three conditions in a specific order: dominant hand, nondominant hand, both hands. The means and standard deviations for the Purdue Pegboard Test performance for each board version are presented in Table 9–19.

A variety of other pegboard performance tests are available. The Wide Range Assessment of Visual-Motor Abilities (Adams and Sheslow, 1995), for example, has a pegboard subtest that allows 90 seconds.

Grip Strength Test

Comparisons of the two sides of the body can also be made using a dynamometer or similar measure of gross motor strength. The Halstead-Reitan procedure requires the child to grip an apparatus, the Smedley Hand Dynamometer,[1] twice with each upper extremity, alternating between dominant hand and nondominant hand side. The mean grip strength for each side is then calculated. There are recent grip strength data that suggest functional motor asymmetries do indeed exist in children, as they do in adults (Emerson, Harrison et al., 2001).

The Findeis and Weight meta-normative study also included grip strength data for 5 to 14 year olds (see Chapter 6 for description of this meta-analysis). The results of these data

[1]The Smedley Hand Dynamometer is purchased through the Stoelting Corporation.

Table 9–18. Purdue Pegboard Test Means and SDs: Wilson et al. Data

Age	N	M/F	RIGHT HAND			LEFT HAND			BOTH HANDS		
			M[1]	SD	Range	M[1]	SD	Range	M[2]	SD	Range
2–6 to 2–11	20	10/10	4.70	1.08	3–7	4.05	1.15	2–7	2.95	1.28	0–5
3–0 to 3–5	24	10/14	5.54	1.62	3–9	5.13	1.42	2–8	3.63	1.53	0–6
3–6 to 3–11	25	10/15	6.80	1.26	4–9	6.00	1.38	3–8	4.20	1.23	2–7
4–0 to 4–5	40	23/17	8.08	1.49	4–11	6.68	1.25	4–9	5.23	1.44	2–8
4–6 to 4.11	46	27/19	9.07	1.58	6–13	8.20	1.56	4–11	6.07	1.20	4–9
5–0 to 5–5	31	15/16	10.16	1.77	7–14	9.19	2.02	6–14	6.81	1.76	4–10
5–6 to 5–11	20	10/10	9.90	1.59	7–13	9.00	1.26	6–11	6.35	1.69	3–9

Source: Wilson et al., 1982; © Swets & Zeitlinger.

[1]Mean number of pegs placed; [2]Mean number of pairs of pegs placed.

Table 9–19. Purdue Pegboard Test Means (*SDs*) by Age and Gender: Tupper Data

Age	Sex	N	NUMBER OF PEGS		
			Dominant Hand	Nondominant Hand	Both Hands
3	Male	15	6.07 (2.31)	5.67 (2.23)	3.53 (1.64)
	Female	15	6.60 (1.30)	6.13 (1.36)	4.13 (0.99)
4	Male	15	8.67 (1.45)	7.67 (1.59)	5.40 (1.64)
	Female	15	8.87 (1.19)	7.67 (1.54)	6.00 (0.76)
5	Male	16	10.31 (1.58)	9.00 (1.63)	7.38 (1.86)
	Female	15	10.60 (1.24)	9.13 (0.99)	6.87 (0.99)
6	Male	23	10.91 (1.41)	10.74 (1.25)	7.70 (1.02)
	Female	19	12.11 (1.79)	10.42 (1.77)	8.68 (1.57)
7	Male	22	12.18 (1.47)	11.00 (1.60)	9.14 (1.21)
	Female	21	12.48 (1.12)	11.48 (1.21)	9.24 (1.14)
8	Male	23	13.83 (2.01)	12.52 (1.93)	9.91 (1.31)
	Female	20	13.95 (1.57)	12.60 (1.57)	9.95 (1.57)

Source: Unpublished data, courtesy of David. E. Tupper (1983), personal communication.

analyses are presented in Table 9–20. Data for a school-referred population of 212 Texas children aged 5 to 8, with academic or behavioral problems, are also presented in Table 9–20 (Gray, Livingston et al., 2000). Normative data for 358 Canadian adolescents (152 male and 206 female), aged 12- to 15 (Christopher Paniak and colleagues, personal communication, unpublished norms) are presented in Table 9–21. Normative data for adolescents and young adults were obtained as part of a broader adult study, and these selected normative data are presented in Table 9–22 (Fromm-Auch and Yeudall, 1983).

PSYCHOMOTOR PROBLEM SOLVING

Tactual Performance Test

The Tactual Performance Test (TPT) utilizes a modification (Halstead, 1947) of the Seguin formboard (Sequin, 1866). It requires the child to be blindfolded and is therefore often stressful and best left to late in the test session due to the risk of upsetting the child and losing cooperation. Once blindfolded, oral instructions indicate that the child should feel for the blocks on the table (6 for young children and 10 for older children) and place each block in its respective formboard hole. The 6-hole form-

Table 9–20. Grip Strength Test Means and *SDs*

Age	DOMINANT HAND[1]			NONDOMINANT HAND[1]			DOMINANT HAND[2]			NONDOMINANT HAND[2]		
	N	Mean	SD	N	Mean	SD	N	Mean	SD	N	Mean	SD
5	156	8.27	1.9	128	7.53	1.9	8	6.12	3.22	8	5.56	2.94
6	142	9.13	2.2	142	8.41	2.2	51	8.76	10.29	51	6.91	2.93
7	208	11.60	2.3	208	10.56	2.1	81	9.03	3.77	81	8.59	3.65
8	140	12.43	2.6	140	11.47	2.3	72	11.40	4.49	72	10.20	4.44
9	27	14.74	1.9	27	14.12	1.9						
10	23	17.14	2.7	23	16.09	3.3						
11	33	19.45	3.4	33	18.86	3.2						
12	53	22.92	3.5	53	21.65	4.3						
13	20	26.65	4.7	20	25.10	4.9						
14	20	36.50	3.9	20	32.48	4.6						

Source: Adapted from [1] = Findeis & Weight (1994); [2] = Gray et al. (2000).

Table 9–21. Grip Strength Test Means (SDs) by Gender: Paniak Data

| | | MALE | | | FEMALE | |
| | | Right Hand | Left Hand | | Right Hand | Left Hand |
Age	N	Mean (SD)	Mean (SD)	N	Mean (SD)	Mean (SD)
12	38	26.88 (5.23)	25.41 (4.36)	56	24.17 (4.48)	21.97 (4.53)
13	39	30.54 (6.20)	28.64 (5.67)	57	25.73 (5.13)	23.95 (5.61)
14	46	35.71 (7.04)	33.23 (7.09)	70	27.96 (5.57)	25.73 (5.28)
15	29	38.31 (6.01)	35.78 (5.78)	23	25.50 (6.37)	23.83 (5.62)

Source: Unpublished data, courtesy of Christopher Paniak, personal communication.

board is positioned horizontally for 5- to 8-year-old children and the 10-hole board is positioned vertically for children 9 and older, directly in front of the seated child with the blocks randomly placed before the board. The first timed trial is for the preferred upper extremity alone, the second trial is for the nonpreferred upper extremity alone, and the third trial allows use of both sides together.

Qualitatively, one should note whether the child still relies predominantly on one side, despite the allowance for use of both sides, or whether the use of two sides results in a more effective search and placement strategy. It is also important to be absolutely sure that the child cannot peek out and see the apparatus, once blindfolded. The ability to see is sometimes evident from the way the child's head tilts. After completion of the three trials, the blocks and board are removed, and the blindfold is then removed. The child is given a sheet of paper and a pencil and instructed to draw the blocks as best as he or she can remember them and in their correct location as they were on the board. Thus, time-to-completion scores are obtained for the preferred side, nonpre-

ferred side, and both sides together. These are also summed for a total time score. A memory score is based on number of correctly drawn shapes. A location score is based on the accuracy with which shapes are recalled in their correct spatial location, that is, position accuracy with respect to two other shapes.

While I found the multifactorial TPT useful, especially for serial monitoring the hydrocephalus and Spina Bifida population, I eventually concluded that the lengthy administration time and stress on the child outweighed the data obtained and that such data could be obtained through other less-threatening means. Nonetheless, the test is still in wide use and provides evidence of impaired or intact interhemispheric communication, a particularly appealing finding associated with the administration of unilateral, and then bilateral trials.

With multiple available early normative data for the TPT, the results of the Findeis and Weight meta-normative analysis of 20 studies are of interest and are presented in Table 9–23 (see Chapter 6 for this analysis's demographic data and a listing of normative data studies). Data are presented for 5- to 8-year-old chil-

Table 9–22. Grip Strength Means (SDs) for Adolescents and Young Adults by Gender

| | | MALE | | | | FEMALE | | |
| | | Preferred Mean | Nonpreferred Mean | | | Preferred Mean | Nonpreferred Mean | |
Age	N	(SD)	(SD)	Range	N	(SD)	(SD)	Range
15–17	17	38.0 (8.4)	35.8 (9.6)	22.2–51.0	15	28.1 (5.0)	26.3 (5.2)	17.8–33.5
18–23	43	49.7 (9.7)	46.6 (9.9)	26.7–73.0	29	28.8 (7.8)	26.4 (6.2)	13.5–38.0

Source: Fromm-Auch & Yeudall (1983); © Swets & Zeitlinger.

Table 9–23. Meta-Norm Means, *SDs*, [*N*] for the Tactual Performance Test

Age	5	6	7	8	9	10	11	12	13
Tactual Performance Test	6.46	5.93	5.17	4.15	4.36	3.67	3.15	3.20	2.44
DH (minutes)—(6 blocks)	3.1	3.1	2.7	2.2	2.4	1.7	1.4	1.6.8	.9
	[191]	[160]	[188]	[101]	[92]	[91]	[96]	[104]	[31]
Tactual Performance Test	5.24	4.74	3.66	3.13	3.08	2.73	2.17	2.20	1.61
NDH (minutes)	3.1	2.8	1.9	3.1	1.7	1.6	.9	1.4	.9
	[191]	[160]	[188]	[166]	[92]	[91]	[96]	[104]	[32]
Tactual Performance Test	3.80	3.11	1.98	1.68	1.28	1.27	1.13	1.03	.80
Both Hands (minutes)	2.6	2.1	1.2	1.1	.7	.7	.6	.5	.3
	[191]	[160]	[188]	[167]	[92]	[91]	[96]	[104]	[32]
Tactual Performance Test	15.50	13.83	10.98	8.79	8.80	7.66	6.36	6.13	4.90
Total Time (minutes)	5.6	6.8	4.5	3.8	4.1	3.3	2.3	2.6	1.5
	[206]	[190]	[218]	[197]	[92]	[91]	[96]	[104]	[32]
Tactual Performance Test	2.47	3.06	4.15	4.44	4.40	4.48	4.53	4.77	5.04
Memory (No. correct)	1.8	1.5	1.2	1.2	1.2	1.2	1.1	.8	.9
	[206]	[190]	[218]	[196]	[92]	[91]	[96]	[104]	[31]
Tactual Performance Test	1.10	1.80	2.69	3.22	3.00	3.07	3.07	3.75	3.00
Location (No. correct)	1.1	1.5	1.7	1.7	1.6	1.5	1.6	1.5	1.3
	[206]	[190]	[218]	[196]	[57]	[49]	[58]	[71]	[10]

Source: Unpublished data, courtesy of the authors, Findeis & Weight (1994).

DH = dominant hand; NDH = non-dominant hand.

dren, using the 6-block formboard, and for 9- to 13-year-old children, using the 10-block formboard. Earlier data were published for adolescents and adults with the 10-block formboard. These normative data by age blocks for 15- to 17-year-olds and 18- to 23-year-olds are presented in Table 9–24.

TPT ecological validity and applicability for 5- to 12-year-old Zairian children was examined using the horizontal board position for the entire sample and comparing their results with those of American and Canadian children and differential patterns of typical performance resulted (Boivin, Giordani et al., 1995). Zairian children did not improve performance between preferred and nonpreferred trials, as did the comparison groups, and younger Zairian children took a longer time per block to compete the task with the nonpreferred hand. Whether developmental lag, nutritional differences, or neuropsychological deficit contributed to their poorer performance was considered. It was concluded that the TPT serves a purpose in monitoring longitudinal brain behavior impact of health interventions for enhancing African childrens' cognitive development, but it is probably not appropriate for direct intercultural comparisons.

Another motor test of interest is the Bruininks-Oseretsky Test of Motor Proficiency (BOTMP; Bruininks, 1978). This test aids in the assessment of gross and fine motor skills, such as balance, running speed and agility, response speed visual motor control, upper limb speed and dexterity. Data are presented in scaled scores with a mean of 15 ($SD = 5$) and short form standard scores with a mean of 50 ($SD = 10$).

SENSORY-PERCEPTUAL TESTS

Five distinct somatosensory association cortices are present in humans, each with a characteristic cytoarchitecture and specific patterns of thalamocortical and corticocortical connectivity. They are the primary somatosensory cortex (SI), ventrolateral association cortices (SII, SIII, and SIV), and the dorsomedial association cortex (supplementary sensory area). The areas are associated with differential sensory deficits when impaired. For example, damage to ventrolateral somatosensory cortex produces *tactile agnosia* (impaired object recognition), and impaired size, shape, and texture discrimination. Dorsomedial association cortex lesions

Table 9–24. Tactual Performance Test Means, SDs, [N] for 15–23 Year Olds

Age	15–17	18–23
Tactual Performance Test DH (minutes)—(6 blocks)	4.6 1.2 [32]	5.1 2.2 [74]
Tactual Performance Test NDH (minutes)	3.3 1.2 [32]	3.5 1.6 [74]
Tactual Performance Test Both Hands (minutes)	1.7 0.5 [32]	2.1 1.3 [74]
Tactual Performance Test Total Time (minutes)	9.5 2.1 [32]	10.6 4.5 [74]
Tactual Performance Test Memory (No. correct)	8.9 1.0 [32]	8.2 1.3 [74]
Tactual Performance Test Location (No. correct)	6.8 2.5 [32]	5.7 2.1 [74]

Source: Fromm-Auch & Yeudall (1983); © Swets & Zeitlinger.

are associated with apraxia and sensorimotor integration deficits (Casseli, 1993; Baron, Fennell et al., 1995). A functional magnetic resonance imaging study of healthy right-handed adults examined the anatomical effects of directing attention during somatosensory processing. Attention to unilateral graphesthetic stimuli produced bihemispheric activation with minimal or no activation of the ipsilateral primary sensorimotor region. Attention to unilateral left hand stimuli produced more cerebral activation than attention to unilateral right hand stimuli. Activity in the somatosensory area contralateral to non-attended stimuli increased during bilateral stimulation irrespective of the side of attentional focus. The direction of attention to the right hand during bilateral stimulation increased activation in the left somatosensory region. The direction of attention to the left hand during bilateral stimulation increased activation in both cerebral hemispheres (Meador, Allison et al., 2002).

Sensory examination of the adult may include testing for extinction, barognosis discrimination (weight discrimination), texture perception, dimension, shapes, and substance and tactile object recognition, but sensory examination for children is not routinely as complex (Baron, Fennell et al., 1995). Perception of pain, temperature, and vibration sense are not routinely evaluated in child neuropsychological evaluations, but touch and kinesthetic information are. This is commonly accomplished with tests of tactile form recognition and limb or body movement and position sense. The neuroanatomical substrates for sensory perception and the systems that allow for precise integration and conscious awareness of somatosensory information are described elsewhere (Casey and Rourke, 1992; Baron, Fennell et al., 1995). While tactile-perceptual tests appear to be less reliable than other neurosychological tests (Brown, Rourke et al., 1989), a limited error range for such tests may explain this lowered test–retest reliability (Casey and Rourke, 1992). Importantly, their clinical usefulness for a child is not lessened by a limited normative error range, and the evidence of strongly lateralized impairment is an important finding that requires further exploration to explain its presence. Tests of graphesthesia (fin-

gertip number writing) or finger recognition perception (finger agnosia tests) are especially useful, and potentially confirm a lesion in somatosensory regions of either cerebral hemisphere posterior to the postcentral gyrus, depending on the number of errors and lateralization. While errors do not always indicate pathology, the child's age along with concurrent results from other measures aid in determining the significance of an error profile.

Reitan-Kløve Sensory Perceptual Examination

Tests of primary sensation (tactile, auditory, and visual extinction) and more intergrative tests of finger recognition perception (finger agnosia), graphesthesia (fingertip symbol writing or number writing perception) and form perception (stereognosis) are administered as part of the HRNTB, entitled the Reitan-Kløve Sensory Perceptual Examination (Reitan, 1984). It is possible to administer these tests to children through pantomime demonstration and with slight administrative modifications. Test–retest reliability data (Brown, Rourke et al., 1989) are reported. There are some normative data for these measures, but qualitative judgments about performance are especially important, as noted above.

Double Simultaneous Stimulation

The examination includes testing of double simultaneous stimulation (DSS) for tactile, auditory, and visual stimuli preparatory to examine more integrative sensory-perceptual functions. These tests of double tactile, auditory, and visual perception enable determination of whether there is suppression in response to simultaneous bilateral stimulation after intact function is observed with a single unilateral stimulus presentation on preliminary trials. Eyes are closed for the tactile and auditory conditions. For example, a tactile stimulus can be presented on a contralateral homologous body area, or ipsilateral extinction can be induced, for example, by presenting a stimulus to the face and hand simultaneously for DSS tactile testing. Contralesional extinction suggests sensory neglect, and lateralized errors across modalities make for a stronger case. In the presence of such errors, one will want to pay special attention to other indicators compatible with this hypothesis. A child may read a word, omitting the far left letter(s). Incidental drawings may be drawn primarily on the right side of the page with a wide left margin remains. Paragraph production may be positioned off-center, also with a wide left margin. Clock drawing may reveal compression of features on the right side of space.

It is likely that the most common error will be extinction of the response to the face stimulus when face and hand are touched simultaneously (Casey and Rourke, 1992). Data suggest that a child can be successful on such testing by 3 to 5 years old (Maiuro, Townes et al., 1984; Roeltgen and Roeltgen, 1990). In a study of normal 3- to 15-year-old children, localization of symmetrical stimuli (hand–hand) was well developed in 3 year olds, but localization of asymmetrical stimuli (hand–face) was only successful for 80% of those 8 years old (Fink and Bender, 1953). Presentation of a soft clicking sound (fingers pulled apart) to each ear independently will precede simultaneous clicking sounds for DSS auditory testing. Single finger movement in each hemispace is compared to bilateral finger movements in each of the upper, middle, and lower visual fields for DSS visual testing.

After DSS testing, the test continues with evaluation of finger recognition ability (finger agnosia test), graphesthesia (Finger-tip Symbol Writing Test for children 5 to 8 years old or Finger-tip Number Writing Test for children 9 years old and older) and astereognosis (Tactile Form Recognition). Such testing requires the child's awareness of body schema involving knowing where fingers are in space and having an ability to identify or name the fingers touched (Benton, 1979).

Finger Recognition Testing

Testing of finger recognition perception is conducted to determine if finger agnosia is present. Finger agnosia is a body schema disorder in which the individual cannot identify or name the fingers. It is often associated with lesions of the left parietal lobe and can be due to sensory deficit, spatial disorientation, or inatten-

tion, as well as to aphasic naming problems. The child's ability to differentiate fingers is nearly fully developed by 5 years old, intersensory integration (pointing to the touched finger) does not plateau until about 9 or 10, and representation thinking then develops between age 12 and adulthood (Casey and Rourke, 1992).

For finger recognition testing, the examiner lightly touches a finger between the first and second joint while the child's eyes are closed. The thumb is number 1, and the pinky finger is number 5. The child must indicate by number or finger name which finger was touched. It is important to confirm when a child says "1" that they do not mean "5". This is especially true for the second, nonpreferred hand trials since the numbers are now in reverse order. For some children, assistance is useful, especially when the child finds it hard to keep eyes closed over trials. It may be necessary to state "close eyes," then touch the finger and say, "Open eyes" for each trial. That is, the numbers 1 to 5 are written separately and placed before each respective outstretched finger. The examiner can then say "Close eyes," touch a finger, say "Open eyes," and then say "Now point to the number in front of the touched finger." This procedure is repeated for each trial. Importantly, examiners must double-check that the child keeps his or her eyes closed for the stimulus presentation and does not become so focused on touching the fingers correctly that he or she forgets to look up to check the child's eyes.

The number of finger recognition errors for the 20 trials per hand is recorded for each upper extremity. Finger recognition test reliability over two years for this procedure was modest (ranging from 0.31 to .0.39) (Brown, Rourke et al., 1989), but this is not surprising, given the impact of developmental maturation. Validity studies are reported for finger recognition testing using this procedure (Reitan, 1971; Boll and Reitan, 1972; Reitan and Boll, 1973; Boll, 1974) and provide evidence of the sensitivity of this sensory-perceptual test for brain dysfunction.

Some examiners are confused by the standard HRNTB finger recognition scoring form. An alternative appeals to those who find it difficult to coordinate testing and respond within the original answer sheet format. The following chart of finger numbers exactly follows the standard test form order, which ensures that two consecutive fingers are not touched and that one does not touch finger 1 and then finger 5, or vice versa. The numbers below refer to the order in which fingers are touched. Each finger is touched once for each line for a total of 20 trials per side. Errors can be indicated by a cross-out and the erroneous response written above the correct number.

Right Hand	13524	Left Hand	13524
	24135		24135
	35241		35241
	41352		41352

Fingertip Symbol Writing Recognition and Fingertip Number Writing Recognition

The fingertip symbol writing or number writing recognition tests require the child to accurately perceive a stimulus written with a pencil tip on the pad of each finger, in succession. Young children (5 to 8 years old) have either an X or an O written with a pencil point. Sometimes it is helpful to place a written X and an O on the table for very young children to assist them in responding accurately. The examiner says, "Close your eyes," writes on the fingertip, and then says, "Open your eyes and point to the X or O mark you felt." The "close eyes-write-open eyes" procedure is easily repeated for each trial and allows for both a verbal or pointing response.

Older children (9 years old and older) have the numbers 3, 4, 5, and 6 written on their fingertips and can respond by verbally stating the number they perceived while keeping their eyes closed. It is important to emphasize in the instructions that only the numbers 3, 4, 5, and 6 will be written. Sometimes a child will respond with "2" or another number. The first time this happens, I will repeat the instructions, saying, "I only write 3, 4, 5, or 6. Which do you think it was?"

There are four stimuli per finger for a total of 20 trials. Lateralized errors on graphesthesia testing is also potentially indicative of left cerebral hemisphere inefficiency due to the symbolic nature of the stimuli or of right hemi-

sphere dysfunction due to the spatial nature of the task. However, as with the finger recognition test, bilateral errors on a test of graphesthesia may also suggest attentional fluctuation. For example, a mild to moderate number of bilateral errors may be a reasonable marker of inattention, particularly when noted in the absence of documented bilateral cerebral dysfunction or any other lateralizing signs and in the presence of other signs of attentional deficit. Such broadly construed etiological possibilities once again emphasize the need for a convergence profile analysis (see Chapter 1).

Tactile Form Recognition

Tactile form recognition testing of the younger child involves the presentation of plastic geometric forms (square, cross, circle, triangle) to a hand and pointing with the contralateral hand to its match on a visual presentation of the four stimului. Tactile form recognition for older children involves the presentation of identical coins to each hand. In both instances, the child must determine whether what is felt in each hand is similar or different. Impairment, or astereognosis, is another marker of contralateral (parietal) cerebral hemisphere dysfunction. Astereognosis is usually unilateral. Errorless performance is to be expected after age 8 (Knights and Norwood, 1980). In the latter study, data were collected on 184 children 5 to 14 years old from two elementary schools. Gender was not reported. The socioeconomic status level was Hollingshead Class II and Class IV. Children from school 1 had a mean IQ of 111 ($SD = 14.5$) and those from school 2 had a mean IQ of 102 ($SD = 10.6$). In another Reitan-Indiana Neuropsychological Test Battery normative study, the error pattern between the right and left upper extremity was not different for young children (Maiuro, Townes et al., 1984).

Benton Finger Localization Procedure

A 60-item evaluation of finger localization was also developed for the upturned hand (Benton, 1955; Benton, Hamsher et al., 1983b). The subject must first name a finger observed being touched at the fingertip with a pencil point, then name the touched finger and identify pairs of fingers touched simultaneously without visual input. A modification decreased the number of items to 20, and was administered to children between 6 and 12 years of age. An exponential increase in scores between 6 and 8 years of age was found, parallel to Benton's data. Around 9 years old, the rate of improvement slowed and reached an asymptote around age 12. Naming with visual input was better than naming without visual input: children 6 years old were able to name 88.4% of fingers under visual monitoring, but only 67.4% without. Children 9 years old scored 99.3% and 92.3%, respectively.

The two-finger task was considerably more difficult (18.7% and 31.3%, at ages 6 and 9, respectively), but involved more complex sensory and attentional components. The outside fingers of the hand were more accurately identified than center fingers in this and other studies (Lefford, Birch et al., 1974). There was also a hierarchy of finger awareness: the thumb was more accurately localized than the little fingers, followed by the index, middle, and the ring fingers. No substantial right–left differences were noted, except in a few children 6 years old. Test–retest reliability was 0.70 for the short-term 20-minute interval retesting and 0.75 for a 10-week interval retesting, using this procedure (Benton, 1955).

Quality Extinction Test

The Quality Extinction Test presents a variety of tactile materials (carpet, velvet, metal, wire grating) mounted on a board and requires verbal responses (Schwartz, Marchok, and Flynn 1977). When given to hemiplegic children and young adults, 23 of 39 patients (58%) manifested extinction (Lenti et al., 1991). Nineteen extinguished the hand contralateral to the damaged hemisphere. Extinction was noted on the right hand in four patients with a right hemiparesis, three of whom had localized left frontal lesions. These authors did not find significantly more subjects with right hemisphere lesions manifesting left sided neglect.

The Behavioural Inattention Test (Wilson, Cockburn et al., 1987) is a standardized test battery to detect unilateral visual neglect. It includes line crossing, star cancellation, letter cancellation, sentence copying, figure copying, representational drawing, and article reading.

The Ishihara Color Plates (Ishihara, 1979) is commonly used for color perception evaluation.

CONCLUSION

Motor and sensory-perceptual examinations contribute significantly to child neuropsychological evaluation. Rather than omitting or incompletely assessing these functions, clinicians need to recognize their utility and learn to adjust their overall impressions based on the resulting patterns of performance. It is especially important that the specific normative data referred to parallel the methodology employed by the clinician. Enormous variability in procedures is encountered in the literature. The value of motor and sensory-perceptual results in longitudinal study is particularly interesting as stage-like developmental progression may be monitored in context with the diverse influence of varied neurological insults and sometimes may prove to be the decisive data that indicate a change in the neurodevelopmental course.

REFERENCES

Adams, W., & Sheslow, D. (1995). *Wide Range Assessment of Visual Motor Abilities-Manual*. Wilmington, DE: Jastak, Inc.

Annett, M. (1971). The growth of manual preference and speed. *British Journal of Psychology, 61*, 545–558.

Baron, I. S., Fennell, E. B., & Voeller, K. K. S. (1995). *Pediatric Neuropsychology in the Medical Setting*. New York: Oxford.

Baron, I. S., & Goldberger, E. (1993). Neuropsychological disturbances of hydrocephalic children with implications for special education and rehabilitation. *Neuropsychological Rehabilitation, 3*, 389–410.

Benton, A. L. (1955b). Development of finger-localization capacity in school children. *Child Development, 26*, 225–230.

Benton, A. L. (1962). Dyslexia in relation to form perception and directional sense. In J. Money

(Ed.), *Reading Disability* (pp. 81–102). Baltimore: The Johns Hopkins Press.

Benton, A. L. (1979). The neuropsychological significance of finger recognition. In M. Bortner (Ed.), *Cognitive growth and development: Essays in memory of Herbert G. Birch* (pp. 85–104). New York: Brunner/Mazel.

Benton, A. L., Hamsher, K., Varney, N. R., & Spreen, O. (1983a). *Pantomime Recognition Test.* New York: Oxford University Press.

Benton, A. L., Hamsher, K., Varney, N. R., & Spreen, O. (1983b). *Contributions to neuropsychological assessment: A clinical manual.* New York: Oxford University Press.

Benton, A. L., Sivan, A. B., Hamsher, K., Varney, N. R., & Spreen, O. (1994). *Contributions to neuropsychological assessment. A clinical manual.* (2nd ed.). New York: Oxford University Press.

Blackburn, L. B., & Spevack, T. V. (2000). Personal communication.

Boivin, M. J., Giordani, B., & Bornefeld, B. (1995). Use of the Tactual Performance Test for cognitive ability testing with African children. *Neuropsychology, 9,* 409–417.

Boll, T. (1974). Behavioral correlates of cerebral damage in children aged 9 through 14. In R. M. Reitan & L. A. Davison (Eds.), *Clinical Neuropsychology: Current Status and Application.* New York: John Wiley & Sons.

Boll, T., & Reitan, R. (1972). Motor and tactile-perceptual deficits in brain-damaged children. *Perceptual and Motor Skills, 34,* 343–350.

Bonda, E., Petrides, M., Frey, S., & Evans, A. (1995). Neural correlates of mental transformations of the body-in-space. *Proceedings of the National Academy of Sciences, 92,* 11180–11184.

Briggs, G., & Nebes, R. (1975). Patterns of hand preference in a student population. *Cortex, 11,* 230–238.

Brown, S. J., Rourke, B. P., & Cicchetti, D. (1989). Reliability of tests and measures used in the neuropsychological assessment of children. *The Clinical Neuropsychologist, 3,* 353–368.

Bruininks, R. H. (1978). *Bruininks-Oseretsky Test of Motor Proficiency: Examiner's Manual.* Circle Pines, MN: American Guidance Service.

Buchanan, R. W., & Heinrichs, D. W. (1989). The Neurological Evaluation Scale (NES): A structured instrument for the assessment of neurological signs in schizophrenia. *Psychiatry Research, 27,* 335–350.

Butterworth, G., & Hopkins, B. (1993). Origins of handedness in human infants. *Developmental Medicine and Child Neurology, 35,* 177–184.

Casey, J. E., & Rourke, B. P. (1992). Disorders of somatosensory perception in children. In I. Rapin

& S. J. Segalowitz (Eds.), *Handbook of Neuropsychology, Vol. 6: Child Neuropsychology* (pp. 477–494). Oxford, England: Elsevier Science Publishers.

Casseli, R. J. (1993). Ventrolateral and dorsomedial somatosensory association cortexdamage produces distinct somesthetic syndromes in humans. *Neurology, 43,* 762–771.

Chapman, L. J., & Chapman, J. P. (1987). The measurement of handedness. *Brain and Cognition, 6,* 175–183.

Christensen, A.-L. (1975). *Luria's Neuropsychological Investigation: Text.* New York: Spectrum Publications, Inc.

Coren, S., Porac, C., & Duncan, P. (1979). A behaviorally validated self-report inventory to assess four types of lateral preference. *Journal of Clinical Neurology, 1,* 55–64.

Coren, S., Porac, C., & Duncan, P. (1981). Lateral preference behaviors in preschool children and young adults. *Child Development, 52,* 443–450.

Costa, L. D., Searola, L. M., & Rapin, I. (1964). Purdue Pegboard scores for normal grammar school children. *Perceptual and Motor Skills, 18,* 748.

Denckla, M. B. (1973). Development of speed in repetitive and successive finger-movements in normal children. *Developmental Medicine and Child Neurology, 15,* 635–645.

Denckla, M. B. (1974). Development of motor coordination in normal children. *Developmental Medicine and Child Neurology, 16,* 729–741.

Denckla, M. B. (1985). Revised Neurological Examination for Subtle Signs. *Psychopharmacology Bulletin, 21,* 773–779.

Deuel, R. K., & Doar, B. P. (1992). Developmental manual dyspraxia: A lesson in mind and brain. *Journal of Child Neurology, 7,* 99–103.

Elliott, T. K., & Watkins, J. M. (1998). Indices of laterality in Turner syndrome. *Child Neuropsychology, 4,* 131–143.

Emerson, C. S., Harrison, D. W., Everhart, E., & Williamson, J. B. (2001). Grip strength asymmetry in depressed boys. *Neuropsychiatry, Neuropsychology, and Behavioral Neurology, 14,* 130–134.

Fennell, E. B. (1986). Handedness in neuropsychological research. In H. J. Hannay (Ed.), *Experimental techniques in human neuropsychology.* New York: Oxford University Press.

Fennell, E. B., Satz, P., & Morris, R. (1983). The development of handedness and dichotic ear listening asymmetries in relation to school achievement: A longitudinal study. *Journal of Experimental Child Psychology, 35,* 248–262.

Findeis, M. K., & Weight, D. G. (1994). *Meta-norms for Indiana-Reitan Neuropsychological Test Bat-*

tery and Halstead-Reitan Neuropsychologial Test Battery for Children, ages 5–14. Unpublished manuscript.

Fink, M. D., & Bender, M. B. (1953). Perception of simultaneous tactile stimulation in normal children. *Neurology, 3,* 27–34.

Finlayson, M. A., & Reitan, R. M. (1976). Handedness in relation to measures of motor and tactile perceptual functions in normal children. *Perceptual and Motor Skills, 43,* 475–481.

Francis, D. J., Fletcher, J., & Rourke, B. P. (1988). Discriminant validity of lateral sensorimotor tests in children. *Journal of Clinical and Experimental Neuropsychology, 10,* 779–799.

Fromm-Auch, D., & Yeudall, L. T. (1983). Normative data for the Halstead-Reitan Neuropsychological Tests. *Journal of Clinical Neuropsychology, 5,* 221–238.

Gardner, R. A., & Broman, M. (1979). The Purdue Pegboard: Normative Data on 1334 school children. *Journal of Clinical and Child Psychology, 1,* 156–162.

Geschwind, N. (1965). Disconnection syndromes in animals and man. I. [Review]. *Brain, 88,* 237–294.

Geschwind, N. (1975). The apraxias: Neural mechanisms of disorders of learned movement. *American Scientist, 63,* 188–195.

Golden, C. J. (1981). The Luria-Nebraska Children's Battery: Theory and formulation. In G. W. Hynd & J. E. Obrzut (Eds.), *Neuropsychological assessment and the school-age child* (pp. 277–302). New York: Grune & Stratton.

Goodglass, H., & Kaplan, E. (1963). Disturbance of gesture and pantomime in aphasia. *Brain, 86,* 703–720.

Goodgold-Edwards, S. A., & Cermak, L. S. (1990). Integrating motor control and motor learning concepts with neuropsychological perspectives on apraxia and developmental dyspraxia. *American Journal of Occupational Therapy, 44,* 431–439.

Gray, R. M., Livingston, R. B., Marshall, R. M., & Haak, R. A. (2000). Reference group data for the Reitan-Indiana Neuropsychological Test Battery for young children. *Perceptual and Motor Skills, 91,* 675–682.

Green, M. F., Satz, P., Smith, C., & Nelson, L. (1989). Is there atypical handedness in schizophrenia? *Journal of Abnormal Psychology, 98,* 57–61.

Haaland, K. Y., & Harrington, D. L. (1996). Hemispheric asymmetry of movement. *Current Opinion in Neurobiology, 6,* 796–800.

Haaland, K. Y., Harrington, D. L., & Knight, R. T. (2000). Neural representations of skilled movement. *Brain, 123,* 2306–2313.

Halstead, W. C. (1947). *Brain and intelligence: A quantitative study of the frontal lobes.* Chicago: University of Chicago Press.

Harrington, D. L., Rao, S. M., Haaland, K. Y., Bobholz, J. A., Mayer, A. R., Binder, J. R., et al. (2000). Specialized neural systems underlying representations of sequential movements. *Journal of Cognitive Neuroscience, 12,* 56–77.

Harris, A. J. (1947). *Harris Tests of Lateral Dominance, manual of directions for administration and interpretation.* New York: The Psychological Corporation.

Harris, L. J. (1982). The human infant as focus in theories of handedness: some lessons from the past. In R. N. Malatesha & L. C. Hartlage (Eds.), *Neuropsychology and cognition, Vol. II* (pp. 8–26). The Hague: Martinus Nijhoff.

Heilman, K. M., Rothi, L. J., & Valenstein, E. (1982). Two forms of ideomotor apraxia. *Neurology, 32,* 342–346.

Instructions and normative data for Model 32020 Purdue Pegboard. (undated). Lafayette, IN: Lafayette Instrument Company.

Ishihara, S. (1979). *Tests for blindness.* Tokio: Kanehara Shuppan.

Kane, J., & Gill, R. P. (1972). Implications of the Purdue Pegboard as a screening device. *Journal of Learning Disabilities, 547,* 36–40.

Kaspar, J. C., & Sokolec, J. (1980). Relationship between neurological dysfunction and a test of speed of motor performance. *Journal of Clinical Neuropsychology, 2,* 13–21.

Klonoff, H., & Low, M. (1974). Disordered brain function in young children and early adolescents: Neuropsychological and electroencephalographic correlates. In R. M. Reitan & L. A. Davison (Eds.), *Clinical Neuropsychology: Current Status and Applications* (pp. 121–178). New York: John Wiley and Sons.

Klove, H. (1963). Clinical neuropsychology. In F. M. Foster (Ed.), *The Medical Clinics of North America.* New York: Saunders.

Knights, R. M. (1966). *Normative data on tests evaluating brain damage in children 5–14 years of age. Research Bulletin No. 20.* London, ON: Department of Psychology, University of Western Ontario.

Knights, R. M. (1970). *Smoothed normative data on tests for evaluation brain damage in children.* Unpublished manuscript. Ottawa, Ontario.

Knights, R. M., & Moule, A. D. (1967). Normative and reliability data on finger and foot tapping in children. *Perceptual and Motor Skills, 25,* 717–720.

Knights, R. M., & Moule, A. D. (1968). Normative data on the Motor Steadiness Battery for Children. *Perceptual and Motor Skills, 26,* 643–650.

Knights, R. M., & Norwood, J. A. (1980). Revised smoothed normative data on the neuropsychological test battery for children. Mimeo. Department of Psychology, Carleton University, Ottawa, ON.

Kolb, B., & Milner, B. (1981). Performance of complex arm and facial movements after focal brain lesions. *Neuropsychologia, 19,* 491–503.

Krams, M., Rushworth, M. F., Deiber, M.-P., Frackowiak, R. S., & Passingham, R. (1998). The preparation, execution and suppression of copied movements in the human brain. *Experimental Brain Research, 120,* 386–398.

Lefford, A., Birch, H. G., & Green, G. (1974). The perceptual and cognitive basis for finger localization and selective finger movement in preschool children. *Child Development, 45,* 335–343.

Lenti, C., Radice, L., Cerioli, M., & Musetti, L. (1991). Tactile extinction in childhood hemiplegia. *Developmental Medicine and Child Neurology, 33,* 789–794.

Levy, J. (1982). Handwriting posture and cerebral organization: How are they related? *Psychological Bulletin, 91,* 589–608.

Levy, J., & Reid, M. L. (1976). Variations in writing posture and cerebral organization. *Science, 194,* 337.

Liepmann, H. (1920). Apraxia. *Erbgn der ges Med, 1,* 516–543.

Llorente, A. M., Satz, P., Brumm, V. L., & Philpott, L. M. (1998). Pathological left handedness: A case report examining the developmental course of the syndrome following head trauma. *Child Neuropsychology, 4,* 98–109.

Maiuro, R., Townes, B. D., Vitaliano, P., & Trupin, E. (1984). Age norms for the Reitan-Indiana Neuropsychological Test Battery for Children. In R. A. Glow & R. J. Prinz (Eds.), *Advances in the Behavioral Measurement of Children, Volume 1* (pp. 159–173). Greenwich, CT: JAI Press.

Meador, K. J., Allison, J. D., Loring, D. W., Lavin, T. B., & Pillai, J. J. (2002). Topography of somatosensory processing: Cerebral lateralization and focused attention. *Journal of the International Neuropsychological Society, 8,* 349–359.

Mozaz, M., Gonzalez-Rothi, L. J., Anderson, J. M., Crucian, G. P., & Heilman, K. M. (2002). Postural knowledge of transitive pantomimes and intransitive gestures. *Journal of the International Neuropsychological Society, 8,* 958–962.

Müller, R. A., Rothermel, R. D., Behen, M. E., Muzik, O., Mangner, T. J., & Chugani, H. T. (1998). Differential patterns of language and motor reorganization following early left hemisphere lesion: A PET study. *Archives of Neurology, 55,* 1113–1119.

Ochipa, C., Rothi, L. J., & Heilman, K. M. (1989). Ideational apraxia: A deficit in tool selection and use. *Annals of Neurology, 25,* 190–193.

Ochipa, C., Rothi, L. J., & Heilman, K. M. (1992). Conceptual apraxia in Alzheimer's disease. *Brain, 115,* 1061–1071.

Oldfield, R. C. (1971). The assessment and analysis of handedness: The Edinburgh Inventory. *Neuropsychologia, 9,* 97–113.

Peigneux, P., & van der Linden, M. (1999). Influence of ageing and educational level on the prevalence of body-part-as-objects in normal subjects. *Journal of Clinical and Experimental Neuropsychology, 21,* 547–552.

Peterson, J. M. (1979). Handedness: Differences between student artists and scientists. *Perceptual and Motor Skills, 48,* 961–962.

Piek, J. P., & Skinner, R. A. (1999). Timing and force control during a sequential tapping task in children with and without motor coordination problems. *Journal of the International Neuropsychological Society, 5,* 320–329.

Porac, C., & Coren, S. (1981). *Lateral preferences and human behavior.* New York: Springer-Verlag.

Psychological Assessment Resources, Inc. (1992). *Finger Tapper Record Form.* Unpublished manuscript, Odessa, FL.

Ramsay, D. S. (1980). Onset of unilmanual handedness in infants. *Infant behavior and development, 3,* 377–385.

Rasmussen, T., & Milner, B. (1977). The role of early left-brain injury in determining lateralization of cerebral speech functions. *Annals of the New York Academy of Sciences, 299,* 355.

Raymer, A. M., Maher, L. M., Foundas, A. L., Heilman, K. M., & Rothi, L. J. (1997). The significance of body part as tool errors in limb apraxia. *Brain and Cognition, 34,* 287–292.

Reitan, R. (1969). *Manual for Administration of Neuropsychological Test Batteries for Adults and Children.* Unpublished manuscript, Indianapolis University Medical Center.

Reitan, R. (1971). Sensorimotor functions in brain-damaged and normal children of early school age. *Perceptual and Motor Skills, 33,* 655–664.

Reitan, R. (1984). *Aphasia and sensory-perceptual deficits in children.* Tucson, Az: Neuropsychology Press.

Reitan, R., & Boll, T. (1973). Neuropsychological correlates of minimal brain dysfunction. *Annals of the New York Academy of Sciences, 205,* 65–88.

Reitan, R., & Davison, L. (1974). *Clinical neuropsychology: Current status and applications.* New York: Hemisphere.

Roeltgen, M. G., & Roeltgen, D. P. (1990). Asymmetrical lateralized attention in children. *Developmental Neuropsychology, 6,* 25–37.

Satz, P. (1972). Pathological left handedness: An explanatory model. *Cortex, 8,* 121–135.

Satz, P., & D'Elia, L. (1989). *The PIN Test.* Odessa, FL: Psychological Assessment Resources, Inc.

Schwartz, A. S., Marchok, P. L., & Flynn, R. E. (1977). A sensitive test for tactile extinction: Results in patients with parietal and frontal lobe disease. *Journal of Neurology, Neurosurgery and Psychiatry, 40,* 228–233.

Sequin, E. (1866). *Idiocy: Its treatment by the physiological methods* (Reprinted from the original 1866 edition). New York: Bureau of Publications, Teachers College, Columbia University, 1907.

Shadmehr, R., & Holcomb, H. H. (1997). Neural correlates of motor memory consolidation. *Science, 277,* 821–825.

Sivan, A. B., & Varney, N. R. (1985). Pantomime recognition in normal and dyslexic children. *Developmental Neuropsychology, 1,* 49–52.

Smith, E., & Jonides, J. J. (1999). Storage and executive processes in the frontal lobes. *Science, 283,* 1657–1661.

Snow, W. G. (1987). Standardization of test administration and scoring criteria: Some shortcomings of current practice with the Halstead-Reitan Test Battery. *The Clinical Neuropsychologist, 1,* 250–262.

Sopher, H. v., Satz, P., Orsini, D. L., & VanGorp, W. G. (1987). Handedness distribution in a residential population with severe or profound mental retardation. *Neuropsychologia, 22,* 511–515.

Spiegler, B. J., & Yeni-Komishian, G. (1983). Incidence of left-handed writing in a college population with reference to family patterns of hand preference. *Neuropsychologia, 21,* 651–659.

Spreen, O., & Gaddes, W. H. (1968). *Developmental norms for 15 neuropsychological tests. Age 6–15.* Unpublished manuscript, Department of Psychology, University of Victoria, Victoria, BC. Unpublished manuscript.

Spreen, O., & Gaddes, W. H. (1969). Developmental Norms for 15 neuropsychological tests age 6 to 15. *Cortex, 5,* 171–191.

Spreen, O., & Strauss, E. (1998). *A compendium of neuropsychological tests: Adminstration, norms, and commentary* (2nd ed.). New York: Oxford University Press.

Tiffin, J., & Asher, E. J. (1948). The Purdue Pegboard: Norms and studies of reliability and validity. *Journal of Applied Psychology, 32,* 234–247.

Trites, R. (1977). *Neuropsychological Test Manual.* Ottawa, ON, Canada: Royal Ottawa Hospital; available from Lafayette Instrument Company.

Tupper, D. E. (1983a). The development of bimanual and unimanual coordination in children 3 to 8: Involvement of one system or two? Unpublished manuscript. Paper presented at the 11th Annual Meeting of the International Neuropsychological Society, Mexico City.

Tupper, D. E. (1983b). The pattern of lateral preference and motor dominance in children ages 3 to 8. Unpublished manuscript, Paper presented at the 11th Annual Meeting of the International Neuropsychological Society, Mexico City.

Waber, D. P., Mann, M., & Merola, J. (1985). Motor overflow and attentional processes in normal school-age children. *Developmental Medicine and Child Neurology, 27,* 491–497.

Welsh, M. C., Pennington, B. F., & Groisser, D. B. (1991). A normative-developmental study of executive function: A window on prefrontal function in children. *Developmental Neuropsychology, 7,* 131–149.

Wilson, B. A., Cockburn, J., & Halligan, P. (1987). *Behavioural Inattention Test: Manual.* Fareham: Thames Valley Test Company.

Wilson, B. C., Iacovello, J.M., Wilson, J.J. and Risucci, P. (1982). Purdue Pegboard performance of normal preschool children. *Journal of Clinical Neuropsychology, 4,* 19–26.

Wolff, P., Gunne, C., & Cohen, C. (1983). Associated movements as a measure of developmental age. *Developmental Medicine and Child Neurology, 25,* 417–429.

10

Visuoperceptual, Visuospatial, and Visuoconstructional Function

Before concluding that higher order sensory-perceptual integrative difficulties are involved, a clinician must be assured that a patient's primary sensory systems are intact. Visual information is but one primary sensory input present early in life. Newborns have immediate vision, which will steadily improve over the first month with use. Equal vision in both eyes is required for normal visual function. The visual system continues to change over the early years with resistance to change evident at about age 9. Full integration between visual, tactile, and proprioceptive information is accomplished around this time, having been well integrated only after the age of 8 (von Hofsten and Rösblad, 1988). The path from early basic perception into complex integrated function is also apparent across many abilities. For example, infants can imitate facial expressions by 12 days old (Meltzoff and Moore, 1977), and the ability to identify facial expressions improves up until 8 to 10 years (Harrigan, 1984). Basic emotions are recognized by age 6, recognition of complex emotions comes later (Markham and Adams, 1992).

Assessment of nonverbal abilities is not as straightforward as many might believe. Tests of visuoperceptual, visuospatial, and visuomotor function comprise substantial portions of commonly administered general intelligence tests and neuropsychology test batteries. Yet, there are relatively few clinical tests of discrete perceptual or expressive function in children and far more of those for which the contribution of multicomponential factors presents serious interpretive complications. It would be ideal to limit the contribution of other factors that directly influence test performance, such as the requirement for intact working memory, motor control, or sustained attention. However, it is especially hard to develop tasks that discretely separate visual and spatial components (Baddeley, 2001) either for research or clinical practice.

The influence of demands for speed, perception of a Gestalt, eye-hand coordination, motor control, attention to visuoperceptual detail, and executive functions such as planning and organization must all be considered for multifactorial tests and, as a result, caution in interpretation is needed. Further, the presence of a primarily nonverbal test within an intelligence test or memory scale does not guarantee its clinical utility in lesion lateralization (Dade and Jones-Gotman, 2001). One must guard against assumptions of laterality that might be erroneously concluded by someone unfamiliar with the child's particular neurodevelopmental course and the known effects of any interference on normal brain development at different stages in development.

OBSTACLES TO INTERPRETATION OF NONVERBAL DEFICIT

Many contributory factors need to be considered when interpreting any test result. Within the nonverbal domain, for example, observed difficulty on a test incorporating visual stimuli requires confirmation of the child's intact visual acuity. While most children will be routinely screened for vision by pediatricians or in preschool, there remains the occasional instance in which vision has not yet been examined. Motor slowness might confound results obtained on timed tests, and rapid response requirements can erroneously lead to a conclusion of a perceptual problem when it is the speeded condition that complicates the child's performance. The presence of visuoconstructional problems might be concluded incorrectly when poor fine motor control interferes with the child's ability to hold a pencil securely or manipulate small test stimuli. Sorting out all of the relevant contributory factors to determine which merit emphasis becomes an active exercise in hypothesis testing, aided by clinical acumen and the availability of a wide variety of test instruments.

A limited source of developmentally appropriate stimuli within the nonverbal test armamentarium further complicates child assessment. The usefulness of some existing clinical and research measures remain questionable or controversial. As is true for tests within many other domains, child normative data for nonverbal tests are often limited or applied to the individual despite weakly related demographics. Those who choose to administer existent standardized global test batteries often find the nonverbal subtests included in the battery allow for only restricted evaluation of relevant component processes, making the addition of supplemental tests or alternative administration strategies necessary to reach a valid conclusion.

QUALITATIVE AND QUANTITATIVE FEATURES

It is well recognized that the information one obtains from a clinical assessment must include qualitative as well as quantitative data. These qualitative observations have often been left to the examiner's discretion and, therefore, depend on experience. Formal specification of behavioral observations is only recently becoming a routine part of test protocol forms and procedures. The development of these structured assists for observing behavior makes it more likely that important and discriminating behaviors will be recognized and recorded. The strategies children employ are receiving even greater clinical attention as an emphasis on qualitative observations becomes codified and the need to inspect data for nonquantitative features is formally highlighted. Recent research has also focused on strategies in a developmental context. For example, one study found that children faced with tasks requiring more advanced types of spatial analysis adopted strategies that were successful when they were younger. These data suggested that while the children had a variety of spatial analytic strategies available by age 6, they selected a strategy that was a function of stimulus complexity and their capabilities (Akshoomoff and Stiles, 1995).

Within the nonverbal domain, it is helpful to observe how easily the child approaches tests that inherently limit verbal cueing strategies. Signs of withdrawal or reluctance to approach tasks that are perceived by the child to be a likely source of failure are often initial clues to perceptual dysfunction. Examples of other qualitative features that should be noted on nonverbal, design-copying tests include whether the child retains visual detail over time or omits such detail in recall drawings but maintains the basic configuration. Observations about pencil grasp and line quality are also essential. It is useful to note whether the child recognizes what puzzle pieces, blocks, or other incomplete stimuli will form a proper alignment. It is also useful to observe whether a developmentally appropriate strategy is demonstrated or an ineffectual trial-and-error approach predominates for manipulative visual analysis and synthesis tasks, that is, those that do not require writing. Often, the child's overt behavior is a clue to critical aspects of his situation that require exploration in the formal evaluation.

ADULT TESTS EXTENDED DOWNWARD VS. TESTS DESIGNED PRIMARILY FOR CHILDREN

Efforts are ongoing to develop appropriate assessment instruments that provide reliable and valid child normative data. Historically, child neuropsychology test development often relied on tests first developed for use with adults rather than being constructed specifically for children. For example, an early test of unfamiliar face learning and long-term retention for face stimuli was initially developed for an adult study (Dade and Jones-Gotman, 2001), as was another facial recognition test and a line orientation test (Benton, Van Allen et al., 1975) (Benton, Varney et al., 1978). Of particular concern, administration procedures developed for adults might not account for the fluidity of behavior within and between age levels, restricting clinical interpretation. As a result of this insensitivity to developmental issues these tests have questionable utility, especially at young ages. Constructs applied from an adult model need to be tested for applicability to children, but unfortunately, this has not always been accomplished. The trend toward tests designed specifically for children is a most welcome advance (Kerns, 2000; Espy, Kaufmann et al., 2001) and it is expected that the continued recognition of the importance of such test development ultimately will positively change child evaluation.

RIGHT HEMISPHERE VS. LEFT HEMISPHERE

The differential influence of the right cerebral hemisphere and the left cerebral hemisphere on visuoperceptual, visuospatial, and visuomotor tasks has long been studied. Research data generally indicate that right cerebral damage has a more profound effect on the spatial distribution of attention (Mesulam, 1985b; Heilman, Watson et al., 1993). Consistent with the literature and clinical observation, a study of adults found left hemisphere injury resulted in difficulty reproducing local level elements, while right hemisphere injury resulted in difficulty with global structure (Delis, Robertson et al., 1986). Subsequently, parallel findings were reported for children with focal lesions (Stiles, Bates et al., 1998).

There is also evidence that fragmentation of visual processing occurs subsequent to either right or left hemisphere damage, but the most distortion is associated with right cerebral brain damage and neglect secondary to such impair-

ment. Ventral and occipitotemporal lesions are especially implicated (Dennis, Fletcher et al., 2002). The requirement for visual closure on a picture fragmentation test was found to be sensitive to the presence of object agnosia (Farah, 1995). Yet, caution in prediction is needed since an intact right hemisphere does not ensure a holistic, synthetic approach to copying complex geometric figures (Binder, 1982). An important role for the right corpus striatum in mental rotation was reported for an adult case study, suggesting the caudate nucleus and putamen may be component regions in a corticosubcortical network necessary to select and maintain an appropriate motor program for performing smooth and accurate mental rotation. These structures receive direct spatial mapping input from parietal regions and appear to integrate both visuospatial and motor information related to the mental rotation process. Also, a dissociation between recognition of rotated objects and mental rotation was found for their clinical case study (Harris, Harris et al., 2002), although this has been a point of some debate in the object recognition literature.

The Rey-Osterrieth Complex Figure (ROCF) test has proven to be a complex measure influenced by multiple factors. It is neither a right nor left hemisphere indicator but, rather, a test that provides varied data that can be analyzed for the component processes that lead to either successful or unsuccessful performance. Nonetheless, ROCF results for both copy and recall conditions can support suppositions about right–left differential processing. In clinical practice, the ROCF productions of left-hemisphere-injured individuals often reveal a characteristic loss of detail, but maintenance of general form or Gestalt, whereas right-hemisphere-injured individuals are more likely to preserve form, but tend to make errors of omission, displacement, or distortion. Of course, this pattern can be observed in other simple to complex visuoconstructional productions that require appreciation for and execution of form and detail. It is now well documented that left hemisphere dysfunction is associated with disorders of pattern segmentation while right hemisphere dysfunction affects integrative ability (Stiles, Moses et al., 2003).

Support for these common clinical observations, well documented in adults, was also obtained for children. A study using the ROCF with right-hemisphere- or left-hemisphere-injured children, compared to controls, found deficits most evident for the youngest lesion group children (6–7 years) but with development (9–10 years) performance improved sufficiently to allow for accurate copies of the ROCF. However, piecemeal processing strategies characterized the productions of both lesion groups. At the older ages (up to 14 years), the copy and memory results of those with right focal injury were similar in terms of content and process, with piecemeal strategies employed to produce detailed figures. In contrast, the memory performance of the left focal injury group revealed adoption of an advanced core rectangle organizational strategy, along with limited detail production (Akshoomoff, Feroleto et al., 2002).

Functional neuroimaging studies provide further insight into differential right and left cerebral hemisphere function and the child's adaptation to brain damage. Late effects of early focal right cerebral hemisphere brain injury were examined in an adolescent who had a documented right parietal skull fracture and associated right temporal lobe hemorrhage at 7 months old. Functional magnetic resonance imaging (fMRI) found left hemisphere activation for a normally right hemisphere mediated spatial task (Levin, Scheller et al. 1996). These data suggested that an active compensation is indeed possible throughout the childhood years after early lesion and leads to the supposition that this is accomplished in an attempt to ensure preservation of essential function. With the benefit of sophisticated neuroimaging techniques, it is therefore possible to hypothesize that in some instances this capacity for plasticity will change the locus of mediation for a function that would otherwise have been mediated through the damaged region.

VERBAL IQ–PERFORMANCE IQ SPLIT

The issue of Verbal–Performance IQ (VIQ–PIQ) differential results is an important one, especially since IQ tests are ubiquitous in cognitive and academic achievement evaluations. A "significant" VIQ–PIQ difference is easily subject to misinterpretation. Caution should be taken in attributing significance to a large difference without verifying that the statistically significant difference is also a *clinically significant* difference. Clinical significance can be verified by referring to the baserate table in the manual that specifies the cumulative percentages of individuals in the normative data sample who obtained a difference of a similar magnitude. Checking will often alter interpretation based on a simple difference. For example, a VIQ–PIQ split of 18 points might appear noteworthy, but the table indicates that as many as 17% of the normative sample would have that large a split, or greater. The WISC-III table also provides cumulative percentages for index score discrepancies. Thus, for example, 23% of the standardization sample had a discrepancy as large or greater for a statistically significant verbal comprehension–perceptual organization discrepancy of 16 points.

Visuoperceptual function weaker than verbal function on an IQ test is common, and the discrepancy occurs independent of etiology or lesion lateralization. It is well recognized that a large verbal IQ > performance IQ split can be associated with many chronic or longstanding neurological or other systemic conditions, including early brain lesions (Aram and Eisele 1992), hydrocephalus (Dennis, Fitz et al., 1981; Donders, Canady et al., 1990; Brookshire, Fletcher et al., 1995), and myelomeningocele (Wills, Holmbeck et al., 1990). Thus, a large split is not necessarily diagnostic of lateralized cerebral dysfunction, although it occasionally is truly indicative of such impairment.

It is often erroneous and simplistic to conclude, for example, that a statistically or clinically significantly lower performance IQ than verbal IQ indicates right cerebral hemisphere dysfunction. Further, since a VIQ–PIQ split in either direction often can be normal, a split in which verbal abilities appear to exceed nonverbal abilities should not be considered abnormal, or indicative of brain impairment, without confirmation from other data sources. More precise delineation of reasons for any weakness on an IQ measure can often be made with judicious neuropsychological evaluation. Independent of the test measure, even with medical evidence of lateralized dysfunction of one cerebral hemisphere, one might be mistaken to conclude that there is lack of competence by the other hemisphere (Rhodes, 1985). Thus, the neuropsychological evaluation must remain an objective hypothesis-testing exploration of cognitive function in order to succeed in its purpose.

EVALUATION OF PERCEPTUAL AND SPATIAL ABILITIES

The importance of evaluating the nonverbal domain routinely is largely intuitive. Besides the potential for identification of specific cognitive weakness, the determination of strengths within this domain directly applies to an appreciation for the child's overall neurocognitive and neurobehavioral profile and to the application of intervention strategies. Modifications to daily routine can be effectively introduced in the school setting as well as at home only when they are based on a clear understanding of strengths and weaknesses. A series of simple, but individually designed, adaptations can make learning easier for a child with auditory/verbal strengths, despite nonverbal weakness (Baron and Goldberger, 1993). For example, recommendation for an auditory/verbal supportive structure and verbal cueing for nonverbal material when spatial, form, or line discrimination is required (e.g., for map reading or interpretation of charts, tables, or graphs) might be useful. The use of appealing writing instruments or colored pens may make writing more attractive to the avoiding child might prove enticing. Tutorial or other supplemental assistance, may be helpful when a negative impact on academic performance is evident in subjects that incorporate highly visual material such as geography, trigonometry, or algebra.

Academic weaknesses are often explained once clinical distinctions are elucidated by the neuropsychological evaluation. For example, one might expect difficulty when a child who has a visuospatial and/or visuoperceptual deficit is faced with highly visual math curriculum, or when it is necessary to interpret charts, graphs, or tables, or to read a map without verbal cues or defined guidelines for performance are unclear. Identification of such a pattern of deficit or relative weakness might well explain a child's reluctance to engage in subject matter requiring nonverbal analysis. It

can also provide a basis for better understanding the child's idiosyncratic response to stress and frustration, level of emotional maturity, and success of interpersonal social skills, and might correlate with the child's ability to interpret gesture and nonverbal communication. The correlation of impairment within this domain with social skill acquisition is an interesting area of investigation that has increasingly had direct influence on treatment and intervention strategies.

PERCEPTUAL AND SPATIAL TESTS

A variety of research and clinical tests fall within the nonverbal domain but, as noted above, normative data for clinical use are sometimes limited or absent. Further, some nonverbal tests have a linguistic component that negates attempts to ascribe poor performance to a lesion in the nondominant-for-language hemisphere, or the nature of the task is such that the distributed neural network underlying successful performance is not easily ascribed to a lateralized summation of which brain regions contribute. Functional neuroimaging studies are revealing more diverse brain regions being activated to modality-specific conditions than was appreciated before such technological advances.

There are various ways to group tests within this domain. Some have divided their experimental tasks into categories of object identification, multistable representations of visual space, and visually guided overt actions (Dennis, Fletcher et al., 2002). Among the test instruments that fall principally within this domain are those that test basic perception and visual discrimination (e.g., sensory-perceptual screening of visual fields and visual imperception, line bisection, and cancellation tests). Others are tests of object-based visual perception, such as face recognition (e.g., Benton Facial Recognition Test), fragmented object recognition and visual closure (e.g., Gollin Figures), visuospatial orientation (e.g., Judgment of Line Orientation Test), and visual illusion perception (e.g., Visual Illusions Test). Some are tests of figure–ground discrimination, route finding, or planning (e.g., WISC-III Mazes; Porteus Mazes), conceptual reorganization or mental rotation (e.g., Money Road Map Test,

Hooper Visual Organization Test, Raven's Matrices, WAIS-III Matrix Reasoning), visuomotor integration (e.g., tests requiring design copying and figure drawing), and symbol or design matching (e.g., WISC-III Symbol Search). Some of these tests are described below, with reference to normative data where available.

LINE BISECTION

Line bisection testing is useful in documenting inattentiveness to visual space or a visual neglect syndrome. Visual neglect is defined as a behavioral disorder signifying a failure to orient, respond, or report to novel or meaningful stimuli presented to the side opposite a brain lesion when there is no motor or sensory defect, such as in space contralateral to right hemisphere brain damage (Heilman, Watson et al., 1993). Developmental changes in visual line bisection were investigated in right-handed children and adults for four age groups, 10–12 years, 13–15 years, 18–21 years, and 24–53 years. The hypotheses—that line bisections with the right hand would shift from a right bias to a strong left bias with increasing age but that left-handed line bisections would show a developmentally stable leftward bias—were upheld. No change was predicted for the two older age groups since maturational changes in corpus callosum size is considered completed by 18 years (Hausmann, Waldie et al., 2003).

It is important to determine if an underlying neurological deficit in perception might account for poor academic or cognitive performance. Manifestations of such a deficit might be detected clinically when a child is observed skipping lines when reading or working with printed material, omitting letters on one side of the written word when reading, or having difficulty aligning visual elements when copying designs or writing letters. Often, these deficits can be subtle and remain undetected to the child's detriment until formal evaluation is obtained. Line bisection and visual search cancellation tests (see Chapter 7 for the latter) are useful measures to detect the presence of a visual neglect syndrome.

Line bisection requires perception of stimulus length in order to respond with a simple

visuomotor response. The child is instructed to draw a line from the top of the page to the bottom that cuts or divides a horizontal line centered on the page in half, so that the same amount of horizontal line is on either side of the vertical dividing line. In some instances, making a mark dividing the line into equal segments is all that is required. A line bisection that is off-center is evaluated for the possibility that the bisecting line displacement is toward the side of a lesion, as commonly seen in individuals with neglect. Neurologically intact adults will make a mark slightly left of true center while those with left hemineglect often mark right of true center (Mesulam, 2000). In the presence of hemianopia the individual is likely to place the bisector to the side contralateral to the lesion (Barton and Black, 1998; Ferber and Karnath, 2001). Prominent contralesional negect is mostly apparent after right hemisphere lesion. However, hemianopia is not necessary or sufficient for the emergence of neglect (Mesulam 2000).

Whether a child has a spatial neglect or form of visuospatial impairment can be screened using such tests or through inspection of other tests that are included as part of a larger test battery, especially, copying and drawing tests. Line bisection and cancellation results can be mutually exclusive since each has different cognitive requirements, and performance on one will not necessarily predict performance on the other (Ferber and Karnath, 2001). The cancellation test requires a visual search of multiple stimuli and a response that confirms the detection of each relevant target stimulus. Clock drawing (see below) is another commonly used visuomotor integration test that also has merit in the detection of neglect, and other visuoperceptual and visuospatial features.

Incidental observation of a visual field defect might be apparent on one of the available cancellation tests requiring the child to cross out or circle a target stimulus each time it appears on the page (see Chapter 7). A line-crossing test consisting of 40 uncrossed lines in seven rows is one such measure (Albert, 1973). In another, distractor items are included in a 60-target item, letter-cancellation test with competing distractor stimuli (Weintraub and Mesulam, 1985). A 56-small-star, target-cancellation test with large stars and capital letters distractors is also in use (Halligan, Marshall et al., 1989), as is the Bells Test with bells interspersed with distractors (Gauthier, Dehaut et al., 1989; Vanier, Gauthier et al., 1990), and the random-letter cancellation test (Mesulam, 2000). (See Chapter 7 for discussion and normative data for the Cancellation of Targets Test, Rudel Denckla et al., 1978.)

VISUOMOTOR CONSTRUCTIONAL TESTS

Structured Drawings

A request that the child draw a picture is often a way to comfortably initiate testing, especially for a young child or one who admits fondness for artistic production. Besides lessening a child's initial anxiety about testing, visuomotor production becomes an additional way to assess neurodevelopmental maturity, perception of interpersonal relationships, self-image, and emotional state. Drawing impairment has long been recognized to be associated with parietal lobe lesions (Goodglass and Kaplan, 1983), but it can offer much more than neurodiagnostic evidence supporting hypotheses of brain disorder.

Drawing can also serve as a screening of emotional integrity since picture drawing helps a child communicate what cannot be easily verbalized. Verbal defenses may be offset by the drawing task's communicative power. This is especially true for all children, but especially when a child has visuoperceptual strengths but verbal weaknesses. For example, draw-a-person and draw-a-family tests often offer insights into the child's perception about self-image and family relationships, respectively, while also enabling determination of developmental level in the acquisition of visuomotor skill, including pencil coordination, maturity of line quality, and figure integration.

These tests are also useful if presented to a parent in an interpretive session, with qualifications about interpretive conclusions drawn only from screening drawings made clear. Directing parents to attend to the size and placement, feeling state conveyed, facial emotions, emphasized or overdrawn features, omitted or distorted body parts, included or excluded sig-

nificant others, for example, enables them to draw on their own knowledge of their child and their specific family circumstances. Parent opinions are often remarkably prescient about the child's self-image as depicted in the person drawing or about the relationships expressed overtly for included figures. They often will offer insight into why certain family members are excluded from the kinetic family drawings and react to the actions in which the figures are engaged or the interpersonal relationships suggested. Sometimes, the meaning is grossly apparent. For example, one child drew the family in the kitchen. Mom was cooking breakfast, the child was sitting at the table eating breakfast, and Dad was sitting across the table reading a newspaper. The newspaper was emphasized, and drawn vertically, blocking the man's view of his child. When shown the picture in the interpretive session, this child's father acknowledged he had not been accessible to his daughter recently, and communication was more absent than strained. (Other examples are presented in Chapter 3.)

Drawings also offer insight into a child's perception of the condition, disorder, illness, or pain. While long recognized that children will communicate emotion, self-perception, and feeling state through drawing, the observer must have the ability to interpret what is drawn. A request to "Draw-the-Pain" is sometimes useful in differentiating between functional and organic etiology. In one study, quantitative analysis of children's drawings about how their headaches felt contributed to good sensitivity (93.1%) and specificity (82.7%), positive predictive value (87.1%), and negative predictive value (90.6%) in differential diagnosis of migraine vs. non-migraine headaches (Stafstrom, Rostasy et al., 2002).

Beery Developmental Test of Visual-Motor Integration

The Beery Developmental Test of Visual-Motor Integration (4th ed.) (VMI) (Beery, 1997) is a widely used paper-and-pencil, design-copying test that can be administered individually or to a group. The untimed test of visuomotor integration, visually guided fine motor coordination, spatial organization and visuoperceptual ability is best characterized as a measure of visuomotor ability developmental level since shape complexity increases with item progression (Demsky, Carone et al., 2000). Included in the fourth edition are supplemental tests of visual perception and motor coordination. It is not necessary to administer all three tests, but the order of administration must be VMI, visual, then motor, if all are given.

The design-copying portion of the test presents a developmental sequence of 24 geometric forms in a format that reduces distraction, glare, and translucency. The full format includes 24 designs and an initial 3 designs that are both imitated and copied for a total of 27 items. A visual motor imitation page can be given to children 3 years old or younger. A table of age norms for very young children describes related behaviors starting at 28 weeks and continuing through 3 years, 6 months. It is intended to assist in the early identification of visuomotor weakness in preschool through primary school children. An 18-item short format for 3 to 8 years old includes the initial three and first 15 VMI forms. Normative data are provided in the form of standard scores with a mean of 100 and a standard deviation of 15 through age 17 years, 11 months. A table of VMI raw score age equivalents is also provided. Demographic data for the fourth revision normative sample are presented in Table 10–1.

The Beery and Wechsler Preschool and Primary Scales of Intelligence-Revised (WPPSI-R) geometric design subtest correlation was high ($r = .60$) in one concurrent validity study

Table 10–1. Beery Developmental Test of Visual-Motor Integration: Demographic Data

Subjects: 2614 children, ranging from 103 to 227 per age group
Age: 3 to 17 years
Gender: 51% males; 49% females
Handedness: not reported
Race: 14% African American, 12% Hispanic, 1 Native American, 3% Oriental-Pacific Island, 70% Other
SES: 19% High, 56% Middle, 23% Low
Geographic Area: 21% East, 24% North Central, 32% South, 23% West
Residence: 11% Rural, 68% Suburban, 21% Urban

(Aylward and Schmidt, 1986). The concurrent and content validity of the Rey-Osterrieth Complex Figure Test (ROCFT) and the Beery Developmental Test of Visual-Motor Integration (3rd rev.) (Beery, 1989) were investigated through correlational analysis and by group administration procedures for 432 children, age 6 to 11 (see Chapter 11 for this sample's demographic data). Children performed better on both measures across age groups, providing support for their sensitivity to the development of visuomotor integration.

Analysis indicated overlap in the content of the two scales. The shared variance depended on age and ranged from 7% to 31%, suggesting they do not measure identical content. Considerable shared variance was reported in the scores of those who took both tests (Demsky, Carone et al., 2000). It should be noted that the Beery (3rd rev.) scoring guidelines (maximum score = 50) differ from the fourth revision (maximum score = 27). A higher point value is assigned for more complex than simple designs in the third revision, while a single point value is assigned for each design in the fourth revision. Normative means and standard deviations for the Beery raw score and standard score for children aged 6 to 11 are presented in Table 10–2.

Matching Figures, Matching V's, Matching Pictures, Star Test, and Concentric Squares Test

Five subtests from the Reitan-Indiana Neuropsychological Test Battery were subject to meta-analysis (Findeis and Weight, 1994; see Chapter 6 for details). The Matching Figures Test requires the child to match printed figures that increase in complexity. It is timed and considered a measure of visual perception. Scores are presented in terms of errors and time. The Matching V's Test requires the child to arrange a sequence of Vs in order based on the degree of angle, from smallest to largest. The Matching Pictures Test is five pages long and requires the child to match pictures at the top of the page with their paired picture at the bottom of the page. The child must respond to equivalent category determination. Both the Star Test and Concentric Squares Test are tests of visual

Table 10–2. Beery° Normative Data for 6 to 11 year olds: Taylor Scoring

DEVELOPMENTAL TEST OF VISUAL-MOTOR INTEGRATION

		RAW SCORE		STANDARD SCORE	
Age	N	Mean	SD	Mean	SD
6	51	12.9	4.7	100.0	15.0
7	83	15.6	5.5	100.0	15.0
8	98	20.1	6.9	100.0	15.0
9	59	20.1	6.8	100.0	15.0
10	80	26.2	8.5	100.0	15.0
11	61	28.9	8.4	100.0	15.0

Source: Adapted from Demsky et al. (2000).

°Beery, 3rd edition (1989).

perception and fine motor coordination. The Star Test requires the child to copy a star figure and is scored for number of errors and completion time. The Concentric Squares Test requires the child to copy a series of squares of varying complexity. The test is scored for errors and completion time. Normative data for all five tests from the meta-analysis are presented in Table 10–3.

Additional data were reported for young children from a school-referred population of 224 children, aged 5 to 8, with academic or behavioral problems from rural or suburban Texas on these same measures (Gray, Livingston et al., 2000). The sample consisted of children with specific learning disability ($N = 125$), emotional disturbance ($N = 38$), Speech Handicap ($N = 50$), and ADHD ($N = 31$). Mean FSIQ was 96, based on data obtained from one of four common intelligence tests. These reference group data are presented by age, with a very limited number of 5-year-olds, but better representation for those 6 to 8 years old (Gray, Livingston et al., 2000). These data are also presented in Table 10–3.

Draw-A-Clock

Clock drawing is a widely used screening test in adult neuropsychology (Freedman, Leach et al., 1994) and one that has something to offer to child neuropsychologists as well. The test taps several diverse capacities, providing information about visuomotor, visuoperceptual, visuoconstructional, linguistic, and executive functioning, the latter including the individual's

ability to plan, organize, and simultaneously process information. Expectations for performance differ, depending on whether neurological dysfunction is cortical or subcortical, anterior or posterior, or in the left or right cerebral hemisphere (Freedman, Leach et al., 1994). Not surprisingly, this multiply determined task was sensitive to impaired executive function in adults with dementia (Libon, Swenson et al., 1993; Libon, Malamut et al., 1996). One must always consider the possibility that visual neglect or aphasia might be contributing to impaired performance.

The most commonly used time settings presented to adults are "10 after 11," "20 after 8," and "3 o'clock," listed here in decreasing order of sensitivity to verbal command and detection of stimulus-bound behavior (Freedman, Leach et al., 1994). Additionally, the latter time setting (3 o'clock) is not particularly sensitive to visual neglect since no hand needs to be drawn in the left hemispace.

This visuoconstructional drawing test and measure of praxis holds interest for both quantitative and qualitative aspects of a child's drawing. For example, it can be sensitive to a visual field defect, spatial neglect, conceptual error related to time, number reversals or immature writing, visuomotor impairment, impaired auditory perception for the verbal command, and incorrect number sequencing, in addition to visuoconstructional or visuospatial perceptual processing disturbance.

While scoring systems for clock drawing have long existed for adults, scoring a child's clock drawing was dependent on clinical judg-

Table 10–3. Reitan-Indiana NTB Meta-Norms and Reference Group Means, (SD), [N] for 5 to 8 years old

		AGE (YEARS)			
	SUBTEST:	5	6	7	8
Findeis Data	Matching Figures (seconds)	41.30 (13.7) [206]	30.70 (9.7) [190]	23.82 (9.0) [218]	21.07 (7.8) [184]
	Matching Figures (errors)	0.48 (0.9) [296]	0.40 (0.8) [160]	0.21 (0.6) [188]	0.15 (0.5) [154]
	Matching V's] (seconds)	52.39 (26.5) [206]	40.22 (16.9) [190]	32.31 (12.6) [218]	28.72 (11.5) [184]
	Matching V's (errors)	2.58 (1.9) [296]	1.91 (1.7) [160]	1.29 (1.6) [188]	1.08 (1.3) [154]
	Star (correct)	3.72 (3.1) [191]	6.03 (2.6) [160]	7.17 (1.4) [188]	7.82 (1.4) [154]
	Star (seconds)	29.63 (23.1) [181]	23.43 (17.1) [136]	19.71 (17.4) [158]	17.65 (9.4) [119]
	Concentric Squares (seconds)	37.48 (21.4) [248]	33.24 (14.8) [136]	32.29 (18.1) [158]	30.22 (15.6) [119]
	Concentric Squares (correct)	2.21 (2.2) [296]	2.75 (2.3) [106]	4.26 (2.8) [158]	5.10 (2.5) [89]
	Matching Pictures (correct)	15.48 (3.2) [311]	18.40 (4.3) [160]	19.98 (1.1) [218]	21.75 (2.6) [184]
Gray Data	Matching Figures (seconds)	39.28 (14.87) [7]	33.72 (17.99) [50]	28.01 (11.94) [78]	22.68 (9.57) [60]
	Matching Figures (errors)	0.28 (0.75) [7]	0.46 (1.09) [50]	0.02 (0.22) [78]	0.06 (0.36) [60]
	Matching V's (seconds)	54.00 (25.54) [7]	40.36 (15.26) [50]	37.95 (18.93) [80]	29.93 (12.32) [62]
	Matching V's (errors)	3.28 (2.42) [7]	2.22 (1.91) [50]	1.61 (1.68) [80]	1.14 (1.53) [62]
	Star (correct)	2.83 (2.56) [6]	4.78 (1.96) [47]	5.49 (1.41) [75]	5.88 (0.45) [61]
	Star (seconds)	15.66 (7.44) [6]	14.44 (6.70) [47]	13.64 (6.80) [75]	12.72 (6.83) [61]
	Concentric Squares (seconds)	22.00 (10.61) [4]	32.76 (27.21) [46]	24.93 (12.94) [76]	28.36 (19.23) [63]
	Concentric Squares (correct)	3.25 (1.70) [4]	4.785 (2.47) [46]	5.88 (2.38) [76]	6.07 (2.10) [63]
	Matching Pictures (correct)	14.12 (1.95) [8]	16.60 (2.36) [53]	16.91 (2.2) [79]	17.53 (1.84) [63]

Source: Unpublished data, courtesy of Michael K. Findeis & David G. Weight, Brigham Young University (1994); Adapted from Gray, Livingston et al. (2000).

ment until publication of a formal scoring system and normative data for 6 to 12 year olds (Cohen, Ricci et al., 2000; see Table 10–4 for this study's demographic characteristics). The authors found developmental progression of the concept of time through age 8 and of clock construction through age 12. Number reversals disappeared by age 7, regardless of handedness, and quadrant neglect disappeared by age 8. However, spacing problems and erasures/second attempts were still present at age 12. Normative data for the concept of time are presented in Table 10–5, and for construction in Table 10–6.

The instructions simply ask the child: "Draw the face of a clock and make the clock say three o'clock." After completion of this task, the child is then presented with two pre-drawn clocks

Table 10–4. Clock Drawing: Cohen et al. Study (2000)

Subjects: 429 children in central Georgia
Age: 6 to 12 years, in 1st through 6th grade public school
Gender: 210 male, 219 female
Handedness: 393 right handed, 36 left handed
Race: Not specified
Inclusion/Exclusion Criteria: Must read at grade level and have no history of grade retention, behavior or learning disorder, or stimulant medication usage

Table 10–6. Clock Drawing: Construction

Age	Mean	SD
6	8.65	2.1
7	9.46	1.73
8	10.84	1.14
9	10.81	1.13
10	11.34	0.98
11	11.39	1.09
12	11.62	0.98

Source: Cohen et al. (2000), © Swets & Zeitlinger.

and asked to indicate the times of 9:30 and 10:20. Performance is scored for concept of time and construction as follows:

Assessment of the Concept of Time:
Maximum score = 5

1 point	the hour hand is distinctly different from the minute hand AND one of the following:
4 points	if the placement of hands is pointing directly to correct numbers, or
3 points	if the placement of hands is off by less than 1 number, or
2 points	if the placement of hands is off by 1 number, or
1 point	if the placement of hands is off by more than 1 number or the hour/minute hands are reversed, or one of the hands is missing

Assessment of the Clock Face Construction:
Maximum Form score = 13

1 point	some indication of the concept of a clock

1 point	hands present, regardless of location or size
1–4 points	1 point for each quadrant of clock face used
1 point	equal spacing of all numbers, 1–12
0–2 points	2 points: all numbers present and in correct sequence
1 point: numbers out of sequence, repeated, or sequence goes beyond 12
0 points: any numbers (1–12) are missing
1 point	numbers 3–9 directly opposite each other
1 point	numbers 12–6 directly opposite each other
0–2 points	2 points if all numbers are in correct spatial orientation
1 point if 1 or more numbers are rotated ≥45°
0 points if 1 or more numbers are reversed

Children's clock drawing was also studied in 126 children in three age groups: 6 to 7 years;

Table 10–5. Clock Drawing to Time

		TIME DRAWN TO THE:					
		HOUR		HALF-HOUR		MINUTE	
Age	N	Mean	SD	Mean	SD	Mean	SD
6	40	3.20	1.65	3.20	1.45	2.15	1.46
7	79	3.97	1.27	3.86	1.26	3.03	1.62
8	70	4.59	0.96	4.35	0.91	4.30	1.18
9	69	4.68	0.76	4.55	0.80	4.57	0.92
10	91	4.56	0.90	4.35	0.99	4.38	1.06
11	54	4.62	0.89	4.51	0.84	4.47	1.09
12	26	4.54	0.86	4.69	0.68	4.65	0.89

Source: Cohen et al. (2000), © Swets & Zeitlinger.

8 to 9 years; and 10 to 12 years. A pre-drawn circle without numbers and a pre-drawn circle with the numbers 3, 6, 9, and 12 drawn were given to the children, and responses were scored qualitatively for organization and planning. By age 8 to 9, the children made few conceptual errors, and significant organizational improvement was observed with increasing age (McLane, Marcotte et al., 2001). The clock drawing capabilities of 41 children with attention deficit hyperactivity disorder (ADHD) were investigated in another child study. The clinical population performed less well than 41 matched controls, but those with Predominately Inattentive Type ADHD performed equivalently to those with Combined Type ADHD. Qualitative analysis suggested errors in the ADHD group were due to executive dysfunction. Supporting this interpretation, multiple regression analysis found that the Wisconsin Card Sorting Test-perseverative errors and failures-to-maintain-set scores were predictive of clock construction performance in children with ADHD (Kibby, Cohen et al., 2002).

PERCEPTUAL TESTS: NON-CONSTRUCTIONAL

The early face recognition and face perception literature attests to the importance of right hemisphere brain regions for perception and recall (Benton and Van Allen, 1968; Benton, Hannay et al., 1975), particularly the right temporal lobe. Hemiface preference study provided further support (Kolb, Milner et al., 1983). Tachistoscopic (Rhodes, 1985), structural imaging (De Renzi, Perani et al., 1994), and functional imaging (Sergent, Ohta et al., 1992; Haxby, Horwitz et al., 1994; Haxby, Hoffman et al., 2000) studies confirmed the importance of temporal and temporo-occipital brain structures and delineated an extrastriatal cortex region of increased activity when faces are viewed, that is, the fusiform face area.

Face perception appears to be an object-based ventral stream process, with single-face stimuli selectively activating inferior temporal cortex and facial expressions activating superior temporal sulcus regions (Andreason, O'Leary et al., 1996). A role for the left hemisphere appears to be evident for processing semantic information about faces, for example, names, social and physical attributes, and perhaps for more familiar than unfamiliar faces (Dade and Jones-Gotman, 2001). Hemispheric perception of emotional valence from facial expression studies have also dissociated visuoperceptual functions of the right and left cerebral hemisphere. Perception of negative valence relied preferentially on the right hemisphere, but positive valence perception relied on both cerebral hemispheres (Jansari, Tranel et al., 2000; Adolphs, Jansari et al., 2001). A familial factor in developmental face recognition deficit was suggested (De Haan, 1999).

There are qualitatively different facial recognition strategies. The perception of a face as a whole is referred to as a holistic or configural processing strategy, while processing of component portions is referred to as a featural strategy approach and commonly used in abstract pattern recognition. A study conducted on 106 children aged 7 and 10 was conducted to determine if speed of information processing might define differences in recognition of faces, emotional expressions, and abstract nonsocial information. These authors found speed, but not accuracy, improves between 7 and 10 years of age and can increase greatly beyond 10 years, as evident from comparison with an adult population. They concluded that speed and accuracy are sensitive parameters in revealing different processing strategies (De Sonneville, Verschoor et al., 2002).

Support for the finding that facial recognition performance is impaired in the presence of right hemisphere lesions is well documented (Hamsher, Levin et al., 1979), and recent neuroimaging data identified functional specialization of right ventral stream posterior regions for face identification and recognition (Sergent, Ohta et al., 1992; Haxby, Grady et al., 1993; Tovée and Cohen-Tovée, 1993). Besides evidence that right parietal and occipital lesions contribute to face recognition and face affect recognition impairment, the literature provides evidence of the influence of bilateral damage and of frontal and temporal lobe lesion contribution to face processing capacity (Braun, Denault et al., 1994; Clarke, Lindemann et al., 1997). Study of neurologically normal adults found both normal atrophic brain changes apparent in MRI evidence of ventricular enlargement and decreased processing speed contributed to individual differences in face discrimination (Schretlen, Pearlson et al., 2001). Schretlen and colleagues have suggested that "facial discrimination invokes a type of cognitive processing that is dependent on perceptual comparison speed . . ." (p. 409).

A functional anatomic dissociation between face recognition and face affect perception is documented in adults, but also in children using a mixed sensory paradigm in a study designed to determine whether there was preferential right hemisphere involvement in face recognition or facial affect processing (Everhart, Shucard et al., 2001). The authors suggested different neuronal systems might be used by prepubertal boys versus girls and speculated that their data supported the hypothesis that sex differences in brain organization are present early in development and do not change with puberty. Specifically, they found sex-related differences in face processing, that is, boys displayed greater right versus left event-related potential amplitude to auditory tone probes during face recognition, and girls had the opposite pattern. Further, boys, but not girls, had positive correlations between event-related potential amplitude during face recognition and facial affect identification testing. These authors used a face recognition test, developed in their laboratory and based on Ekman and Friesen standardized facial affect pictures (Ekman and Friesen, 1978).

Benton Facial Recognition Test

The Benton Facial Recognition Test (BFRT; Benton, Hamsher et al., 1983) is a matching-to-sample unfamiliar face discrimination test. As such, it is commonly thought of as indicative of right cerebral hemisphere function, but this is not always the case (Benton, 1980; Sergent, 1982). The BFRT consists of 22 target black-and-white photographic stimulus pictures, each presented to the child with six multiple choice pictures printed below the target. The first seven items require selection of the one full frontal face that exactly matches the target face. The subsequent items (7–22) require selection of three non-frontal faces with various position and luminance conditions that exactly match the target face. The maximum total score is 52 points. An abbreviated short-form version requires responses to the first six items and the next seven items, for a maximum total score of 27 points, which can then be prorated (Levin, Hamsher et al., 1975). The long form is generally administered to children, but if the scores are well into the normal range and there are few errors, it is permissible to administer the short form and prorate the long-form score. It has been suggested that the BFRT is relatively free of racial bias since it has a low correlation with IQ and appears relatively unaffected by demographic variables such as minority status (Roberts and Hamsher, 1984).

In clinical practice, the Benton Facial Recognition Test has wide acceptance, but normative data for children are limited. Data from a study of 266 children (224 aged 6 to 11, and 42 aged 13 and 14) are presented in Table 10–7 (Benton, Hamsher et al., 1983; 1994). The

Table 10–7. Facial Recognition Test: Means and SDs

Age	BENTON ET AL. DATA		PAQUIER ET AL. DATA		
	N	Mean: Long Form	N	Mean	SD
6	22	33.0			
7	59	37.2	10	35.0	4.5
8	33	37.6	10	37.0	3.0
9	27	38.1	11	38.9	5.8
10	50	40.6	11	41.2	4.4
11	33	41.3	9	39.8	5.1
12	X	X	9	41.5	4.3
13	23	43.0	10	41.9	3.0
14	19	45.1	11	41.4	4.4

Source: Adapted from Benton et al. (1983; 1994); Paquier et al. (1999)

mean long-form scores by age are presented without standard deviations. The BFRT was administered to 81 control subjects aged 7 to 14 as part of a study of children from the Netherlands with unilateral cerebral lesions (18 children with acquired left cerebral lesions and 14 with acquired right cerebral lesions). The data for the control subjects are presented in Table 10–7 as well. The reader should note how few subjects there are at each age level.

A study of sixty 7-year-olds, fifty-three 10-year-olds and fifty-five 13-year-olds provided additional data (Lindgren, 1977, unpublished doctoral dissertation). Means and standard deviations are presented in Table 10–8. The original adult norms (Benton, Hamsher et al., 1983) apply for those aged 16 to 18 and older. No age correction need be applied.

Face recognition subtests are also part of the Rivermead Behavioural Memory Test for Children. This face recognition subtest presents the child with five individual pictures of faces at a rate of one every 5 seconds. The child is asked to indicate if the picture is of a man or woman, and if the person is young, middle-aged, or old. Delayed recognition memory testing occurs for the five faces among five distractors.

The Kaufman Assessment Battery for Children (K-ABC) facial recognition subtest (Kaufman and Kaufman, 1983) is a 15 item task that requires brief visual memory in addition to recognition skill. A Memory for Faces subtest is part of the NEPSY (Korkman, Kirk et al., 1997). This subtest assesses the ability to recognize 16 faces after a single exposure in an immediate memory condition (from among two foils) and after a 30-minute interference for the delayed memory condition.

Judgment of Line Orientation Test

The Judgment of Line Orientation Test (JLOT; Benton, Varney et al., 1978; Benton, Hamsher et al., 1983) was developed as a nonverbal test of visuospatial perceptual ability. Unlike some other visuoperceptual tests, it does not require a motor response. Early adult studies found line-position perception in two-dimensional space to be impaired in the presence of posterior right hemisphere lesions, especially right parietal lesions (Warrington and Rabin, 1970; Benton, Hannay et al., 1975; Benton, Varney et al., 1978; Hannay, Falgout et al., 1987; Riccio and Hynd, 1992). Regional cerebral blood flow study found the JLOT task activating the temporo-occipital cortex (Hannay, Falgout et al., 1987), possibly because the items can be solved as shape discriminations (Dennis, Fletcher et al., 2002).

Besides being sensitive to right cerebral hemisphere dysfunction, the JLOT was found to be sensitive to diffuse brain damage in adults (Eslinger and Benton, 1983), and it is sensitive to attentional problems, including sustained attention (Meador, Moore et al., 1993). In a diagnostically mixed adult neuropsychiatric sample, the unabbreviated test form had a coefficient alpha value of 0.84, above the recommended value of 0.80 (Winegarden, Yates et al., 1998). Retesting with an alternate form over a short 20-minute time interval did not result in obvious practice effects in adults with Parkinson's disease (Montse, Pere et al., 2001). A recommended short form for adults is a 20 item Form V, items 11 through 30, and score conversions from short form to long form are published (Winegarden, Yates et al., 1998).

The JLOT procedure includes five practice stimuli with full-length lines, followed by 30 test stimulus pictures of line segments, whose positions can be matched to two of 11 full-length lines in 18-degree intervals, drawn in sequen-

Table 10–8. Facial Recognition Test Means and SDs

Age	N	Mean (SD)
Males		
7	29	37.7 (5.2)
10	27	41.7 (4.0)
13	29	44.3 (3.4)
Females		
7	31	39.0 (3.9)
10	26	42.2 (5.2)
13	26	43.4 (4.8)
All Children		
7	60	38.4 (4.6)
10	53	41.9 (4.6)
13	55	43.8 (4.1)

Source: Courtesy of Scott Lindgren (1977), Dissertation Abstracts.

Table 10–9. Judgment of Line Orientation: Lindgren & Benton Study (1980)

Subjects: 221 Washington, Iowa children, some retested
  1 year later for a total of 315
Age: 7 to 14 years
Gender: 153 males; 162 females
Handedness: Not reported
Race: Not reported
SES: Predominantly middle class
Inclusion Criteria: Prorated WISC-R VIQ ranged from
  81–127, $M = 106.77$ ($SD = 10.88$)

---

tial array below the target lines. All items are presented and a score of 1 is given for each set of two lines correctly discriminated, for a maximum score of 30. There are two versions, Form H and Form V, which have the same items but in a different ascending order of difficulty.

A developmental study of line orientation perception in children was conducted using Form V of the Benton JLOT (Lindgren and Benton, 1980; see Table 10–9 for demographic characteristics). Corrected split-half reliability coefficients at each age level ranged from .61–.87 with a trend toward increased reliability at upper ages. Long-term test reliability was assessed for 94 children and a correlation of .64 ($p < .001$) was found for the total group, with 0.39 for grade 1 to grade 2 children ($p < .01$) and .78 for grade 4 to grade 5 children ($p < .001$). Boys performed superior to girls (Lindgren and Benton, 1980) at all ages, with

a statistically significant difference only at ages 13 and 14. Critical scores were computed, see Table 10–10, marking particularly poor performance for a child who earns a lower score. Verbal intelligence estimates were only slightly related to JLOT performance, consistent with the idea that language dysfunction does not impair performance on this test. Those 13 years old showed a level of performance comparable to that of same gender adults (Benton, Varney et al., 1978).

The JLOT test was also included in a study of children from the Netherlands with acquired unilateral cerebral lesions to determine if it is useful in detecting right cerebral hemisphere lesions in children (Paquier, Van Mourik et al., 1999). The JLOT and Facial Recognition Test performances of 18 children with acquired left cerebral lesions and 14 children with acquired right cerebral lesions were examined, and these did not predict the presence of cerebral pathology in a group unselected for age, sex, or etiology with demonstrated unilateral cerebral lesions. These tests did not contribute to prediction of lesion laterality. Therefore, the clinical utility or discriminative validity of either test with brain-damaged children was not supported. The results of JLOT administration for 81 control subjects aged 7 to 14 are presented in Table 10–10. The reader should note how few subjects there are at each age level.

Table 10–10. Judgment of Line Orientation Test M, SD, and Critical Scores: Two Studies

	LINDGREN AND BENTON DATA								PAQUIER ET AL. DATA		
	MALE				FEMALE				ALL SUBJECTS		
Age	N	Critical Score[°]	M	SD	N	Critical Score[°]	M	SD	N	M	SD
7	24	9	16.8	4.5	23	7	15.3	5.4	10	17.3	3.1
8	23	12	19.0	4.3	27	11	17.6	3.7	10	21.8	4.9
9	18	13	21.7	4.1	19	12	19.7	4.2	11	22.1	3.4
10	17	13	20.6	6.6	19	12	19.3	5.2	11	23.1	3.5
11	20	13	22.8	5.3	24	12	21.7	5.1	9	22.0	4.9
12	20	17	24.7	3.8	22	16	22.7	4.0	9	24.6	3.8
13	18	18	26.1	3.5	18	16	22.7	4.2	10	24.4	2.9
14	13	19	26.3	2.7	10	17	23.1	4.0	11	24.8	3.1

Sources: Adapted from Lindgren & Benton (1980); Paquier et al. (1999).

[°]Critical score represents score exceeded by 89%–100% of children at given age and gender.

Table 10–11. Judgment of Line Orientation Test: Riva & Benton Study (1993)

Subjects: 150 children
Age: 8 to 12 years
Gender: 75 males; 75 females
Handedness: Not reported
Nationality: Italian
SES: Not reported
Inclusion Criteria: Prorated WISC VIQ ranged from 90–110; age appropriate school grade

Qualitative errors made by the child should be noted, such as a tendency to omit lines falling within a visual field or the distance between the target and reported line falling more than one line apart. Patients with suspected or known unilateral visual neglect are often not able to take this test in its original format because of the spread of line positions into the neglected visual hemispace. An error-type analysis proposed to distinguish normal elderly from early Alzheimer's disease coded JLOT errors (Ska, Poissant et al., 1990) and was also included in Parkinson's disease studies (Finton, Lucas et al., 1998; Montse, Pere et al., 2001). While not examined in any child study to-date, the usefulness of the authors' four error types and additional subtypes might be of interest to the reader who wishes to quantify error severity and examine differential error profiles between groups.

The 11 error types are summarized below. It is noted that a quadrant refers to either JLOT lines 2 to 5, or lines 7 to 10.

QO: Intraquadrant Oblique Error: errors between lines of same quadrant

QO1—different by one spacing of 18
QO2—different by two or three spacings of 18
QO3—both lines displaced to one or two spacings in same direction respecting the initial spacing
QO4—both lines displaced without maintenance of initial spacing
Vertical or Horizontal Error
V—Vertical Error—incorrect for line 6
H—Horizontal Error—incorrect for line 1 or line 11
VH—Vertical and Horizontal errors with simultaneous incorrect identification of line 6 and any horizontal line
IQO: Interquadrant Oblique Error
IQO—displacement of a line from one quadrant to another
Combined Oblique Interquadrant and vertical or horizontal errors
IQOH—combination of IQO error and H error
IQOV—combination of IQO error and V error

Independent normative data were subsequently reported for a sample of 150 8-to 12-year-old Italian children (see Table 10–11) and compared to the 209 U.S. school children in the Lindgren and Benton study (Lindgren and Benton, 1980) of similar age and with VIQ scores of 81 to 123 (Riva and Benton, 1993). These data are presented in Table 10–12.

Hooper Visual Organization Test

The Hooper Visual Organization Test (HVOT) was constructed to be a measure of visual analysis and synthesis, conceptual reorganization and mental rotation, that in its standard administration format also requires a naming response (Hooper, 1958; Hooper, 1983; Spreen and Strauss, 1998). It was originally intended

Table 10–12. Judgment of Line Orientation Test: Italian Children Data

	MALE			FEMALE		
Age	N	Mean	SD	N	Mean	SD
8	15	18.3	6.2	15	18.1	5.8
9	13	19.3	5.0	17	17.8	6.2
10	18	20.6	5.2	12	21.3	3.7
11	15	24.0	5.3	15	22.7	3.5
12	14	23.1	2.7	16	20.6	3.9

Source: D. Riva and A. Benton (1993), Visuospatial judgment: A crossnational comparison. *Cortex* (29): 141–143, Adapted from Table 1, p. 142.

to differentiate those 13 years and older with and without brain damage, but developmental studies of the Hooper were subsequently reported (Hilgert and Treloar, 1985; Kirk, 1992; Seidel, 1994). Limitations are evident in clinical application of this test in children, and it can often be omitted without substantial loss of essential information about visuospatial integration. A recent adult study confirmed these clinical impressions of limited usefulness when it found the HVOT should be considered a measure of global visual-spatial intelligence, similar to WAIS-R PIQ subtests, since it loaded on this global factor and had the highest correlation with these subtests (Johnstone and Wilhelm, 1997). This finding was similar to the results found in a child study (Seidel, 1994). It was also suggested that face validity suggests that the HVOT measures the same abilities as the Wechsler Adult Intelligence Scale-Revised (WAIS-R) object assembly subtest and noted that the HVOT might be preferable to the Wechsler Adult Intelligence Scale-Revised Performance IQ for those compromised by limited motor function or impaired processing speed (Johnstone and Wilhelm, 1997).

The HVOT test consists of a series of 30 line drawings of familiar objects that have been divided into fragments. The child must mentally reassemble the fragments to determine the object's identity. The score is the total number correct. The test has long been considered a gross measure of general impairment and is not significantly related to lesion lateralization in adults (Boyd, 1981). It may be sensitive to focal right hemisphere dysfunction secondary to perceptual impairment (Rathbun, 1982), but it was suggested that it is also affected by language-dominant hemisphere problems, perhaps due to the requirement for oral naming. More recent investigation in an adult vascular dementia population does not support this notion since it was found that more than 60% of the variance in HVOT performance was accounted for by the WAIS-R block design subtest performance while Boston Naming Test performance did not contribute substantially (Paul, Cohen et al., 2001). Its limitations in being interpreted in isolation from other measures for rehabilitation or educational planning are noted (Johnstone and Wilhelm, 1997).

Importantly, the Hooper total score appears to be influenced by age and intelligence (full-scale IQ) (Hilgert and Treloar, 1985). The influence of gender is less clear (Kirk, 1992; Seidel, 1994), although, for these studies, the school populations and exclusion criteria differed. While the Hooper might be as reliable for children as for adults, with an internal consistency reliability of 0.72, (Seidel, 1994), it is not necessarily as clinically useful as other measures in child assessment. The test does not discriminate well between specific neurological populations. Further, it is largely measuring what the WISC Perceptual Organization factor measures, is loaded with "visual-spatial" tasks, and is especially highly correlated with the block design subtest (Seidel, 1994). Thus, the HVOT alone is not singularly useful, but it might contribute as part of a comprehensive battery.

It should also be noted that there is a both a visuospatial and language requirement in the HVOT. Because it requires a naming response, adults with anomia, in particular, might be disadvantaged on this test. To examine this further, a multiple-choice format version was developed and administered to 14 right-handed adults with either stroke or traumatic cerebral contusion to determine if reducing the task-naming demands would allow for better assessment of the visuospatial aspects. The authors concluded that HVOT performance improved under a multiple-choice format that reduced the naming demands among those with a naming deficit, and improvement was noted for those with both right- and left-hemisphere impairment (Schultheis, Caplan et al., 2000).

A normative study was conducted of 207 5- to 11-year-old children with a prorated verbal IQ of at least 70. The demographic data for these children are presented in Table 10–13, and the means and standard deviations are presented by age level in Table 10–14.

Standardized Road Map Test of Directional Sense (Money Road Map Test)

The Standardized Road Map Test of Directional Sense, or Money Road Map Test (Money, Alexander et al. 1965; Money, 1976) as it is also known, is of interest particularly

Table 10–13. Hooper Visual Organization Test: Seidel Study (1994)

Subjects: Normative: 211 English speaking children minus 4 children with VIQ < 70 = 207 children.
Clinical: 49 children, various neurological disorders.
Age: 5 to 11 years
Gender: Normative: 102 males; 109 females; Clinical: 41 males; 8 females
Handedness: Normative: not given; Clinical: 41 right handed; 8 left handed
Race: Not specified
SES: From 4 public schools that represent a wide SES range
Inclusion Criteria: No exclusion criteria used

when the child has questionable ability to discriminate right from left or there is concern about the child's ability to spatially orient. There are clear age effects for direction sense maturation (Money, Alexander et al., 1965).

The test is printed on a single page. A short practice route and longer test route are traced before the child begins the test. After practice, the child is instructed to retrace the path "up the street" and then "down the street," indicating at each of 32 corners whether a right or left turn must be made to stay on the designated path. There are eight different types of turns, that is, turning right or left after proceeding up, down, right or left. The examiner writes R (for right) or L (for left) at each turn as instructed by the child.

Right–left disorientation is associated with dominant parietal dysfunction, and the right parietal lobe is necessary for the mediation of cross-modal associations and mental manipulation of space or rotation (Butters, Barton et al.,

1970). In more recent investigations, poor Money Road Map test performance was found to have a greater association with parietal lesions than with frontal lesions (Vingerhoets, Lannoo et al., 1996), and evidence of parietal activation was found on functional imaging studies requiring mental rotation of visual stimuli (Cohen, Kosslyn et al., 1996; Alivisatos and Petrides, 1997).

Clinically, it is noted that the child experiencing spatial orientation problems may be more likely to err when coming "down the street," which requires mentally rotating space, while making no, or a minimal number of, errors traveling "up the street." Children with attention problems may be more likely to make errors in both directions, or fail to sustain attention toward the end of the task.

The original normative data were obtained on 1044 children between ages 7 and 18 in Anne Arundel County, Maryland (Money, Walker et al., 1965). Subjects ranged in social class, intelligence, and achievement, but elementary school students were predominantly from middle- and upper-class families. Between the ages of 7 and 10 (152 male, 193 female), errors were distributed on a normal curve. There was a bimodal distribution for those 11 to 14 years old (203 male, 201 female). Most scores for those 15 to 18 years old were quite good. Early data were presented for three conditions in which impaired directional sense was predicted: Turner syndrome, Gerstmann's syndrome, (those with parieto-occipital area dysfunction), and specific developmental dyslexia (Alexander, Walker et al., 1964).

Clinical experiences suggests perfect performance is not necessarily to be expected, even into the teen years, but a difference between number of errors made while traveling in each direction or errors made on both sides of the page, and particularly when mental rotation was necessary, deserve special attention. A difference of three errors between the two sides appears to be a more rare occurrence and should received clinical attention.

Children's Size-Ordering Task

The Children's Size-Ordering Task (CSOT, Kerns and McInerney, 2001) was developed re-

Table 10–14. Hooper Visual Organization Test: Seidel Data

Age (Years)	N	Mean No. Correct	SD
5	21	18.4	3.1
6	34	19.4	3.8
7	32	21.1	3.1
8	28	23.4	2.0
9	28	23.7	2.9
10	34	24.0	2.5
11	30	24.1	2.9

Source: Seidel (1994), © Swets & Zeitlinger.

cently, and while its validity has yet to be established, it is mentioned here as an alternative test of spatial ability that might be of interest to the reader. It is available directly from the authors. The test requires the child to order words with respect to their size. For example, if the child hears "cow, nickel," the correct response would be "nickel, cow". This is clarified in the instructions below.

Instructions: "I am going to tell you the names of some things. Listen carefully, and when I stop, I want you to think about how big the things are, and then say them back to me from the smallest to biggest. For example, if I say 'Mountain–Horse,' what would you say?" If the child is correct, say, "That's right! A horse is smaller than a mountain so first you would say 'horse.' A mountain is bigger than a horse, so next you would say 'mountain.' And the whole answer would be 'Horse-Mountain.'" If the child is incorrect, say, "No, you would say 'Horse-Mountain.' A horse is smaller than a mountain, so first you would say horse. A mountain is bigger than a horse so next you would say 'mountain.' And the whole answer would be 'Horse-Mountain.' Remember, you have to say them back to me from smallest to biggest." (Repeat example, rewording as necessary).

"Let's try another example. If I say 'Apple-Train-Car,' what would you say?" If the child is correct, say: "That's right! An apple is smaller than a car, so first you say 'Apple.' A car is bigger than an apple but smaller than a train, so next you say 'car.' And last you say 'train,' because it's the biggest one of all. The whole answer would be 'Apple-Car-Train.' If the child is incorrect, say: "No, you would say 'Apple-Car-Train.' An apple is smaller than a car, so you say 'Apple' first. A car is bigger than an apple but smaller than a train, so next you say 'Car.' And last you say 'Train,' because it's the biggest one of all. The whole answer would be 'Apple-Car-Train.' Remember, you have to say them back to me from smallest to biggest." Repeat and reword as necessary.

"OK, we're going to begin the real game now. As the game goes on, I'll be saying more and more things, so listen carefully!"

The sequences range in length from two to seven items. There are two trials at each difficulty level, as for the WISC-III digit span. Each correct word pair in a sequence receives a point. Thus, the maximum number of points at level 1 is 2, that is, 1 point for each two-item trial. The maximum number of points at level 6 is 12, that is, 6 points for each 7-item trial. The maximum total score is 42. Preliminary normative data were obtained on 82 control and 59 attention deficit hyperactivity disorder children between the ages of 7 and 13. Children were recruited through flyers, advertisements, and brochures sent to local physicians. The sample was mostly Caucasian (about 95%). All children were from local elementary schools in Victoria, B. C., Canada. The control subjects included 21 females and 61 males without a history of significant developmental, neurological, or behavioral problems, a history of a significant fall or head injury, and if they did not meet diagnostic criteria for ADHD. The ADHD sample included 10 females and 49 males, all medication-free for at least 24 hours.

Children in the ADHD group were considered for study if they were formally diagnosed with ADHD by a health care professional. Of the 30 children in the first of two ADHD study groups, there was a 73% return rate for the Conners' Parent Questionnaire. Of the forms returned, 91% scored greater than 1.5 standard deviations above the mean (equal to or greater than the 93rd percentile) on both the impulsivity-hyperactivity and ADHD scales. Finally, the parent or guardian of prospective participants completed the Diagnostic Interview for Children and Adolescents-Fourth Edition (DICA-IV) by telephone. Children with ADHD were admitted to the study only if they met diagnostic criteria for ADHD (Combined Type) according to the DICA-IV and at least one other diagnostic method. The Diagnostic Interview Schedule for Children (DISC) was used for a second ADHD study group rather than the DICA-IV. Preliminary normative data were pooled from the two studies, and the results are presented in Table 10–15.

The Kaufman Assessment Battery for Children Gestalt Closure subtest also requires identification of incomplete figures and assesses visual closure (Kaufman and Kaufman, 1983).

Table 10–15. Children's Size-Ordering Test Normative Data

Control Subjects

Age	N	M	SD
7	15	19.27	4.25
8	12	20.17	3.88
9	11	25.09	3.45
10	18	23.50	5.16
11	13	23.92	6.18
12	13	27.08	3.07

ADHD Subjects

Age	N	M	SD
7	12	11.92	5.79
8	8	16.38	7.91
9	7	17.71	6.07
10	13	18.85	6.11
11	10	19.70	5.60
12	6	20.17	9.45
13	3	24.33	5.69

Source: Kimberly Kerns and Robert McInerny, personal communication.

VISUAL PLANNING AND ORGANIZATION: MAZES

Wechsler Mazes and Porteus Mazes

Maze tests assess route planning and route finding along with visuomotor control. There are a number of such tests, including the Wechsler IQ series Mazes subtests (Wechsler, 1991) that assess route finding and the Porteus Maze Test, which assesses route planning (Porteus, 1959; Porteus, 1965). In adult studies, route-finding performances were more impaired in the presence of parietal lobe lesions than for lesions of other cerebral regions (Semmes, Weinstein et al., 1963). The test was found to be especially sensitive to traumatic brain injury severity and to volume of circumscribed prefrontal lesions (Levin, Song et al., 2001).

For the supplementary Wechsler IQ Mazes subtest, the child uses a pencil to quickly draw a path from a central starting point out to the circumference for a series of increasingly complex mazes. Instruction is given not to draw the line into a dead end or cross over the route-border lines. The number of errors determines the point value of each item.

The Porteus Maze Test is an untimed nonverbal test in which the child plans paths through a series of increasingly more difficult mazes. Trial and error is not useful, and planning is necessary (Porteus, 1959; 1965). A single error results in presentation of the next maze. Normative data are available for children 3 to 12 years old and 14 years old (Krikorian and Bartok, 1998). (See Chapter 6 for more detail on Porteus mazes and these normative data.)

Other Nonverbal Measures

The reader might also be interested in several other nonverbal measures and their research and clinical applicability. The Gollin Incomplete Figures test (Gollin, 1960; Warrington and Rabin, 1970) requires identification of 20 familiar objects, presented to the child in five degrees of fragmentation, with a maximum score of 100 possible. The score is the number of guesses required until correct identification with a higher score representing a poorer performance. This visual closure task was incorporated into a study of visual perception in children with spina bifida and hydrocephalus (Dennis, Fletcher et al., 2002).

The Visual Illusions Test (Dennis, Rogers et al., 2001) is an object-based visual perception task. Stereopsis was assessed in a study of children with spina bifida and hydrocephalus (Dennis, Fletcher et al., 2002) using the Randot Preschool Stereoacuity Test (Birch, 1999). This test presents a series of 18 binocularly disparate random dot patterns through polarizing glasses and requires the child to name the objects over six disparity levels. The Motor-Free Visual Perception Test (rev.) (Colarusso and Hammill, 1995) for children 4 to 11 years old is a brief individually administered test of five visuoperceptual subdomains for children with fine or gross motor impairment. Items assess *(1)* spatial relationship or the ability to orient in space and perceive an object's position, *(2)* visual discrimination, *(3)* figure-ground, *(4)* visual closure, and *(5)* visual memory.

REFERENCES

Adolphs, R., Jansari, A., & Tranel, D. (2001). Hemispheric perception of emotional valence from facial expressions. *Neuropsychology, 15,* 516–524.

Akshoomoff, N. A., Feroleto, C. C., Doyle, R. E., & Stiles, J. (2002). The impact of early unilateral brain injury on perceptual organization and visual memory. *Neuropsychologia, 40,* 539–561.

Akshoomoff, N. A., & Stiles, J. (1995a). Developmental trends in visuospatial analysis and planning: I. Copying a complex figure. *Neuropsychology, 9,* 364–377.

Albert, M. (1973). A simple test of visual neglect. *Neurology, 23,* 658–664.

Alexander, D., Walker, H. T., & Money, J. (1964). Studies in direction sense: I. Turner's syndrome. *Archives of General Psychiatry, 10,* 337–339.

Alivisatos, B., & Petrides, M. (1997). Functional activation of the human brain during mental rotation. *Neuropsychologia, 35,* 111–118.

Andreason, N. C., O'Leary, D. S., Arndt, S., Cizadlo, T., Jurtig, R., Rezai, K., et al. (1996). Neural substrates of facial recognition. *Journal of Neuropsychiatry and Clinical Neurosciences, 12,* 139–146.

Aram, D., & Eisele, J. A. (1992). Plasticity and recovery of higher cognitive functions following early brain injury. In I. Rapin & S. J. Segalowitz (Eds.), *Handbook of neuropsychology: Volume 6. Child neuropsychology* (pp. 73–92). Oxford, England: Elsevier Science Publishers.

Aylward, E. H., & Schmidt, S. (1986). An examination of three tests of visuomotor integration. *Journal of Learning Disabilities, 19,* 328–330.

Baddeley, A. D. (2001). Is working memory still working. *American Psychologist, 56,* 851–864.

Baron, I. S., & Goldberger, E. (1993). Neuropsychological disturbances of hydrocephalic children with implications for special education and rehabilitation. *Neuropsychological Rehabilitation, 3,* 389–410.

Barton, J. J. S., & Black, S. E. (1998). Line bisection in hemianopia. *Journal of Neurological Neurosurgical Psychiatry, 64,* 660–662.

Beery, K. E. (1989). *The VMI Developmental Test of Visual-Motor Integration: Administration, scoring, and teaching manual* (3rd ed.). Cleveland, OH: Modern Curriculum Press.

Beery, K. E. (1997). *The Beery-Buktenica Developmental Test of Visual-Motor Integration: Administration, Scoring and Teaching Manual* (4th ed.). Parsippany, NJ: Modern Curriculum Press.

Benton, A. L. (1980). The neuropsychology of facial recognition. *American Psychologist, 35,* 176–186.

Benton, A. L., Hamsher, K., & Sivan, A. B. (1994). *Multilingual Aphasia Examination: Manual of instructions* (3rd ed.). Iowa City: AJA Associates, Inc.

Benton, A. L., Hamsher, K., Varney, N. R., & Spreen, O. (1983c). *Contributions to neuropsychological assessment: A clinical manual.* New York: Oxford University Press.

Benton, A. L., Hannay, H. J., & Varney, N. R. (1975a). Visual perception of line direction in patients with unilateral brain disease. *Neurology, 25,* 907–910.

Benton, A. L., & Van Allen, M. W. (1968). Impairment in facial recognition in patients with cerebral disease. *Cortex, 4,* 344–358.

Benton, A. L., Van Allen, M. W., Hamsher, K., & Levin, H. S. (1975b). *Test of facial recognition.* Iowa City: Department of Neurology, University of Iowa Hospitals.

Benton, A. L., Varney, N. R., & Hamsher, K. (1978). Visuospatial judgment: A clinical test. *Archives of Neurology, 35,* 364–367.

Binder, L. M. (1982). Constructional strategies on complex figure drawings after unilateral brain damage. *Journal of Clinical Neuropsychology, 4,* 51–58.

Birch, E. (1999). *Randot Preschool Stereoacuity Test.* Chicago: Stereo Optical Company.

Boyd, J. L. (1981). A validity study of the Hooper Visual Organization Test. *Journal of Consulting and Clinical Psychology, 49,* 15–19.

Braun, C. M., Denault, C., Cohen, H., & Rouleau, I. (1994). Discrimination of facial identity and facial affect by temporal and frontal lobectomy patients. *Brain and Cognition, 24,* 198–212.

Brookshire, B. L., Fletcher, J., Bohan, T. P., Landry, S. H., Davidson, K., & Francis, D. J. (1995). Verbal and nonverbal skill discrepancies in children with hydrocephalus: A five-year longitudinal follow-up. *Journal of Pediatric Psychology, 20,* 785–800.

Butters, N., Barton, M., & Brody, B. A. (1970). Role of the right parietal lobe in the mediation of cross-modal associations and reversible operations in space. *Cortex, 6,* 174–190.

Clarke, S., Lindemann, A., Maeder, P., Borrault, F.-X., & Assal, G. (1997). Face recognition and posterior-inferior lesions. *Neuropsychologia, 35,* 1555–1563.

Cohen, M. J., Ricci, C. A., Kibby, M. Y., & Edmonds, J. E. (2000). Developmental progression of clock face drawing in children. *Child Neuropsychology, 6,* 64–76.

Cohen, M. S., Kosslyn, S. M., Breiter, H. C., DiGirolamo, G. J., Thompson, W. L., Anderson, A. K., et al. (1996). Changes in cortical activity during mental rotation: A mapping study using functional MRI. *Brain, 119,* 89–100.

Colarusso, R., & Hammill, D. D. (1995). *Motor-Free Visual Perception Test-Revised.* Los Angeles: Western Psychological Service.

Dade, L. A., & Jones-Gotman, M. (2001). Face Learning and Memory: The Twins Test. *Neuropsychology, 15,* 525–534.

De Haan, E. H. F. (1999). A familial factor in the development of face recognition deficits. *Journal of Clinical and Experimental Neuropsychology, 21,* 312–315.

Delis, D., Robertson, L. C., & Efron, R. (1986). Hemispheric specialization of memory for visual hierarchical stimuli. *Neuropsychologia, 24,* 205–214.

Demsky, Y., Carone, D. A. J., Burns, W. J., & Sellers, A. (2000). Assessment of visual-motor coordination in 6- to 11-yr.-olds. *Perceptual and Motor Skills, 91,* 311–321.

Dennis, M., Fitz, C. R., Netley, C. T., Harwood-Nash, D. C. F., Sugar, J., Hendrick, E. G., et al. (1981). The intelligence of hydrocephalic children. *Archives of Neurology, 38,* 607–615.

Dennis, M., Fletcher, J., Rogers, T., Hetherington, R., & Francis, D. J. (2002). Object-based and action-based visual preception in children with spina bifida and hydrocephalus. *Journal of the International Neuropsychological Society, 8,* 95–106.

Dennis, M., Rogers, T., & Barnes, M. A. (2001). Children with spina bifida perceive visual illusions but not multistable figures. *Brain and Cognition, 46,* 108–113.

De Renzi, E., Perani, D., Carlesimo, G. A., Silveri, M. C., & Fazio, F. (1994). Prosopagnosia can be associated with damage confined to the right hemisphere—An MRI and PET study and a review of the literature. *Neuropsychologia, 32,* 893–902.

De Sonneville, L. M. J., Verschoor, C. A., Njiokiktjien, C., Op het Veld, V., Toorenaar, N., & Vranken, M. (2002). Facial identity and facial emotions: Speed, accuracy, and processing strategies in children and adults. *Journal of Clinical and Experimental Neuropsychology, 24,* 200–213.

Donders, J., Canady, A., & Rourke, B. P. (1990). Psychometric intelligence after infantile hydrocephalus: A critical review and reinterpretation. *Child's Nervous System, 6,* 148–154.

Ekman, P., & Friesen, W. (1978). *Pictures of facial affect.* Palo Alto, CA: Consulting Psychologists Press.

Eslinger, P. J., & Benton, A. (1983). Visuoperceptual performances in aging and dementia: Clinical and theoretical implications. *Journal of Clinical Neuropsychology, 5,* 213–220.

Espy, K. A., Kaufmann, P., Glisky, M., & McDiarmid, M. D. (2001). New procedures to assess executive functions in preschool children. *The Clinical Neuropsychologist, 15,* 46–58.

Everhart, D. E., Shucard, J. L., Quatrin, T., & Shucard, D. W. (2001). Sex-related differences in event-related potentials, face recognition and facial affect processing in prepubertal children. *Neuropsychology, 15,* 329–341.

Farah, M. (1995). *Visual agnosia.* Cambridge, MA: MIT Press.

Ferber, S., & Karnath, H.-O. (2001). How to assess spatial neglect-line bisection or cancellation tasks? *Journal of Clinical and Experimental Neuropsychology, 23,* 599–607.

Findeis, M. K., & Weight, D. G. (1994). *Meta-norms for Indiana-Reitan Neuropsychological Test Battery and Halstead-Reitan Neuropsychologial Test Battery for Children, ages 5–14.* Unpublished manuscript.

Finton, M. J., Lucas, J. A., Graff-Radford, N. R., & Uitti, R. J. (1998). Analysis of visuospatial errors in patients with Alzheimer's disease or Parkinson's disease. *Journal of Clinical and Experimental Neuropsychology, 20,* 186–193.

Freedman, M., Leach, L., Kaplan, E., Winocur, G., Shulman, K. I., & Delis, D. (1994). *Clock drawing: A neuropsychological analysis.* New York: Oxford University Press.

Gauthier, L., Dehaut, F., & Joanette, Y. (1989). The bells test: A quantitative and qualitative test for visual neglect. *International Journal of Clinical Neuropsychology, 11,* 49–54.

Ghent, L. (1956). Perception of overlapping and embedded figures by children of different ages. *American Journal of Psychology, 69,* 575–587.

Gollin, E. (1960). Developmental studies of visual recognition of incomplete objects. *Perceptual and Motor Skills, 11,* 289–298.

Goodglass, H., & Kaplan, E. (1983). *Assessment of aphasia and related disorders* (2nd ed.). Philadelphia: Lea and Febiger.

Gray, R. M., Livingston, R. B., Marshall, R. M., & Haak, R. A. (2000). Reference group data for the Reitan-Indiana Neuropsychological Test Battery for young children. *Perceptual and Motor Skills, 91,* 675–682.

Halligan, P., Marshall, J. C., & Wade, D. T. (1989). Visuospatial neglect: Underlying factors and test sensitivity. *The Lancet, 14,* 908–911.

Hamsher, K. d., Levin, H. S., & Benton, A. L. (1979). Facial recognition in patients with focal brain lesions. *Archives of Neurology, 36,* 837–839.

Hannay, H. J., Falgout, J. C., Leli, D. A., Katholi, C. R., Halsey, J. H., & Wills, E. L. (1987). Focal right temporo-occipital blood flow changes associated with judgment of line orientation. *Neuropsychologia, 25,* 755–763.

Harrigan, J. (1984). The effects of task order on children's identification of facial expressions. *Motivation and Emotion, 8,* 157–169.

Harris, I. M., Harris, J. A., & Caine, D. (2002). Mental-rotation deficits following damage to the right basal ganglia. *Neuropsychology, 16,* 524–537.

Hausmann, M., Waldie, K. E., & Corballis, M. C. (2003). Developmental changes in line bisection: A result of callosal maturation? *Neuropsychology, 17,* 155–160.

Haxby, J. V., Grady, C. L., Horwitz, B., Salerno, J., Ungerleider, L. G., Mishkin, M., et al. (1993). Dissociation of object and spatial visual processing pathways in human extrastriate cortex. In B. Gulyas, D. Ottoson & P. E. Roland (Eds.), *Functional organization of the human visual cortex.* Oxford, England: Pergamon Press.

Haxby, J. V., Hoffman, E. A., & Gobbini, M. I. (2000). The distributed human neural system for face perception. *Trends in Cognitive Science, 4,* 223–233.

Haxby, J. V., Horwitz, B., Ungerleider, L. G., Maisog, J. M., Peietrini, P., & Grady, C. L. (1994). The functional organization of human extrastriate cortex: A PET-rCBF study of selective attention to faces and locations. *Journal of Neuroscience, 14,* 6336–6353.

Heilman, K. M., Watson, R. T., & Valenstein, E. (1993). Neglect and related disorders. In K. M. Heilman & E. Valenstein (Eds.), *Clinical Neuropsychology* (pp. 279–336). New York: Oxford University Press.

Hilgert, L. D., & Treloar, J. H. (1985). The relationsip of the Hooper Visual Organization Test to sex, age, and intelligence in elementary school children. *Measurement and Evaluation in Counseling and Development, 17,* 203–206.

Hooper, H. E. (1958). *The Hooper Visual Organization Test: Manual.* Los Angeles, CA: Western Psychological Services.

Hooper, H. E. (1983). *Hooper Visual Organization Test.* Los Angeles: Western Psychological Services.

Jansari, A., Tranel, D., & Adolphs, R. (2000). A valence-specific lateral bias for discriminating emotional facial expressions in free field. *Cognition and Emotion, 14,* 341–353.

Johnstone, B., & Wilhelm, K. L. (1997). The construct validity of the Hooper Visual Organization Test. *Assessment, 4,* 243–248.

Kaufman, A. S., & Kaufman, N. L. (1983). *Kaufman assessment battery for children: Interpretive Manual.* Circle Pines, MN: American Guidance Service.

Kerns, K. A. (2000). The CyberCruiser: An investigation of development of prospective memory in children. *Journal of the International Neuropsychological Society, 6,* 62–70.

Kerns, K. A., & McInerney, R. J. (2001). *The Children's Size-Ordering Task.* Victoria, BC: Canada. Unpublished manuscript.

Kibby, M. Y., Cohen, M. J., & Hynd, G. W. (2002). Clock face drawing in children with attention-deficit/hyperactivity disorder. *Archives of Clinical Neuropsychology, 17,* 531–546.

Kirk, U. (1992a). Evidence for early acquisition of visual organization ability: A developmental study. *The Clinical Neuropsychologist, 6,* 171–177.

Kolb, B., Milner, B., & Taylor, L. (1983). Perception of faces by patients with localized cortical excisions. *Canadian Journal of Psychology, 37,* 8–18.

Korkman, M., Kirk, U., & Kemp, S. (1997). *NEPSY: A developmental neuropsychological assessment.* San Antonio: The Psychological Corporation.

Krikorian, R., & Bartok, J. (1998). Developmental data for the Porteus Maze Test. *The Clinical Neuropsychologist, 12,* 305–310.

Levin, H. S., Hamsher, K. d., & Benton, A. (1975). A short form of the test of facial recognition. *Journal of Psychology, 91,* 223–228.

Levin, H. S., Scheller, J., Rickard, T., & Grafman, J. (1996). Dyscalculia and dyslexia after right hemisphere injury in infancy. *Archives of Neurology, 53,* 88–96.

Levin, H. S., Song, J., Ewing-Cobbs, L., & Roberson, G. (2001). Porteus maze performance following traumatic brain injury in children. *Neuropsychology, 15,* 557–567.

Libon, D. J., Malamut, B. L., Swenson, R., Sands, L. P., & Cloud, B. S. (1996). Further analyses of clock drawings among demented and nondemented older subjects. *Archives of Clinical Neuropsychology, 11,* 193–205.

Libon, D. J., Swenson, R., Barnoski, E. J., & Sands, L. P. (1993). Clock drawing as an assessment tool for dementia. *Archives of Clinical Neuropsychology, 8,* 405–415.

Lindgren, S. D., & Benton, A. (1980). Developmental patterns of visuospatial judgment. *Journal of Pediatric Psychology, 5,* 217–225.

Markham, R., & Adams, K. (1992). The effect of type of task on children's identification of facial expressions. *Journal of Nonverbal Behavior, 16,* 21–39.

McLane, M. S., Marcotte, A. C., Stern, C., Kibby, M. Y., Wilson, J. W., Rice, K., et al. (2001). Children's clock drawings: A new scoring system and developmental trends [abstract]. *The Clinical Neuropsychologist, 15,* 255–256.

Meador, K. J., Moore, M. E., Nichols, O. L., Abney, H. S., Taylor, H. S., Zamrini, E. Y., et al. (1993). The role of cholinergic systems in visuospatial processing and memory. *Journal of Clinical and Experimental Neuropsychology, 15,* 832–842.

Meltzoff, A. N., & Moore, M. K. (1977). Imitation of facial and manual gestures in human neonates. *Science, 198,* 75–78.

Mesulam, M.-M. (1985b). Attention, confusional states and neglect. In M.-M. Mesulam (Ed.), *Principles of behavioral neurology.* Philadelphia: F. A. Davis Co.

Mesulam, M.-M. (2000). *Principles of behavioral and cognitive neurology.* New York: Oxford University Press.

Money, J. A. (1976). *A standardized road map test of directional sense. Manual.* San Rafael, CA: Academic Therapy Publications.

Money, J. A., Alexander, D., & Walker, H. T. (1965). *A standardised road map test of directional sense.* Baltimore: Johns Hopkins Press.

Money, J. A., Walker, H. T. J., & Alexander, D. (1965). Development of direction sense and three syndromes of impairment. *Slow Learning Child, 11,* 145–155.

Montse, A., Pere, V., Carme, J., Francesc, V., & Eduardo, T. (2001). Visuospatial deficits in Parkinson's disease assessed by Judgment of Line Orientation Test. *Journal of Clinical and Experimental Neuropsychology, 23,* 592–598.

Paquier, P. F., Van Mourik, M., Van Dongen, H. R., Catsman-Berrevoets, C. E., Creten, W. L., & Stronks, D. L. (1999). Clinical utility of the judgment of line orientation test and facial recognition test in chidren with acquired unilateral cerebral lesions. *Journal of Child Neurology, 14,* 243–248.

Paul, R., Cohen, R., Moser, D., Ott, B., Zawacki, T., & Gordon, N. (2001). Performance on the Hooper Visual Organizational Test in patients diagnosed with subcortical vascular dementia: Relation to naming performance. *Neuropsychiatry, Neuropsychology, and Behavioral Neurology, 14,* 93–97.

Porteus, S. D. (1959). *The maze test and clinical psychology.* Palo Alto, CA: Pacific Books.

Porteus, S. D. (1965). *Porteus Maze Test: Fifty years' application.* New York: The Psychological Corporation.

Rathbun, J., & Smith, A. (1982). Comment on the validity of Boyd's validation of the Hooper Visual Organization Test. *Journal of Consulting and Clinical Psychology, 50,* 281–283.

Rhodes, G. (1985). Lateralized processes in face recognition. *British Journal of Psychology, 76,* 249–271.

Riccio, C. A., & Hynd, G. W. (1992). Validity of Benton's judgment of line orientation test. *Journal of Psychoeducational Assessment, 10,* 210–218.

Riva, D., & Benton, A. (1993). Visuospatial judgment: A crossnational comparison. *Cortex, 29,* 141–143.

Roberts, R. J., & Hamsher, K. d. (1984). Effects of minority status on facial recognition and naming performance. *Journal of Clinical Psychology, 40,* 539–545.

Rudel, R. G., Denckla, M. B., & Broman, M. (1978). Rapid silent response to repeated target symbols by dyslexic and nondyslexic children. *Brain and Language, 6,* 52–62.

Schretlen, D. J., Pearlson, G. D., Anthony, J. C., & Yates, K. O. (2001). Determinants of Benton Facial Recognition Test performance in normal adults. *Neuropsychology, 15,* 405–410.

Schultheis, M. T., Caplan, B., Ricker, J. H., & Woessner, R. (2000). Fractioning the Hooper: A multiple-choice response format. *The Clinical Neuropsychologist, 14,* 196–201.

Seidel, W. T. (1994). Applicability of the Hooper Visual Organization Test to pediatric populations: Preliminary findings. *The Clinical Neuropsychologist, 8,* 59–68.

Semmes, J., Weinstein, S., Ghent, L., & Teuber, H. L. (1963). Correlates of impaired orientation in personal and extrapersonal space. *Brain, 86,* 747–772.

Sergent, J. (1982). About face: Left-hemisphere involvement in processing physiognomies. *Journal of Experimental Psychology: Human Perception and Performance, 8,* 1–14.

Sergent, J., Ohta, S., & MacDonald, B. (1992). Functional neuroanatomy of face and object processing. A positron emission tomography study. *Brain, 115,* 15–36.

Ska, B., Poissant, A., & Joanette, Y. (1990). Line orientation judgment in normal elderly and subjects with dementia of Alzheimer's type. *Journal of Clinical and Experimental Neuropsychology, 12,* 695–702.

Spreen, O., & Strauss, E. (1998). *A compendium of neuropsychological tests: Adminstration, norms, and commentary* (2nd ed.). New York: Oxford University Press.

Stafstrom, C. F., Rostasy, K., & Minster, A. (2002). The usefulness of children's drawings in the diagnosis of headache. *Pediatrics, 109,* 460–472.

Stiles, J., Bates, E., Thal, D. J., Trauner, D., & Reilly, J. (1998). Linguistic, cognitive, and affective development in children with pre-and perinatal focal brain injury: A ten-year overview from the San Diego Longitudinal Project. In C. Rovee-Collier, L. P. Lipsitt & H. Hayne (Eds.), *Advances in infancy research* (pp. 131–163). Stamford, CT: Ablex Publishing Corporation.

Stiles, J., Moses, P., Roe, K., Trauner, D., Hesselink, J., Wong, E., et al. (2003). Alternative brain organization after prenatal cerebral injury: Convergent fMRI and cognitive data. *Journal of the International Neuropsychological Society.*

Tovée, J. J., & Cohen-Tovée, E. M. (1993). The neural substrates of face processing models: A review. *Cognitive Neuropsychology, 10,* 505–528.

Vanier, M., Gauthier, L., Lambert, J., Pepin, E., Robillard, A., Dubouloz, C., et al. (1990). Evaluation of left visuospatial neglect: Norms and discrimination power of two tests. *Neuropsychology, 4,* 87–96.

Vingerhoets, G., Lannoo, E., & Bauwens, S. (1996). Analyses of the Money Road Map Test performance in normal and brain-damaged subjects. *Archives of Clinical Neuropsychology, 11,* 1–9.

von Hofsten, C., & Rösblad, B. (1988). The integration of sensory information in the development of precise manual pointing. *Neuropsychologia, 26,* 805–821.

Warrington, E. K., & Rabin, P. (1970). Perceptual matching in patients with cerebral lesions. *Neuropsychologia, 8,* 475–487.

Wechsler, D. (1991). *Wechsler Intelligence Scale for Children* (3rd ed.). San Antonio, TX: The Psychological Corporation.

Weintraub, S., & Mesulam, M.-M. (1985). Mental state assessment of young and elderly adults in behavioral neurology. In M.-M. Mesulam (Ed.), *Principles of behavioral neurology* (pp. 71–123). Philadelphia: F. A. Davis.

Wills, K., Holmbeck, G. N., Dillon, K., & McLone, D. G. (1990). Intelligence and achievement in children with myelomeningocele. *Journal of Pediatric Psychology, 15,* 161–176.

Winegarden, B. J., Yates, B. L., Moses, J. A., Benton, A., & Faustman, W. O. (1998). Development of an optimally reliable short form for Judgment of Line Orientation. *The Clinical Neuropsychologist, 12,* 311–314.

11

Learning and Memory

As child neuropsychologists are acutely aware, a presenting complaint of "memory problems" often reflects a restricted understanding of the broad range of reasons why a child might appear to experience poor information recall. Conditions that produce true amnestic disorder, or even a dementia (Shapiro and Balthazor, 2000), can certainly present in childhood, but these are often relatively uncommon and may manifest differently than in the adult. Specific amnestic disorders of childhood might be seen as sequelae of epilepsy (Williams and Sharp, 1999), space occupying lesions, focal cerebral trauma, cancer, central nervous system prophylaxis treatment, hypoxia, toxic exposure, and metabolic disorder, among other possibilities. Memory impairment, when generalized, is likely due to diffuse axonal injury, multiple ischemic lesions, and secondary injury due to excitotoxicity (Levin, 1990). Concern about memory is well founded when the neural pathways or networks that mediate encoding, consolidation, storage, and/or retrieval are clearly compromised as a result of neurological dysfunction.

This specific information, however, is often unknown at the start of many outpatient clinical evaluations, and alternative hypotheses about the basis for memory complaints must be carefully considered. Further, memory disorder is rarely observed as a component of a developmental disorder.

Other explanatory etiologies for "memory disorder" often need to be considered. Impairment might be due to poor planning and disorganization associated with an executive function (EF) disorder. Emotional factors such as anxiety or phobia might compromise a child's ability to acquire and therefore retain information. A potentially reversible, but undiagnosed, medical etiology may mimic the presentation of memory disturbance or result in true memory impairment. Related subject factors such as inattention and poor motivation may be highly relevant and could compromise learning, resulting in later retrieval difficulties due to inefficient or incomplete encoding. Poor strategic use of mnemonics, poor working memory, or language disorder with impaired comprehension could each be explanatory. It is therefore essential that the broad range of possibilities be considered in the differential diagnosis and tested in response to expressed concern about "memory" problems. This is especially important if one is to offer appropriate intervention strategies and well-coordinated treatment planning.

Conceptualizations about memory and speculation about its neuroanatomical substrate have led to a preponderance of models and terms associated with various aspects of learning and memory. A number of excellent sources for detailed description of normal and abnormal memory are available, (Atkinson and Shiffrin, 1968; Craik and Lockhart, 1972; Tulving, 1983; Baddeley, 1986; Squire, 1987; Cowan, 1988; Squire, Knowlton et al., 1993; Schacter and Tulving, 1994; Craik, Govoni et al., 1996). One should also be familiar with the concept of *levels of processing,* a framework that is intended to explain how what the individual encodes is linked to whether the material is shallow (e.g., requiring perceptual identification) or deep (e.g., requiring semantic elaboration) (Craik and Lockhart, 1972; Lockhart and Craik, 1990). The reader is also directed to some sources specific to development of memory in childhood (Kail, 1984; Schneider and Pressley, 1988; Nelson, 1995; Cowan, 1997). The investigations of these researchers and others have demonstrated that children are able to make reliable explicit judgments about the functioning and capacities of their basic memory systems, that rudimentary memory awareness is present in preschool children, and that specific strategies for memory and learning are mostly developed by approximately 12 years.

MEMORY TERMS

Memory terms are classified in a number of ways. Among these are reference to whether there is conscious awareness of recall (explicit or declarative memory vs. implicit or procedural memory); central stages or features (encoding, consolidation, storage, retrieval); consideration of a time-interval span (immediate, short-term, or long-term, the latter including recent and remote memory); specific memory impairment (anterograde amnesia, retrograde amnesia); or by characteristics related to the recall (prospective memory, source memory). These are considered briefly below to prime the reader for the discussion of tests and normative data that follows.

Explicit or Declarative Memory

Explicit (Schacter, 1992) or declarative (Squire, 1987) memory refers to a conscious awareness of recall and subsumes both *episodic* memory and *semantic* memory. Consensus about the neural substrates of these two memory subsystems has not been reached, but numerous studies on brain-impaired populations attempt to better explicate the role of different brain structures. These studies highlight the impor-

tance of an intact hippocampal system, including the perirhinal and parahippocampal cortices, subiculum, CA fields, dentate gyrus, and entorhinal cortex (Yancey and Phelps, 2001). Despite controversial viewpoints, data also point to the importance of the mammillary bodies in episodic memory (Hildebrandt, Müller et al., 2001), although their role is somewhat different than the hippocampal system.

Episodic memory is defined as the conscious memory for events or facts, that is, the memory of specific personally experienced events (Tulving 1972; 1983). The adult literature suggests that memory decline in the normal elderly may be primarily a result of a decline in episodic memory. The mesial temporal lobe system plays a critical role in episodic memory. This system includes the amygdala, hippocampus, and adjacent anatomically related cortices, including the entorhinal, perirhinal, and parahippocampal cortices. An interhemispheric processing basis for episodic memories has been suggested (Christman and Propper, 2001), whereas semantic memories may be more unilaterally localized (Tulving, Kapur et al., 1994).

Some clinical measures that are useful in assessing episodic memory include list-learning, story-learning, and design-learning tests. These tests assist in evaluating encoding or learning of novel information and consolidation or retention of information. Retrieval techniques of free recall, cued recall, and recognition priming help dissociate different types of memory impairment. Free recall capacity increases noticeably with increasing age in childhood (Rich, Yaster et al., 1999). Techniques that often prove useful to improving episodic memory include mnemonic strategies, elaboration of semantic memory, and increasing metacognitive knowledge of one's memory abilities.

It is of interest that magnetic resonance imaging (MRI) measured lesion size in prefrontal regions was associated with residual impaired learning and memory in children with severe traumatic brain injury (TBI) (i.e., lowest post-resuscitation Glasgow Coma Scale score of 8 or less, during entire hospital stay) (Di Stefano, Bachevalier et al., 2000). These authors found a lack of consistent volumetric differences in the hippocampal formation for both mild and severe TBI children, but their data highlighted the importance of the frontal regions for memory and learning and their particular vulnerability when injured in childhood.

Semantic memory refers to factual knowledge that is part of long-term memory. It contains the permanent representation of our knowledge of concepts, words, and their meaning, giving meaning to our sensory experience (Squire, 1987). Some measures that are useful in assessing semantic memory include tests of word fluency or category fluency, vocabulary, naming, and free association. Several of these provide scores that reflect organizational strategies employed in learning novel information, such as the California Verbal Learning Test (CVLT) semantic clustering score and the serial clustering score (see below) or indices from the Selective Reminding Test. One can have both episodic and semantic memory impairment. This is well documented in the adult literature describing those with Alzheimer's disease.

Implicit or Procedural Memory

The hallmark characteristic of *implicit* (procedural, nondeclarative) memory is that the subject is unaware of both this memory system and the fact that he or she is using the information present within the system (Cermak, 1996). Implicit memory is inferred from performance that reflects prior exposure, but it does not reference a prior learning episode (Roediger, 1990). It is less sensitive to age effects than explicit memory and might precede explicit memory developmentally (Graf, 1990). Unlike explicit memory, implicit memory is not impaired by hippocampal or related medial temporal lobe structural lesion. Rather, implicit memory appears to be mediated by neural systems that include the neostriatum: the caudate nucleus and putamen in the basal ganglia (Poldrack, Prabhakaran et al., 1999). Learning is mediated by premotor cortex and the striatum (Saint-Cyr and Taylor, 1992), and striatal involvement is visualized with functional activation studies (Grafton, Hazeltine et al., 1995; Poldrack, Prabhakaran et al., 1999). It has also been suggested that the basal ganglia play a more general role than previously acknowledged in the acquisition of novel skills, including motor but also nonmotor and cognitive skill learning (Poldrack, Prabhakaran et al., 1999).

Implicit memory can be assessed across modalities. Examples of tests of implicit memory for visuomotor function include motor sequence learning, mirror tracing, and rotary pursuit learning. Such tasks have been used in studies of children such as the rotary pursuit test with children with Attention Deficit Hyperactivity Disorder (ADHD) (Leavell, Ackerson et al., 1995; Colvin, Fennell et al., 1997; Leavell, Bowers et al., 1999). Implicit memory for verbal material can be assessed, using repetition and priming techniques with lexical-semantic information, such as lexical-decision, word-fragment, and word-stem completion tasks.

Nonverbal implicit memory can be assessed with pictorial priming such as fragment picture naming, that is, identification of degraded pictures tasks (Snodgrass, 1989). Measurement variables suggestive of successful priming include increased accuracy of identification and decreased latency to response. Priming itself can be further subdivided into perceptual priming and conceptual priming. *Perceptual priming* refers to analysis of the stimulus's perceptual form and is modality-specific while *conceptual priming* requires analysis of the stimulus's meaning and is not sensitive to modality such as category exemplar production and word-associate production (Vaidya, Gabrieli et al., 1999).

Encoding conditions in explicit and implicit memory have been studied, and that research found implicit memory to exhibit a modality-specific characteristic (Roediger and Blaxton, 1987). It appears that implicit memory is affected by encoding conditions to a greater extent than explicit memory (Graf, Shimamura et al., 1985). Successful *transfer appropriate processing* (TAP; Morris, Bransford et al., 1977) refers to when priming is greatest for processing operations at test (retrieval) that are most similar to those engaged in during the learning stage.

It was also found that complex figure recall was dependent on executive strategizing at the encoding stage, with poor strategy resulting in poor recall in healthy adults who otherwise had intact spatial information processing and nonverbal memory (Newman and Krikorian, 2001). The latter study supports clinical impressions that failure to approach, or "attack," the task effectively can only be expected to result in future recall inefficiency. Therefore, it makes interpretation of "poor memory performance" difficult and confounds the issue of true etiology for the observed poor performance. A clinician must, therefore, be especially careful about diagnosing a memory disorder when a child's delayed recall is impaired if she has not evaluated and made a determination about the child's efficiency in the initial encoding and learning stages.

Studies of the distinction between explicit and implicit learning and memory in normal children support the validity of dissociation already well documented for adults (Graf and Masson, 1993; Naito and Komatsu, 1993; DiGiulio, Seidenberg et al., 1994). Yet, there are relatively few developmental investigations of procedural or implicit memory in either normal or clinical child populations. Several studies of development and dissociation of explicit from implicit memory in normal children have been reported, the majority utilizing priming for visual rather than lexical stimuli (Carroll, Byrne et al., 1985; Parkin and Streete, 1988; Greenbaum and Graf, 1989; Naito, 1990; Russo, Nichelli et al., 1995).

Studies of clinical populations are particularly sparse. There are reports of implicit memory investigation for children with moderate head injury (Guger, 2000; Guger and Rich, 2001), learning disabilities (Lorsbach and Worman, 1989; Lorsbach, Sodoro et al., 1992), traumatic brain injury (Shum, Jamieson et al., 1999), ADHD (Leavell, Ackerson et al., 1995; Colvin, Fennell et al., 1997; Leavell, Bowers et al., 1999), and brain tumor (Dennis, Hetherington et al., 1998). For example, a fragmented picture-completion procedure (Snodgrass, Smith et al., 1987) was used in the study of implicit memory in children with traumatic brain injury (Shum, Jamieson et al., 1999). The test includes a series of stimulus pictures in three sets. Each stimulus picture has eight stages, from most degraded to a complete picture at the eighth stage. Normative data on the average level of identification are provided for each set, and these did not differ significantly (Snodgrass and Corwin, 1988): 4.94 (SD = 0.93) for Set A, 4.61 (SD = 0.92) for Set B, and

4.23 (SD = 0.83) for Set C. Such investigations are likely to become more common with greater recognition of the considerable value inherent to such study, for example, the potential development of novel rehabilitative strategies subsequent to neurological illness or injury.

Registration, Acquisition, and Encoding

Encoding is considered a neuroanatomic-cognitive process and is different than acquisition, a functional behavior that can be observed and measured. Encoding is the first stage of mnemonic processing (Yancey and Phelps, 2001). It is the process by which the cognitive system builds up a stimulus representation into memory (Loring, 1999). Cognitive deficits can interfere with successful registration, acquisition, and encoding, or learning new information. Examples of such deficits include poor ability to attend to and register new information, process information , and divide attention. Encoding new information into long-term memory is presumed to occur with successive presentations of stimulus material, and the degree to which this occurs can be measured as an index of encoding.

Consolidation and Storage

Consolidation refers to the elaboration of information over time (Squire, 1982), that is, the maintenance, elaboration, and storage of new information in long-term memory after it is encoded (Vanderploeg, Crowell et al., 2001). Problems in memory consolidation (retention) are evident on inspection of the difference between initial acquisition or immediate learning and performance after a delay (Glosser, Cole et al., 2002). Thus, consolidation problems are evident when there is rapid forgetting, poor retrieval, and poor delayed recognition memory. Currently, there are no reliable neuroimaging methods that enable study of this intermediate stage as a process distinct from either encoding or retrieval (Yancey and Phelps, 2001).

Retrieval and Recognition

Retrieval, the final stage of memory, may be best assessed by a comparison of free recall with recognition memory. Recognition is a better indicator of memory disorder and poor recognition often suggests more severe impairment (Squire, 1986); inclusion of a recognition trial, along with free recall, increases the sensitivity of a memory test (Fastenau, 1996). Not all memory tests, however, include both free recall and recognition trials to enable these comparisons, and the clinician's test modifications to incorporate these conditions may complicate interpretation due to the absence of normative data. Some existing test procedures do include both recall and recognition conditions, but in the absence of a recognition trial, it may be worthwhile to adapt the task demands to include this trial.

Recognition memory is assessed in various ways, including selection from a multiple-choice array or forced-choice decision. The Selective Reminding Test provides a score for long-term storage (LTS) that is an index of information acquired into long-term storage and for consistent long-term retrieval (CLTR) that is a measure of retrieval efficiency for information already stored. Phonemic cued recognition and multiple-choice cueing conditions are part of the Selective Reminding Test procedure. Early study of design recognition (Vanderplas and Garvin, 1959) led to the development of random designs that are helpful in investigating visual short-term memory since they are not encoded with verbal labels. Recognition memory trials are also included as part of the Rivermead Behavioural Memory Test for Children (Wilson, Ivani-Chalian et al., 1991).

Short-Term Memory

Short-term memory (STM) refers to the ability to hold information in a buffer for a short period of time, usually seconds (the registration of information), and then to encode and retain this information. Some conceptualize STM as consisting of two distinct processes: *immediate memory* or primary memory and *rehearsal* (Trahan and Larrabee, 1988). Immediate memory refers to the immediate registration of information perceived from the environment, and the ability to maintain the information in conscious awareness (Loring, 1999).

Digit span forward and block span forward are classic examples of clinical immediate memory measures, although this has been disputed by some. Preservation of such span tests in the presence of memory disorder and closed-head injury (Levin, Benton et al., 1982) has reinforced the notion that forward span is a measure of immediate memory. In contrast, backward span requires strategic auditory/verbal rehearsal. The rehearsal stage prevents rapid decay of information and increases the likelihood that information will be encoded and stored on a more permanent basis, in long-term memory. It is well documented that short-term memory can be impaired while long-term memory remains unaffected (Shallice and Warrington, 1970).

Besides span tests, STM is commonly assessed with other tests such as paragraph passage recall, the immediate, or 3-minute, recall of the Rey-Osterrieth Complex Figure Test, and the Benton Visual Retention Test. A dual-task paradigm that requires working in STM might be used. Researchers may employ more complex designs that allow for manipulation of association value and reduced verbal encoding, such as the Vanderplas random designs (Vanderplas and Garvin, 1959). Distractor techniques are also used, such as in the Auditory Consonant Trigrams Test (see Chapter 7).

Long-Term Memory

Long-term memory (LTM), or secondary memory, refers to the ability to consolidate and store information, enabling retrieval when needed at a future time. Neocortical brain areas are thought to be the repositories of long-term memory (Squire, Knowlton et al., 1993), although this is still an area of active investigation. Positron emission tomography (PET) study of adult humans found activation of the left ventrolateral frontal cortex during verbal recall from long-term memory (Petrides, Alivisatos et al., 1995). LTM is typically assessed clinically by requesting recall after a temporal delay, and after intervening or competing stimulus material is presented. Patients with brain stem lesions had difficulty with long-term recall and retention, suggesting a failure to focus on new information. Yet, acquisition following successive trials was intact (Heu-brock, 1995). Such patients have difficult maintaining vigilance, that is, sustaining attention over a time course (Crosson, 1992). Examples of tests of LTM include delayed recall for word lists, delayed paragraph recall, and delayed design replication.

Anterograde Memory

Anterograde memory refers to the ability to learn and recall novel information from a point in time forward. Anterograde amnesia refers to a deficit in the formation of new and lasting memories or a loss of memory for events that occurred after the onset of amnesia, that is, recall of events that occur after a point in time (Squire, 1982). Examples of tests used to assess anterograde verbal memory/learning include digit-sequence learning, and list-learning tests such as the Rey Auditory Verbal Learning Test, the Selective Reminding Test, and the California Verbal Learning Test. Examples of anterograde visual memory/learning tests include the Benton Visual Retention Test and the Rey-Osterrieth Complex Figure Test.

Retrograde Memory and Remote Memory Impairment

Retrograde memory refers to memory for information previously stored or learned (Loring, 1999). It is not a unitary dimension. Retrograde amnesia and remote memory impairment refer to a deficit recalling already acquired memories, including those undergoing consolidation and elaboration when the injury occurred (Squire, 1982). Memory can be lost for events in a preceding period of time without affecting more remote memories, that is, those more distant in time from the present, suggesting that memory becomes more resistant to loss with greater elapsed time and that remote memory dysfunction might involve brain regions besides those directly affected with specific amnesia syndromes (Squire, 1982). Subcomponents of retrograde memory include memory for personal events (autobiographical memory), memory for famous people and well-known events, memory for facts and meanings

(semantic memory), and memory for skills (implicit or procedural memory). Tests or procedures that aid in evaluating retrograde memory include the Boston Remote Memory Test, the Recognition of Famous Faces, a recall questionnaire, and recognition memory testing.

Prospective Memory

Prospective memory is described as "remembering to remember." It is associated with an emphasis on performance of action, not just recall. Extending the definition of prospective memory beyond action to include self-initiated search and retrieval processes and the strategies involved in planning, monitoring, and organizing memory was proposed in context with the evaluation of frontal lobe patients (Shimamura, Janowsky et al., 1991). The frontal lobes are hypothesized to be particularly involved in prospective memory (Glisky, 1996). It is also suggested that prospective memory may be even more impaired in abnormal aging than retrospective memory (Maylor, 1996).

Time-based, event-based, and activity-based prospective memory are all receiving attention in the adult literature (Einstein and McDaniel, 1990). Time-based prospective memory requires the individual to remember to do something at a specified time. Event-based prospective memory refers to remembering to interrupt one's activity in order to do something in response to an external cue. Activity-based prospective memory involves remembering to take an action, but it does not require interruption of an activity (Kvavilashvili and Ellis, 1996) and is therefore considered easier than either time- or event-based prospective memory (Shum, Valentine et al., 1999).

The capacity to remember to carry out specific actions in the future can be evaluated informally, for example, telling the child to remember to do something specific at the end of the testing session and seeing if the child carries out the action as instructed when testing concludes. In general, prospective memory in children has received little attention until recent years. However, prospective memory is formally examined in the Rivermead Behavioral Memory Test for Children. An inventive computerized and standardized test of prospective memory in children—the CyberCruiser (Kerns, 2000)—was recently developed.

Source Memory

Source memory is memory for the context or episode during which information was learned or presented (Johnson, Hashtroudi et al., 1993), that is, remembering where the knowledge came from. Source memory can refer to who presented the information or where the individual was when it was presented. It can be obtained incidentally or be learned intentionally. Source memory may be facilitated by emotional valence. That is, memory for item and source information may be enhanced by autonomic and limbic activity, and the effects may be related to whether the emotionally valenced conditions are related to personally relevant memories (autobiographical clustering) (Doerksen and Shimamura, 2001). Neuroimaging studies suggest a role for prefrontal cortex, especially with respect to source memory (Janowsky, Shimamura et al., 1989). Source memory appears more sensitive than item memory to frontal lesions and requires more strategic processing, engaging more attentional resources and effort than needed for item information processing (Troyer, Winocur et al., 1999). Primate experiments showed dorsolateral prefrontal cortex involvement in retention of information over a temporal delay (Fuster, 1989).

MEMORY AND RACE/ETHNICITY

Relatively little attention has been directed toward examining the influence of race and ethnicity on memory test performance in childhood, but one adult study found verbal learning and memory performance of older persons was influenced by age, education, and gender, but not by race. The authors suggested that race-adjustment is likely unnecessary in the norming of memory tests (Grober et al., 1998).

MEMORY BATTERIES

Memory batteries for children have been developed, largely by including downward ex-

tensions of tasks from adult memory tests rather than by constructing tests with developmental principles in mind. As a result, these memory batteries receive criticism by clinicians who find this practice questionable and who dispute the validity of these battery subtests. Criticism centers on the purported factors derived from statistical analyses, the methodology used in test development that might lessen clinical utility and make overestimates or underestimates likely, and the inclusion of subtests into global scales despite clinical or psychometric utility not being demonstrated for such placement. Need-based selection of individual subtests rather than administration of a full battery may be a more ideal way to examine a child, while recognizing some statistical properties may be diminished under these circumstances.

Also of concern is the requirement within a battery approach that some less useful individual subtests be included, when time constraints limit full battery assessment and other tests may contribute more to delineation of the individual child's cognitive strengths and weaknesses. Inconsistency in function suggested by one test when compared to another of related content may be a more useful comparison even if one must administer a subtest from within another battery or assess performance on an individual test that has potentially greater promise for the particular child. The downward extension of adult models for memory assessment to children also raises concern about the dependence of these tasks on social, verbal, or nonverbal skill acquisition that is not yet sufficiently well developed in the child. The failure to norm multimodal memory measures on the same representative sample also is a complicating factor for the child clinician.

The Rivermead Behavioural Memory Test for Children, the Children's Memory Scale, the Wide Range Assessment of Memory and Learning, and Tests of Memory and Learning are four memory batteries that might be considered. The reader will need to consult the respective detailed manuals to obtain detailed age-stratified normative data. Also noted here are the five learning and memory subtests included within the broader range of cognitive functions assessed by the NEPSY battery.

Rivermead Behavioural Memory Test for Children Aged 5 to 10 Years Old

The Rivermead Behavioural Memory Test (RBMT) was developed to assess the construct of everyday memory in adults. It was subsequently modified for young children as the Rivermead Behavioural Memory Test for Children, aged 5 to 10 years old (RBMTC; Wilson, Ivani-Chalian et al., 1991). The RBMT is also appropriate for use with adolescents, 11 to 14 years old (Wilson, Forester et al., 1990). Demographic data for the younger children are presented in Table 11–1 and for a small clinical sample in Table 11–2. Developmental changes are incorporated into scoring systems for each age group; these are described in the manual (Wilson, Ivani-Chalian et al., 1991). Good interrater reliability was found. Interrater agreement was 100% on a Standardized Profile Score (SPS), a score determined from raw scores and set at 2 for normal, 1 for borderline, and 0 for abnormal. The SPS uses a 90% cut-off so that a score of 2 would include 90% of children for the child's respective age group.

Good parallel-form reliability for the four versions was reported and supported the equivalence of these versions. The overall Spearman rank correlation coefficient was .77 for scores on first and second testing, ($p < .0001$). Agreement between the six test combinations ranged from .55 ($p < .0001$) to .89 ($p < .0001$). Practice effects are minimal. Validity data for RBMTC scores and houseparents' ratings resulted in a correlation of .71. It should be noted that the test makes greater demands on intellectual capacity at the younger ages, whereas the test's memory demands exert greater influence on the older children's performance (Aldrich and Wilson, 1991; Wilson, Ivani-

Table 11–1. Rivermead Behavioral Memory Test: Normal Sample

Subjects: 335 children in Hampshire, England
Age: 5 to 10 years 11months
Gender: 170 boys, 165 girls
Handedness: Not specified
Race: Not specified
Inclusion criteria: In mainstream rural and urban schools without obvious learning difficulty

Table 11–2. Rivermead Behavioral Memory Test: Clinical Sample

Subjects: 36 children with epilepsy in Surrey, England
Age: 8.3 to 15.9 years (M = 12.48; SD = 2.00 years)
Gender: 26 boys, 10 girls
Full scale IQ ranged from 37 to 108 (M = 62; SD = 21)
Handedness: Not specified
Race Not specified
Inclusion: All children communicated verbally and had no major behavioral problems

Chalian et al., 1993). Additional data confirmed the applicability of the RBMT adult version for 85 children from mainstream schools without obvious learning difficulties (42 male, 43 female) 11 to 14 years, 11 months (Wilson, Forester et al. 1990; Wilson, Ivani-Chalian et al., 1991; Wilson, Ivani-Chalian et al., 1993). No significant differences between four alternate versions were found, or between males and females or first and second assessments for this age group.

The RBMTC consists of 11 subtests. Remembering a Name requires the child to look at a woman's picture while being told her first and last name. The child must recall the name later. Remembering the Hidden Belonging is a prospective memory test that requires the child to remember at the test's conclusion where a packet of gold stars was hidden. For Remembering an Appointment the examiner sets an alarm to sound in 20 minutes and rehearses with the child a question to ask when the alarm sounds. Picture Recognition involves presentation of 10 line drawings for 5 seconds each for the child to name, followed by a filled delay, and later recognition selection from among 20 choices. Immediate Prose Recall of an oral story about a presented picture involves immediate free recall, then prompting with 10 specific questions. After a free delayed recall, prompting questions are asked only for those questions answered incorrectly.

Face Recognition presents individual pictures of five faces at a rate of 1 every 5 seconds. The child must indicate if the face is of a man or woman, and if the person is young, middle-aged, or old. Testing of recognition memory for the five faces among five distractors occurs after a delay. Remembering a Short

Route requires the child to imitate a short walk around the testing room with five specified locations, earning 1 point for each stage of the route followed in correct sequence. The child must also leave a message envelope at the fourth stage. Delayed route recall is also assessed. For Remembering to Deliver a Message the child is expected to deliver the message at the stage of the route according to the examiner's instructions, and again in the delayed recall condition. Orientation Questions includes 11 personal questions about the child.

There are four parallel forms and also prose paragraphs especially for older children in American English. Tables present standardized profile scores for normal, borderline, and impaired performance. An appendix includes tables of percentages for each age group's raw score performance, cut-off scores, and cumulative percentage scores for obtaining the cut-off scores.

Children's Memory Scale

The Children's Memory Scale (CMS; Cohen, 1997) has updated norms since 1997 and is based on 1995 U.S. census survey data. It was standardized on 1000 children and includes data on race/ethnicity, parent education, geographic region, and an equal male : female ratio. The age range is 5 to 16 years, 11 months. The CMS has been co-normed with the Wechsler Intelligence Scale for Children—III (WISC-III). This allows for interpretation of a predicted memory score on a statistical basis rather than merely a discrepancy score. Split-half reliability for immediate recall is .74, for delayed recall is .75, and for delayed recognition is .75. The standard error of measurement is 1.5 for all three conditions, immediate recall, delayed recall, and delayed recognition.

The CMS is, in some respects, a downward extension of the Wechsler Memory Scale (WMS) series for adults. The CMS subtest stimuli are similar to the WMS adult stimuli. The CMS is therefore criticized for appearing to neglect how a child's cognitive and memory difficulties might differ from those of an adult. Summary scores of the CMS include Verbal Immediate, Verbal Delayed, Visual Immediate, Visual Delayed, General Memory, Learning,

Delayed Recognition, and Attention/Concentration indexes. Immediate, delayed recall, and delayed recognition scores are converted to scaled scores. Core auditory/verbal subtests include Stories and Word Pairs, with Word Lists as a supplemental subtest. There are three different story sets, two incrementally more difficult paragraphs for each of three age groups: 5 to 8 years; 9 to 12 years; and 13 to 16 years, each providing immediate, delayed, and delayed recognition scores.

The CMS includes theme scoring along with detail recall scoring. The Word Pairs subtest provides scores for learning, long delay free recall, and delayed recognition recall. The delay condition elicits delayed free recall of the word pairs. There are no delayed cued recall or delayed recognition trials. Core attention/concentration subtests include Numbers and Sequences, with Picture Locations as a supplement. Numbers is identical to the WISC-III digit span subtest. Visual/nonverbal core subtests of Dot Locations and Faces can be supplemented with Family Pictures. The Dot Locations subtest scores learning and long delay. There is a 3×4 grid with six chips for ages 5 to 8 and a 4×4 grid with eight chips for those 9 to 16 years old. Faces includes an immediate and delayed condition. Both Faces and Dot Locations are criticized for the strong floor effect for the youngest children, as average scaled scores can be obtained for chance responding.

Wide Range Assessment of Memory and Learning

The Wide Range Assessment of Memory and Learning (WRAML; Sheslow and Adams, 1990) is appropriate for children aged 5 to 17 years, 11 months. Based on the 1980 U. S. census survey data, it was standardized on 2363 children and includes data on race/ethnicity, parent education, geographic region, and an equal male : female ratio. Immediate recall reliability study resulted in a coefficient alpha of 0.86. The standard error of measurement for immediate recall is 2.7. Immediate recall scores are converted to scaled scores, but delayed recall and delayed recognition scores are not. There are nine subtests with a mean of 10

(*SD* = 3): Picture Memory, Design Memory, Verbal Learning, Story Memory, Finger Windows, Sound Symbol, Sentence Memory, Visual Learning, Number/Letter Memory. A General Memory Index with a mean of 100 (*SD* = 10) is computed from these scores. Structural equation model analysis of the WRAML in the standardization sample (Burton, Donders et al., 1996) and in a clinical sample (Burton, Mittenberg et al., 1999) found support for a 3-factor model, including verbal memory, visual memory, and attention and concentration factors. These data supported the notion that attention is an important component of memory as measured by the WRAML, but these data did not support the Learning Index.

Test of Memory and Learning

The Test of Memory and Learning (TOMAL; Reynolds and Bigler, 1994) is standardized for ages 5 to 19 years, 11 months. It was standardized on 1342 children and based on 1990 U. S. census survey data. It includes data on race/ethnicity, geographic region, socioeconomic status (SES), urban/rural, and an equal male : female ratio, but not parent education. An immediate recall reliability study resulted in a coefficient alpha of .86, and delayed recall had a coefficient alpha of .85. Immediate and delayed recall scores are converted to scaled scores. There is no delayed recognition. The standard error of measurement is 1.1 for immediate recall and 1.2 for delayed recall. There are 10 core subtests, 5 verbal and 5 nonverbal. Memory for Stories is a verbal subtest requiring immediate and delayed recall. Word Selective Reminding requires verbal free recall. Object Recall involves paired verbal and nonverbal stimuli and verbal recall. Paired Recall is verbal immediate recall and learning. Facial Memory is a nonverbal subtest requiring recognition and identification of faces from a set of distractors. Visual Selective Reminding is a nonverbal analogue to Word Selective Reminding. Abstract Visual Memory requires immediate recall of meaningless abstract geometric figures. Visual Sequential Memory requires recall of an array of geometric abstract forms in correct order. There is also a Memory for Location subtest.

Index scores are computed for a composite memory index (CMI), verbal memory index (VMI), nonverbal memory index (NMI), and delayed memory index (DMI).

NEPSY Learning and Memory Subtests

The NEPSY includes five subtests under the learning and memory domain. Narrative memory is administered to children 3 to 12 years old. It requires the child to repeat an oral story. There are free and cued recall conditions. Sentence Repetition is administered to children 3 to 12 years old. It requires the child to recall four sentences if 6 years old or younger, and a maximum of 17 increasingly more complex sentences if 7 to 12 years old. There are procedures for qualitative scoring of the number of times the child asks for repetition and for scoring off-task behavior.

Memory for Faces is administered to children 5 to 12 years old. It requires the child to choose a face from a three-face array. There is a 30-minute delayed recognition of the target faces from new distractors. Memory for Names is administered to children 5 to 12 years old. It requires the child to learn the names of eight children (six children, if the child is 5 years old) over three trials. There is a 30-minute delayed recall. List Learning (using the Rey Auditory Verbal Learning Test procedure) requires the child to learn a 15-word list of single words over five trials, followed by the presentation of an interference 15-word list. The child must then recall the first list. There is also a 30-minute delayed recall of the first list. Repetition of responses, novel intrusions, and interference list intrusions are scored error types, for which there are normative data. Total score is calculated differently than for other list-learning tests, that is, the total raw score is the sum of correct word recall for trials 1 to 5 plus delayed recall number correct.

VERBAL LEARNING AND MEMORY

A variety of verbal learning and memory tests are commonly included in child neuropsychological evaluations. Word list-learning tests, such as the Verbal Selective Reminding Test

(VSRT), the California Verbal Learning Test—Children (CVLT–C) and the Rey Auditory Verbal Learning Test (RAVLT) are commonly used and involve processing unstructured, supraspan, noncontextual information. These list-learning tests are sensitive to episodic memory dysfunction (Delis, Filoteo et al., 1994). Paragraph recall tests, such as the Wechsler series Logical Memory (LM) subtests, involve retention of meaningful stimuli, have inherent organization and less demand for active semantic processing. An MRI study found verbal memory related to frontal lobe lesion size in head-injured children (Levin, Culhane et al., 1994). The frontal lobes likely aid memory processing by providing useful organizational strategies, and frontal lobe damage interferes with strategic encoding and information retrieval (Di Stefano, Bachevalier et al., 2000).

Reminding or list-learning tests have the advantage of providing varied clinical data about memory strategies contributing to free recall, that is, how efficiently the child organizes list items for recall. For example, one can note linking of list words as a "chunking" strategy, how well early trial recall predicts subsequent trial recall, how common is a primacy or recency effect or serial order effects, or if the child is subject to intrusion or perseverative errors. Excessive intrusions may indicate a failure of self-inhibition. Intrusion errors, such as producing words from a prior novel word list, demonstrate storage of recent information by virtue of the person obviously retaining the information over time (Squire, 1982). A gender effect in adults has been suggested, that is, adult males made more intrusion errors than adult females on the Selective Reminding Test (SRT) (Hannay and Levin, 1985).

Developmental factors need to be considered in evaluating strategic planning since clear strategy differences can exist between adults and children. For example, one cannot extrapolate the implications of semantic clustering data from adults to children and assume a similar process underlies behavior in both groups (Cowan, 1997). Also, semantic reorganization of the verbal material to be learned has been shown to differ between clinical groups and normal subjects (Tager-Flusberg, 1989). For example, autistic subjects with impaired lan-

guage pragmatics repeated words exactly as presented, failing to reorganize the words into semantic categories as did normal subjects (Hermelin and O'Conner, 1970).

Cautions about interpreting some qualitative indices of word list-learning tests have been published, including the concern that some computational formulae for qualitative indices are spuriously correlated with recall level and that some computed indices directly affect the computation of another (Schmidt, 1997). An adjusted ratio of clustering (ARC) index was proposed as preferable. Qualitative indices investigated included position effects of recall from first to last response (primacy to recency), recall consistency (recall of the same word over trials), clustering (recall of words from a semantic category, paired by the subject) and seriation (consecutive list words recalled consecutively). Clustering and seriation are indices that reflect organizational strategy.

Verbal Selective Reminding Test

The Verbal Selective Reminding Test (VSRT) is a word-list learning test (Buschke, 1973; Buschke, 1974a; Levin, 1981; Hannay and Levin, 1985; Fletcher, 1985) that has evolved to include four distinct parts: list learning, cued recall, recognition recall, and delayed recall. The examiner reads aloud a lengthy word list at a 2-per-second rate. The words selected occur frequently in English usage (Carroll, Davies et al., 1971). The child names as many list words as possible in any order while the examiner records these in numerical order of recall on an answer sheet. At the conclusion of each trial, the examiner orally states the omitted words and requests recall of the entire word list on the next trial.

This procedure continues until the entire list is stated correctly (for two consecutive trials for some administrations; three consecutive trials for others), or the maximum number of allowed trials is reached. The subject is then presented with an untimed cued recall task, to determine whether partial information facilitates recall (Warrington and Weiskrantz, 1970). The cues are presented one by one, with the first two letters of each list word printed individually on eleven 5 × 7 cards (one list word is not amenable to two-letter cueing). The cards are presented in the same order as they were read on the list, and a total correct score obtained. Cueing is known to benefit all subjects (Squire, 1982). A recognition task was added (Levin, Benton et al., 1982) that consists of twelve 5×7 cards, printed with a four-word set for each target list word (list word, homonym, synonym, unrelated distractor) and requiring the subject to indicate which word was on the list, and resulting in a maximum score of 12. Delayed recall is obtained 30 minutes later. Test–retest reliability was somewhat lower than desirable for psychological tests, with an index of consistency ranging from 0.484 to 0.654 (Hannay and Levin, 1985). Alternate forms were constructed for adults: each form matched word-for-word with identical serial orders, that is, the second word of each form matches the second word of another form for word frequency, initial letter, word length.

The procedure of selective cueing allows for examination of acquisition, storage, and recall of novel verbal stimuli. Measurement of items recalled but not presented on every trial enables determination of long-term storage (LTS) and short-term recall (STR) (Hannay and Levin, 1985). Several crucial scores are obtained (Levin, Benton et al., 1982). The LTS score is the total number of items per trial recalled at least once from memory. That is, a word that is retrieved on two subsequent trials is considered to be in LTS. Long-term retrieval (LTR) is when a word is recalled from LTS. A word in LTS that is recalled on every subsequent learning trial is in consistent long term retrieval. The consistent long term retrieval (CLTR) score is the sum total number of words per trial consistently retrieved from LTS on every trial until the test concludes.

Other scores are also obtained (Buschke and Fuld, 1974), such as the final Trial 12 recall, delayed recall, multiple choice recognition, and delayed multiple choice. Intrusion or perseverative errors can be quantified for clinical interpretation. The validity of SRT measures of short-term recall, random long-term recall (RLTR), and CLTR for the standard 12-trial, 12-word test was examined in multiple sclerosis patients and normal controls. The results provided evidence that the operational defini-

tions of these measures have predictive validity (Beatty, Krull et al., 1996).

More recently, it was recognized that some additional summary scores could be obtained that are useful to the clinician, and these are similar to variables obtained on the CVLT. A new scoring method was introduced that included primacy/recency, learning across trials, consistency of item recall, semantic and phonological errors, and contrast measures. The method allows for measurement of perseverative errors, interval between presentation and recall, clustering score, proportion of presented and unpresented words correctly recalled, and discrimination, without adding time or modifying the original administration procedure (Pluth, Hannay et al., 2002). The percentage of words recalled from the first third, middle third, and last third of the word list for the 12 learning trials represents primacy, middle and recency respectively.

Slope, or learning over trials, is calculated by dividing the increment of correctly recalled words by the number of trials. Consistency of item recall is the count of the number of times a word recalled on one trial is also recalled on the following trial, divided by the number of words recalled on all trials. Contrast measures included delayed recall/delayed multiple choice, delayed recall/trial 12, and delayed recall/multiple choice. Intrusion errors can be coded as semantic, phonemic or other for errors of semantically related, phonemically related, or unrelated errors, respectively. Intrusion error and perseveration error totals are computed. A recalled presentation proportion variable refers to the proportion of times that words presented by the examiner over the 12 trials was subsequently recalled on the delayed recall trial. The unrecalled presentation proportion variable refers to the proportion of times that words presented by the examiner over the 12 trials were not subsequently recalled on the delayed recall trial. The proportion of correct responses on the multiple-choice trial can result in d' values generated from a table based on forced choice among four orthogonal alternatives (Pluth, Hannay et al., 2002).

Proven effective in examination of those with epilepsy lateralizing effects, traumatic brain injury (TBI), dementia, and the effects of medication on memory in adults (Drane, Loring et al., 1998), the VSRT has been included in the study of memory function of young children pre- and post-anesthesia (Morgan, Furman et al., 1981; Morgan, 1982). It has been studied in children (Buschke, 1974) (Clodfelter, Dickson et al., 1987) and in adolescents (Levin and Grossman, 1976), with normative study in 5- to 16-year-old children (Gaither, 2002, personal communication; Roman, Gaither et al., 1994), and 9- to 15-year-old Canadian children (Christopher Paniak, 2002, personal communication). The use of SRT normative data without considering intellectual level may result in overestimation of memory deficit in low-average IQ individuals (Bishop, Dickson et al., 1990).

A variety of methodologies are employed. Both shortened or original 12-trial versions exist. A 6-trial format did not result in significant loss of sensitivity for left temporal lobe impaired adults (Drane, Loring et al., 1998). While 12-word lists are common for adults, list length and number of trials are shortened for children. Six-, 8-, and 10-word versions exist, and there are versions with 6, 8, or 10 trials. Four alternate forms consisting of 10 words with a maximum of 10 learning trials were developed for an adult study (Dikmen, Heaton et al., 1999). These authors included the usual 30-minute recall, but added a 4-hour recall.

The Selective Reminding Test was adapted for young children to determine its efficacy with this age range (Morgan, 1982). Alternate test forms within a repeated testing paradigm were used over the course of 4 to 5 hours and test–retest consistency and practice effects were also assessed. Demographic data for this study are presented in Table 11–3. The mean age in months of the 5- and 6-year-old group was 70.0 ($SD = 7.5$) and the mean age of the 7- and 8-year-old group was 96.6 months ($SD = 7.6$). The sum of the age-scaled scores on the WISC Information and Similarities subtests (the index of intellectual level) was 20.1 ($SD = 5.3$) for the 5- and 6-year-old group and 21.4 ($SD = 6.9$) for the 7- and 8-year-old group. Three forms were examined (see Table 11–4). Data were presented for LTS, LTR, CLTR, and recall/trial for all 66 children. No delayed recall was obtained.

Table 11–3. Selective Reminding Test Demographic Data for 5- to 8-years old: Morgan Study (1982)

Subjects: 66 children; mean age = 82.5 months ($SD = 15.4$); 36 prior to minor surgery with anesthesia and 30 normal controls

Age: 5–8 years old

Gender: 34 male and 32 female

Handedness: Not specified

Race: Not specified

Intellectual level: Mean combined age scaled WISC Information and Similarities score of 20.7 ($SD = 6.1$)

Inclusion criteria: "Normal school children"

List words were presented to the children at a 2-per-second rate. The test continued for six trials, or until two consecutive perfect trials were completed. No time limits were imposed. Form B was associated with lower performances relative to Forms A and C; mean LTS score for Form A was 32.5 ($SD = 11.5$), Form B was 27.9 ($SD = 10.5$), and Form C was 35.4 ($SD = 7.0$). Summary data for only the 30 control subjects divided into two age groups were also presented. The stability coefficients for test–retest correlations ranged from 0.55 to 0.66. Practice effects over 4 to 5 hours were not found. A strong relationship was found between age and performance, leading to a recommendation for a larger collection of normative data for more age divisions if clinical use with individual subjects is intended. The normative data means and standard deviations for 5 to 8 year olds are presented in Table 11–5.

Young children were also the subject of a larger normative study of two age groups

Table 11–4. Selective Reminding Test Word Lists for 5–8 year olds: Morgan Study

Form A	Form B	Form C
Dog	Balloon	Apple
Horse	Crayons	Meat
Turtle	Doll	Egg
Lion	Bicycle	Candy
Squirrel	Paints	Carrot
Bear	Baseball	Cereal
Elephant	Clay	Bread
Rabbit	Book	Banana

Source: Morgan, (1982), © Swets & Zeitlinger.

Table 11–5. Verbal Selective Reminding Test Means and *SD*s for 5- to 8-Year-Old Children

Measure	5 & 6 YEARS OLD (N = 16)		7 & 8 YEARS OLD (N = 14)	
	Mean	SD	Mean	SD
Recall/Trial	5.3	1.2	6.1	1.1
LTS	28.6	10.1	35.7	9.1
LTR	25.7	9.9	33.4	10.2
CLTR	18.9	11.3	27.7	13.2

Source: Morgan (1982), © Swets & Zeitlinger.

(Gaither, 2002, personal communication; Roman, Gaither et al., 1994). An 8-trial, 8-toy-related word form used for 131 children, 5 to 8 years old, was identical to the Morgan study Form B. In addition, a 10-trial, 10-unrelated-word-form was administered to sixty-two 9- to 16-year-old children (see Table 11–6). The data were collected from a database of over 400 children referred to a hospital evaluation center for suspected academic problems. The author indicated that while not clearly normal, the children from competitive school systems were referred for relatively poor performance rather than a more traditional question about learning disabilities for referred urban children.

Demographic data for the Gaither study are presented in Table 11–7. Full-scale IQ was reported for each age group, and ranged from 105.30 to 109.14 for the younger group, and from 102.90 to 105.85 for the older group. Data for total recall, LTS, CLTR, delayed recall, rate of forgetting at delay relative to the last learning trial and to the maximum recall trial are presented in Table 11–8. Data were also collected for STR, LTR, number of words recalled at trial one, intrusion errors, number of words recalled at delay that were in LTS, CLTR, or neither, maximum recall on a single learning trial, and number of words recalled on each trial immediately following a reminder.

Normative data for twenty-six 6 year olds, twenty-six 8 year olds, thirty-one 10 year olds, and fifty 13 to 18 year olds were collected, but unpublished for the Buschke version of the SRT (Harvey Levin, 1981, personal communication). In the latter group there were 23 males and 27 females: 6 males and 6 females, aged 13 to 14; 5 males and 12 females, aged 15 to 16, and 12 males and 9 females, aged 17 to 18. These data were collected in one geographical region of Texas. Children under 12 were administered 12 four-footed animal names for a maximum of 8 trials. Those 13 years old and older were administered 12 words for a maximum of 12 trials. Table 11–9 lists these word lists. In a study of 20 male and 20 female adult subjects, Form I was found to be significantly

Table 11–6. Selective Reminding Test Word Lists: Gaither Study

Age 5–8	Age 9–16
Balloon	Book
Crayons	Event
Doll	Woods
Bicycle	Flower
Paints	Method
Baseball	Artist
Clay	Opinion
Book	Coast
	Shame
	House

Table 11–7. Selective Reminding Test Demographic Data: Gaither Study

Subjects: 193 children in Illinois: 131 5 to 8 years old; 62 9 to 16 years old
Age: 5–16 years old
Gender: Not specified
Handedness: Not specified
Race: Not specified
SES: Middle to upper middle class
Inclusion criteria: Full-scale IQ scores of 80 or above, no neurological impairment

Source: Rebecca Gaither (unpublished Master's thesis).

Table 11–8. Selective Reminding Test Means (*SD*s): Gaither Study

						Maximum Recall	Last Trial
Age	N	LTS (*SD*)	CLTR (*SD*)	Total Recall (*SD*)	Delayed Recall	minus Delay	minus Delay
5	21	39.76 (13.71)	21.00 (14.06)	42.38 (9.12)	5.43 (1.78)	1.52 (1.44)	0.71 (1.55)
6	34	44.18 (12.06)	28.79 (16.96)	45.79 (9.00)	5.76 (2.05)	1.56 (1.44)	0.85 (1.44)
7	34	43.62 (14.22)	29.38 (17.97)	46.94 (9.81)	5.82 (1.75)	1.47 (1.16)	1.06 (1.35)
8	42	49.88 (11.53)	40.76 (15.59)	52.24 (9.39)	5.62 (1.25)	1.12 (0.89)	0.76 (1.01)

5 TO 8 YEARS OLD (N = 131)

Source: Rebecca Gaither (unpublished Master's Thesis).

more difficult than the other three forms, and Forms II, III, and IV were equivalent in difficulty (Hannay and Levin, 1985). Therefore, either Form II, III, or IV is the optimal initial administration form, with either or both of the remaining two forms serving as retest forms.

In another study, two SRT word list forms were developed for children 9 to 12 years old (Clodfelter, Dickson et al., 1987), and examined along with the same 12 four-footed animal categorical version used by Levin. The newer and more difficult lists were constructed to offset ceiling effects associated with the animal list in this age group and serve to provide alternate forms since significant learning effects are seen on retest. The 12-word lists were administered for a maximum of eight learning trials or until there was perfect recall for two consecutive trials. The available demographic information omits race and the incidence of right-handedness appears slightly low (over 80%), given normal population incidence of about 11% left-handedness (Spiegler and Yeni-Komishian, 1983).

WISC-III block design and vocabulary subtest standard scores are reported, along with digits forward and FAS fluency scores. There were no significant differences between younger (9–10 years) and older (11–12 years) children on these descriptive measures. On the SRT, LTS, and CLTR indices, Form A at initial testing was correlated with Form B at retest, and Form B at initial testing with Form A at retest. Thus, the alternate forms were judged suitable for serial evaluation (Pearson *r*, range = 0.56 to 0.85). The word lists for Form A, Form B, and for the animal version, Form C, are presented in Table 11–10. Demographic

Table 11–9. Hannay & Levin Selective Reminding Test Word Lists for <12 (child) and >12 years

Child	Form 1	Form 2	Form 3	Form 4
Dog	Bowl	Shine	Throw	Egg
Fox	Passion	Disagree	Lily	Runway
Horse	Dawn	Fat	Film	Fort
Lion	Judgment	Wealthy	Discreet	Toothache
Elephant	Grant	Drunk	Loft	Drown
Bear	Bee	Pin	Beef	Baby
Rat	Plane	Grass	Street	Lave
Racoon	County	Moon	Helmet	Damp
Goat	Choice	Prepare	Snake	Pure
Squirrel	Seed	Prize	Dug	Vote
Beaver	Wool	Duck	Pack	Strip
Turtle	Meal	Leaf	Tin	Truth

Source: Hannay and Levin (1985), © Swets & Zeitlinger.

Table 11–10. Selective Reminding Test Word Lists for ages 9–12: Clodfelter et al. Study

List A	List B	List C
Garden	Market	Dog
Doctor	Palace	Fox
Metal	Flower	Horse
City	Picture	Lion
Money	Dollar	Elephant
Cattle	River	Bear
Prison	Cotton	Rat
Clothing	Sugar	Raccoon
Water	College	Goat
Cabin	Baby	Squirrel
Tower	Temple	Beaver
Bottle	Butter	Turtle

Source: Clodfelter et al. (1987), © Swets & Zeitlinger.

data are presented in Table 11–11 and normative data are presented in Table 11–12.

Fewer words, but more trials, was the procedure used in a study mentioned earlier (Rebecca Gaither, 2002, personal communication; Roman, Gaither et al., 1994). A 10-word list (see Table 11–7) was administered to sixty-two 9- to 16-year-old children, and the variables noted above for young children were analyzed for older children. Selected data about long term storage, consistent long term retrieval, total recall, delayed recall, maximum recall minus delayed recall, and last trial maximum minus delayed recall are reported in Table 11–13.

SRT data, stratified according to the Canadian Cognitive Abilities Test IQ level, that is, low-average to average IQ (110 or below) or high IQ (above 110), were presented (Miller, Murphy et al., 1996) and published for 9- to 15-year-old children (Spreen and Strauss,

Table 11–11. Demographic Data: Clodfelter et al. Study (1987)

Subjects: 58 initially; 51 at retesting 8 days later
Age: 28 9–10 years old, 30 11–12 years old initially;
    22 and 29 respectively at retesting
Gender: 12 male and 21 female middle SES; 11 male,
    14 female lower SES
Handedness: "Over 80% were right handed"
Race: Not specified
SES: Lower and middle SES
Inclusion Criteria: No history of head injury or
    cerebral disease

1998). These low- and high-IQ SRT data were subsequently merged by age level and gender (Christopher Paniak, 2002, personal communication). The 13- to 15-year-old children were administered Form I of the Hannay-Levin list words (see Table 11–9), but with 8 learning trials rather than 12. The 9- to 12-year-old children were administered the same words as Form A in the Clodfelter study (see Table 11–10). These previously unpublished normative data are presented in Table 11–14.

Normative data on military dependents in South Carolina and Landstuhl, West Germany, were also collected but unpublished (C. A. Hopewell, 2002, personal communication). Data for LTR, LTS, and CLTR for 120 6- to 8-year-olds administered the 8-trial version of the Levin stimulus words are presented in Table 11–15. Data on mean number of intrusion errors were also collected and are presented for children aged 6 to 11, by gender.

Rey Auditory Verbal Learning Test

The Rey Auditory Verbal Learning Test (RAVLT) is a word list learning and memory test that provides a learning curve and assesses interference effects on recall (Taylor, 1959; Rey, 1964; Geffen, Moor et al., 1990). Children with learning problems may have a flat learning curve over the trials, while children with attentional disorder may demonstrate inconsistent performance (Bishop, Knights et al., 1990). The test takes 10 to 15 minutes to administer and is considered simpler than the CVLT (Bishop, Knights et al., 1990). Besides a learning curve and scores for delayed recall after interference and recognition memory (Ryan, Rosenberg et al., 1983), data may be obtained about phonetic and semantic substitution, repetition, or fabrication (Bishop, Knights et al., 1990). Older normative data are available for Swiss children (Rey, 1964), but are judged to be too high for child populations with current administration procedures and lists (Bishop, Knights et al., 1990). Modifications of list words (Wiens, Crossen et al., 1988) further invalidated the already weak original Rey data. Data for a 16- to 19-year-old age block are included in a study of adults through 86 years old (Geffen, Moor et al., 1990). Child normative

Table 11–12. Mean SRT, LTS, and CLTR scores (*SD*) for Initial Testing of 9–12 Year Olds

Age	N	LTS Form A	LTS Form B	LTS Form C	CLTR Form A	CLTR Form B	CLTR Form C	INTRUSION ERRORS Form A	INTRUSION ERRORS Form B	INTRUSION ERRORS Form C
9–10	22	61.92 (13.92)	59.32 (18.29)	72.00 (14.42)	42.07 (21.11)	41.71 (22.32)	54.25 (18.55)	1.50 (2.63)	2.85 (3.19)	4.00 (4.19)
11–12	29	67.10 (18.65)	65.80 (19.81)	76.00 (16.57)	49.40 (23.09)	51.10 (25.66)	64.27 (23.50)	1.03 (2.07)	.93 (1.85)	1.23 (2.32)

Source: Clodfelter et al. (1987), © Swets & Zeitlinger.

LTS = Long Term Storage; CLTR = Consistent Long Term Retrieval

data for the RAVLT were also published for 80 children, 7- to 15-years-old (Forrester and Geffen, 1991) and 943 children 8- to 17-years-old, using a Hebrew version (Vakil, Blachstein et al., 1998).

An English list of words (Taylor, 1959) is published (Lezak, 1983) along with recommended directions and list words from two other sources (Crawford, Stewart et al., 1989). The recommended procedure consists of orally reciting 15 words (List A) at a rate of 1 per second, and then asking the child to retrieve as many words as possible. Four additional learning trials are given with the reminder that the entire list should be recalled, and then a novel list (List B) is presented for a single recall (trial 5). Free recall of List A is then required again (trial 6). A delayed recall is recommended 30 minutes later.

Another version (Bishop, Knights et al., 1990) modifies these directions to include administration of nonverbal tests for 30 minutes after trial 6, followed by a delayed recall trial for List A words and then a recognition trial.

Using this version, performance on the RAVLT was examined in 252 English and French Canadian (195 anglophones, 57 francophones) patients (179 male, 73 female) aged 5 to 16 who had an IQ of at least 70. IQ correlated moderately with RAVLT performance, males and females had equivalent performance, and French children did less well than English children, with IQ a confounding variable. Small sample size prevented matching of male and female on age, IQ, language, and diagnosis.

A RAVLT procedure was also used to collect normative data on 391 children between 7- and 13-years-old (Anderson, Lajoie et al., 1995). These authors used the Taylor list words (Taylor, 1959), read at the rate of 1 per second for the usual five trials. Words were checked off as retrieved by the child without feedback regarding correct or erroneous responses provided. Word repetitions were noted by extra checkmarks, and intrusion errors (non-list words) were recorded. After Trial 5, a story recall test was administered. A recall of list words, "Recall A," was requested immediately after

Table 11–13. Selective Reminding Test Means (*SD*): Gaither Study

				9 TO 16 YEARS OLD (*N* = 62)			
Age	N	LTS (*SD*)	CLTR (*SD*)	Total Recall (*SD*)	Delayed Recall	Maximum Recall minus Delay	Last Trial minus Delay
9–10	21	64.76 (15.98)	44.19 (21.57)	72.00 (10.92)	6.24 (1.84)	2.81 (1.12)	2.10 (1.64)
11–12	18	70.28 (20.47)	51.94 (21.88)	76.83 (11.40)	6.67 (1.65)	2.67 (1.03)	2.11 (1.08)
13–14	13	73.38 (15.07)	48.23 (16.96)	76.62 (9.46)	6.85 (1.52)	2.62 (1.26)	2.15 (1.46)
15–16	10	77.50 (12.07)	62.40 (19.24)	81.20 (9.82)	7.30 (2.58)	2.40 (2.32)	2.10 (2.13)

Source: Courtesy of Rebecca Gaither (unpublished Master's Thesis).

Table 11–14. Selective Reminding Test Means (*SDs*): Paniak, Miller and Murphy Data

Age	N	LTS	CLTR	Total Recall	LTR	STR4:3 1 PM	Cued Recall	Multiple Choice	Delay Recall	Delay Cued	Savings Percent
9	81	72.81 (10.41)	52.21 (17.96)	72.86 (9.14)	67.17 (12.10)	5.70 (3.83)	9.80 (1.61)	11.96 (0.19)	9.95 (1.87)	10.01 (1.70)	95.00 (16.76)
10	140	73.36 (10.73)	58.01 (18.31)	75.46 (8.37)	69.24 (12.24)	6.22 (4.68)	10.13 (1.77)	11.94 (0.27)	10.21 (1.66)	10.49 (1.64)	92.44 (12.47)
11	132	71.90 (11.92)	52.88 (18.17)	73.73 (8.39)	66.98 (12.66)	6.78 (5.03)	9.97 (1.73)	11.95 (0.27)	10.14 (1.71)	10.33 (1.73)	95.66 (15.33)
12	122	77.16 (9.84)	61.37 (17.23)	78.12 (7.88)	73.13 (11.26)	5.0 (4.15)	10.57 (1.37)	12.00 (0.00)	10.72 (1.40)	10.97 (1.38)	96.09 (11.87)
13	96	73.50 (10.58)	58.33 (16.44)	76.56 (7.42)	69.62 (11.58)	6.94 (4.80)	9.30 (1.74)	11.8 (0.38)	59.82 (1.95)	9.49 (1.85)	89.71 (16.00)
14	116	76.02 (10.24)	64.59 (17.37)	79.13 (7.76)	73.20 (11.50)	5.93 (4.37)	9.72 (1.47)	11.90 (0.33)	10.57 (1.47)	10.15 (1.45)	94.10 (11.58)
15°	52	74.46 (11.09)	60.31 (17.25)	77.10 (8.18)	70.73 (12.54)	6.37 (5.25)	9.60 (1.62)	11.90 (.36)	10.27 (2.20)	9.96 (1.78)	92.82 (16.51)

Source: Reprinted with permission of Chris Paniak, Harry Miller, and Deirdre Murphy, personal communication.
[1]Vocabulary scaled score of 9; caution advised.

Table 11–15. Selective Reminding Test Means (*SDs*): Hopewell Data

				LONG-TERM RETRIEVAL					
Age	N	Trial 1	Trial 2	Trial 3	Trial 4	Trial 5	Trial 6	Trial 7	Trial 8
6	40	2.45(1.60)	3.92(2.39)	5.00(2.61)	5.75(2.81)	6.87(2.87)	6.52(2.99)	7.52(2.48)	7.10(2.68)
7	40	3.73(1.88)	4.80(2.19)	5.93(2.02)	7.00(2.31)	7.29(2.35)	7.97(2.23)	8.15(2.18)	8.61(1.99)
8	40	3.55(1.62)	5.38(1.98)	6.60(1.98)	7.38(2.01)	7.92(1.83)	8.48(1.96)	8.98(1.67)	8.83(1.95)
				LONG-TERM STORAGE					
6	40	2.45(1.60)	3.92(2.43)	5.55(2.69)	6.55(2.74)	7.57(2.89)	8.40(2.71)	8.83(2.44)	8.83(2.44)
7	40	3.07(1.88)	4.85(2.19)	6.73(2.27)	7.92(2.27)	8.66(2.26)	9.34(2.02)	9.97(1.77)	9.97(1.77)
8	40	3.63(1.66)	5.38(1.98)	7.05(2.02)	8.15(2.19)	8.88(1.95)	9.58(1.88)	9.78(2.38)	9.78(2.38)
				CONSISTENT LONG-TERM RETRIEVAL					
6	40	1.17(1.37)	1.62(1.58)	2.40(1.92)	3.27(2.29)	3.82(2.33)	4.60(2.45)	5.90(2.59)	5.90(2.59)
7	40	1.34(1.51)	2.29(2.06)	3.05(1.97)	3.83(2.44)	4.61(2.44)	5.44(2.39)	6.93(2.18)	6.93(2.18)
8	40	2.25(1.43)	3.25(1.98)	3.83(2.04)	4.75(2.17)	5.63(2.26)	6.53(2.31)	7.83(1.97)	7.83(1.97)
				INTRUSIONS (MALE; FEMALE)					
6		4.77 (3.78); 4.77(3.78)							
7		1.35 (1.69); 1.67(2.38)							
8		1.89 (2.32); 1.38(2.42)							
9		1.52 (1.88); 1.96(2.65)							
10		1.64 (2.25); 2.07(4.99)							
11		1.00 (1.76); 1.25(1.42)							

Source: Courtesy of C. Alan Hopewell, personal communication.

completion of the story recall. A recognition trial consisted of a recognition story sheet placed in front of the child, with the instruction that the child should read the story and "put a circle around all the words that were in the list we just read." The examiner read the story if the child could not comply with the directions and instructed the child to indicate all list words as they were heard. Scores are obtained for number of words per trial, total number of words recalled on a spontaneous recall trials, number of intrusion errors, number of repetition errors, and recognition accuracy. These normative data are presented in Table 11–16.

California Verbal Learning Test–Children's Version

The California Verbal Learning Test—Children's Version (CVLT-C; Delis, Kramer et al., 1994) is a downward extension of the adult version California Verbal Learning Test (CVLT; Delis, Kramer et al. 1987). It is nationally normed for children 5 to 16 years old, while the CVLT normative data begin at 16 years. It is co-normed with the Children's Category Test (Boll, 1993). The CVLT-C is another supraspan list-learning test of explicit (declarative)

memory that requires sustained auditory attention, immediate memory, and delayed recall. It also utilizes repetition of stimuli, but differs from the SRT list-learning tests by including words that have semantic associations, that is, the words fall within three semantic categories. This may initiate working memory and provide an assistive strategy (Williams, Phillips et al., 2001). Recent reanalysis of the standardization sample data using confirmatory factor analysis resulted in a 5-factor model of learning and memory for this measure. These were Attention Span (for supraspan stimuli), Learning Efficiency (active use of organized or consistent levels of processing), Delayed Free Recall (recall after distractor intervention), Delayed Cued Recall (prompted recall), and Inaccurate Recall (target from distractor discrimination) (Donders, 1999). Using this model, intact verbal memory skills were found for children with well-controlled idiopathic or cryptogenic epilepsy and no comorbid conditions, and significant differences were not found for seizure type or length of diagnosis and treatment (Williams, Phillips et al., 2001).

The normative data were derived from a standardization sample that was based on the 1988 U. S. Census survey data, including vari-

Table 11–16. Rey Auditory Verbal Learning Test Means (*SD*s): Anderson et al. data

						REY AUDITORY VERBAL LEARNING TEST						Delay
Age	N	Trial 1	Trial 2	Trial 3	Trial 4	Trial 5	Intrusion	Repetition	Total	Recall	Recog	Rec
7	56	5.05 (1.8)	7.23 (2.0)0	9.20 (2.71)	9.34 (2.9)	9.84 (2.9)	1.5	3.2	39.64 (10.0)	9.02 (2.8)	12.86 (3.0)	8.76 (2.9)
8	56	5.48 (1.6)	8.27 (2.33)	9.20 (2.71)	9.75 (3.25)	11.05 (2.71)	0.7	4.5	43.38 (9.8)	10.26 (2.3)	13.87 (1.4)	10.62 (2.4)
9	61	6.03 (1.8)	8.80 (2.2)	10.21 (2.6)	10.21 (2.6)	11.87 (2.3)	0.8	5.4	48.03 (9.1)	11.63 (2.2)	14.03 (1.1)	11.57 (2.3)
10	62	6.42 (1.6)	8.89 (2.0)	10.66 (2.2)	11.27 (2.5)	11.87 (2.4)	0.7	5.0	48.69 (9.5)	11.26 (2.5)	13.98 (1.3)	11.46 (2.4)
11	51	6.31 (1.8)	9.16 (2.1)	10.80 (1.9)	11.82 (2.1)	12.08 (1.9)	0.8	5.1	50.14 (7.5)	11.62 (2.0)	14.33 (0.8)	11.16 (2.0)
12	54	6.82 (1.6)	9.56 (1.9)	11.26 (1.9)	12.28 (1.9)	12.33 (1.7)	0.9	5.9	52.24 (6.7)	11.83 (1.7)	14.41 (0.8)	11.54 (2.2)
13	51	7.35 (1.9)	10.04 (2.3)	11.37 (2.1)	12.20 (2.1)	12.55 (2.1)	0.7	4.7	53.31 (8.5)	12.31 (1.8)	14.45 (1.2)	11.98 (2.4)

Source: Unpublished manuscript (1995), courtesy, V. Anderson, G. Lajoie, and R. Bell.

ables of age, gender, race/ethnicity, geographic region, and four levels of parent education. The authors used a stratified random sampling plan to ensure a representative proportion of children from each demographic group. The sample included 920 children aged between 5 and 16 in 12 age groups, with 70 to 80 children included at each age range. There were 459 females and 461 males, with approximately equal representation in each age group.

A varimax rotated factor structure found 6 factors for 19 CVLT-C indices, the same factor structure that underlies the adult version (Delis, Kramer et al., 1987). Internal consistency for across-trial consistency (odd–even correlations from .84 to .91 and coefficient alpha from .81 to .88) and internal consistency for across-word consistency (odd–even correlation of .83 and coefficient alpha correlation of .81) were moderately strong. Across-semantic-category consistency correlations averaged .72. Test–retest reliability correlations, with a median interval of 28 days, ranged from .38 to .90 for 8 year olds, .17 to .77 for 12 year olds, and from .31 to .85 for 16 year olds. Children aged 8 and 12 improved performance about 1 word per trial, while 16 year olds improved about 2 words per trial. Correlations between the CVLT-C List A Trials 1–5 raw score total and the Wechsler Intelligence Scale for Children-Revised (WISC-R) vocabulary subtest ranged from 0.32 to 0.40, indicative of a significant but mild relationship. Only 9% to 16% of the variance was shared by the two tests, suggesting that the CVLT-C measures an aspect of cognition distinct from verbal IQ.

Normative data for 4-year-olds are reported separately (Goodman, Delis et al., 1999). The demographic data for this study are presented in Table 11–17. The authors found an average first trial recall score of 3.6 that increased to 5.2 on the fifth trial. Total words recalled across the five learning trials was 24.2 words. They found 61% of the words were recalled consistently across these trials, 29.1% from primacy regions, 37.8% from middle regions, and 33.1% from recency regions. The 4-year-olds had similar semantic (1.4) and serial (1.6) cluster scores compared to 5-year-olds; these only slightly above chance levels. Short delay free recall averaged 3.1 words, and semantic cueing in-

Table 11–17. CVLT-C Normative Sample for Children 4 Years-old: Goodman et al. Study (1999)

Subjects: 80 children recruited from community
Age: 4 years old (each month represented)
Gender: 40 male, 40 female
Race: 13.75% Non-Caucasian (1 African American, 4 Hispanics, 2 Native American, 4 mixed ethnic background, 4 unknown
SES: 76% of the sample coded for mean Hollingshead score of 50.7
Inclusion: All children spoke English as first language; screened with maternal questionnaire

---

creased this to 3.8 words. Long-delay free recall averaged 3.5, and long delay cued recall averaged 3.4. Data are also presented for recognition testing, error responding, and response pattern. This sample made a disproportionately large number of intrusion errors, or non-list words. It was also noted that detection of moderate or greater memory impairment in this age group may be limited for some variables due to floor effects. Overall, there was support for the use of the CVLT-C for such young children.

There are also a number of studies that examined clinical populations using the CVLT-C as a verbal learning and recall measure. Language-impaired children had poorer new learning and increased perseverative responses but equivalent delayed recall and intrusion errors compared to normal controls (Shear, Tallal et al., 1992). Mild head-injured children recalled fewer words after a delay, but had intact new learning and recognition, and severe head-injured children demonstrated poorer new learning, delayed recall, and recognition than normative data controls and made more intrusion errors (Yeates, Blumenstein et al., 1995). Children with myelomeningocele, but without shunted hydrocephalus, were equivalent to normal controls and had better long-delay free recall than children with myelomeningocele and shunted hydrocephalus. The latter group had equivalent immediate recall on the first trial, but poorer new learning over trials and poorer delayed recall than normal controls, but equivalent recognition (Yeates, Enrile et al., 1995). Verbal learning and recognition were intact for children with idiopathic or cryptogenic epilepsy and no comorbid problems, their generalized or partial complex seizures well controlled with monotherapy (Williams, Phillips et al., 2001). A small number of children could be classified according to lateralization of seizure focus, but results did not result in differences in memory performance. Other clinical groups include studies of autism (Minshew and Goldstein, 1993), epilepsy (Williams, Phillips et al., 2001), and fetal alcohol syndrome (Mattson, Riley et al., 1996).

CVLT performance in adults was associated with EF impairment to a greater degree than for the Wechsler Memory Scale-Revised Logical Memory subtest (Tremont, Halpert et al., 2000). These authors recommended inclusion of the LM subtest along with CVLT to better discriminate between EF impairment (i.e., direct effects of frontal systems dysfunction) and direct memory dysfunction since these are not interchangeable measures. They further suggested that LM may be a more direct measure of temporal and hippocampal integrity, while list-learning tests like the CVLT require active structuring and encoding of auditorily presented information and therefore, the prefrontal cortex, anterior cingulate, and cerebellum might be more involved.

Interestingly, they found no significant difference in retention rates between EF-impaired groups for either the CVLT or LM, suggesting that memory retention may be unaffected by executive dysfunction and therefore potentially a "pure" measure of memory. They also did not find significant reduction of semantic clustering associated with increasing executive dysfunction. The relationship of CVLT performance and EF abilities was also examined in another adult study (Vanderploeg, Schinka et al. 1994) and a 5-factor structure was found, validating previous findings.

In addition to information about learning and episodic memory, the CVLT-C also allows for quantifying the strategies and error types displayed while learning new verbal information, the "process" by which the child integrates and expresses novel information. The CVLT *semantic clustering score* is considered indicative of conceptually driven organization. A semantic clustering ratio can be calculated: number of instances of two consecutively re-ported words from the same semantic category/expected number of possible clustered responses, based on total number of words produced and number of different categories represented on any trial (Glosser, Gallo et al., 2002). This score provides useful information for adults but does not appear to be as useful an index for children.

A *serial clustering score* is indicative of a "a passive, low-level, concrete approach to recall, which does not involve any new transformation or organization of presented information and is believed to be related to worse memory performance." (Glosser, Gallo et al., 2002, p. 193). It can be computed by dividing the number of times two words that were recalled in succession also appeared in the same order on the word list by the expected number of serial-order clusters (Glosser, Gallo et al., 2002). Such strategy commonly does not emerge prior to adolescence (Delis, Filoteo et al., 1994).

It has been reported that intelligence level plays a mediating role on CVLT-C performance (Denckla 1996), but it might be a stronger covariate of the relationship between CVLT-C and EF among younger children than for older children or adolescents (Riccio, Hall et al., 1994; Beebe, Ris et al., 2000). The results of one child study found only a weak correlation between the CVLT-C total score with the Children's Category Test, a multifactorial executive function measure (Donders, 1998). Intelligence (measured by WISC-III vocabulary and block design scores) was only a weak mediator in a study of adolescents and did not relate to any CVLT-C indices that correlated with EF (Beebe, Ris et al., 2000). Gender might be predictive of performance, with girls tending to outperform boys (Kramer, Delis et al., 1997; Beebe, Ris et al., 2000).

The process variables are purported to be ways to further examine EF (Levin, Culhane et al., 1991). However, empirical data do not fully support this contention. The predicted correlation between having brain dysfunction and demonstration of increased impairment in semantic clustering, serial clustering, recall consistency, perseverations and/or intrusions on the CVLT-C was not found for children with myelomeningocele and hydrocephalus (Yeates, Enrile et al., 1995) or traumatic brain injury

(Roman, Delis et al., 1998; Yeates, Blumenstein et al., 1995). The distinction between learning and process on the CVLT-C was examined in a sample of community-dwelling adolescents. The authors concluded that clinical interpretation of the process indices did not reflect EF (Beebe, Ris et al., 2000).

Administration and Scoring

The CVLT-C procedure requires the child to repeat a set list of 15 nouns from three exemplary semantic categories over five immediate-recall learning trials (List A), and then repeat a new, competing 15-noun list free recall (interference List B), which can elicit evidence of proactive interference in impaired individuals. Short-delay recall and semantic-cued recall of List A are then requested. After 20 minutes, long-term delay free recall and semantic-cued recall trials are elicited. Finally, a yes–no recognition memory trial including 15 target words, 12 List B words, and 18 distractor words is presented.

The CVLT-C allows for calculation of a number of variables. Learning outcome measures enable clinical determination of the ability to encode, store, and retrieve the novel information. Immediate free recall is the total number of words recalled for List A across learning trials 1 to 5. Short-delay (5-minute) free recall is the total number of List A words recalled after presentation of List B. Short-delay cued recall is the total number of List A words recalled after presentation of List B when semantic categories are specified. Long-delay free recall is the total number of List A words recalled after a 20-minute delay. Long-delay cued recall is the total number of List A words recalled after a 20-minute delay when semantic categories are specified. A recognition trial presents list words and distractors, and the score is the number of correctly identified List A words.

Learning strategies can also be scored. *Recall perseverative error* (indicative of poor self-monitoring) refers to the number of repeated responses on trials 1 to 5. *Recall intrusion errors*, indicative of impulsivity or poor inhibition, refer to the total number of off-list items reported on trials 1 to 5. Semantic or serial learning strategies are also quantified. A *semantic cluster ratio index* refers to the total number of words recalled over the five trials immediately after word recall from the same semantic category. A *serial cluster ratio index* score refers to the degree to which the child consecutively recalls list words in the same order they were presented. Recall of the same words across consecutive learning trials results in a percent recall consistency score. A false positive index refers to the number of incorrect words endorsed during delayed recognition. Susceptibility to interference is indicated by the number of words recalled immediately after List B. Computer scoring assistance is available (Fridlund and Delis, 1994).

The indication of release from proactive inhibition (PI; Wickens, 1970) is interesting since failure to release from PI can indicate frontal dysfunction (Moscovitch, 1981), but need not be interpreted as indicative of memory disorder (Squire, 1982). It has also been proposed that sensitivity to PI might be a consequence of deficient suppression of irrelevant information at retrieval secondary to defective inhibitory attentional mechanisms, in a study of anterior communicating artery aneurysm patients (Van der Linden, Bruyer et al., 1993). A child's attentiveness over the learning trials may be discerned as contributing to overall functioning. For example, inconsistent responding over the learning trials, but a relatively strong performance on Trial 5, may highlight the clinical importance of attentional factors.

Hopkins Verbal Learning Test

The Hopkins Verbal Learning Test (HVLT; Brandt, 1991) and its revision that includes delayed recall and recognition following a 20-minute delay period (HVLT-R; Benedict, Schretlen et al., 1998) is generally considered an adult test. However, it holds interest for child neuropsychologists as well, and there is now a report of adolescent data (Barr, 2003), an age group for which many gaps exist in available normative data. The HVLT-R includes three trials to recall a 12-word list sequence presented orally by the examiner at a 2-second interstimulus interval. At the conclusion of the third trial, there is a 20-minute delay, then a free recall. Finally, a yes/no recognition probe is included with 12 distractor words interspersed with the

12 target-list words. Scores are obtained for each trial recall, for the total recall for the three trials, for the free recall condition, and for the recognition probe. Learning (the higher of trial 2 or trial 3 minus trial 1) and percent retained (the better of trials 2 and 3 divided by trial 4 recall times 100) can also be calculated. A discrimination index is calculated by subtracting recognition errors from the total correct recognition (true positives minus false positives) (Benedict, Schretlen et al., 1998). There are six alternate forms (Brandt, 1991).

Male and female adolescent data were reported for 100 high school athletes (8 freshman, 15 sophomores, 46 juniors, and 31 seniors) from suburban New York City. (See Table 4–13 for demographic data; note no differences were found for athletes with or without preexisting concussion or learning disability.) The HVLT normative data were obtained along with data from selected Wechsler Adult Intelligence Scale-III subtests (digit span, digit symbol, symbol search) allowing for calculation of a WAIS-III Processing Speed Index (PSI), the Controlled Oral Word Association Test (COWAT), and the Trail Making Test. The HVLT data presented in Table 11–18 are for three dependent measures: total learning over

the three trials, delayed recall, and the discrimination index, by gender. The neuropsychological test scores for Test 1 and Test 2 (test–retest) in a sample of 48 subjects, tested approximately 60 days apart, are presented in Table 11–19. Test–retest reliabilities were low, ranging from $r = 0.389$ to $r = 0.784$, and there was no gender difference. No significant practice effects increases were found for the HVLT, using alternate forms, although these were found for the WAIS-III, PSI, Trail Making Test, and COWAT, despite the use of alternate forms for the latter. In a very desirable presentation, one that portends the presentation of results for future normative data studies, the adjusted reliable change indices were calculated for the common 90%, less conservative 80%, and 70% confidence intervals followed by the percent of sample with scores falling below the lower limit. These data are presented in Table 11–20.

In clinical interpretation, the percentage values represent the level of decline required to exceed what is expected, based on normal error variance and practice effects. For example, if a digit-span total raw score declines 4 points on second testing, reference to Table 11–20 indicates that the lowered score exceeds the

Table 11–18. Neuropsychological Test Scores: Total Sample

	TOTAL SAMPLE ($N = 100$)	MALES ($N = 60$)	FEMALES ($N = 40$)	MALES V. FEMALES	
	M (SD)	M (SD)	M (SD)	t (98 df)	P
WAIS-III Digit Span					
Forward—Raw Score	11.0 (1.9)	10.9 (1.9)	11.1 (1.9)	0.51	.609
Backward—Raw Score	6.8 (2.3)	7.0 (2.5)	6.5 (1.8)	0.97	.332
Total—Raw Score	17.8 (3.4)	17.9 (3.4)	17.7 (3.1)	0.36	.717
WAIS-III PSI	106.7 (14.8)	104.6 (11.4)	109.8 (18.4)	1.73	.086
Digit Symbol—Raw Score	84.8 (13.1)	80.1 (12.6)	91.9 (10.4)	4.91	.001
Symbol Search—Raw Score	38.8 (6.4)	37.8 (6.4)	40.3 (6.0)	1.94	.055
Trailmaking Test					
Part A (seconds)	22.5 (6.7)	23.2 (7.6)	21.4 (4.9)	1.32	.190
Part B (seconds)	52.5 (17.1)	56.1 (18.9)	47.2 (12.4)	2.60	.010
COWAT—Total Words	35.3 (9.8)	33.1 (8.8)	38.7 (10.3)	2.93	.004
Hopkins Verbal Learning Test					
Total Learning (Trials 1–3)	25.8 (4.8)	25.7 (4.3)	25.9 (5.5)	0.25	.805
Delayed Recall	9.4 (1.9)	9.2 (2.1)	9.7 (1.7)	1.21	.228
Discrimination Index	11.7 (0.7)	11.6 (0.7)	11.7 (0.6)	0.62	.537

Source: Barr, W. (2003). Reprinted from *Archives of Clinical Neuropsychology*, Vol 18, Neuropsychological testing of high school athletes: Preliminary norms and test-retest indices, 91–101, © 2003, with permission from Elsevier Science.

Table 11–19. Neuropsychological Test Scores at Time 1 and Time 2

T1–T2	TIME 1	TIME 2	T2–T1
r SE_m S_{Diff}	M (SD)	M (SD)	M (SD)
WAIS-III Digit Span			
Forward—Raw Score	10.8 (1.8)	11.0 (2.1)	+0.21 (1.7)
.602 1.12 1.58			
Backward—Raw Score	7.2 (2.2)	7.7 (2.4)	+0.50 (1.8)
.634 1.32 1.87			
Total—Raw Score	17.9 (3.2)	18.6 (4.1)	+0.70 (2.9)
.703 1.73 2.45			
WAIS-III Processing Speed Index	106.7 (14.8)	114.6 (13.6)	+7.86 (8.6)
.784 6.85 9.70			
Digit Symbol—Raw Score	84.2 (14.6)	89.4 (16.1)	+5.19 (11.4)
.726 7.61 10.76			
Symbol Search—Raw Score	39.1 (6.6)	43.1 (6.4)	+4.00 (5.9)
.583 4.28 6.05			
Trailmaking Test			
Part A (seconds)	21.4 (5.4)	19.3 (5.4)	−2.14 (5.9)
.410 4.16 5.88			
Part B (seconds)	50.1 (17.3)	44.9 (15.6)	−5.83 (13.8)
.651 10.22 14.45			
COWAT—Total Words	36.3 (9.0)	39.7 (9.4)	+3.42 (7.4)
.680 5.09 7.20			
Hopkins Verbal Learning Test			
Total Learning (Trials 1–3)	27.0 (3.4)	27.3 (4.3)	+0.27 (3.9)
.536 2.63 3.72			
Delayed Recall	9.6 (1.8)	9.8 (2.1)	+0.19 (1.9)
.563 1.21 1.71			
Discrimination Index	11.6 (0.9)	11.7 (0.7)	−0.01 (0.9)
.389 0.73 1.03			

Source: Barr, W. (2003). Reprinted from *Archives of Clinical Neuropsychology*, Vol 18, Neuropsychological testing of high school athletes: Preliminary norms and test-retest indices, 91–101, © 2003, with permission from Elsevier Science.

lower limit (−3) of the traditional 90% confidence interval (CI) and was found in less than 5% of the test–retest sample. The overall results from this study indicate caution is necessary in interpreting test data from high school athletes, raise questions about test–retest reliability, and suggest that separate norms for males and females are warranted in the evaluation of performance, for example, following concussion.

Sentence Memory

There are a wide variety of sentence memory tests, also known as sentence repetition or sentence span tests, both individual tests and those that are part of larger test batteries. Developmental norms for a Sentence Repetition Test (Spreen and Benton, 1963) were published for 6- to 13-year-old children (Spreen and Gaddes, 1969). Subsequently, the same sentences were used in a normative study with a larger sample of 1081 children ranging in age from 3 to 13 in the central interior of British Columbia, Canada (Carmichael and MacDonald, 1984). The sentences increase in syllable length from 1 to 26 syllables. Administration is discontinued when there are five consecutive failures. The Spreen and Gaddes norms refer to a procedure in which the sentences are played on a tape-

Table 11–20. Adjusted Reliable Change Indices Calculated for 90%, 80%, and 70% Confidence Intervals (CI) Followed by Percent of Sample with Scores Falling Below the Lower Limit

	90% CI	80% CI	70% CI
WAIS-III Digit Span			
Forwards—Raw Score	−2, +3 (14.5%)	−2, +2 (14.6%)	−1, +2 (31.3%)
Backwards—Raw Score	−3, +4 (6.3%)	−2, +3 (14.6%)	−1, +2 (27.1%)
Total—Raw Score	−3, +5 (4.2%)	−2, +4 (14.6%)	−2, +3 (14.6%)
WAIS-III PSI	−8, 124 (6.3%)	−5, 120 (10.4%)	−2, 118 (16.7%)
Digit Symbol—Raw Score	−12, +23 (4.2%)	−9, +19 (8.3%)	−6, +16 (10.4%)
Symbol Search—Raw Score	−6, +14 (4.2%)	−4, +12 (4.2%)	−2, +10 (10.4%)
Trailmaking Test			
Part A (seconds)	−12, +8 (4.2%)	−10, +5 (12.5%)	−8, +4 (12.5%)
Part B (seconds)	−30, +18 (0%)	−24, +13 (4.2%)	−21, +9 (14.2%)
COWAT—Total Words	−8, 115 (6.3%)	−6, 113 (10.4%)	−4, 111 (16.7%)
Hopkins Verbal Learning Test			
Total Learning (Trials 1–3)	−6, +6 (2.1%)	−4, +5 (18.8%)	−4, +4 (18.8%)
Delayed Recall	−3, +3 (8.3%)	−2, +2 (14.6%)	−2, +2 (14.6%)
Discrimination Index	−2, +2 (8.3%)	−1, +1 (14.6%)	−1, +1 (14.6%)

Source: Barr, W. (2002). Reprinted from *Archives of Clinical Neuropsychology,* Vol 18, Neuropsychological testing of high school athletes: Preliminary norms and test-retest indices, 91–101, © 2002, with permission from Elsevier Science.

recording. For oral recitation administration, they suggest adjusting the means one point higher. However, the Carmichael and MacDonald results differed from the Spreen and Gaddes norms, and the 1-point adjustment to compensate for an audiotaped presentation advantage might skew results even more. The differences were attributed to sample size, population characteristics, and a greater effect of oral compared to audiotape presentation than suggested by Spreen and Gaddes. The data from both of these studies are presented in Table 11–21.

Table 11–21. Sentence Repetition Test Means and *SD*: A Comparison of Two Studies

	CARMICHAEL & MacDONALD DATA									SPREEN AND GADDES DATA								
	MALES			FEMALES			ALL			MALES			FEMALES			ALL		
Age	*N*	*M*	*SD*	*N*	*M*	*SD*	*N*	*M*	*SD*	*N*	*M*	*SD*	*N*	*M*	*SD*	*N*	*M*	*SD*
3	20	5.2	2.7	23	6.4	3.0	43	5.8	2.9									
4	28	8.9	2.0	28	8.7	1.8	56	8.8	1.9									
5	54	9.0	2.7	60	9.0	2.6	114	9.0	2.7									
6	59	10.9	3.0	52	10.9	2.6	111	10.9	2.8	22	9.3	.9	30	9.3	2.0	52	9.3	1.6
7	45	12.4	3.1	57	12.3	2.6	102	12.3	2.8	27	9.5	2.2	24	10.5	1.7	51	10.0	2.0
8	67	13.3	3.1	50	13.4	2.9	117	13.3	3.0	25	14.8	1.5	23	11.2	1.1	48	11.5	1.3
9	57	14.4	2.5	44	14.7	2.2	101	14.6	2.4	23	11.9	.9	30	11.5	2.5	53	11.7	2.0
10	53	14.7	2.9	41	14.4	3.5	94	14.5	3.2	25	12.5	1.4	25	12.6	1.6	50	12.5	1.5
11	48	15.8	2.5	62	15.8	2.5	110	15.8	2.5	22	13.3	1.8	22	13.1	1.7	44	13.2	1.7
12	51	17.0	3.2	47	16.6	3.2	98	16.8	3.2	13	13.7	1.4	13	13.5	2.4	26	13.6	1.9
13										17	13.8	1.6	12	13.9	1.2	29	13.8	1.4

Adapted from Carmichael & MacDonald (1984) and Spreen and Gaddes (1969).

Table 11–22. Multilingual Aphasia Examination Sentence Repetition Means and SDs

Mean Age	N	Grade	Mean	SD
6.3	35	K	7.0	1.5
7.3	34	1	7.2	1.5
8.2	32	2	8.3	1.5
9.3	43	3	9.0	1.7
10.2	33	4	8.9	1.5
11.3	31	5	9.7	2.0
12.3	21	6	9.6	1.9

Source: Schum, Sivan and Benton (1989), © Swets & Zeitlinger.

Multilingual Aphasia Examination: Sentence Repetition

The Multilingual Aphasia Examination (MAE) sentence repetition subtest (Schum, Sivan et al., 1989) has two equivalent forms available, each consisting of 14 sentences from 3 to 18 words in length. The total score is the sum of each score of 1 for correct repetitions, with 0 recorded for sentences containing any error. Misarticulation is disregarded in scoring. The directions are, "I will say some sentences. Listen carefully and when I have finished, repeat the sentence exactly as I have said it. Remember, do not begin until I have given you the whole sentence."

The sentences for Form I and II are below. The normative data by grade are presented in Table 11–22, and the percentiles for children for grades K through 6 are presented in Table 11–23. Additional normative data for 65 teenagers in grades 7 and 8 were collected, and these unpublished data are presented in Table 11–24, courtesy of Steven Zorich and Kerry Hamsher.

Form I

1. Take this home
2. Where is the child?
3. The car will not run
4. Why are they not living here?
5. The band played and the crowd cheered
6. Where are you going to work next summer?
7. He sold his house and they moved to the farm
8. Work in the garden until you have picked all the beans
9. The artist painted many of the beautiful scenes in this valley
10. This doctor does not travel to all the towns in the country
11. He should be ale to tell us exactly when she will be performing here
12. Why do members of that group never write to their representatives for aid?
13. Many men and women were not able to get to work because of the severe snow storm
14. The members of the committee have agreed to hold their meeting on the first Tuesday of each month

Form II

1. They never work
2. Who is not here?

Table 11–23. Multilingual Aphasia Examination Sentence Repetition–Percentiles for Children by Grade

Score	K	1	2	3	4	5	6	Score
15								15
14						99	99	14
13					99	95	95	13
12				99	95	90	90	12
11			99	96	90	85	85	11
10		99	95	80	70	65	65	10
9	99	90	85	60	60	45	40	9
8	80	80	60	40	40	35	30	8
7	60	50	25	15	20	15	10	7
6	35	35	5	5	5	5	5	6
5	20	10	1	1	1	1	1	5
4	4	1						4
3	1							3

Source: Schum, Sivan and Benton (1989), © Swets & Zeitlinger.

Table 11–24. Multilingual Aphasia Examination Sentence Repetition Normative data: 7th and 8th Grade

Age	N	Grade	Mean	SD
13	32	7	9.9	1.6
14	33	8	10.4	1.8

Source: Unpublished data: Courtesy of Steven Zorich and Kerry Hamsher.

3. He asked but they refused
4. Give that dirty dog a bath
5. The child is playing in his room
6. He will come when the bell rings
7. Will you send some to all the people on this list?
8. Put all your problems behind you during this time of joy
9. The birds were carried to the south but they found their way back
10. You must be sure that you understand the rules which they have made.
11. Which one of those three horses is not going to be entered in the next race?
12. She no longer brings her class of young artists to the museum with her
13. Will the winner of the contest go up on the stage to receive the trophy?
14. My mother wants a loaf of bread, a pound of cheese and two quarts of milk

Other Word and Sentence Memory Tests

As noted above, the Wide Range Assessment of Memory and Learning (see Table 11–25) and the NEPSY also include sentence memory subtests. The Das-Naglieri Cognitive Assessment System (CAS) has a 20-item subtest with sentences composed of color words to reduce "simultaneous" processing and emphasize the serial relationships among words and the use of syntax, such as "the red is greening." The Das-Naglieri CAS also includes a Word Series 27-item subtest that has nine single-syllable, high-frequency words. It requires the child to listen to a series of 2 to 9 words, read at a rate of 1 word per second, and repeat the words in the exact serial order. A Recalling Sentences subtest is also included in the Clinical Evaluation of Language Fundamentals (3rd ed.) battery (Semel, Wiig et al., 1995).

Table 11–25. WRAML Sentence Memory Raw Scores for Average Range

Age	Scaled Score of 10	Scaled Score 8 to 11
5.0–5.5	9	6–11
5.6–5.11	10–11	8–12
6.0–6.5	11–12	9–13
6.6–6.11	12–13	10–14
7.0–7.5	14	11–15
7.6–7.11	15	11–17
8.0–8.5	15–16	12–17
8.6–8.11	16–17	13–18
9.0–9.5	17–18	14–19
9.6–9.11	18–19	15–21
10.0–10.5	18–19	15–21
10.6–10.11	20	17–22
11.00–11.5	20–21	17–23
11.6–11.11	21	17–23
12.0–12.05	22	18–24
12.6–12.11	21–22	18–24
13.0–13.5	22–23	18–25
13.6–13.11	23	19–25
14.0–14.11	23–24	20–26
15.0–15.11	23–24	20–26
16.0–17.11	24–25	20–26

Source: Adapted from Shelslow & Adams (1990).

Paired Associate Learning

Paired associate learning (PAL) has been examined in children to a lesser degree than in adults. It is another way to assess verbal memory, with only a small amount of the variance accounted for by linguistic abilities (Halperin, Healey et al., 1989). In a study of 240 6- to 12-year-old children, the Wechsler Memory Scale (Wechsler, 1945) PAL subtest was administered along with other language tests. Girls performed better than boys for easy, but not hard, paired associates. Rather than performance increasing with age as with some other tests in this study, performance reached a plateau quickly, by 9 years old, and a clear developmental curve was not found (Halperin, Healey et al., 1989). Table 11–26 presents mean scores for easy and hard associations, and total correct by age.

It has been suggested that episodic memory information is unorganized, requiring deliberate or conscious effort to access its content (i.e., low associate pairs) and that information in semantic memory is organized and content is accessed more automatically (i.e., high associate

Table 11–26. Paired Associate Learning Normative Data

Age	N	EASY		HARD		TOTAL SCORE	
		Mean	SD	M	SD	M	SD
6	34	14.53	2.0	6.44	2.7	13.71	3.2
7	40	15.60	1.9	7.53	2.2	15.33	2.8
8	38	15.74	1.9	7.53	2.6	15.40	3.33
9	44	16.98	1.1	8.66	2.2	17.15	2.5
10	38	16.76	1.1	7.84	2.6	16.17	2.8
11	36	16.50	1.6	8.19	2.2	16.44	2.6
12	10	17.00	1.1	7.80	1.6	16.30	1.9

Source: Halperin et al. (1989), © Swets & Zeitlinger.

pairs) (Tulving, 1983). An adult normative study of the meaningfulness of observed differences between Wechsler Memory Scale I high-associate and low-associate scores was conducted, and a difference of 15 to 16 points was found to be exceedingly rare (des Rosiers and Ivison, 1986). The study was intended to emphasize the importance of looking at the two conditions independently, due to their potential utility with respect to the two different aspects of memory functioning.

Wechsler Memory Scale-Revised Logical Memory

As noted above, paragraph recall tests involve retention of meaningful stimuli, have inherent organization and less demand for active semantic processing than list learning tests. The Wechsler Memory Scale-Revised Logical Memory subtest (Paniak, Murphy et al., 1998) along with the Visual Reproduction subtest (Wechsler, 1987) were administered to 714 9- to 15-year-old Canadian children. The demographic data are presented in Table 11–27 and the normative data are presented in Table

Table 11–27. Wechsler Memory Scale-Revised: Paniak et al. Study (1988)

Subjects: 714 children in Edmonton, Canada
Age: 9–15 years old
Gender: 326 male and 388 female
Handedness: Not specified
Race: Not specified
SES: Not specified
Inclusion Criteria: Screened for biasing neurological, behavioral, and linguistic issues

11–28, i.e., means, standard deviations and percent savings scores.

Story Recall

Story Recall is a verbal, short-term memory test in which the child must recall two stories modified from the Luria Neuropsychological Test Battery (Christensen, 1979). The child tells each story in his or her own words. Each story is divided into 22 chunks, and a point is given each correct chunk recalled or 0.5 point for partial recall. Normative data for 391 Australian children aged 7 to 13 were collected for Story A recall, Story B recall, Story A and B recall, Delayed Story A recall, Delayed Story B recall, and Delayed Story A and B recall, i.e., number of story segments recalled for each condition. These data are presented as means and standard deviations in Table 11–29.

NONVERBAL LEARNING AND MEMORY

Nonverbal learning and memory tests include those that require drawing. They include the Wechsler Memory Scale-Revised Visual Reproduction subtest, the Benton Visual Retention Test, the Rey-Osterrieth Complex Figure Test, and the Extended Complex Figure Test. Those that do not require a visuomotor response include the Continuous Recognition Memory Test, the Nonverbal Selective Reminding Test, and the Biber Figural Learning Test, the latter a test for adults but of potential interest to the reader and therefore described below.

Table 11–28. Wechsler Memory Scale-Revised Means, *SD*s and Percentiles: Paniak et al. Data

Age		LM I	LM II	LMII/I%	VRI	VR II	VR II/I%
				WMS-R VARIABLE			
9	M	19.7	17.3	88.0	29.3	23.8	81.6
	SD	7.7	7.6	21.2	4.3	6.1	18.0
	5%	6.0	6.0	57.3	20.0	14.1	47.8
	16%	11.0	8.1	72.0	26.0	18.1	65.5
	50%	20.0	18.0	88.9	30.0	24.0	81.6
	84%	27.8	24.0	103.5	34.0	29.0	99.7
	95%	34.8	30.0	116.3	36.9	33.9	107.2
10	M	21.2	18.6	86.6	29.8	26.3	88.8
	SD	7.3	7.5	14.5	4.3	5.5	16.8
	5%	9.0	7.0	56.4	22.0	17.0	61.3
	16%	14.0	11.0	72.1	25.0	21.0	72.4
	50%	21.0	18.0	87.6	30.0	27.0	89.2
	84%	29.0	27.0	100.0	34.0	31.0	103.8
	95%	34.9	31.0	109.4	37.0	34.0	115.0
11	M	23.2	20.2	86.4	31.2	27.1	87.0
	SD	7.4	6.9	13.3	4.7	5.8	15.0
	5%	11.0	9.0	59.6	23.0	17.6	61.6
	16%	16.0	13.0	73.0	27.0	22.0	70.4
	50%	23.0	20.0	87.8	31.0	28.0	88.5
	84%	31.0	27.0	100.0	36.0	33.0	100.0
	95%	36.0	31.4	104.9	38.0	36.0	110.6
12	M	24.9	22.3	89.5	33.3	30.7	92.4
	SD	6.8	6.8	11.6	3.6	4.5	11.1
	5%	14.0	12.0	70.3	26.2	22.6	72.5
	16%	17.0	15.0	80.0	30.0	26.8	81.3
	50%	25.0	21.0	89.7	33.0	31.0	94.6
	84%	32.0	30.0	100.0	37.0	35.0	103.0
	95%	35.0	33.0	106.6	39.0	37.8	107.7
13	M	25.3	22.2	86.7	34.4	31.4	91.1
	SD	6.9	6.9	12.5	3.3	5.1	11.9
	5%	13.0	9.8	60.8	27.8	21.0	65.1
	16%	18.0	14.5	76.8	31.0	25.0	80.0
	50%	25.0	23.0	87.2	35.0	32.0	94.2
	84%	33.0	29.0	100.0	38.0	37.4	102.7
	95%	38.0	34.2	103.7	39.0	38.0	103.9
14	M	27.8	24.7	88.3	35.5	33.7	94.5
	SD	6.4	6.8	11.3	2.6	3.8	9.1
	5%	16.8	13.8	69.4	30.8	25.8	78.0
	16%	21.0	18.0	77.4	32.6	30.0	85.2
	50%	28.0	25.0	88.7	36.0	34.0	97.1
	84%	34.4	31.0	100.0	38.0	37.4	102.7
	95%	38.2	36.2	104.8	39.0	38.0	106.1
15	M	28.8	25.6	87.7	35.4	33.4	94.1
	SD	6.9	7.5	12.9	2.4	4.0	8.9
	5%	16.4	8.4	51.2	31.0	23.9	75.4
	16%	20.6	20.3	77.7	32.6	29.6	81.2
	50%	30.0	27.0	91.0	35.5	34.0	97.1
	84%	36.1	32.0	100.0	38.0	38.0	102.7
	95%	40.1	38.1	100.0	39.6	39.0	106.0

Source: Paniak et al. (1998), courtesy of Lawrence Erlbaum Associates.

Table 11–29. Story Recall Means (SDs)

					STORY RECALL		
Age	N	Story A	Story B	Story A & B	Delay Recall A	Delay Recall B	Delay A & B
7	56	9.95 (3.3)	11.71	21.65 (7.0)	8.88 (3.6)	11.32 (5.3)	20.21 (8.0)
8	56	11.50 (3.7)	13.29 (5.0)	24.20 (8.3)	10.34 (3.8)	12.88 (5.0)	23.21 (7.9)
9	61	12.29 (3.2)	26.95 (7.2)	26.95 (7.2)	11.37 (3.3)	14.96 (5.0)	26.32 (7.4)
10	62	13.30 (3.2)	29.66 (5.7)	29.66 (5.7)	12.64 (3.0)	16.03 (3.9)	28.30 (6.8)
11	51	13.98 (2.9)	31.63 (4.9)	31.63 (4.9)	12.56 (3.4)	11.93 (3.6)	13.50 (3.4)
12	54	12.84 (3.2)	29.15 (5.6)	29.15 (5.6)	11.93 (3.6)	16.21 (3.4)	17.59 (3.4)
13	51	13.90 (3.3)	31.32 (5.9)	31.32 (5.9)	13.50 (3.4)	17.59 (3.4)	31.09 (6.0)

Source: Unpublished manuscript (1995), courtesy of V. Anderson, G. Lajoie, and R. Bell.

As noted above, the many possible contributions to memory dysfunction need to be dissociated before a clinician can comfortably ascribe a memory disorder to a child. For example, there has been support for the notion that the degree of organization and of active executive strategizing at encoding were important determinants of recall ability for complex spatial information, and possibly, for memory functioning at a more general level. Recall of a complex two-dimensional nonrepresentational figure was significantly better for those normal young adults applying a prescribed organized strategy compared to those applying a prescribed disorganized strategy (Newman and Krikorian, 2001). Spatial information processing or IQ differences did not influence these results. The circumstances under which there is memory failure or intact function need to be evaluated, including any distinction evident across modalities.

Wechsler Memory Scale–Revised Visual Reproduction

The Wechsler Memory Scale-Revised Visual Reproduction (WMS-R VR) subtest requires the child to view a design for 10 seconds, and then immediately draw the design when it is removed (VR I). There are four designs. A delayed recall drawing of each design is requested approximately 30 minutes later (VR II). The WMS-R VR subtest (Paniak, Murphy et al., 1998) along with the Logical Memory subtest mean scores, SDs, and percent savings scores are presented in Table 11–28, and demographic data for the 714 9- to 15-year-old

Canadian children are presented in Table 11–27.

Benton Visual Retention Test (5th ed.)

The Benton Visual Retention Test (5th ed.) (BVRT; Benton, 1974; Sivan, 1992) assesses visuospatial perception, visuomotor and visuoconstructive abilities, and visual memory in persons 8 years old to adulthood. It also involves executive control due to its requirement for encoding design features (Sergent and Scholten, 1983). It is a test of immediate memory when design recall is requested immediately after design presentation (Administration A). It is sensitive to the effects of adult cerebral dysfunction due to disease, injury, and maldevelopment, and omission and size errors are prominent in these populations (Sivan, 1992). The BVRT correlates moderately with IQ (Benton, 1974), with correlations between BVRT and intelligence measures ranging from .46 to .71 (Sivan, 1992). Administration A performance increased from age 8, and reached a plateau at 14 to 15 years. The demographic data are presented in Table 11–30.

Table 11–30. Benton Visual Retention Test: Demographic Data for BVRT, Form C: Sivan Study (1992)

Subjects: 236 children in public schools in Iowa and Wisconsin
Age: 6 years, 6 months to 13 years, 5 months
Gender: No significant differences; data combined
Handedness: Not specified
Race: Not specified
Inclusion Criteria: Wechsler Full Scale IQ in range from 85–115

Table 11–31. Benton Visual Retention Test: Expected Number Correct Score by Age in Years

Estimated IQ	8	9	10	11	12	13–14
105 and >	4	5	6	7	8	8
95–104	3	4	5	6	7	7
80–94	2	3	4	5	6	7
70–79	1	2	3	4	5	6
69 and <	0	1	2	3	4	5

Source: Sivan (1992).

Normative standards were based on the performances of over 600 adults and children with the following restrictions: *(a)* no evidence or history of psychosis; *(b)* with the exception of the mentally defective subjects, no evidence of cerebral injury or disease; *(c)* no serious physical depletion as a consequence of somatic disease. A majority of the children were tested at schools in Iowa City and Des Moines, Iowa. Normative data found the BVRT to be less discriminatory for children than adults but still of clinical utility, with 15% of normal children falling within borderline or defective limits compared to the 55% of children with cerebral injury who fall within these ranges (Sivan, 1992).

There are three parallel forms of comparable difficulty, Forms C, D, and E (Sivan, 1992). The test is standardized for four administration procedures. Administration A is commonly selected. This procedure requires the child to view each of 10 stimulus pictures of one or more geometric forms for 10 seconds, and then to draw the designs immediately after the stimulus picture is withdrawn. Administration B is the same as Administration A but allows only 5 seconds viewing before immediate repro-

duction. Administration C allows the person to draw the design while it remains in view. This is especially useful when very poor performance leads to concern about a visuoconstructional deficit or impaired visual acuity (Benton, 1955). Administration D presents the stimulus design for 10 seconds; after a 15-second delay the reproduction is requested. There are no recognition trials. Intrerater reliabiity is high ($r = .95$ to $.97$).

The designs are scored for *(1)* number of entirely correct productions (1–10), and, *(2)* number of errors totaled across all 10 stimuli, including errors of omission, distortion, perseveration, misplacement, rotation, and size. Errors can also be examined with respect to right or left hemifield patterns, with the assumption made of contralateral cerebral hemisphere dysfunction. Interpretation is based on comparison of observed and expected (based on estimated premorbid IQ) performance, with a 2-point difference raising a question of disability and a 3-point or greater difference suggestive of such disability (Sivan, 1991). Normative data for number correct are presented in Table 11–31 and for number of errors in Table 11–32.

Table 11–32. Benton Visual Retention Test: Expected Number Error Score by Age in Years

Estimated IQ	8	9	10	11	12	13–14
105 and >	8–9	7–8	6	5	4	3
95–104	10–11	9–10	7–8	6	5	4
80–94	12–13	11–12	9	7–8	6	5
70–79	14	13	10–11	9	7–8	6–7
69 and <	15	14	12	10	9	8

Source: Sivan (1992).

Rey-Osterrieth Complex Figure Test and its Derivations

The Rey-Osterrieth Complex Figure Test (ROCFT) is a constructional copying test that also measures visual organizational skill, general planning ability, and memory for complex visual information when delay recall trials are included (Rey, 1941; Osterrieth, 1944; see Corwin and Bylsma, 1993 for an English translation). The ROCFT is an especially useful clinical test for both adults and children, given its many cognitive demands. Interpretation of test performance is complicated for these same reasons and because the test crosses domains of attention, executive function, visuomotor, visuoperceptual, and visuospatial function, and learning and memory. Because it is a "drawing" test and one that employs colored pens that are attractive to children, I find it a useful test to administer early (see Chapter 4). This test produces a great deal of information and raises various hypotheses that can be further assessed as the test session progresses.

Intelligence has been found to be a moderator variable in adult studies, with the visuospatial demands of the ROCFT copy trial more salient for those with high average or better intelligence and the organizational demands more salient for those with average intelligence or lower (Fujii, Lloyd et al., 2000). However, IQ was not determinant of performance in samples of children with learning disabilities (Waber and Bernstein, 1995; Kirkwood, Weiler et al., 2001). The diversity of explanations for poor performance makes the ROCFT a valuable test, but a complex one to interpret. One must dissociate which component process contributes most to a poor performance, that is, whether memory disorder or executive dysfunction underlies problematic production. It has been suggested that the diversity of component processes may detract from the ability to implicate EF as sufficiently explanatory (Tranel, Anderson et al., 1994). The ROCFT test procedures are useful for a wide variety of child clinical populations, including autism (Prior and Hoffmann, 1990) and dyslexia (Klicpera, 1983), and are very useful in evaluating the organizational style, copy performances, and recall ability of all children.

Administration

The ROCFT has no administration time limits, but time may be monitored for additional qualitative appraisal. Common administration procedure involves the subject's sequential use of colored pens or pencils to enable the examiner's later inspection of organizational style. Number of colors and time per color vary by procedure. The color order recommended by Bernstein and Waber (Bernstein and Waber, 1996) is green, blue, black, yellow, red. Their recommended time intervals per color are 60 seconds for 5 to 7 years (Kindergarten–Grade 2), 45 seconds for 8- to 11-years-old (Grade 3–6), and 30 seconds for 12- to 14-years-old (Grade 7 and higher). They do allow for examiner judgment of an appropriate time interval that will make it likely that all colors are used.

Various administration procedures are also followed. This has made comparing research studies difficult and has also affected selection of normative data. Some examiners administer the copy trial, wait 3 minutes, and administer a short-term recall. Others administer the copy trial, request an immediate recall without interference, and request a delayed recall approximately 20 to 30 minutes later, after intervening verbal tasks. This step is considered an incidental recall since the subject is unaware that a delayed recall will be elicited. Thus, any reevaluation with this design, or an alternative form, may no longer be considered a measure of incidental recall. Still other clinicians choose to obtain a copy performance and a delayed recall drawing, without an immediate recall or short-term recall production. Selectively, some choose to test recognition for structural elements after assessing delayed memory retrieval capacity.

Some examiners present the subject with an $8\frac{1}{2}'' \times 11''$ sheet of paper on which the Rey-Osterrieth figure is printed on the top half; the subject is then asked to copy the form on the bottom half of the page. This procedure is not recommended. The figure should be placed above the empty sheet of paper, and the child should have a full page in which to produce his or her drawing.

Alternate Designs

In view of the likelihood of strong practice effects should retesting be necessary, along with an average 10% improvement in percent recall scores (Spreen and Strauss, 1998), an alternate figure is recommended for retesting. However, even with alternate designs, the delayed recall performance can improve, irrespective of which design is given first (Hubley and Tremblay, 2002). The Taylor Complex Figure is a common alternative that has been judged comparable to the ROCF for copy performance, but less difficult than the ROCF for memory in young adults (Strauss and Spreen, 1990; Peirson and Jansen, 1997). Some suggest the Taylor figure is more susceptible to verbal mediation, however, than the ROCF (Casey, Winner et al., 1991) and is encoded more efficiently than the ROCF by adults (Tombaugh and Hubley, 1991), is easier to organize (Hamby, Wilkins et al., 1993), and recalled with greater accuracy and in less time (Peirson and Jansen, 1997). Copy time required is believed to be relatively equivalent between the ROCFT and Taylor figure test (Tombaugh and Hubley, 1991). Thus, comparability of the two designs remains questionable.

In an attempt to provide an improved alternate complex figure, a modification of the Taylor figure was constructed along with an 18-unit scoring system that scores for accuracy and position for a maximum 36 points, as is standard for the Taylor scoring method (see below). The new design was studied in adults from 17 to 41 years (mean = 21 years), with the result that comparability was found (Hubley and Tremblay, 2002). No significant differences were found between the two figures for copy, immediate recall, or delayed recall total score when the designs were administered to different subjects using a common incidental memory procedure. Nor were differences for learning, immediate recall, or delayed recall total score found for different groups of subjects using an intentional procedure or for the same subjects one week apart in counterbalanced order and with an intentional learning procedure. Other recommendations for equivalent figures from the adult literature include the figures developed at the Medical College of Georgia (Meador, Loring et al., 1991) and the Mack Complex Figure Test (Frazier, Adams et al., 2001).

Such investigations must be interpreted cautiously for child populations as data and conclusions reached in adult studies may not apply similarly to children. For example, in contrast to adult comparability studies, a study of comparability with ADHD and normal child populations found no differences between the ROCFT and Taylor designs, for copy, immediate recall, or 20-minute recall (Sadeh, Ariel et al., 1996). It should be noted that these authors employed an intentional learning paradigm rather than the more common incidental learning paradigm. That is, they informed subjects about the memory trial on the first testing to make test and retest conditions equivalent and eliminate the influence of the subject's anticipation of a second session memory trial. This procedure was recommended for test–retest situations due to the subject's tendency to utilize a different encoding strategy during retest copy performance under standard procedures than used in the initial copy trial (Tombaugh and Hubley, 1991).

Standard ROCFT administration was compared to a structured format for encoding that highlighted the design's organizational framework in a study of 202 children referred for learning disabilities (Kirkwood, Weiler et al., 2001). The authors found the metacognitive assistive encoding procedure aided recall for most children, but not for those who had visuoorganizational, perceptual impairment. These results were of particular interest as an explanation for prior data showing learning-disabled children exhibiting limited improvement on the ROCFT from age 8 into adolescence (Waber and Bernstein, 1995). These results also supported the *dynamic assessment* literature that encourages a practitioner to determine what enables the child to perform successfully as a means of determining which cognitive processes are not fully operational rather than focusing on the traditional level of difficulty approach that seeks to determine when performance breaks down.

Qualitative Interpretation

Quantitative scoring methods are increasingly supplemented by an appreciation for the qualitative characteristics that are both useful and discriminative between populations such as those with right cerebral hemisphere dysfunction, bilateral lesions, temporal lobe epilepsy, or dementia. The literature suggests those with right cerebral dysfunction have a characteristic tendency to distort the image, make alignment errors, and fail to include elements in the left hemispace (Binder, 1982). Left hemisphere dysfunction tends to result in segmental strategies, divided configural elements, loss of the Gestalt or whole, and fragmentation (Binder, 1982). Frontal lesion patients are prone to repeat elements or perseverate, convert nonrepresentational elements into recognizable objects, add to the drawing, or omit important features. Temporal lobe epilepsy studies report recall distortion errors. Schizophrenic patients may insert bizarre elements.

In one study, an analysis of qualitative aspects for 750 normal subjects, aged 4 to 8, was conducted from a systematized registration of possible copy and memory errors. The frequency of the different types of errors in each of the nine units was calculated for each age group, and results were presented in percentiles for their psychometric handling. This was done so that the qualitative parameters that determine quality of execution in relation to the child's population remained established in order to know in which particular aspect his execution deviated from the norm (Salvador, Cortes et al., 1997).

Validity Data

A study of construct validity with adolescents found copy and delayed recall scores loaded on a visuospatial factor (Poulton and Moffitt, 1995), consistent with adult construct validity studies. These authors also reported strong correlation ($r = .49$) with the WISC-R performance scale, with block design and object assembly subtests accounting for most of the variance. Concurrent validity was examined in a recent study, with 6- to 11-year-old children (Demsky, Carone et al., 2000). The authors found better performance on both the Beery and ROCF tests across groups of increasing age, and considerable shared variance for children who took both tests. They also found that race and sex were not significantly related to either test. Independent correlational analyses indicated there were no significant differences among the correlations between test scores by age. Validity was also examined in a study of

brain-injured children (Matthews, Anderson et al., 2001). The diagnostic utility of the ROCFT was supported for brain injured children. Children with generalized damage had poor results on three measures: accuracy, recall and organizational strategy variables derived from the ROCF. These data were interpreted as evidence of global cognitive impairment. Children with frontal lesions had reduced organizational strategy scores, and productions were fragmented and poorly planned. The scores of children with temporal lesions were similar to those of the control subjects on accuracy and strategic process, but their recall scores were impaired.

Developmental Trends

Analyses in the child literature are tempered by the need to consider developmental trends. In one study, children between 6- and 9-years-old tended to break the figure into simple components, but figure integration and drawing of larger portions (e.g., halves, quadrants) improved with age, with an advanced copying strategy and organization around the core rectangle evident at age 12. The younger children demonstrated a similar pattern of performance when copying the main features of the ROCF in isolation from the full design. The authors suggested that children adopt strategies proven successful when they were younger when faced with tasks requiring more advanced types of spatial analysis. Their youngest children had a variety of spatial analytic strategies available, but used a strategy that was a function of pattern complexity and the child's capabilities (Akshoomoff and Stiles, 1995).

Scoring Systems

Different scoring systems exist, and some of the more common appropriate for children are mentioned here. The quantitative E. M. Taylor scoring method (Taylor, 1959) was adapted from Osterrieth (Osterrieth, 1944) and is commonly used, especially as it is the most simple. Each drawing is scored for each of 18 configural elements. A 0.0 to 2.0 point value is assigned for each element for a maximum total of 36 points for each drawing. The Osterrieth scoring system and E. M. Taylor scoring modification were subsequently published (Lezak,

1983). While more stringent scoring criteria are described explicitly for both the original ROCFT figure and the alternate L. B. Taylor Complex Figure, (Spreen and Strauss, 1998, pp. 350–351), child normative studies often use the earlier E. M. Taylor scoring (Sadeh, Ariel et al., 1996; Demsky, Carone et al., 2000). However, the L. B. Taylor scoring criteria were used in a study of Canadian children 6 to 15 years old (see Table 11–33). A clinically useful savings score calculation is easily made with either method to interpret retention of stimulus material independent of initial copy accuracy and proficiency: (Recall Score/Copy Score × 100), although child normative data often omit this useful calculation.

Scoring Hemi-inattention

A scoring system for assessing hemi-inattention in adults adapted the E. M. Taylor scoring system (Rapport, Dutra et al., 1995). For this method, in addition to the standard total scores, each Rey was assigned four additional scores. Rey Omissions-Left (ROL) and Rey Omissions-Right (ROR) were the number of omitted items identified as belonging to the left and right hemispace, respectively. Scoring items 2, 3, 4, and 5 were not included since they were at midline or assigned to both sides. Rey Quality-Left (RQL) and Rey Quality-Right

(RQR) were accuracy scores for the average number of points per item obtained for items attempted on the left and right, respectively.

Developmental Scoring System

The organizational method employed is of interest as a measure of EF, that is, planning, strategy, and decision making, and some scoring procedures provide a structured way to assess organizational style. One scoring system emphasizes both developmental trajectory and organizational skill, the Developmental Scoring System for the Rey-Osterrieth Complex Figure (Bernstein and Waber, 1996). The ROCF productions are scored for four components: organization, accuracy, style, and mistakes. This system emphasizes development of visual integration capacity and de-emphasizes accuracy of detail (Waber and Holmes, 1985; Waber and Holmes, 1986; Bernstein and Waber, 1996). The organization scoring approach relies heavily on graphomotor skill precision (Sadeh, Ariel et al., 1996), and thus places children with graphomotor difficulties at a disadvantage. The organization score from the copy condition of the R-O is considered a measure of EF (Waber and Holmes, 1985). Organization was also the focus of other investigators (Anderson, Anderson et al., 2001). Comparison of qualitative scoring systems was also reported (Troyer and Wishart, 1997).

Boston Qualitative Scoring System

The Boston Qualitative Scoring System (BQSS) (Stern, Singer et al., 1994; Stern, Javorsky et al., 1999) was developed for children, adolescents and adults. It allows for calculation of qualitative scores across the lifespan and for scoring variables of interest for a specific population so that one may tailor the focus of interest for a child or population group. Unlike the developmental scoring system that emphasizes features relevant to the developing child, the BQSS scores were designed to be applicable to the full age range—adolescents and adults as well as children. Scores are obtained for 17 dimensions: configural presence, configural accuracy, cluster presence, cluster accuracy, cluster placement, detail presence, detail placement, fragmentation, planning, reduction, vertical expansion, horizontal expan-

Table 11–33. Rey-Osterrieth Complex Figure Test Means and SDs: L. Taylor Scoring

		REY-OSTERRIETH COMPLEX FIGURE TEST NORMS: KOLB AND WHISHAW			
Age	N	Copy Score	SD	30-min Recall	SD
6	192	16.66	7.97	10.53	5.80
7	353	21.29	7.67	13.57	6.28
8	347	23.64	8.00	16.34	6.77
9	329	24.46	6.94	18.71	6.61
10	301	27.20	7.58	19.73	6.71
11	280	28.61	7.31	22.59	6.65
12	225	30.21	6.69	23.20	6.38
13	237	32.63	4.35	24.59	6.29
14	180	33.53	3.18	26.24	5.40
15	116	33.60	2.98	26.00	6.35

Source: Adapted from Spreen and Strauss (1998); Kolb and Whishaw (1990).

sion, rotation, perseveration, confabulation, neatness, and asymmetry. A set of criteria, templates, and exemplary productions assist in scoring. The scores assess qualitative features and the processes employed in producing the figure. The BQSS was part of a study of normal children (Akshoomoff and Stiles, 1995) and of children with ADHD (Cahn, Marcotte et al., 1996). Its usefulness as a measure of executive function has begun to be empirically documented (Somerville, Tremont et al., 2000).

Rey Complex Figure Test and Recognition Trial

Another scoring system that uses a 36-point system extends normative data through adolescence and into adulthood, the Rey Complex Figure Test and Recognition Trial (RCFT). This administration version also includes a recognition trial immediately after the delayed recall trial that includes details taken from the Taylor figure as foils. Norms are available for 505 children and adolescents, in 6-month increments from 6 to 8 years, and yearly through 18 years (Meyers and Meyers, 1996). Test–retest reliability is reported to be .76 to .89, and interrater reliability ranged from .93 to .99.

Normative Data

Normative data for 2560 6- to 15-year-old Canadian children using the L. B. Taylor scoring criteria for a copy trial and a 30-minute delayed recall trial were previously published (Spreen and Strauss, 1998) and are presented in Table 11–33.

Local Southern U.S. norms for the ROCF with group administration procedures and using the scoring approach of E. M. Taylor (1959), including standard scores, were reported for 432 children aged 6 to 11 (Demsky, Carone et al., 2000). The demographic data for this sample are presented in Table 11–34, the normative data in Table 11–36, and a table of standard score norms in Table 11–35.

Copy and delay normative data under individual administration conditions have been reported (Spreen and Strauss, 1998). It has been common to refer to Osterrieth's original ROCFT normative data for subjects 16 years old and older. These data were normed on populations 16 to 60 years old. The percentile

Table 11–34. Rey-Osterrieth Complex Figure Test: Demsky et al. study (2000)

Subjects: 432 children from urban public school in southern United States
Age: 6 to 11 years old (see distribution in Table 36)
Gender: 204 boys; 228 girls
Race/Ethnicity: 242 White, 50 Black, 117 Hispanic, 23 Others
SES: Household median income of $35, 942/year
Inclusion/Exclusion Criteria: not specified

norms for the copy trial are presented in Table 11–37, and the percentile norms for the recall drawings in Table 11–38.

Special Population Data: Rey-Osterrieth and Deaf Children

Special child populations require that additional caution be applied in the interpretation of neuropsychological test results and the acceptance of available norms. Often, population-specific normative data are not available for these children, and a clinical judgment must be made about the validity of existing data for the child. In such instances, one must consider the possibility of different functional organization, such as for those with sensory impairment (Kammerer, Gardner et al., 1988).

In some instances, neuropsychological data for a special population are reported. For example, a study of the ROCF drawings of deaf children with different etiologies of deafness was presented (Kammerer, Gardner et al., 1988). The authors adopted the Waber and Holmes scoring method, looking at organization level and style (Waber and Holmes, 1985). The children first copied the ROCF and then reproduced the design from memory after 15 minutes. Demographic data for these profoundly or severely prelingually deaf children fluent in American Sign Language with a mean hearing loss of 96.7 decibels are presented in Table 11–39. The at-risk group had a significantly lower mean IQ (103.53) than the "hereditary" group (115.27).

A distribution of subjects by organizational level found an expected progression of better performance at older ages, see Table 11–40. Memory production scores did not differ significantly between the deaf and hearing popu-

Table 11–35. Rey-Osterrieth Complex Figure Test: Standard Scores for Ages 6 to 11 years

STANDARD SCORES FOR THE REY-OSTERRIETH COMPLEX FIGURE TEST

Raw Score	AGE						Raw Score	AGE					
	6	7	8	9	10	11		6	7	8	9	10	11
36.0	143	145	139	132	127	129	18.0	104	97	92	89	79	71
35.5	142	144	137	131	126	128	17.5	103	95	91	87	78	69
35.0	141	142	136	130	124	126	17.0	102	94	90	86	76	68
34.5	140	141	135	129	123	124	16.5	101	92	88	85	75	66
34.0	139	140	134	128	122	123	16.0	100	91	87	84	74	64
33.5	137	138	132	126	120	121	15.5	99	90	86	82	72	63
33.0	136	137	131	125	119	119	15.0	98	88	85	81	71	61
32.5	135	135	130	124	118	118	14.5	97	87	83	80	70	60
32.0	134	134	128	123	116	116	14.0	96	86	82	79	68	58
31.5	133	133	127	121	115	115	13.5	95	84	81	78	67	56
31.0	132	131	126	120	114	113	13.0	94	83	79	76	66	55
30.5	131	130	125	119	112	111	12.5	93	82	78	75	64	53
30.0	130	129	123	118	111	110	12.0	91	80	77	74	63	51
29.5	129	127	122	116	110	108	11.5	90	79	75	73	61	50
29.0	128	126	121	115	108	106	11.0	89	78	74	71	60	48
28.5	127	125	119	114	107	105	10.5	88	76	73	70	59	47
28.0	126	123	118	113	106	103	10.0	87	75	72	69	57	45
27.5	125	122	117	112	104	102	9.5	86	74	70	68	56	43
27.0	124	121	115	110	103	100	9.0	85	72	69	67	55	42
26.5	122	119	114	109	102	98	8.5	84	71	68	65	53	40
26.0	121	118	113	108	100	97	8.0	83	70	66	64	52	38
25.5	120	117	112	107	99	95	7.5	82	68	65	63	51	37
25.0	119	115	110	106	98	94	7.0	81	67	64	62	49	35
24.5	118	114	109	104	96	92	6.5	80	66	63	60	48	34
24.0	117	113	108	103	95	90	6.0	79	64	61	59	47	32
23.5	116	111	106	102	94	89	5.5	78	63	60	58	45	30
23.0	115	110	105	101	92	87	5.0	76	62	59	57	44	29
22.5	114	109	104	100	91	85	4.5	75	60	57	56	43	27
22.0	113	107	103	98	89	84	4.0	74	59	56	54	41	25
21.5	112	106	101	97	88	82	3.5	73	58	55	53	40	24
21.0	111	105	100	96	87	81	3.0	72	56	54	52	39	22
20.5	110	103	99	95	86	79	2.5	71	55	52	51	37	21
20.0	109	102	97	93	84	77	2.0	70	53	51	50	36	19
19.5	107	101	96	92	83	76	1.5	69	52	50	48	35	17
19.0	106	99	95	91	82	74	1.0	68	51	48	47	33	16
18.5	105	98	94	90	80	72	0.5	67	49	47	46	32	14

Source: Demsky, Y., Carone, D. A., Jr., Burns, W.J., & Sellers, A. Assessment of visual-motor coordination in 6- to 11-yr. olds. *Perceptual and Motor Skills, 91,* 311–321 © Perceptual and Motor Skills 2000.

lations, nor between the hereditary and at-risk subgroups and their matched hearing control subjects. These normative data for the deaf and normative hearing sample are presented in Table 11–41. Comparisons of style scores and differences between the deaf and hearing found the deaf children showing a less differentiated style than control subjects reselected, based on age and level of organization. The figure-copying scores for deaf subjects were significantly below those of hearing subjects in both deaf subgroups, despite their average intelligence. Memory was not significantly different, attesting to accurate encoding. These data were interpreted to be consistent with the hypothesis of different processing systems.

The interested reader is referred to another paper for neuropsychological test results obtained on 7- to 17-year-old deaf children for the following measures: WISC-R Performance IQ

Table 11–36. Rey-Osterrieth Complex Figure
Test Means and SDs: Demsky et al. Data

		RAW SCORE		STANDARD SCORE	
Age	N	Mean	SD	Mean	SD
6	51	16.0	7.0	100.0	15.0
7	83	19.3	5.6	100.0	15.0
8	98	21.0	5.8	100.0	15.0
9	59	22.7	6.2	100.0	15.0
10	80	25.9	5.6	100.0	15.0
11	61	27.0	4.6	100.0	15.0

REY-OSTERRIETH COMPLEX FIGURE TEST

Source: Demsky, Y., Carone et al. Assessment of visual-
motor coordination in 6- to 11-yr. olds. *Perceptual and Motor Skills*, 2000, *91* 311–321 © Perceptual and Motor Skills
2000.

and scaled scores, Rey Auditory Verbal Learning Test, Hiskey Visual Attention Span Test,
Knox Cubes Test, Trail Making Test, Stroop
Color Word Test, ROCFT, Benton Line Orientation Test, and Beery Buktenica Developmental Test of Visual Motor Integration. Data
were also presented for a timed motor examination that included the Purdue Pegboard Test
and for two emotional/behavioral measures, the
Meadow Kendall Social Emotional Assessment
Inventory and the Conners Teacher Rating
Scale (Wolff, Kammerer et al., 1989). These authors concluded that many different cognitive
styles can subserve adaptive functioning and
that norms from the hearing population cannot
be routinely applied to the deaf.

Extended Complex Figure Test

The Extended Complex Figure Test (ECFT;
Fastenau and Manning, 1992; Fastenau and
Denburg, 1994; Fastenau, 1996) adds recognition and matching trials to the ROCFT. These
are administered following the standard copy,

immediate recall, and delayed recall trials. The
recognition memory trial requires the selection
of the true design element from among five
choices. The matching trial requires selection
of the element that looks exactly the same as
the target model before the subject. The
ECFT's development, pilot versions, revisions,
preliminary normative data, and clinical validation study are described (Fastenau, 1996).
Updated normative data for 211 adults using
30 recognition items for the Total Scale and
matching items for 10 of the 30 recognition
items along with data for the ROCF copy, immediate, and delayed recall trials were subsequently reported (Fastenau, Denburg et al.,
1999).

This extension was subsequently applied
to children, and there are now preliminary
developmental data for children aged 6 to 18
(Sasher and Fastenau, 2001). Demographic
data are presented in Table 11–42. The means
and SDs for the standard copy, immediate recall, and delayed recall appear to match up well
with other published studies, suggesting that
this sample is comparable and that the reference data for the Recognition and Matching
trials are representative (Philip Fastenau, 2002,
personal communication). These preliminary
ECFT data for children aged 6 to 18 are presented in Table 11–43 (note the especially
small cell size for the upper age ranges). The
authors found an increase in scores with age
for copy, immediate recall, delayed recall
($r = .48 - .67, p < 0.005$), recognition ($r = .55$,
$p < 0.005$), and matching ($r = .58, p < 0.005$),
but no significant gender differences. They
found recognition and matching improved
steadily until about age 13, when a plateau or
slight score decrease became evident. As predicted, matching correlated significantly with
copying ($r = .58, p < .0005$) and recognition
correlated significantly with free recall ($r =
.63-.66, p < .0005$). They concluded that these

Table 11–37. Percentile Norms: Adult Accuracy Scores on Rey-Osterrieth
Complex Figure Test-Copy Trial

Percentile	10	20	30	40	50	60	70	80	90	100
Score	29	30	31	32	32	33	34	34	35	36

Adapted from Osterrieth (1944).

Table 11–38. Percentile Norms: Adult Accuracy Scores on Rey-Osterrieth Complex Figure Test-Memory Trials

Percentile	10	20	30	40	50	60	70	80	90	100
Score	15	17	19	21	22	24	26	27	28	31

Adapted from Osterrieth (1944).

data supported the construct validity of the ECFT for use with younger children.

Continuous Recognition Memory Test and its Derivations

The Continuous Recognition Memory Test (CRMT) places minimal demand on verbal or visuomotor skill. It consists of a series of line drawings of familiar categories of living things, rather than the geometric or nonsense figures of other recognition memory tests. It was designed to be sensitive to memory and attentional deficits consequent to diffuse cerebral insult. Principal factor analysis study in adults supported the construct validity of CRMT hits as a measure of learning and memory and led to consideration that the false alarms are a measure of attention to visual detail rather than the expected divided attention factor (Fuchs, Hannay et al., 1999). The CRMT was not related to education level in adults (Hannay, Levin et al., 1979).

The test is based on signal detection theory, which assumes that the distribution of sensory input produced on noise-only trials (when new stimuli are presented) overlaps with the distribution of sensory input resulting from signal-plus noise trials (when old stimuli are presented). Therefore, the stimulus situation is ambiguous. Noise (new) stimuli should sometimes be easy and sometimes difficult to discriminate from signal-plus noise (old) stimuli, such that the subject will have difficulty deciding whether stimuli are from the noise distribution or from the signal plus noise distribution part of the time. The subject is assumed to set a response criterion (c) for making decisions about whether a stimulus is noise or signal plus noise. The stimulus situation is made ambiguous by creating some new stimuli that vary in their perceptual similarity to particular old stimuli (Hannay and Levin, 1989).

The CRMT (Hannay, Levin et al., 1979; Hannay and Levin, 1989) consists of 120 $5'' \times 7''$ cards (6 blocks of 20 cards), each containing a black-and-white line drawing of an animal or plant. Some of the drawings are included in the deck only a single time while others are repeated several times. The child's task is to recognize a recurring picture each time it occurs.

The order of administration is practice items, test stimuli and then discrimination stimuli. After practice and confirmation that the child understands the tasks, each test card is presented in sequence for up to 3 seconds. If the child takes more than 3 seconds to decide, the card is removed and the child asked to make a guess. The examiner should not en-

Table 11–39. Rey-Osterrieth Complex Figure Test: Kammerer Study

Subjects: 93 deaf children in Washington, DC region
Age: 7 to 17 years; Mean age = 12.63
IQ: 72 to 146; Mean = 107.59 (SD = 18.02)
Gender: N/A
Race or SES: N/A
Etiology Groups: 1) At-Risk = history of pre- or perinatal, or early childhood complications resulting in deafness; 2) Hereditary = family history, no known complications; 3) Unknown = no discernible etiology
Exclusion Criteria:

Table 11–40. Rey-Osterrieth Complex Figure Test Distribution of Children by Organizational Level: Kammerer et al. Data

Organization Level	N	Mean Age	Age Range
1	16	10.656	7.25–15.33
2	23	11.928	7.83–17.75
3	23	12.362	8.16–17.75
4	19	14.289	8.33–17.00
5	8	15.510	12.08–17.83

Source: Unpublished data courtesy of Betsy Kammerer.

Table 11–41. Deaf and Hearing Organizational Level Means and SD: Kammerer et al. Data

Age	DEAF POPULATION			HEARING NORMS	
	N	Mean	*SD*	Mean	*SD*
7	4	2.50	1.29	4.79	3.71
8	8	6.50	3.38	4.82	3.43
9	8	5.38	2.50	7.20	4.10
10	9	5.11	2.26	8.61	3.99
11	9	6.11	2.80	8.62	4.01
12	9	8.78	3.23	8.07	4.25
13	6	5.33	3.50	9.19	4.07
14	8	7.87	3.52	9.51	3.93
15	11	10.91	2.30		
16	8	9.25	2.96		
17	7	9.71	3.35		

Source: Unpublished data courtesy of Betsy Kammerer.

courage the child by indicating a response is correct. The instructions are:

I am going to show you a series of drawings. Look at each drawing carefully. I want you to tell me if it is a "new" drawing, one that I am showing you for the first time or an "old" drawing, a drawing *exactly* like one you've already seen in this deck of cards. Do you understand? I want you to call each of the drawings either "old" or "new." Since each drawing is presented for only 3 seconds, you must tell me if it is old or new right away.

Administration of practice items precedes test items. The test begins after making sure the child understands and can follow the instructions. The examiner can say, "Have I shown you this picture before?" if the new/old concept is not understood. Each response is recorded on the scoring sheet.

On Trial 40, say, "Be sure the picture is exactly like the one you have seen before in or-

der to call it old." If by Trial 60, the child does not understand the test (e.g., the child responds "old" for each item) then discontinue. Otherwise, continue to the end. Discrimination accuracy is assessed with eight printed pages, each with a different target stimulus at the top and a multiple-choice array at the bottom. The examiner asks, "Which one of these six pictures is exactly like the one at the top?" or adjusts this statement for age.

Scores obtained include the number of hits (the number of times an old item is called an old item on trials 21–120), the number of false alarms (the number of times a new item is called an old item on trials 21–120), and the total number of correct responses (hits + 60 minus false alarms). Trials 1–20 present 20 different designs, including the target designs that will recur. These trials are not scored.

Normative data for three age blocks of children (6, 8, and 10 years) are presented in Table 11–46, along with normative data for 13- to 18-year-old adolescents, obtained in a study of closed-head-injured adolescents that supported the efficacy of the test with this population (Hannay and Levin, 1989).

Table 11–42. Extended Complex Figure Test Demographic Data

Subjects: 76 children in grades 1–12 at 6 sites across the U.S.A.; 71% grades 1 to 6

Age: Mean = 10.1 years, Median = 9.0 years, SD = 3.3 years; 51% 6 to 9 years

Gender: 44 male (58%); 32 female (42%)

Race and SES: Not specified

Exclusion Criteria: Learning disability and mental retardation

Continuous Recognition Memory–Preschool

The Continuous Recognition Memory-Pre (CRM-Pre) was modeled after the CRMT of

Table 11–43. Extended Complex Figure Test Means and SD

		COPY		IMMEDIATE		DELAYED		RECOGNITION		MATCHING	
Age (Years)	N	M	SD	M	SD	M	SD	M	SD	M	SD
6 to 7	22	16.2	7.5	10.5	5.7	10.2	6.1	8.1	2.6	6.3	1.7
8 to 9	17	22.8	6.5	13.9	6.3	14.6	6.0	10.2	4.0	7.9	2.0
10 to 11	11	26.5	6.9	15.9	8.0	16.4	7.2	16.0	4.9	8.6	1.1
12 to 13	12	27.3	4.5	17.8	8.1	17.4	7.0	17.3	5.2	9.0	0.9
14 to 15	9	30.7	3.4	18.4	18.4	18.0	7.1	14.3	4.3	9.1	1.2
16 to 18	5	32.4	2.7	21.1	7.9	21.6	7.1	15.2	6.3	9.0	1.0

Hannay and Levin and designed to be sensitive to age and individual performance differences in very young children (Espy, McDiarmid et al., 2001). Verbal/semantic (animals) and nonverbal (spacemen) stimuli were utilized. The general procedures are similar to those described above for the adult and older-child versions. A 5-card preparatory session precedes the actual test items and is repeated as often as necessary until the child achieves complete accuracy on the training cards. Following practice, 78 task stimuli are presented at a rate of 2 per second. Included are 30 target stimuli (15 verbal and 15 nonverbal) and 18 distractors. Target stimuli are repeated once, after 1 to 5 other picture card presentations. Each delay interval has 6 intermixed stimuli (3 verbal and 3 nonverbal). Preliminary data were obtained on 49 preschool children recruited from local birth announcements and from three preschools in Illinois. The group consisted of 17 3 year olds, 15 4 year olds, and 17 5 year olds, 54% male and 46% female, and mostly Caucasian. Sex was equivalently distributed across ages. Mean maternal education was 17.6 years, and the children in this early study were from mostly upper-middle-class families. All children weighed more than 2500 grams at birth and had achieved developmental milestones at age-appropriate times. The CRM-Pre was found to be sensitive to performance differences across age groups, with an increasing number of correct responses observed with increasing age along with fewer false positives. Verbal–nonverbal response differences were restricted to children 3 years old. Minimal delay interval effects were found. Further empirical studies are needed to evaluate this test's usefulness with other socioeconomic status groups and for clinical populations, but it appears to have promise and adds to the limited number of memory measures appropriate for the younger ages. The initial data for performance by age group are presented in Table 11–44.

Brown-Scott Continuous Picture-Recognition Test

The Continuous Picture-Recognition Test procedure (Brown and Scott, 1971) was part of a

Table 11–44. Continuous Recognition Memory-Pre Means and SDs by Age

	3-YEARS OLD		4-YEARS OLD		5-YEARS OLD	
	M	SD	M	SD	M	SD
Correct	18.24	7.59	26.27	3.53	26.47	3.36
False Alarms	5.35	5.57	2.07	2.66	2.18	2.43

Source: Kimberly Espy et al. 2001, personal communication.

Table 11–45. Picture Recognition Normative Data

		NO. CORRECT	
Age	N	Mean	SD
3	10	93.2	6.58
4	10	97.4	1.84
5	10	97.4	1.71
6	10	98.0	1.49
7	10	97.5	2.92
8	10	98.4	.843
9	10	98.6	1.58
10	10	98.4	2.27
11	10	98.5	1.58
12	10	98.9	1.45

Source: Welsh et al, 1991, Courtesy of Lawrence Erlbaum Associates.

Total $n = 100$

study of prefrontal function in children (Welsh, Pennington et al., 1991). For the latter, 100 cards with pictures from four categories were presented to the child. The categories were Smurfs, animals, houses and people. Twenty-two cards appeared only once in the deck. Eighty-eight cards were presented a second time and these were separated from the initial presentation by 0, 5, 10, 25, or 50 cards. The child had to respond to each card, indicating whether the picture was seen before. The maximum score was 100, one point for each correct response. Normative data for 3- to 12-year-olds are presented in Table 11–45. It is apparent from the means, compared to that of adults, that children as young as 4 years old had already obtained adult-level performance.

Continuous Visual Memory Test

The Continuous Visual Memory Test (CVMT) was originally developed for adults (Trahan and

Larrabee, 1988), but later extended downward for children. Preliminary normative data (see Table 11–47 for demographic data) were published by grade (Ullman, McKee et al., 1997) for U. S. children 7- to 11-years-old (see Table 11–48), and the CVMT manual also reports these data as percentile rankings. Percentile rankings for 640 9- to 15-year-old Canadian girls and boys of low average to average IQ (110 and below) or high IQ (above 110), according to the Canadian Cognitive Abilities Test, are also published in the test manual (Trahan and Larrabee, 1997). Scores by low and high IQ stratification for this sample were presented preliminarily (Miller, Murphy et al., 1996). The low and high IQ groups were subsequently merged and the data analyzed by age and gender only (Christopher Paniak, 2002, personal communication). See Table 11–49 for demographic data, and the results on 712 Canadian children are presented in Table 11–50.

The test consists of a series of black-and-white, two-dimensional geometric designs, followed by a recognition memory portion in which the child must identify the recurring target stimulus from a multiple-choice array. There is also a matching portion in which the child selects the design that matches each of the seven target stimuli from seven multiple-choice options. Alternate form development and examination of the equivalence of the two forms were reported for adults (Trahan, Larrabee et al., 1996), but not for children.

The CVMT manual makes several important points. Demographic factors and sampling characteristics need to be considered since the U.S. and Canadian samples differ, with the Canadian children doing less well than their U.S. age peers. The U.S. sample came from families that generally were of above average

Table 11–46. Continuous Recognition Memory Test Normative Data

		HITS			FALSE ALARMS			TOTAL CORRECT		
Age	N	Mean	SD	Range	Mean	SD	Range	Mean	SD	Range
6	26	37.1	3.5	25–40	9.7	6.4	2–31	87.4	6.7	67–98
8	26	37.1	3.1	28–40	7.7	5.3	1–20	89.3	4.2	80–95
10	31	38.4	2.4	29–40	4.8	2.9	0–11	93.6	3.3	86–99
13–18°	46	38.13	2.27	30–40	6.63	3.756	1–17	91.5	3.96	80–98

Source: °Hannay & Levin, 1989, © Swets & Zeitlinger.

Table 11–47. Continuous Visual Memory Test: United States Normative Data: Ullman et al. Study (1997)

Subjects: 138 children in grades 1 through 5 in a midwestern town
Age: Mean by grade ranged from 7 years 2 months to 11 years 2 months
Gender: 71 male; 67 female. No gender differences found; data combined.
Race: 94% Caucasian, 3% Hispanic, 2% African American, 1% other
SES: Median household income of $27,000; Hollingshead clases from high to low = 37%, 38%, 17%, 5%, 2%.
Exclusion Criteria: Not specified

Table 11–49. Continuous Visual Memory Test: Paniak Study

Subjects: 712 children from large western Canadian city
Age: 9 to 15 years old
Gender: 325 male; 387 female. Gender differences found, data presented separately
Race: Not specified
SES: Not specified
Exclusion Criteria: Failure in one or more grades, hospitalization for brain injury or behavior problems, placement in self-contained LD classrooms, English not the main language spoken at home

Source: Christopher Paniak, Harry Miller & Deirdre Murphy, 2002, Personal communication.

socioeconomic status and from a university town of about 30,000 people. The Canadian sample included children from a number of schools within a large urban population whose families were of average socioeconomic status. Therefore, the appropriate database for a child from average of lower socioeconomic status might be the Canadian, and the U.S. norms might be best for a child from above average socioeconomic status.

Another caution relates to the younger ages. These data suggest that children under 8 years can perform the CVMT, but a percentage of these children did not succeed, i.e., 10% to 15% of these children had total scores that suggested impairment. Therefore, while average or better performance indicates good visual recognition memory, interpretation of impairment is questionable for the young child who is not successful, and corroboration with other visual learning measures is needed.

Nonverbal Selective Reminding Test

The Nonverbal Selective Reminding Test (NSRT; Fletcher, 1985) was developed as a measure of memory for spatial locations analogous to the Verbal Selective Reminding Test. It also assesses EF as a measure of strategic thinking and working memory. It is presented to the child as a "dot game." The child is shown eight boxes with an array of dots, four boxes on two lines. The examiner touches one "special" dot in each box and then asks the child to show the examiner all the special dots touched. The bottom-line, left box is touched first, then the remaining dots from left to right on that line followed by the four boxes on the upper line. The child is then reminded of the dots that were missed and asked to respond again. The boxes are touched in the original order, and only the dots in boxes that were missed are then touched by the examiner, saying, "The dot to remember in this box is here."

Table 11–48. Continuous Visual Memory Test: Ullman et al. Data by Grade

Grade ($\bar{X}$ age)	N (No. M/No. F)	ACQUISITION TASK				
		Hits	False Alarms	Total Score	Delayed Recognition	Visual Discrim.
1 (7y 2m)	29 (15/14)	33.6 (6.1)	18.0 (8.6)	69.6 (8.7)	4.1 (1.5)	6.9 (0.3)
2 (8y 2m)	27 (14/13)	36.5 (4.6)	13.0 (8.3)	77.6 (8.5)	4.9 (1.6)	6.9 (0.3)
3 (9y 2m)	30 (15/15)	37.2 (3.0)	14.0 (5.7)	77.1 (6.0)	5.0 (1.2)	6.9 (0.3)
4 (10y 2m)	27 (14/13)	37.5 (3.3)	15.6 (6.2)	75.9 (7.3)	5.6 (0.9)	7.0 (0.0)
5 (11y 2m)	25 (13/12)	37.5 (2.6)	12.4 (5.1)	79.2 (5.4)	5.2 (1.3)	7.0 (0.0)

Source: Ullman et al. (1997), © Swets & Zeitlinger.

Table 11–50. Continuous Visual Memory Test Means (*SDs*): Paniak Data

		MALES					FEMALES			
Age	N	Hits	False Alarm	Total Score	Delay Recog°	N	Hits	False Alarm	Total Score	Delay Recog°
9	35	31.46 (5.64)	18.91 (7.34)	66.54 (9.06)	3.94 (1.45)	45	31.62 (5.84)	20.67 (6.71)	64.96 (8.44)	3.55 (1.37)
10	64	32.48 (5.45)	19.17 (7.09)	67.37 (9.64)	4.09 (1.59)	76	30.70 (6.31)	21.13 (8.89)	63.57 (9.20)	3.32 (1.71)
11	76	33.22 (4.54)	18.84 (7.09)	68.51 (8.52)	4.14 (1.65)	54	32.02 (5.41)	18.62 (7.36)	67.22 (9.47)	3.81 (1.51)
12	50	36.60 (3.92)	13.40 (5.69)	77.20 (7.86)	5.26 (1.27)	73	35.04 (5.02)	13.68 (6.45)	75.38 (8.73)	5.22 (1.34)
13	40	37.77 (2.98)	14.05 (6.57)	77.73 (7.37)	5.20 (1.29)	56	36.52 (3.79)	12.37 (5.13)	78.14 (5.82)	5.43 (1.22)
14	45	38.24 (2.72)	12.40 (5.29)	79.89 (6.14)	5.44 (1.25)	70	37.04 (3.53)	12.37 (5.95)	78.67 (6.54)	5.37 (1.36)
15	15	37.93 (2.76)	11.67 (5.72)	80.27 (5.22)	5.60 (1.06)	13	36.31 (3.28)	11.62 (4.39)	78.69 (4.82)	5.31 (.95)

Source: Courtesy of Christopher Paniak, Harry Miller & Deidre Murphy, 2002, personal communication.

°Delay Recog = Delayed Recognition

Examiner proficiency with dot placement is essential to accurate administration and scoring. A total of eight trials are allowed, or the test is terminated after perfect performance on three consecutive trials. Scoring is similar to that of the Verbal Selective Reminding Test. A factor analysis found the NSRT loading on a speculative factor of planning-sequencing (Taylor, Schatschneider et al., 1996), along with the Beery VMI, Microcomputer Test of Attention (Murphy-Berman and Wright, 1987) and Token Test, Part V (DiSimoni, 1978). These data were interpreted as providing support for use of the test despite an absence of normative data (Taylor, Albo et al., 1987). The NSRT was one measure in a study of children with Acute Lymphocytic Leukemia (Pfefferbaum-Levine, Copeland et al., 1984). It was also included in studies of children with *Haemophilus influenzae* Type b meningitis (Taylor, Barry et al., 1993; Taylor, Schatschneider et al., 1996; 2000) and its sensitivity to the effects of meningitis, provided evidence of test validity, but reliability studies are not available. Of note, factor analysis found it loading more on an executive function factor than with WISC Performance subtests (Taylor, Schatschneider et al., 1996).

Unpublished norms for the NSRT consisting of the means and *SDs* for the long-term storage and consistent long-term retrieval scores for 94 unaffected siblings of the postmeningitis children, 6- to 16-years-old, are presented in Table 11–51 (H. G. Taylor, 2001, personal communication). The families were recruited for large metropolitan areas in Canada (Toronto, Montreal, and Ottawa).

Biber Figural Learning Test

The Biber Figure Learning Test (BFLT; Glosser, Goodglass et al., 1989) was originally developed for use with stroke patients, especially aphasics. The test was subsequently modified into the Biber Figure Learning Test—Extended (BFLT-E) for use with younger neurologically impaired patients, specifically to assess long-term visuospatial memory epilepsy surgery candidates (Glosser, Ryan et al., 1992; Glosser, Cole et al., 2002). Two alternate forms of the BFLT-E are available. While of interest in the study of explicit (declarative) memory

Table 11–51. Non-Verbal Selective Reminding Test: Means and *SDs*

Variable	Age	N	Mean	SD	Range
N LTS					
	6.0–7.5	5	30.40	10.26	
	7.6–8.11	10	33.60	10.88	
	9.0–10.11	25	41.88	11.57	
	11.0–12.11	23	42.39	13.19	
	13.0–14.11	18	45.50	9.73	
	15.0–16.11	13	45.23	12.63	
N CLTR					
	6.0–7.5	5	15.60	5.50	
	7.6–8.11	10	19.40	10.69	
	9.0–10.11	25	28.64	14.09	
	11.0–12.11	23	30.34	14.79	
	13.0–14.11	18	34.77	13.96	
	15.0–16.11	13	35.38	16.01	

Source: Courtesy of H. Gerry Taylor, 2002, personal communication.

in adult populations (Glosser, Gallo et al., 2002), and criterion validity data are available (Glosser, Cole et al., 2002), the authors reaffirm that the test is multifactorial and therefore likely sensitive to both material-specific and more general cognitive dysfunction. The BFLT has not yet received attention as a learning and memory test for children, and no systematic data collection on childrens' learning test performance are reported. However, modification as noted below makes it a possible contributor to the armamentarium of child neuropsychologists, with the original 10-item test useful for children between 7 and 13, and the extended 15-item test for children 14 and older (G. Glosser, 2002, personal communication).

The BFLT procedure involves learning trials, immediate recognition, delayed free recall, delayed recognition, immediate reproduction, and design copying. The test involves presentation of 10 novel geometric designs, serially, in a fixed order over five learning trials. This 10-item version contrasts with the 15 figures of the BFLT-E. Free recall is assessed after each of the five learning trials. Immediate forced choice recognition is tested for each target design with three distractor or unrelated stimuli. Free delayed recall is assessed after 20 minutes of noncompeting interference.

Table 11–52. Reitan-Indiana NTB Meta-norms Means, *(SD)*, *[N]* for Target Test

SUBTEST:	AGE (YEARS)			
	5	6	7	8
Target Test (correct)	7.36 (3.3) [311]	9.60 (3.6) [190]	13.63 (2.5) [218]	12.89 (2.5) [184]

Source: Unpublished data courtesy of Michael K. Findeis & David G. Weight, Brigham Young University (1994).

A delayed recognition trial consists of the target design along with three new distractor designs. Immediate reproduction follows, which presents each test design for 3 seconds for immediate drawing, and for each incorrect drawing, the target stimulus is presented again and left in full view for copy production. Performance also can be evaluated for primacy and recency factors, learning slope as an indicator of encoding, savings score as a measure of consolidation or forgetting, and response to proactive interference with some modification. These are parallel to the data from verbal explicit memory tests such as the RAVLT, CVLT, SRT or other supraspan verbal list-learning tests (Glosser, Gallo et al., 2002). They thus hold additional promise for aiding in distinguishing between a child's visuospatial working memory or visuoconstructional abilities and nonverbal long-term memory.

Drawings are scored on a 0- to 3-point-scale, one point for correctly drawing each of the two component shapes and one additional point for maintaining the correct spatial and size relationships. Recognition-memory scoring sums correct target items (hits), incorrect distractor or unrelated items (false alarms), and a discrimination measure computed as number of correct targets minus proportion of false alarm errors.

Target Test

Another test of immediate visual memory is the Target Test from the Reitan-Indiana Neuropsychological Test Battery for 5- to 8-year-old children (Reitan, 1969). This test requires the child to reproduce visuospatial configurations of increasing complexity, following the pattern tapped by an examiner on a target sheet. There are 20 patterns. Normative data from a meta-analysis (Findeis and Weight, 1993; see Chapter 6 for details) are presented in Table 11–52.

REFERENCES

Akshoomoff, N. A., & Stiles, J. (1995a). Developmental trends in visuospatial analysis and planning: I. Copying a complex figure. *Neuropsychology, 9,* 364–377.

Aldrich, F., & Wilson, B. A. (1991). Rivermead Behavioural Memory Test for Children: A preliminary evaluation. *British Journal of Clinical Psychology, 30,* 161–168.

Anderson, P., Anderson, V., & Garth, J. (2001). Assessment and development of organizational ability: The Rey Complex Figure Organizational Strategy Score (RCF-OSS). *The Clinical Neuropsychologist, 15,* 81–94.

Anderson, V., Lajoie, G., & Bell, R. (1995). *Neuropsychological Assessment of the School-Aged Child.* Melbourne: University of Melbourne.

Atkinson, R. C., & Shiffrin, R. M. (1968). Human Memory: A proposed system and its control processes. In K. W. Spence (Ed.), *The psychology of learning and motivation: Advances in research and theory* (pp. 89–195). New York: Academic Press.

Baddeley, A. D. (1986). *Working Memory.* New York: Oxford University Press.

Barr, W. B. (2003). Neuropsychological testing of high school athletes: Preliminary norms and test-retest indices. *Archives of Clinical Neuropsychology, 18,* 91–101.

Beatty, W. W., Krull, K. R., Wilbanks, S. L., Blanco, C. R., Hames, K. A., & Paul, R. (1996). Further validation of constructs from the Selective Reminding Test. *Journal of Clinical and Experimental Neuropsychology, 18,* 52–55.

Beebe, D. W., Ris, M. D., & Dietrich, K. N. (2000). The relationship between CVLT-C process scores and measures of executive functioning: Lack of support among community-dwelling adolescents. *Journal of Clinical and Experimental Neuropsychology, 22,* 779–792.

Benedict, R. H. B., Schretlen, D. J., Groninger, L., & Brandt, J. (1998). Hopkins Verbal Learning Test-Revised: Normative data and analysis of inter-form and test-retest reliability. *The Clinical Neuropsychologist, 12,* 43–55.

Benton, A. L. (1955). Cerebral disease in a child. In A. Burton & R. E. Harris (Eds.), *Clinical studies in personality.* New York: Harper.

Benton, A. L. (1974). *Revised Visual Retention Test: Clinical and experimental applications* (4th Ed.). New York: The Psychological Corporation.

Bernstein, J. H., & Waber, D. P. (1996). *Developmental scoring system for the Rey-Osterrieth Complex Figure. Professional Manual.* Odessa, FL: Psychological Assessment Resources, Inc.

Bernstein, J. H., Waber, D. P. (1990). Developmental neuropsychological assessment: The systemic approach. In A. A. Boulton, G. B. Baker & M. Hiscock (Eds.), *Neuromethods: Vol. 17. Neuropsychology* (pp. 311–371). Clifton, NJ: Humana Press.

Binder, L. (1982). Constructional strategies on complex figure drawings after unilateral brain damage. *Journal of Clinical Neuropsychology, 4,* 51–58.

Bishop, E. G., Dickson, A. L., & Allen, M. T. (1990). Psychometric intelligence and performance on selective reminding. *The Clinical Neuropsychologist, 4,* 141–150.

Bishop, J., Knights, R. M., & Stoddart, C. (1990). Rey Auditory-Verbal Learning Test: Performance of English and French children aged 5 to 16. *The Clinical Neuropsychologist, 4,* 133–140.

Boll, T. (1993). *Children's Category Test.* San Antonio, TX: Psychological Corporation.

Brandt, J. (1991). The Hopkins Verbal Learning Test: Development of a new memory test with six equivalent forms. *The Clinical Neuropsychologist, 5,* 125–142.

Brown, A. L., & Scott, S. S. (1971). Recognition memory for pictures in preschool children. *Journal of Experimental Child Psychology, 11,* 401–412.

Burton, D. B., Donders, J., & Mittenberg, W. (1996). A structural equation analysis of the Wide Range Assessment of Memory and Learning in the standardization sample. *Child Neuropsychology, 2,* 39–47.

Burton, D. B., Mittenberg, W., Gold, S., & Drabman, R. (1999). A structural equation analysis of the Wide Range Assessment of Memory and Learning in a clinical sample. *Child Neuropsychology, 5,* 34–40.

Buschke, H. (1973). Selective reminding for analysis of memory and learning. *Journal of Verbal Learning and Verbal Behavior, 12,* 543–550.

Buschke, H. (1974). Two stages of learning by children and adults. *Bulletin of the Psychonomic Society, 2,* 392–394.

Buschke, H. (1974a). Components of verbal learning in children. Analysis by selective reminding. *Journal of Experimental Child Psychology, 18,* 488–496.

Buschke, H., & Fuld, P. A. (1974b). Evaluating storage, retention, and retrieval in disordered memory and learning. *Neurology, 24,* 1019–1025.

Cahn, D. A., Marcotte, A. C., Stern, R. A., Arruda, J. A., Akshoomoff, N. A., & Leshko, I. C. (1996). The Boston qualitative scoring system for the Rey-Osterrieth Complex Figure: A study of children with attention deficit hyperactivity disorder. *The Clinical Neuropsychologist, 10,* 397–406.

Carmichael, J. A., & MacDonald, J. W. (1984). Developmental norms for the sentence repetition test. *Journal of Consulting and Clinical Psychology, 52,* 476–477.

Carroll, J. B., Davies, P., & Richman, B. (1971). *The American heritage word frequency book.* Boston: Houghton Mifflin.

Carroll, M., Byrne, B., & Kirsner, K. (1985). Autobiographical memory and perceptual learning: A developmental study using picture recognition, naming latency and perceptual identification. *Memory and Cognition, 13,* 273–279.

Casey, M. B., Winner, E., Hurwitz, I., & DaSilva, D. (1991). Does processing style affect recall of the Rey-Osterrieth or Taylor Complex Figures? *Journal of Clinical and Experimental Neuropsychology, 13,* 600–606.

Cermak, L. S. (1996). Current Issues in the Neuropsychology of Memory Disorders: Handout. International Neuropsychological Society Continuing Education Course, Honolulu, HI.

Christensen, A.-L. (1979). *Luria's neuropsychological investigation.* Munksgaard: Schmidts Bogtrykkeri Vojens.

Christman, S. D., & Propper, R. E. (2001). Superior episodic memory is associated with inter-hemispheric processing. *Neuropsychology, 15,* 607–616.

Clodfelter, C. J., Dickson, A. L., Wilkes, C. N., & Johnson, R. B. (1987). Alternate forms of selective reminding for children. *The Clinical Neuropsychologist, 1,* 243–249.

Cohen, M. J. (1997). *Children's Memory Scale.* New York: The Psychological Corporation.

Colvin, A., Fennell, E. B., & Bauer, R. M. (1997). Rotary pursuit performance in children with attention-deficit hyperactivity disorder. *[Abstract] The Clinical Neuropsychologist, 11,* 305.

Corwin, J., & Bylsma, F. W. (1993). Translations of excerpts from Andre Rey's *Psychological Examination of Traumatic Encephalopathy* and P. A. Osterreith's *The Complex Figure Copy Test. The Clinical Neuropsychologist, 7,* 3–21.

Cowan, N. C. (1988). Evolving conceptions of memory storage, selective attention, and their mutual constraints within the human information processing system. *Psychological Bulletin, 104,* 163–191.

Cowan, N. C., & Hulme, C. (1997). *The development of memory in childhood.* Hove East Sussex, UK: Psychology Press.

Craik, F. I. M., Govoni, R., Naveh-Benjamin, M., & Anderson, N. D. (1996). The effects of divided attention on encoding and retrieval processes in human memory. *Journal of Experimental Psychology: General, 125,* 159–180.

Craik, F. I. M., & Lockhart, R. S. (1972). Levels of processing: A framework for memory research. *Journal of Verbal Learning and Verbal Behavior, 11,* 671–684.

Crawford, J. R., Stewart, L. E., & Moore, J. W. (1989). Demonstration of savings on the AVLT and development of a parallel form. *Journal of Clinical and Experimental Neuropsychology, 11,* 975–981.

Crosson, B. (1992). *Subcortical functions in language and memory.* New York: Guilford Press.

Delis, D., Filoteo, J. V., Massman, P. J., Kaplan, E., & Kramer, J. (1994). The clinical assessment of memory disorders. In L. S. Cermak (Ed.), *Neuropsychological explorations of memory and cognition: Essays in honor of Nelson Butters. Critical issues in neuropsychology* (pp. 223–239). New York: Plenum Press.

Delis, D., Kramer, J. H., Kaplan, E., & Ober, B. A. (1987). *California Verbal Learning Test: Adult Version.* San Antonio, TX: The Psychological Corporation.

Delis, D., Kramer, J. H., Kaplan, E., & Ober, B. A. (1994). *California Verbal Learning Test-Children's Version.* San Antonio, TX: Psychological Corporation.

Demsky, Y., Carone, D. A. J., Burns, W. J., & Sellers, A. (2000). Assessment of visual-motor coordination in 6- to 11-yr.-olds. *Perceptual and Motor Skills, 91,* 311–321.

Denckla, M. B. (1996b). A theory and model of executive function: A neuropsychological perspective. In G. R. Lyon & N. A. Krasnegor (Eds.), *Attention, memory, and executive function* (pp. 263–278). Baltimore: Paul H. Brookes.

Dennis, M., Hetherington, C. R., & Spiegler, B. J. (1998). Memory and attention after childhood brain tumors. *Medical and Pediatric Oncology, Suppl. 1,* 25–33.

desRosiers, G., & Ivison, D. (1986). Paired associate learning: Normative data for differences between high and low associate word pairs. *Journal of Clinical and Experimental Neuropsychology, 8,* 637–642.

DiGiulio, D. V., Seidenberg, M., O'Leary, D. S., & Raz, N. (1994). Procedural and declarative memory: A developmental study. *Brain and Cognition, 25,* 79–91.

Dikmen, S., Heaton, R. K., Grant, I., & Temkin, N. R. (1999). Test-retest reliability and practice effects of Expanded Halstead-Reitan Neuropsychological Test Battery. *Journal of the International Neuropsychological Society, 5,* 346–356.

Di Stefano, G., Bachevalier, J., Levin, H. S., Song, J., Scheibel, R. S., & Fletcher, J. (2000). Volume of focal brain lesions and hippocampal formation in relation to memory function after closed head injury in children. *Journal of Neurology, Neurosurgery and Psychiatry, 69,* 210–216.

Doerksen, S., & Shimamura, A. P. (2001). Source memory enhancement for emotional words. *Emotion, 1,* 5–11.

Donders, J. (1998). Performance discrepancies between the Children's Category Test (CCT) and the California Verbal Learning Test-Children's version (CVLT-C) in the standardization sample. *Journal of the International Neuropsychological Society, 4,* 242–246.

Donders, J. (1999c). Structural equation analysis of the California Verbal Learning Test-Children's Version in the standardization sample. *Developmental Neuropsychology, 15,* 395–406.

Drane, D. L., Loring, D. W., Lee, G. P., & Meador, K. J. (1998). Trial-length sensitivity of the Verbal Selective Reminding Test to lateralized temporal lobe impairment. *The Clinical Neuropsychologist, 12,* 68–73.

Einstein, G. O., & McDaniel, M. A. (1990). Normal aging and prospective memory. *Journal of Experimental Psychology: Learning, Memory and Cognition, 16,* 717–726.

Espy, K., McDiarmid, M. A., & Glisky, M. L. (2001). A continuous recognition memory test for preschool children. *Journal of the International Neuropsychological Society, 7,* 200.

Fastenau, P. S. (1996). Development and preliminary standardization of the "Extended Complex Figure Test" (ECFT). *Journal of Clinical and Experimental Neuropsychology, 18,* 63–76.

Fastenau, P. S., & Denburg, N. L. (1994). *Reliability and validity of the Extended Complex Figure*

Test (ECFT). Paper presented at the International Neuropsychological Society meeting, Cincinatti, OH.

Fastenau, P. S., Denburg, N. L., & Hufford, B. J. (1999). Adult Norms for the Rey-Osterrieth Complex Figure Test and for Supplemental Recognition and Matching Trials from the Extended Complex Figure Test (ECFT). *The Clinical Neuropsychologist, 13*, 30–47.

Fastenau, P. S., & Manning, A. A. (1992). Development of a recognition task for the Complex Figure Test [abstract]. *Journal of Clinical and Experimental Neuropsychology, 14*, 43.

Findeis, M. K., & Weight, D. G. (1993). *Meta-norms for Indiana-Reitan Neuropsychological Test Battery and Halstead-Reitan Neuropsychologial Test Battery for Children, ages 5–14.* Unpublished manuscript.

Fletcher, J. (1985). Memory for verbal and nonverbal stimuli in learning disability subgroups: Analysis by selective reminding. *Journal of Experimental Child Psychology, 40*, 244–259.

Forrester, G., & Geffen, G. (1991). Performance measures of 7- to 15-year-old children on the Auditory Verbal Learning Test. *The Clinical Neuropsychologist, 5*, 345–359.

Frazier, T. W., Adams, N. L., Strauss, M. E., & Redline, S. (2001). Comparability of the Rey and Mack forms of the Complex Figure Test. *The Clinical Neuropsychologist, 15*, 337–344.

Fridlund, A. J., & Delis, D. (1994). *California Verbal Learning Test-Children's version: The (CVLT-C) Scoring Assistant software.* San Antonio, TX: The Psychological Corporation.

Fuchs, K. L., Hannay, H. J., Huckeba, W. M., & Espy, K. A. (1999). Construct validity of the Continuous Recognition Memory Test. *The Clinical Neuropsychologist, 13*, 54–65.

Fujii, D. E., Lloyd, H. A., & Miyamoto, K. (2000). The salience of visuospatial and organizational skills in reproducing the Rey-Osterrieth Complex Figure in subjects with high and low IQs. *The Clinical Neuropsychologist, 14*, 551–554.

Fuster, J. M. (1989). *The prefrontal cortex: Anatomy, physiology and neuropsychology of the frontal lobe* (2nd ed.). New York: Raven Press.

Geffen, G., Moor, K., O'Hanlon, A., Clark, D., & Geffen, L. (1990). Performance Measures of 16- to-86 year-old males and females on the Auditory Verbal Learning Test. *The Clinical Neuropsychologist, 4*, 45–63.

Glisky, E. L. (1996). Prospective memory and the frontal lobes. In M. Brandimonte, G. O. Einstein & M. A. McDaniel (Eds.), *Prospective memory: Theory and applications* (pp. 249–266). Mahwah, NJ: Lawrence Erlbaum Associates.

Glosser, G., Cole, L., Khatri, U., DellaPietra, L., & Kaplan, E. (2002). Assessing nonverbal memory with the Biber Figural Learning Test-Extended in temporal lobe epilepsy patients. *Archives of Clinical Neuropsychology, 17*, 25–35.

Glosser, G., Gallo, J. L., Clark, C. M., & Grossman, M. (2002). Memory encoding and retrieval in Frontotemporal Dementia and Alzheimer's disease. *Neuropsychology, 16*, 190–196.

Glosser, G., Goodglass, H., & Biber, C. (1989). Assessing visual memory disorders. *Psychological Assessment, 1*, 82–91.

Glosser, G., Ryan, L., & Fedio, P. (1992). *Validation of a new visual memory test in post temporal lobectomy patients.* Paper presented at the National Academy of Neuropsychology Meeting, Pittsburgh, PA.

Goodman, A., Delis, D., & Mattson, S. N. (1999). Normative data for 4-year-old children on the California Verbal Learning Test-Children's Version. *The Clinical Neuropsychologist, 13*, 274–282.

Graf, P. (1990). Life-span changes in implicit and explicit memory. *Bulletin of the Psychonomic Society, 28*, 353–358.

Graf, P., & Masson, M. E. J. (Eds.). (1993). *Implicit memory: New directions in cognition, development and neuropsychology.* Hillsdale, NJ: Lawrence Erlbaum.

Graf, P., Shimamura, A. P., & Squire, L. R. (1985). Priming across modalities and priming across category levels: Extending the domain of preserved function in amnesia. *Journal of Experimental Psychology: Learning, Memory and Cognition, 11*, 386–396.

Grafton, S. T., Hazeltine, E., & Ivry, R. (1995). Functional mapping of sequence learning in normal humans. *Journal of Cognitive Neuroscience, 7*, 497–510.

Greenbaum, J. L., & Graf, P. (1989). Preschool period development of implicit and explicit remembering. *Bulletin of the Psychonomic Society, 27*, 417–420.

Grober, E., Lipton, R. B., Katz, M., & Sliwinski, M. (1998). Demographic influences on free and cued selective reminding performance in older persons. *Journal of Clinical and Experimental Neuropsychology, 20*, 221–226.

Guger, S. (2000). *Implicit and explicit memory in children with moderate closed head injuries.* Unpublished doctoral dissertation, York University, Toronto, ON.

Guger, S., & Rich, J. B. (2001). Implicit and explicit memory in children with moderate closed head injury [abstract]. *Journal of the International Neuropsychological Society, 7*, 132.

Halperin, J. M., Healey, J. M., Zeitchik, E., Ludman, W. L., & Weinstein, L. (1989). Developmental aspects of linguistic and mnestic abilities in normal children. *Journal of Clinical and Experimental Neuropsychology, 11,* 518–528.

Hamby, S. L., Wilkins, J. W., & Barry, N. S. (1993). Organizational quality on the Rey-Osterrieth and Taylor Complex Figure Tests: A new scoring system. *Psychological Assessment, 5,* 27–33.

Hannay, H. J., & Levin, H. S. (1985). Selective Reminding Test: An examination of the equivalence of four forms. *Journal of Clinical and Experimental Neuropsychology, 7,* 251–263.

Hannay, H. J., & Levin, H. S. (1989). Visual continuous recognition memory in normal and closed-head-injured adolescents. *Journal of Clinical and Experimental Neuropsychology, 11,* 444–460.

Hannay, H. J., Levin, H. S., & Grossman, R. G. (1979). Impaired recognition memory after head injury. *Cortex, 15,* 264–283.

Hermelin, B., & O'Conner, N. (1970). *Psychological experiments with autistic children.* Oxford: Pergamon Press.

Heubrock, D. (1995). Error analysis in neuropsychological assessment of verbal memory and learning. *European Journal of Psychological Assessment, 11,* 21–28.

Hildebrandt, H., Müller, S., Bussmann-Mork, B., Goebel, S., & Eilers, N. (2001). Are some memory deficits unique to lesions of the mammillary bodies? *Journal of Clinical and Experimental Neuropsychology, 23,* 490–501.

Hubley, A. M., & Tremblay, D. (2002). Comparability of total score performance on the Rey-Osterrieth Complex Figure and a Modified Taylor Complex Figure. *Journal of Clinical and Experimental Neuropsychology, 24,* 370–382.

Janowsky, J. S., Shimamura, A. P., & Squire, L. (1989). Source memory impairment in patients with frontal lobe lesions. *Neuropsychologia, 8,* 1043–1056.

Johnson, M. K., Hashtroudi, S., & Lindsay, D. S. (1993). Source monitoring. *Psychological Bulletin, 114,* 3–28.

Kail, R. V. (1984). *The Development of Memory in Children* (2nd ed.). San Francisco: Freeman.

Kammerer, B. L., Gardner, J. K., & Wolff, A. B. (1988). *Rey-Osterrieth Complex Figure drawings of deaf children with different etiologies of deafness.* Paper presented at the International Neurological Society meeting, New Orleans, LA.

Kerns, K. A. (2000). The CyberCruiser: An investigation of development of prospective memory in children. *Journal of the International Neuropsychological Society, 6,* 62–70.

Kirkwood, M. W., Weiler, M. D., Bernstein, J. H., Forbes, P. W., & Waber, D. P. (2001). Sources of poor performance on the Rey-Osterrieth Complex Figure Test among children with learning difficulties: A dynamic assessment approach. *The Clinical Neuropsychologist, 15,* 345–356.

Klicpera, C. (1983). Poor planning as a characteristic of problem-solving behavior in dyslexic children: A study with the Rey-Osterrieth Complex Figure Test. *Acta Paedopsychiatrica, 49,* 73–82.

Kramer, J., Delis, D., Kaplan, E., O'Donnell, L., & Prifitera, A. (1997). Developmental sex differences in verbal learning. *Neuropsychology, 11,* 577–584.

Kvavilashvili, L., & Ellis, J. (1996). Varieties of intention: Some distinctions and classifcations. In M. Brandimonte, G. O. Einstein & M. A. McDaniel (Eds.), *Prospective memory: Theory and applications.* Vol. 6 (pp. 183–207). Amsterdam: Elsevier.

Leavell, C. A., Ackerson, J. D., & Fischer, R. F. (1995). Procedural learning difficulties in children with attention and/or overactivity: Is it motor skill or motor acquisition? [Abstract]. *Journal of the International Neuropsychological Society, 1,* 154.

Leavell, C. A., Bowers, C. A., & Karp, M. P. (1999). Procedural learning in children with problems in attention and learning is dissociable from declarative learning. [Abstract]. *Journal of the International Neuropsychological Society, 5,* 99.

Levin, H. S. (1981). *Instructions for Selective Reminding Memory Test.* Unpublished manuscript.

Levin, H. S. (1990). Memory deficit after closed head injury. *Journal of Clinical and Experimental Neuropsychology, 12,* 129–153.

Levin, H. S., Benton, A., & Grossman, R. G. (1982). *Neurobehavioral consequences of closed head injury.* New York: Oxford University Press.

Levin, H. S., Culhane, K. A., Fletcher, J., & al., e. (1994). Dissociation between delayed alternation and memory after pediatric head injury: Relationship to MRI findings. *Journal of Child Neurology, 9,* 81–89.

Levin, H. S., Culhane, K. A., Hartmann, J., Evankovich, K., Mattson, A. J., Harward, H., et al. (1991). Developmental changes in performance on tests of purported frontal lobe functioning. *Developmental Neuropsychology, 7,* 377–395.

Levin, H. S., & Grossman, R. G. (1976). Storage and retrieval. *Journal of Pediatric Psychology, 1,* 38–42.

Lezak, M. (1983). *Neuropschological assessment,* (2nd ed.). New York: Oxford University Press.

Lockhart, R. S., & Craik, F. I. M. (1990). Levels of processing: A retrospective commentary on a framework for memory research. *Canadian Journal of Psychology, 44,* 87–112.

Loring, D. (Ed.). (1999). *INS dictionary of neuropsychology.* New York: Oxford University Press.

Lorsbach, T. C., Sodoro, J., & Brown, J. S. (1992). The dissociation of repetition priming and recognition memory in language/learning disabled children. *Journal of Experimental Child Psychology, 54,* 121–146.

Lorsbach, T. C., & Worman, L. J. (1989). The development of explicit and implicit forms of memory in learning disabled children. *Contemporary Educational Psychology, 14,* 67–76.

Matthews, L., Anderson, V., & Anderson, P. (2001). Assessing the validity of the Rey Complex Figure as a diagnostic tool: Accuracy, recall and organisational strategy scores in children with brain insult. *Clinical Neuropsychological Asessment, 2,* 85–99.

Mattson, S. N., Riley, E. P., Delis, D., Stern, C., & Jones, K. L. (1996). Verbal learning and memory in children with Fetal Alcohol Syndrome. *Alcoholism: Clinical and Experimental Research, 20,* 810–816.

Maylor. (1996). Prospective memory in normal ageing and dementia. *Neurocase, 1,* 285–289.

Meador, K. J., Loring, D. W., Allen, M. E., Zamrini, E. Y., Moore, E. E., Abney, O. L., et al. (1991). Comparative cognitive effects of carbamazepine and phenytoin in healthy adults. *Neurology, 41,* 1537–1540.

Meyers, J. E., & Meyers, K. R. (1996). *Rey Complex Figure Test and Recognition Trial (RCFT).* Odessa, FL: Psychological Assessment Resources, Inc.

Miller, H. B., Murphy, D., Paniak, C. E., LaBonte, M., & Spackman, L. (1996). *Continuous Visual Memory Test: Norms for ages 9 to 15.* Paper presented at the 24th Annual Meeting of the International Neuropsychological Society, Chicago, IL.

Minshew, N., & Goldstein, G. (1993). Is autism an amnesic disorder? Evidence from the California Verbal Learning Test. *Neuropsychology, 7,* 209–216.

Morgan, S. F. (1982). Measuring Long-Term Memory Storage and Retrieval in Children. *Journal of Clinical Neuropsychology, 4,* 77–85.

Morgan, S. F., Furman, E. B., & Dikmen, S. (1981). Psychological effects of general anesthesia on five- to eight-year old children. *Anesthesiology, 55,* 386–391.

Morris, C. D., Bransford, J. D., & Franks, J. J. (1977). Levels of processing versus transfer appropriate processing. *Journal of Verbal Learning and Verbal Behavior, 16,* 519–533.

Moscovitch, M. (1981). Multiple dissociations of function in amnesia. In L. S. Cermak (Ed.), *Human memory and amnesia* (pp. 337–370). Hillsdale, NJ: Lawrence Erlbaum Associates.

Murphy-Berman, V. A., & Wright, G. (1987). Measures of attention. *Perceptual and Motor Skills, 64,* 1139–1143.

Naito, M. (1990). Repetition priming in children and adults: Age-related dissociation between implicit and explicit memory. *Journal of Experimental Child Psychology, 50,* 462–484.

Naito, M., & Komatsu, S. (1993). Processes involved in childhood development of implicit memory. In P. Graf & M. Masson (Eds.), *Implicit memory: New directions in cognition, development, and neuropsychology* (pp. 231–260). Hillsdale, NJ: Lawrence Erlbaum Associates.

Nelson, C. A. (1995). The ontogeny of human memory: A cognitive neuroscience perspective. *Developmental Psychology, 31,* 723–738.

Newman, P. D., & Krikorian, R. (2001). Encoding and complex figure recall. *Journal of the International Neuropsychological Society, 7,* 728–733.

Osterrieth, P. A. (1944). Le test de copie d'une figure complexe. Contribution a l'etude de la perception et de la memoire. *Archives de Psychologie, 30,* 206–353.

Paniak, C. E., Murphy, D., Miller, H., & Lee, M. (1998). Wechsler Memory Scale-Revised Logical Memory and Visual Reproduction Norms for 9 to 15 year-olds. *Developmental Neuropsychology, 14,* 555–562.

Parkin, A., & Streete, S. (1988). Implicit and explicit memory in young children and adults. *British Journal of Psychology, 79,* 361–369.

Peirson, A. R., & Jansen, P. (1997). Comparability of the Rey-Osterrieth and Taylor forms of the complex figure test. *The Clinical Neuropsychologist, 11,* 244–248.

Petrides, M., Alivisatos, B., & Evans, A. (1995). Functional activation of the human ventrolateral frontal cortex during mnemonic retrieval of verbal information. *Proceedings of the National Academy of Sciences, 92,* 5803–6807.

Pfefferbaum-Levine, B., Copeland, D. R., Fletcher, J., Ried, H., Jaffe, N., & McKinnon, W. R. (1984). Neuropsychological assessment of long-term survivors of childhood leukemia. *American Journal of Pediatric Hematology/Oncology, 6,* 123–128.

Pluth, S., Hannay, H. J., Massman, P. J., & Contant, C. F. J. (2002). *Selective Reminding Test: Novel measures of performance in a CHI population.* Paper presented at the 30th Annual International Neuropsychological Society Meeting, Toronto.

Poldrack, R. A., Prabhakaran, V., Seger, C. A., & Gabrieli, J. D. E. (1999). Striatal activation during acquisition of a cognitive skill. *Neuropsychology, 13*, 564–574.

Poulton, R. G., & Moffitt, T. E. (1995). The Rey-Osterrieth Complex Figure Test: Norms for young adolescents and an examination of validity. *Archives of Clinical Neuropsychology, 10*, 47–56.

Prior, M., & Hoffmann, W. (1990). Neuropsycological testing of autistic children through an exploration with frontal lobe tests. *Journal of Autism and Developmental Disorders, 20*, 581–590.

Rapport, L. J., Dutra, R. L., Webster, J. S., Charter, R., & Morrill, B. (1995). Hemispatial deficits on the Rey-Osterrieth Complex Figure drawing. *The Clinical Neuropsychologist, 9*, 169–179.

Reitan, R. (1969). *Manual for Administration of Neuropsychological Test Batteries for Adults and Children.* Unpublished manuscript. Indianapolis University Medical Center.

Rey, A. (1941). L'examen psychologique dans les cas d'encephalopathie traumatique. *Archives de Psychologie, 28*, 286–340.

Rey, A. (1964). *L'Examen Clinique en Psychologie.* Paris: Presses Universitaires de France.

Reynolds, C. R., & Bigler, E. D. (1994). *Test of Memory and Learning Examiner's Manual.* Austin, TX: Pro-Ed.

Riccio, C. A., Hall, J., Morgan, A., Hynd, G. W., Gonzalez, J. J., & Marshall, R., M. (1994). Executive function and the Wisconsin Card Sorting Test: Relationship with behavioral ratings and cognitive ability. *Developmental Neuropsychology, 10*, 215–229.

Rich, J. B., Yaster, M., & Brandt, J. (1999). Anterograde and retrograde memory in children anesthetized with propofol. *Journal of Clinical and Experimental Neuropsychology, 21*, 535–546.

Roediger, H. L. I. (1990). Implicit memory: retention without remembering. *American Psychologist, 45*, 1043–1056.

Roediger, H. L. I., & Blaxton, T. A. (1987). Retrieval modes produce dissociations in memory for surface information. In D. S. Gorfein & R. R. Hoffman (Eds.), *Memory and cognitive processes: The Ebbinghaus centennial conference* (pp. 349–379). Hillsdale, NJ: Lawrence Erlbaum.

Roman, M. A., Gaither, R. A., & Hoeppner, J. (1994). Developmental norms for two versions of the Selective Reminding Test. *The Clinical Neuropsychologist, 8*, 335–336.

Roman, M. J., Delis, D., Willerman, L., Magulac, M., Demadura, T. L., de la Pena, J. L., et al. (1998). Impact of pediatric traumatic brain injury on components of verbal memory. *Journal of Clinical and Experimental Neuropsychology, 20*, 245–258.

Russo, R., Nichelli, P., Gibertoni, M., & Cornia, C. (1995). Developmental trends in implicit and explicit memory. *Journal of Experimental Child Psychology, 59*, 566–578.

Ryan, J. J., Rosenberg, S. J., & Mittenberg, W. (1983). Factor analysis of the Rey Auditory-Verbal Learning Test. *International Journal of Clinical Neuropsychology, 6*, 239–241.

Sadeh, M., Ariel, R., & Inbar, D. (1996). Rey-Osterrieth and Taylor Complex Figures: Equivalent measures of visual organization and visual memory in ADHD and normal children. *Child Neuropsychology, 2*, 63–71.

Saint-Cyr, J. A., & Taylor, A. E. (1992). The mobilization of procedural learning: The "key signature" of the basal ganglia. In L. Squire & N. Butters (Eds.), *Neuropsychology of memory* (2nd ed.) (pp. 188–202). New York: Guilford Press.

Salvador, J., Cortes, J. F., & Galindo y Villa, G. (1997). Propiedades cualitativas de la ejecucion en la Figura Compleja de Re Para ninos a lo largo del desarrollo en poblacion abierta. *Salud Mental, 20*, 9–14.

Sasher, T. M., & Fastenau, P. S. (2001). Preliminary child normative data for the Extended Complex Figure Test (ECFT) [Abstract]. *The Clinical Neuropsychologist, 15*, 258.

Schacter, D. L. (1992). Understanding implicit memory: A cognitive neuroscience approach. *American Psychologist, 47*, 559–569.

Schacter, D. L., & Tulving, E. (1994). *Memory systems.* Cambridge, MA: The MIT Press.

Schmidt, M. (1997). Some cautions on interpreting qualitative indices for word-list learning tests. *The Clinical Neuropsychologist, 11*, 81–86.

Schneider, W., & Pressley, M. (1988). *Memory Development Between 2 and 20.* New York: Springer-Verlag.

Schum, R. L., Sivan, A. B., & Benton, A. (1989). Multilingual Aphasia Examination: Norms for Children. *The Clinical Neuropsychologist, 3*, 375–383.

Semel, E., Wiig, E. H., & Secord, W. (1995). *Clinical Evaluation of Language Fundamentals-Third Edition.* San Antonio, TX: The Psychological Corporation.

Sergent, J., & Scholten, C. A. (1983). A stages-of-information approach to hyperactivity. *Journal of Child Psychology and Psychiatry (& Allied Disciplines), 24*, 49–60.

Shallice, T., & Warrington, E. K. (1970). Independent functioning of verbal memory stores: A neuropsychological study. *Quarterly Journal of Experimental Psychology, 22*, 261–273.

Shapiro, E. G., & Balthazor, M. (2000). Metabolic and neurodegenerative disorders. In K. Yeates,

M. D. Ris & H. G. Taylor (Eds.), *Pediatric neuropsychology: Research, theory, and practice* (pp. 171–205). New York: The Guilford Press.

Shear, P. K., Tallal, P., & Delis, D. (1992). Verbal learning and memory in language impaired children. *Neuropsychologia, 5,* 451–458.

Sheslow, D., & Adams, W. (1990). *Wide Range Assessment of Memory and Learning.* Wilmington, DE: Jastak.

Shimamura, A. P., Janowsky, J. S., & Squire, L. R. (1991). What is the role of frontal lobe damage in memory disorders? In H. S. Levin, H. M. Eisenberg & A. L. Benton (Eds.), *Frontal lobe function and dysfunction.* New York: Oxford University Press.

Shum, D., Jamieson, E., Bahr, M., & Wallace, G. (1999). Implicit and explicit memory in children with traumatic brain injury. *Journal of Clinical and Experimental Neuropsychology, 21,* 149–158.

Shum, D., Valentine, M., & Cutmore, T. (1999). Performance of individuals with severe long-term traumatic brain injury on time-, event-, and activity-based prospective memory tasks. *Journal of Clinical and Experimental Neuropsychology, 21,* 49–58.

Sivan, A. B. (1992). *Benton Visual Memory Test, Fifth Edition.* San Antonio: The Psychological Corporation.

Snodgrass, J. G. (1989). Sources of learning in the picture fragment completion task. In S. Lewandowsky, J. Dunn & K. Kirsner (Eds.), *Implicit memory: Theoretical Issues* (pp. 259–282). Hillsdale, NJ: Erlbaum.

Snodgrass, J. G., Smith, B., Feenan, K., & Corwin, J. (1987). Fragmenting pictures on the Apple Macintosh computer for experimental and clinical applications. *Behavior Research Methods, Instruments, and Computers, 19,* 270–274.

Somerville, J., Tremont, G., & Stern, R. A. (2000). The Boston Qualitative Scoring System as a measure of executive functioning in Rey-Osterrieth Complex Figure peformance. *Journal of Clinical and Experimental Neuropsychology, 22,* 613–621.

Spiegler, B. J., & Yeni-Komishian, G. (1983). Incidence of left-handed writing in a college population with reference to family patterns of hand preference. *Neuropsychologia, 21,* 651–659.

Spreen, O., & Benton, A. (1963). *Sentence Repetition Test: administration, scoring, and preliminary norms.* Unpublished manuscript, University of Iowa.

Spreen, O., & Gaddes, W. H. (1969). Developmental Norms for 15 neuropsychological tests age 6 to 15. *Cortex, 5,* 171–191.

Spreen, O., & Strauss, E. (1998). *A compendium of neuropsychological tests: Adminstration, norms, and commentary* (2nd ed.). New York: Oxford University Press.

Squire, L. R. (1982). The neuropsychology of human memory. *Annual Review of Neuroscience, 5,* 241–273.

Squire, L. R. (1986). The neuropsychology of memory dysfunction and its assessment. In I. Grant & K. M. Adams (Eds.), *Neuropsychological assessment of neuropsychiatric disorders* (pp. 268–299). New York: Oxford University Press.

Squire, L. R. (1987). *Memory and Brain.* New York: Oxford University Press.

Squire, L. R., Knowlton, B., & Musen, G. (1993). The structure and organization of memory. *Annual Review of Psychology, 44,* 453–495.

Stern, R. A., Javorsky, D. J., Singer, E. A., Singer Harris, N. G., Somerville, J. A., Duke, L. M., et al. (1999). *The Boston Qualitative Scoring System for the Rey-Osterrieth Complex Figure.* Odessa, FL: Psychological Assessment Resources, Inc.

Stern, R. A., Singer, E. A., Duke, L. M., Singer, N. G., Morey, C. E., Daughtrey, E. W., et al. (1994). The Boston qualitative socring system for the Rey-Osterrieth Complex Figure: Description and interrater reliability. *The Clinical Neuropsychologist, 8,* 309–322.

Strauss, E., & Spreen, O. (1990). A comparison of the Rey and Taylor Figures. *Archives of Clinical Neuropsychology, 5,* 417–420.

Tager-Flusberg, H. (1989). A psycholinguistic perspective on language development in the autistic child. In G. Dawson (Ed.), *Autism: Nature, diagnosis, and treatment* (pp. 92–109). New York: Guilford.

Taylor, E. M. (1959). *Psychological appraisal of children with cerebral deficits.* Cambridge, MA: Harvard University Press.

Taylor, H. G., Albo, V., Phebus, C., Sachs, B., & Bierl, P. (1987). Postirradiation treatment outcomes for children with acute lymphoblastic leukemia: Clarification of risks. *Journal of Pediatric Psychology, 12,* 395–411.

Taylor, H. G., Barry, C. T., & Schatschneider, C. (1993). School-age consequences of *Haemophilus influenzae* Type b meningitis. *Journal of Clinical Child Psychology, 22,* 196–206.

Taylor, H. G., Schatschneider, C., & Minich, N. (2000). Longitudinal outcomes of *Haemophilus influenzae* Meningitis in School-age children. *Neuropsychology, 14,* 509–518.

Taylor, H. G., Schatschneider, C., Petrill, S., Barry, C. T., & Owens, C. (1996). Executive dysfunction in children with early brain disease: Outcomes post *Haemophilus Influenzae* Meningitis. *Developmental Neuropsychology, 12,* 35–51.

Tombaugh, T. N., & Hubley, A. M. (1991). Four studies comparing the Rey-Osterrieth and Taylor complex figures. *Journal of Clinical and Experimental Neuropsychology, 13,* 587–599.

Trahan, D. E., & Larrabee, G. J. (1988). *The Continuous Visual Memory Test.* Odessa, FL: Psychological Assessment Resources, Inc.

Trahan, D. E., & Larrabee, G. J. (1997). *Continuous Visual Memory Test: Supplemental normative data for children and older adults.* Odessa, FL: Psychological Assessment Resources, Inc.

Trahan, D. E., Larrabee, G. J., Fritzsche, B., & Curtiss, G. (1996). Continuous Visual Memory Test: Alternate form and generalizability estimates. *The Clinical Neuropsychologist, 10,* 73–79.

Tranel, D., Anderson, S. W., & Benton, A. (1994). Development of the concept of "executive function" and its relationship to the frontal lobes. In F. Boller & J. Grafman (Eds.), *Handbook of Neuropsychology,* vol. 9, 125–148. Amsterdam: Elsevier.

Tremont, G., Halpert, S., Javorsky, D. J., & Stern, R. A. (2000). Differential impact of executive dysfunction on verbal list learning and story recall. *The Clinical Neuropsychologist, 14,* 295–302.

Troyer, A. K., Winocur, G., Craik, F. I. M., & Moscovitch, M. (1999). Source memory and divided attention: Reciprocal costs to primary and secondary tasks. *Neuropsychology, 13,* 467–474.

Troyer, A. K., & Wishart, H. A. (1997). A comparison of qualitative scoring systems for the Rey-Osterrieth Complex Figure Test. *The Clinical Neuropsychologist, 11,* 381–390.

Tulving, E. (1972). Episodic and semantic memory. In E. Tulving & W. Donaldson (Eds.), *Organization of memory* (pp. 381–403). New York: Academic Press.

Tulving, E. (1983). *Elements of Episodic Memory.* New York: Oxford University Press.

Tulving, E., Kapur, S., Craik, F. I. M., Moscovitch, M., & Houle, S. (1994). Hemispheric encoding/retrieval symmetry in episodic memory: Positron emission tomography findings. *Proceedings of the National Academy of Sciences, 91,* 2016–2020.

Ullman, D. G., McKee, D. T., Campbell, K. E., Larrabee, G. J., & Trahan, D. E. (1997). Preliminary children's norms for the continuous visual memory test. *Child Neuropsychology, 3,* 171–175.

Vaidya, C. J., Gabrieli, J. D. E., Monti, L. A., Tinklenberg, J. R., & Yesavage, J. A. (1999). Dissociation between two forms of conceptual priming in Alzheimer's disease. *Neuropsychology, 13,* 516–524.

Vakil, E., Blachstein, H., & Sheinman, M. (1998). Rey AVLT: Developmental norms for children and the sensitivity of different memory measures to age. *Child Neuropsychology, 4,* 161–177.

Van der Linden, M., Bruyer, R., Roland, J., & Schils, J. P. (1993). Proactive interference in patients with amnesia resulting from anterior communicating artery aneurysm. *Journal of Clinical and Experimental Neuropsychology, 15,* 525–536.

Vanderplas, J. M., & Garvin, E. A. (1959). The association value of random shapes. *Journal of Experimental Psychology, 57,* 147–154.

Vanderploeg, R. D., Crowell, T. A., & Curtiss, G. (2001). Verbal learning and memory deficits in traumatic brain injury: Encoding, consolidation, and retrieval. *Journal of Clinical and Experimental Neuropsychology, 23,* 185–195.

Vanderploeg, R. D., Schinka, J. A., & Retzlaff, P. (1994). Relationships between measures of auditory learning and executive functioning. *Journal of Clinical & Experimental Neuropsychology, 16,* 243–252.

Waber, D. P., & Bernstein, J. H. (1995). Performance of learning-disabled and non-learning-disabled children on the Rey-Osterrieth Complex Figure: Validation of the Developmental Scoring System. *Developmental Neuropsychology, 11,* 237–252.

Waber, D. P., & Holmes, J. M. (1985). Assessing children's copy productions of the Rey-Osterrieth Complex Figure. *Journal of Clinical and Experimental Neuropsychology, 7,* 264–280.

Waber, D. P., & Holmes, J. M. (1986). Assessing children's memory productions of the Rey-Osterrieth Complex Figure. *Journal of Clinical and Experimental Neuropsychology, 8,* 563–580.

Warrington, E. K., & Weiskrantz, L. (1970). Amnesic syndrome: Consolidation or retrieval. *Nature, 228,* 628–630.

Wechsler, D. (1945). A standardized memory scale for clinical use. *The Journal of Psychology, 19,* 87–95.

Wechsler, D. (1987). *Wechsler Memory Scale-Revised manual.* San Antonio, TX: The Psychological Corporation.

Welsh, M. C., Pennington, B. F., & Groisser, D. B. (1991). A normative-developmental study of executive function: A window on prefrontal function in children. *Developmental Neuropsychology, 7,* 131–149.

Wickens, D. D. (1970). Encoding categories of words: An empirical approach to meaning. *Psychological Review, 77,* 1–15.

Wiens, A. N., Crossen, J. R., & McMinn, M. R. (1988). Rey Auditory-Verbal Learning Test: Development of norms for healthy young adults. *The Clinical Neuropsychologist, 2,* 67–87.

Williams, J., Phillips, T., Griebel, M. L., Sharp, G. B., Lange, B., Edgar, T., et al. (2001). Patterns of memory performance in children with controlled epilepsy on the CVLT-C. *Child Neuropsychology, 7*, 15–20.

Williams, J., & Sharp, G. B. (1999). Epilepsy. In K. O. Yeates, M. D. Ris & H. G. Taylor (Eds.), *Pediatric Neuropsychology: Research, theory and practice* (pp. 47–73). New York: Guilford.

Wilson, B. A., Forester, S., Bryant, T., & Cockburn, J. (1990). Performance of 11- to 14-year-olds on the Rivermead Behavioural Memory Test. *Clinical Psychology Forum, 30*, 8–10.

Wilson, B. A., Ivani-Chalian, R., & Aldrich, F. (1991). *The Rivermead Behavioural Memory Test for Children Aged 5–10 years: Manual.* Bury St. Edmunds, UK: Thames Valley Test Company, Ltd.

Wilson, B. A., Ivani-Chalian, R., Besag, F. M. C., & Bryant, T. (1993). Adapting the Rivermead Behavioural Memory Test for use with children aged 5 to 10 years. *Journal of Clinical and Experimental Neuropsychology, 15*, 474–486.

Wolff, A. B., Kammerer, B. L., & Thatcher, R. W. (1989). Brain-behavior relationships in deaf children: The Gallaudet Neurobehavioral Project. *Journal of the American Deafness and Rehabilitation Association, 23*, 19–33.

Yancey, S. W., & Phelps, E. A. (2001). Functional neuroimaging and episodic memory: A perspective. *Journal of Clinical and Experimental Neuropsychology, 23*, 32–48.

Yeates, K. O., Blumenstein, E., Patterson, C. M., & Delis, D. (1995). Verbal learning and memory following pediatric closed-head injury. *Journal of the International Neuropsychological Society, 1*, 78–97.

Yeates, K. O., Enrile, B. G., Loss, N., Blumenstein, E., & Delis, D. (1995). Verbal learning and memory in children with myelomeningocele. *Journal of Pediatric Psychology, 20*, 801–815.

Test Index

Subject Index